Understanding Rheumatoid Arthritis

Understanding Rheumatoid Arthritis

Edited by Travis Reagan

AMERICAN
MEDICAL PUBLISHERS
www.americanmedicalpublishers.com

American Medical Publishers,
41 Flatbush Avenue,
1st Floor, New York,
NY 11217, USA

Visit us on the World Wide Web at:
www.americanmedicalpublishers.com

ISBN: 978-1-63927-478-9

Cataloging-in-Publication Data

Understanding rheumatoid arthritis / edited by Travis Reagan.
p. cm.
Includes bibliographical references and index.
ISBN 978-1-63927-478-9
1. Rheumatoid arthritis. 2. Rheumatism. 3. Arthritis. I. Reagan, Travis.
RC933 .U53 2022
616.72--dc23

Table of Contents

Preface

In my initial years as a student, I used to run to the library at every possible instance to grab a book and learn something new. Books were my primary source of knowledge and I would not have come such a long way without all that I learnt from them. Thus, when I was approached to edit this book; I became understandably nostalgic. It was an absolute honor to be considered worthy of guiding the current generation as well as those to come. I put all my knowledge and hard work into making this book most beneficial for its readers.

Rheumatoid arthritis (RA) is an autoimmune disorder which affects the joints, and causes pain and stiffness. These symptoms typically worsen after rest. Generally, the joints of the cervical spine, hands and feet are affected. However, larger joints may also be involved. Over time, polyarthritis sets in, and as the disease progresses, the inflammatory activity of the body causes tendon erosion and tethering, and leads to the destruction of the joint surface. This leads to deformity and limits the range of movement. RA can also cause inflammation around the lungs and the heart, and low red blood cell count. People with RA are susceptible to atherosclerosis, myocardial infarction, stroke and lung fibrosis. The diagnosis is made on the basis of the presenting signs and symptoms, laboratory testing and X-ray results. There is no known strategy to prevent the disease from occurring or treat the condition when it has set in. Treatments are designed to slow disease progression and control symptoms, such as pain and swelling. This book aims to shed light on some of the unexplored aspects of rheumatoid arthritis and the recent researches in this condition. It provides comprehensive insights into the study of rheumatoid arthritis. This book, with its detailed analyses and data, will prove immensely beneficial to professionals and students involved in this area at various levels.

I wish to thank my publisher for supporting me at every step. I would also like to thank all the authors who have contributed their researches in this book. I hope this book will be a valuable contribution to the progress of the field.

Editor

1

ADAM-17 is expressed on rheumatoid arthritis fibroblast-like synoviocytes and regulates proinflammatory mediator expression and monocyte adhesion

Sho Ishii[1], Takeo Isozaki[1*], Hidekazu Furuya[1], Hiroko Takeuchi[1], Yumi Tsubokura[1], Katsunori Inagaki[2] and Tsuyoshi Kasama[1]

Abstract

Background: To examine the expression of ADAM-17 in rheumatoid arthritis (RA) biological fluids and the role it plays in monocyte adhesion to RA fibroblast-like synoviocytes (FLSs).

Methods: ADAM-17 expression was measured by enzyme-linked immunosorbent assays (ELISAs) in serum from normal (NL) subjects, osteoarthritis (OA) patients, and RA patients. We also analyzed the correlation between ADAM-17 and disease activity score 28 (DAS28) in RA. To determine expression of ADAM-17 in RA synovial tissues (STs) and RA FLS, we performed immunofluorescence analyses. To determine the role of ADAM-17 in RA, we transfected RA FLSs with small interfering RNA (siRNA) against ADAM-17. THP-1 adhesion to ADAM-17 siRNA-transfected RA FLSs was measured. Finally, adhesion molecules on ADAM-17 siRNA-transfected RA FLSs were measured using cell surface ELISAs.

Results: ADAM-17 in RA serum was significantly higher than that in NL and OA serum and correlated with DAS28. ADAM-17 in RA synovial fluids was higher than that in OA synovial fluids. ADAM-17 was expressed on RA cells lining STs and RA FLSs. THP-1 adhesion to ADAM-17 siRNA-transfected RA FLSs was decreased compared with that to control siRNA-transfected RA FLSs. ICAM-1 on TNF-α-stimulated ADAM-17 siRNA-transfected RA FLSs was significantly decreased compared with that on control siRNA-transfected RA FLSs.

Conclusions: These data indicate that ADAM-17 is expressed on RA STs and plays a role in RA inflammation by regulating monocyte adhesion to RA FLSs. ADAM-17 might be an important inflammatory mediator in inflammatory diseases such as RA.

Keywords: ADAM-17, Rheumatoid arthritis, Cell adhesion, Cytokines

Background

Rheumatoid arthritis (RA) is a systemic disorder and common autoimmune disease characterized by chronic synovial inflammation that leads to joint destruction and bone erosion [1]. Although the pathogenesis of RA is only partially understood, inflammatory cells, macrophages, lymphocytes, and fibroblasts are known to produce several cytokines and chemokines in RA inflammation [2]. Determining the cytokine and chemokine networks in RA will help elucidate the pathogenesis of RA and can contribute to development of treatments [3]. In recent decades, RA therapies have changed and have shown improved outcomes. One of the most effective current therapies is biologic disease-modifying therapies, which are designed to block tumor necrosis factor α (TNF-α) and interleukin (IL) -6 [4, 5]. Anti-CD20 therapies which deplete B-cell and T-cell regulation therapies by binding cytotoxic lymphocyte antigen-4 are also highly effective treatments for RA [6, 7]. Although these therapies have been shown to be effective in RA patients, they sometimes

* Correspondence: t.isozaki@med.showa-u.ac.jp
[1]Division of Rheumatology, Department of Medicine, Showa University School of Medicine, 1-5-8 Hatanodai, Shinagawa-ku, Tokyo 142-8666, Japan
Full list of author information is available at the end of the article

fail or produce only partial responses [8–10]. Currently, studies using antibodies to other chemokines or chemokine inhibitors have been conducted in animal models of arthritis [11]. Discovering specific chemokine or chemokine receptor targets may contribute to the development of RA treatment with other molecules.

A disintegrin and metalloproteases (ADAMs) are a family of surface-expressed and secreted proteins that contain metalloproteinase domains [12]. In this family, ADAM-17 is known as a TNF-α-converting enzyme, which is the principal protease involved in the activation of pro-TNF-α. ADAM-17 also has shedding functions and plays a role in a broad range of cell surface molecules. In particular, ADAM-17 has been shown to be involved in generation of the active forms of epidermal growth factor receptor (EGFR) ligands; cytokine receptors, such as IL-6 receptors, and TNF receptors; and adhesion proteins, such as intercellular adhesion molecule (ICAM)-1 [13–15]. Through these molecules, ADAM-17 affects immune and inflammatory responses and cancer development [16]. In addition, ADAM-17 has been related to various diseases, including lung cancer, polycystic kidney, Alzheimer's disease, and autoimmune diseases, such as RA [17–20]. However, the role of ADAM-17 in RA inflammation is still unclear. In this study, we showed that ADAM-17 is expressed on RA synovial tissues (STs) and fibroblast-like synoviocytes (FLSs) and mediates monocyte adhesion and production of proinflammatory cytokines in RA.

Methods

Patients

RA STs were obtained from patients undergoing arthroplasty or synovectomy. RA and osteoarthritis (OA) synovial fluids (SFs) were obtained from patients. RA, OA, and normal (NL) serum were collected. All specimens were obtained with informed consent and collected following approval from the Showa University Institutional Review Board.

Cell culture

Fresh STs were minced and digested in tissue enzyme digestion solution as described previously [21]. FLSs were maintained in RPMI 1640 medium supplemented with 10% fetal bovine serum (FBS). Cells were seeded in six-well plates (BD Biosciences, Bedford, MA, USA) at a density of 1×10^5 cells per well and were maintained in complete medium. After overnight serum starvation, the cells were treated with TNF-α (R&D Systems, Minneapolis, MN, USA).

THP-1 cells (a human acute monocytic leukemia cell line) were purchased from the American Type Culture Collection (Manassas, VA, USA). THP-1 cells were cultured in RPMI 1640 medium supplemented with 10% FBS.

Enzyme-linked immunosorbent assays (ELISAs) of ADAM-17, fractalkine/CX3CL1, and CXCL16

ELISAs were performed as described previously [22]. The ADAM-17 levels in serum and SFs were measured following the manufacturer's protocol (R&D Systems). Briefly, 96-well plates were coated with mouse anti-ADAM-17 antibody. Next day, RA, NL serum or recombinant ADAM-17, which was used as a standard biotinylated anti-human ADAM-17 antibody (R&D Systems) was added as a detection antibody, followed by streptavidin-HRP (BD Biosciences). The plates were developed using tetramethylbenzidine substrate (TMB, Sigma-Aldrich, St Louis, MO, USA) and were read on a microplate reader at 450 nm.

Fractalkine/CX3CL1 and CXCL16 in RA FLS-conditioned medium were measured using an R&D Duo kit (R&D Systems). ADAM-17 or control siRNA-transfected RA FLS were stimulated with TNF-α (10 ng/ml) for 24 h.

Immunofluorescence

For analysis of ADAM-17 expression in RA STs and RA FLSs, rabbit anti-ADAM-17 was used as the primary antibody. (High-activity STs were selected from RA STs using hematoxylin and eosin stain.) (To measure the secretion of ADAM-17 in RA ST synovial fibroblasts, mouse anti-human collagen-1 and rabbit anti-ADAM-17 were used as primary antibodies.) RA FLSs were plated at a density of 20,000/well in eight-well Labtek chamber slides. The next day, the cells were washed with PBS and fixed. RA ST slides were fixed with cold acetone for 20 min and washed with PBS. Then, the slides were blocked with 20% FBS and 5% donkey serum for 1 h at 37 °C. Rabbit anti-human ADAM-17 antibody (10 μg/ml, Abcam, Cambridge, MA, USA) and mouse anti-human collagen-1 antibody (1 μg/ml, Abcam) was used. Alexa Fluor 488-conjugated donkey anti-rabbit antibody and Alexa Flour 555-conjugated donkey anti-mouse antibody were purchased from Life Technologies (Carlsbad, CA, USA). For nuclear staining, 4′,6-diamidino-2-phenylindole (DAPI) was used. Images were taken at ×200 magnification.

RNA isolation and quantitative PCR (qPCR)

RA FLS were incubated in six-well plates in 0.1% BSA RPMI medium overnight, before stimulation with TNF-α (R&D Systems, 10 ng/ml). Total RNA was isolated from RA FLS using RNAeasy mini RNA isolation kits in conjunction with QIAshredders (Qiagen, Valencia, CA, USA) following the manufacturer's protocol. Following isolation, RNA was quantified and checked for purity using a spectrophotometer (Nanodrop Technologies, Wilmington, DE, USA). cDNA was then prepared using a Verso cDNA kit (Thermo Fisher Scientific, Waltham, MA, USA) as per the manufacturer's protocol. Quantitative PCR (qPCR) was performed using Platinum SYBR

Green qPCR SuperMix-UDG (Invitrogen, Carlsbad, CA, USA) following the manufacturer's protocol. All samples were run in duplicate and using Eppendorf software.

Transfection of RA FLSs with ADAM-17 small interfering RNA (siRNA)

RA FLSs were seeded in six-well plates at a density of 1 × 10^5 cells per well. siRNA (100 nM) against ADAM-17 or control siRNA was mixed with TransIT-TKO transfection reagent (Mirus, Madison, WI, USA) according to the manufacturer's instructions and overlaid on the cells. The cells were incubated with the siRNA/TransIT-TKO for 24 h at 37 °C. The ADAM-17 and control siRNAs were purchased from Santa Cruz Biotechnology (Dallas, TX, USA). Knockdown of ADAM-17 secretion was confirmed using Western blotting. Western blotting was performed as described previously [23]. Membranes were probed with rabbit anti-human ADAM-17 antibody (Abcam, Cambridge, MA, USA) and anti-βactin.

In vitro cell adhesion assay

The adhesion of THP-1 cells to control siRNA-treated or ADAM-17 siRNA-treated RA FLSs grown to confluence in 96-well plates was examined. RA FLSs were serum-starved overnight. The next day, the cells were treated with TNF-α (10 ng/ml) for 24 h. THP-1 cells were collected and labeled with calcein AM fluorescent dye (Life Technologies, 5 μM) for 30 min. After being washed twice, 1 × 10^5 THP-1 cells were added to each well and incubated for 30 min at room temperature. Nonadherent cells were washed away, and the fluorescence was measured using a Synergy HT fluorescence plate reader (BioTek Instruments, Winooski, VT, USA).

Cell surface ELISA for adhesion molecule expression

Control siRNA-transfected or ADAM-17 siRNA-transfected RA FLSs (1 × 10^5/well) were seeded in 96-well plates. Confluent RA FLSs were serum-starved overnight prior to stimulation with TNF-α (10 ng/ml) for 24 h. The cells were fixed with 3.7% formalin in PBS for 30 min. Mouse anti-human antibodies specific for intercellular adhesion molecule 1 (ICAM-1, 10 μg/ml, R&D Systems) or vascular cell adhesion molecule 1 (VCAM-1) were incubated for 1 h. Subsequently, biotinylated anti-mouse antibody and streptavidin-HRP were added for 1 h, and the concentration of the samples was measured at 450 nm after reaction with the tetramethylbenzidine substrate.

Statistical analysis

The data were analyzed using Student's t test assuming equal variances. The relationship between ADAM-17 in RA serum and a disease activity score of 28 (DAS28) was evaluated using Spearman's rank correlation. Data are reported as the mean ± SEM. P values less than 0.05 were considered statistically significant.

Results

Expression of ADAM-17 in RA serum and SFs

Table 1 shows the characteristics of the patients. A total of 78.3% patients were RF positive and 65.2% of patients were ACPA positive. To determine whether ADAM-17 was expressed in serum, we examined ADAM-17 levels in RA, OA, and NL sera using ELISAs. ADAM-17 levels in RA serum ($n = 23$) were significantly higher than those in OA serum ($n = 16$) and NL serum ($n = 7$) (2093 ± 539 pg/ml, 121 ± 53 pg/ml and 0 ± 0 pg/ml, $p < 0.05$, respectively, Fig. 1a). We also examined ADAM-17 levels in RA and OA SFs. ADAM-17 in RA SFs ($n = 10$) was elevated compared to that in OA SFs (n = 7) (1644 ± 952 pg/ml and 4.6 ± 4.3 pg/ml, $p < 0.05$, respectively, Fig. 1b).

To confirm the relationship between ADAM-17 and RA disease activity, we performed correlation analysis with DAS28 erythrocyte sedimentation rate (ESR). We found that ADAM-17 in RA serum showed a significant positive correlation with DAS28 ($r = 0.64$, $p < 0.05$, $n = 58$ patients, Fig. 1c).

These results indicate that the serum level of ADAM-17 is involved in RA disease activity.

Expression of ADAM-17 in RA STs and FLSs

We then measured expression of ADAM-17 in RA and OA STs using immunofluorescence analyses. We found that ADAM-17-positive cells were expressed on RA cells lining STs (Fig. 2a). However, ADAM-17 was little expressed on OA STs (Fig. 2b). Next, we isolated FLSs from RA STs to assess ADAM-17 expression using immunofluorescence. We demonstrated that ADAM-17 was expressed in RA FLSs (Fig. 2c and d). In addition,

Table 1 Summary of patient characteristics (mean ± SE)

	RA ($n = 23$)	OA ($n = 16$)	Healthy control ($n = 7$)
Age	56.6 ± 3.4	64.2 ± 6.2	46 ± 4.6
Female, n (%)	17 (74)	13 (81)	3 (43)
Methotrexate dose (mg/week)	7.9 ± 1.2		
Glucocorticoid dose (mg/day)	1.33 ± 0.5		
DAS28 (ESR)	4.81 ± 0.3		
Duration (years)	5.2 ± 1.0		
RF positive (%)	78.3		
ACPA positive (%)	65.2		
Stage (I/II/III/IV)	(7/8/4/4)		
Number of previous biologics	1.0 ± 0.3		

ACPA anti-citrullinated protein antibodies, *DAS28* disease activity score 28, *ESR* erythrocyte sedimentation rate, *ICAM-1* intercellular adhesion molecule 1, *RF* rheumatoid factor

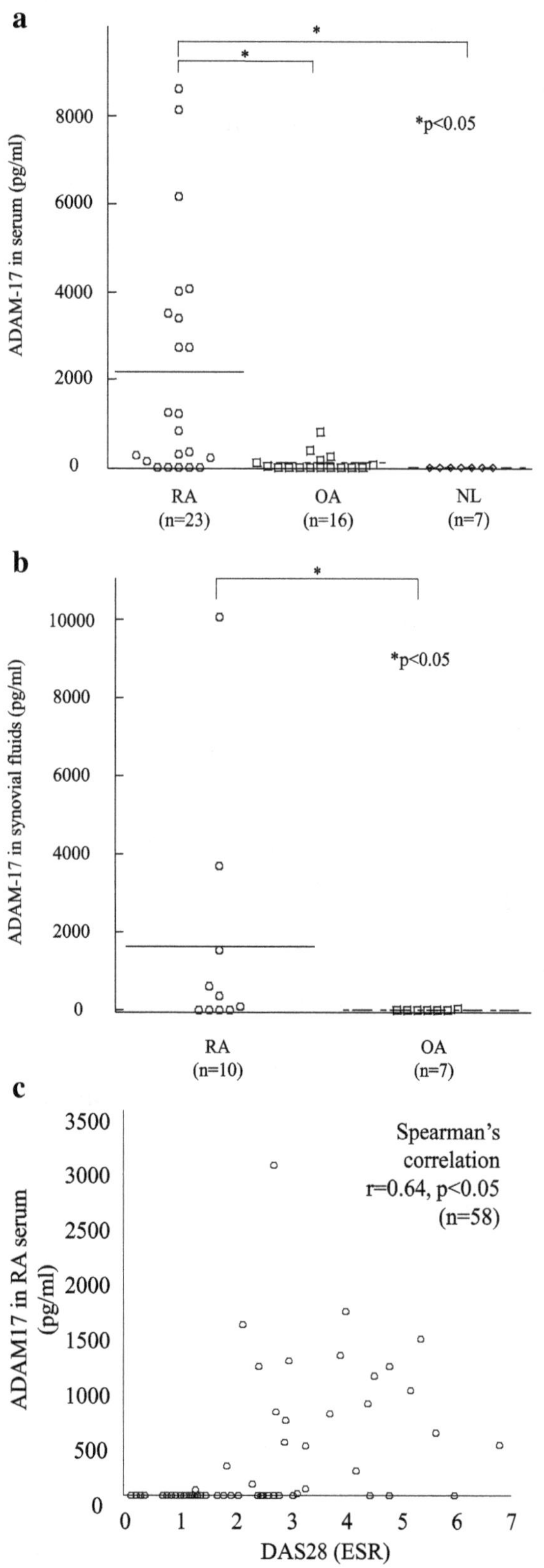

Fig. 1 Expression of ADAM-17 in RA serum and SFs. **a** ADAM-17 is higher in RA serum than OA and NL serum. **b** ADAM-17 expression is also higher in RA SFs than OA SFs. **c** The level of ADAM-17 in RA serum is correlated with disease activity. (n = number of patients). *ADAM* a disintegrin and metalloprotease family protein, *DAS28* disease activity score 28, *ESR* erythrocyte sedimentation rate, *NL* normal, *OA* osteoarthritis, *RA* rheumatoid arthritis

we found the expression of ADAM-17 mRNA was induced by stimulation with TNF-α, and elicited a 2.4-fold increase in ADAM-17 levels within 4 h (Fig. 2e). These results indicate that ADAM-17 is involved in RA inflammation.

The role of proinflammatory mediators in blocking ADAM-17 in RA FLSs

To confirm the function of ADAM-17 in RA FLSs, we transfected RA FLSs with siRNA against ADAM-17. Specific knockdown of ADAM-17 was confirmed by Western blotting, and the ADAM-17 protein levels in ADAM-17 siRNA-transfected RA FLSs were decreased compared with those in control siRNA-transfected RA FLSs (Fig. 3a).

We examined that the expression of fractalkine/CX3CL1 and VEGF in TNF-α-stimulated RA FLS-conditioned medium because these are important cytokines for RA inflammation and angiogenesis. The expression of fractalkine/CX3CL1 was significantly decreased in TNF-α-stimulated ADAM-17 siRNA-transfected RA FLS-conditioned medium compared with TNF-α-stimulated control siRNA-transfected RA FLS-conditioned medium (Fig. 3b). However, VEGF in TNF-α-stimulated ADAM-17 siRNA-transfected RA FLS-conditioned medium was not changed. These results suggest that ADAM-17 in FLSs is involved proinflammatory cytokine secretion in RA inflammation.

Blocking ADAM-17 in RA FLSs reduces THP-1 adhesion

To examine the adhesive function of ADAM-17 in RA FLSs, we used RA FLSs that were transfected with ADAM-17 siRNA or control siRNA. To determine whether ADAM-17 mediates THP-1 adhesion to RA FLSs, we performed in vitro adhesion assays. THP-1 adhesion to ADAM-17 siRNA-transfected RA FLSs was significantly decreased compared with that to control siRNA-transfected RA FLSs (Fig. 4a). In addition, we performed a cell surface ELISA to determine whether cell adhesion molecules were decreased on ADAM-17 siRNA-transfected RA FLSs. ICAM-1, but not VCAM-1, on TNF-α-stimulated ADAM-17 siRNA-transfected RA FLSs was significantly decreased compared with that on control siRNA-transfected RA FLSs (Fig. 4b). These results indicate that ADAM-17 inhibition regulates TNF-α-induced fibroblast adhesion for THP-1 and ICAM-1 expression in RA.

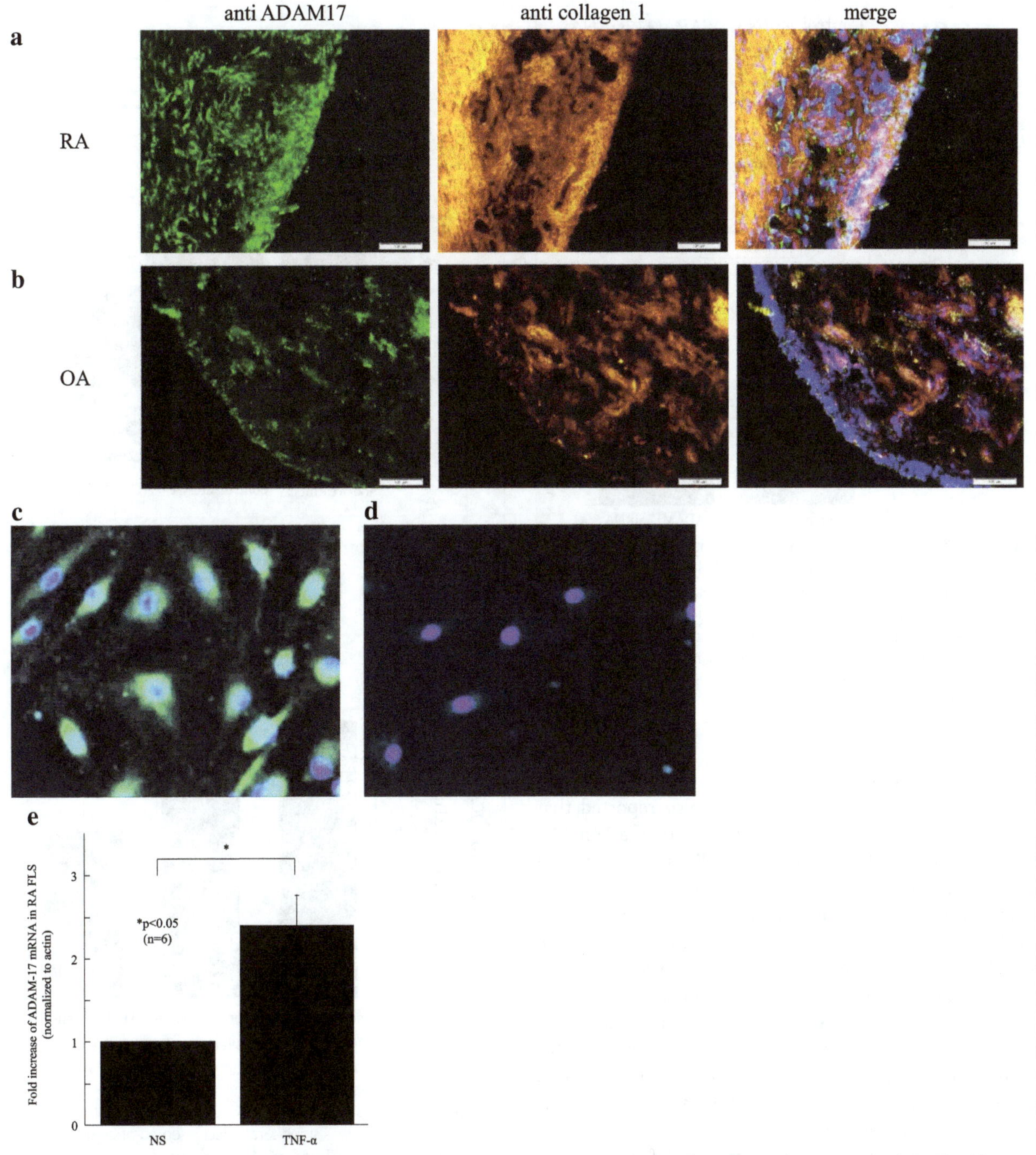

Fig. 2 Expression of ADAM-17 in RA STs and FLSs. **a** Representative photomicrographs of synovial tissues (STs) from patient with RA. The *left panel* shows ST staining with rabbit anti-ADAM-17. The *middle panel* shows staining with mouse anti-collagen-1. The *right panel* shows merging of the *left panel* and *middle panel*. The *yellow color* indicates ADAM-17 associated with ST synovium. **b** Representative photomicrographs of ST samples from patient with OA. **c** and **d** Representative photomicrographs of RA fibroblast-like synoviocytes (FLSs). Cryosections and culture cells were stained for ADAM-17 (**c**) or control IgG (**d**). (Original magnification ×200 (**a** and **b**) ×400 (**c** and **d**)) **e** ADAM-17 mRNA in TNF-α stimulated RA FLSs is increased 2.4-fold compared with nonstimulated RA FLSs. *ADAM* a disintegrin and metalloprotease family, *FLSs* fibroblast-like synoviocytes, *OA* osteoarthritis, *RA* rheumatoid arthritis

Discussion

ADAM-17 is believed be associated with inflammation in RA. In this study, we showed that ADAM-17 is expressed on RA STs and FLSs. Charbonneau et al. reported that ADAM-17 was upregulated in both fibroblast- and macrophage-like synovial cells, along with

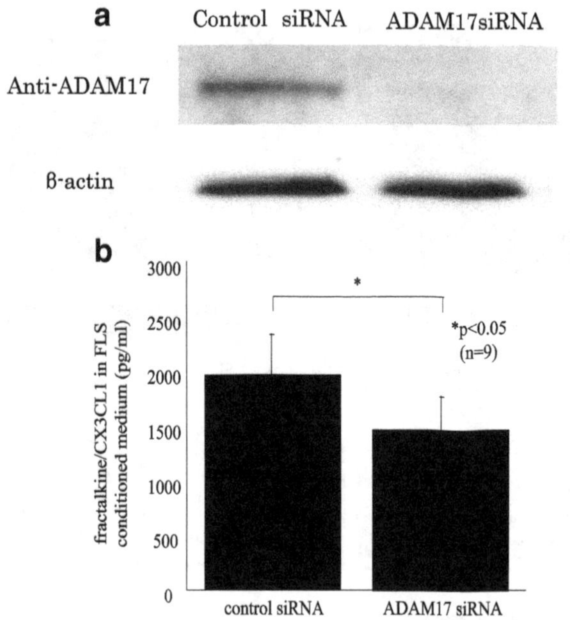

Fig. 3 The expression of proinflammatory mediators blocking ADAM-17 in RA FLSs. **a** ADAM-17 siRNA inhibited ADAM-17 expression in RA FLSs. **b** The expression of fractalkine/CX3CL1 was significantly decreased in TNF-α-stimulated ADAM-17 siRNA-transfected RA FLS-conditioned medium compared with TNF-α-stimulated control siRNA-transfected RA FLS-conditioned medium. (n = number of replicates). *ADAM* a disintegrin and metalloprotease family protein, *FLSs* fibroblast-like synoviocytes, *siRNA* small interfering RNA

elevated expression of both hypoxia inducible factor-1 and TNF-α in mice [24]. Ohta et al. also reported that ADAM-17 on RA STs was stronger than that on OA STs by immunohistochemistry. In addition, they showed that ADAM-17-expressing cells were mainly CD68+ macrophage-like synovial cells [25]. Our data supported ADAM-17 expression in RA. On the other hand, ADAM-17 was not presented in OA synovial tissues. (This result indicates ADAM-17 might be involved in joint destruction.) We clearly demonstrated that ADAM-17 expression is higher in RA serum than NL serum and is related to disease activity. Taken together, these results indicate that ADAM-17 expression is involved in RA inflammation.

Chemokines are believed to be important in RA inflammation. Fractalkine/CX3CL1 is one of these chemokines and is secreted by ADAM-17 [26]. We found that the expression of fractalkine/CX3CL1 was significantly decreased in TNF-α-stimulated ADAM-17 siRNA-transfected RA FLS-conditioned medium compared with TNF-α-stimulated control siRNA-transfected RA FLS-conditioned medium. Whereas ADAM-17 was expressed on virtually all FLS and was efficiently knocked down to zero/below threshold, only a slight reduction in the expression of fractalkine/CX3CL1 was measured. We previously reported

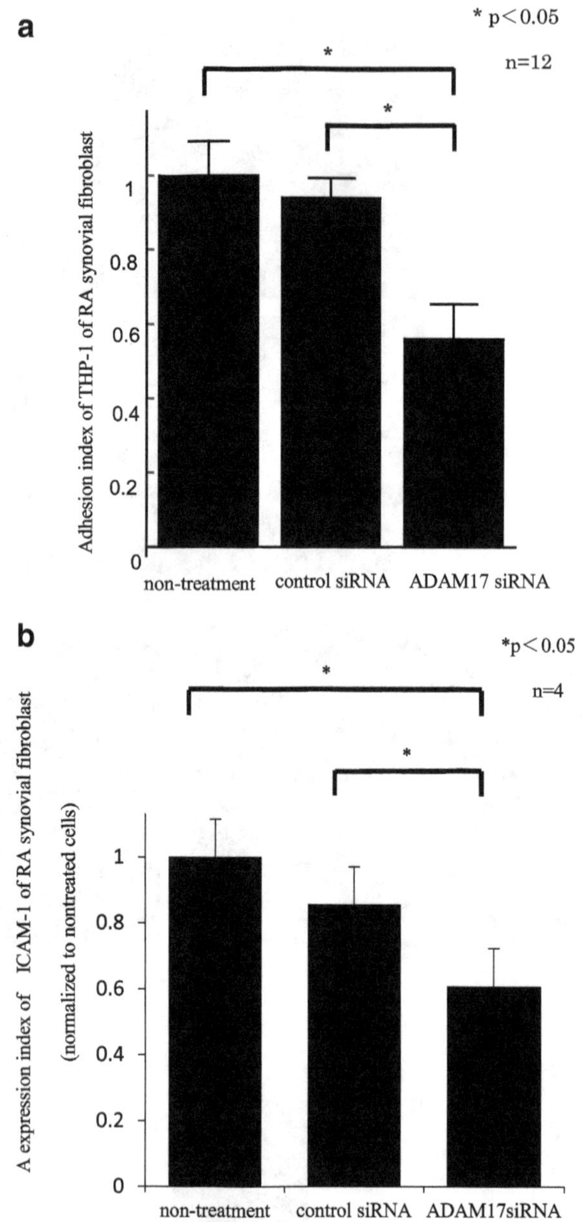

Fig. 4 Blocking ADAM-17 in RA FLSs reduces THP-1 adhesion. **a** THP-1 adhesion to ADAM-17 siRNA-transfected RA FLSs was significantly decreased compared with that to control siRNA-transfected RA FLSs. **b** ICAM-1 on TNF-α-stimulated ADAM-17 siRNA-transfected RA FLSs was significantly decreased compared with that on control siRNA-transfected RA FLSs. (n = number of replicates). *ADAM* a disintegrin and metalloprotease family protein, RA rheumatoid arthritis, *siRNA* small interfering RNA

ADAM-10 mediated fractalkine/CX3CL1 and CXCL16 secretion from RA FLS. These results suggest not only ADAM-17 but ADAM-10 regulates membrane-bound chemokines.

Ruth et al. reported that fractalkine/CX3CL1 and its receptor, CX3CR1, were expressed in RA and a rat adjuvant-induced arthritis model, and soluble fractalkine/

CX3CL1 was upregulated in RA synovitis [27]. Furthermore, the serum level of fractalkine/CX3CL1 was elevated in patients with RA and was correlated with disease activity [22]. Umemura et al. reported that ADAM17 level was positively correlated with fractalkine/CX3CL1 in RA serum [28]. These results indicate that ADAM-17 in FLSs is involved in RA inflammation by regulating fractalkine/CX3CL1 expression.

ADAM-17 regulates the shedding of a number of transmembrane substrates, including several receptors and/or their ligands, such as VEGF [12]. We showed that VEGF in TNF-α-stimulated ADAM-17 siRNA-transfected RA FLS-conditioned medium was not changed compared with that in TNF-α-stimulated control siRNA-transfected RA FLS-conditioned medium. The VEGF level in conditioned medium from several FLS lines decreased, but the VEGF level in other FLS-conditioned medium increased. These results indicated that VEGF in FLSs could be involved in other proinflammatory mediators or metalloproteases.

We next focused on the influence of ADAM-17 on monocyte adhesion in RA FLSs. We found that THP-1 adhesion to ADAM-17 siRNA-transfected RA FLSs was decreased compared with that to control siRNA-transfected RA FLSs. Additionally, we clearly demonstrated that ICAM-1 on TNF-α-stimulated ADAM-17 siRNA-transfected RA FLSs was decreased compared with that on control siRNA-transfected RA FLSs. ICAM-1 is an adhesion molecule that mediates inflammatory and immune responses and is cleaved on the cell surface by ADAM-17 [29]. On the other hand, ICAM-1 showed only 40% reduction after treatment with ADAM-17 siRNA in RA-FLS. ADAM-17 is one of the cleaving enzymes of ICAM-1 from RA-FLS, and other ADAM family might cleave ICAM-1. This study suggests that ADAM-17 promotes ICAM-1 expression on the cell surface and monocyte adhesion in RA FLSs. However, we found that VCAM-1 on TNF-α-stimulated ADAM-17 siRNA-transfected RA FLSs was not decreased compared with that on control siRNA-transfected RA FLSs. Garton et al. reported that shedding of VCAM-1 is mediated by ADAM-17 in murine endothelial cells [30]. Singh et al. also reported that VCAM-1 was released by ADAM-17 from endothelial cells [31]. In addition, they showed that VCAM-1 ectodomain release was regulated by tissue inhibitor of metalloproteinase-3 in endothelial cells. Meanwhile, we clearly demonstrated that ADAM-17 in FLSs enhances monocyte adhesion via upregulation of ICAM-1, but not VCAM-1, expression. These results indicated that ADAM-17 in FLSs might play a role in inflammation through expression of ICAM-1.

In summary, ADAM-17 is expressed on RA STs and FLSs and is correlated with disease activity in RA. ADAM-17 in FLSs mediates monocyte adhesion and production of proinflammatory cytokines, such as fractalkine/CX3CL1 and ICAM-1. TNF-α activation prior to the assay and thus, ADAM17 might also play an important role in TNF-α mediated cell activation. We next need to demonstrate more functional approach to address the role of ADAM-17 in RA. Taken together, ADAM-17 might be a potential target in inflammatory diseases such as RA.

Conclusions

Our study demonstrated that ADAM-17 was expressed in RA biological fluids and is correlated with disease activity. ADAM-17 was also expressed in RA synovium and FLS. Blocking expression of ADAM-17 in RA FLS reduced cell adhesion due to inhibition of adhesion and proinflammatory mediator production. We propose that ADAM-17 plays roles in mediating arthritis by this multistep process.

Abbreviations

ADAM: A disintegrin and metalloprotease family protein; DAB: Chromogen 3,3′-diaminobenzidine; DAPI: 4′,6-diamidino-2-phenylindole; DAS28: Disease activity score 28; ELISA: Enzyme-linked immunosorbent assay; FBS: Fetal bovine serum; FLSs: Fibroblast-like synoviocytes; ICAM-1: Intercellular adhesion molecule 1; IL: Interleukin; NL: Normal; OA: Osteoarthritis; qPCR: Quantitative polymerase chain reaction; RA: Rheumatoid arthritis; SF: Synovial fluid; siRNA: Small interfering RNA; ST: Synovial tissue; TNF-α: Tumor necrosis factor-α; VCAM-1: Vascular cell adhesion molecule 1

Acknowledgements

We thank Dr. Toyoshima for providing synovial tissues.

Authors' contributions

SI performed all assays with assistance from TI, HF, HT, YT, and KI also assisted with the acquisition of data. SI and TI performed the statistical analysis. TI and TK conceived of the study, and participated in its design and coordination. TI assisted SI with drafting the manuscript. All authors read and approved the final manuscript.

Competing interests

The authors declare that they have no competing interests.

Author details

[1]Division of Rheumatology, Department of Medicine, Showa University School of Medicine, 1-5-8 Hatanodai, Shinagawa-ku, Tokyo 142-8666, Japan. [2]Department of Orthopedic Surgery, Showa University School of Medicine, Tokyo, Japan.

References

1. Firestein GS. Evolving concepts of rheumatoid arthritis. Nature. 2003; 423(6937):356–61.
2. Choy EH, Panayi GS. Cytokine pathways and joint inflammation in rheumatoid arthritis. N Engl J Med. 2001;344(12):907–16.

3. Huber LC, Distler O, Tarner I, Gay RE, Gay S, Pap T. Synovial fibroblasts: key players in rheumatoid arthritis. Rheumatology (Oxford). 2006;45(6):669–75.
4. Kulp W, Corzillus M, Greiner W, Pientka L, Siebert U, von der Schulenburg JM, et al. Influence of tumor necrosis factor alpha in rheumatoid arthritis. GMS Health Technol Assess. 2005;1:Doc12.
5. Nishimoto N. Interleukin-6 in rheumatoid arthritis. Curr Opin Rheumatol. 2006;18(3):277–81.
6. Porter D, van Melckebeke J, Dale J, Messow CM, McConnachie A, Walker A, et al. Tumour necrosis factor inhibition versus rituximab for patients with rheumatoid arthritis who require biological treatment (ORBIT): an open-label, randomised controlled, non-inferiority, trial. Lancet. 2016;388(10041):239–47.
7. Schiff M, Weinblatt ME, Valente R, van der Heijde D, Citera G, Elegbe A, et al. Head-to-head comparison of subcutaneous abatacept versus adalimumab for rheumatoid arthritis: two-year efficacy and safety findings from AMPLE trial. Ann Rheum Dis. 2014;73(1):86–94.
8. Gomez-Reino JJ, Rodriguez-Lozano C, Campos-Fernandez C, Montoro M, Descalzo MA, Carmona L, et al. Change in the discontinuation pattern of tumour necrosis factor antagonists in rheumatoid arthritis over 10 years: data from the Spanish registry BIOBADASER 2.0. Ann Rheum Dis. 2012;71(3):382–5.
9. Plasencia C, Pascual-Salcedo D, Garcia-Carazo S, Lojo L, Nuno L, Villalba A, et al. The immunogenicity to the first anti-TNF therapy determines the outcome of switching to a second anti-TNF therapy in spondyloarthritis patients. Arthritis Res Ther. 2013;15(4):R79.
10. Jones G, Sebba A, Gu J, Lowenstein MB, Calvo A, Gomez-Reino JJ, et al. Comparison of tocilizumab monotherapy versus methotrexate monotherapy in patients with moderate to severe rheumatoid arthritis: the AMBITION study. Ann Rheum Dis. 2010;69(1):88–96.
11. Garcia S, Hartkamp LM, Malvar-Fernandez B, van Es IE, Lin H, Wong J, et al. Colony-stimulating factor (CSF) 1 receptor blockade reduces inflammation in human and murine models of rheumatoid arthritis. Arthritis Res Ther. 2016;18:75.
12. Edwards DR, Handsley MM, Pennington CJ. The ADAM metalloproteinases. Mol Asp Med. 2008;29(5):258–89.
13. Lee DC, Sunnarborg SW, Hinkle CL, Myers TJ, Stevenson MY, Russell WE, et al. TACE/ADAM17 processing of EGFR ligands indicates a role as a physiological convertase. Ann N Y Acad Sci. 2003;995:22–38.
14. Yan I, Schwarz J, Lucke K, Schumacher N, Schumacher V, Schmidt S, et al. ADAM17 controls IL-6 signaling by cleavage of the murine IL-6Ralpha from the cell surface of leukocytes during inflammatory responses. J Leukoc Biol. 2016;99(5):749–60.
15. Fontani F, Domazetovic V, Marcucci T, Vincenzini MT, Iantomasi T. Tumor necrosis factor-alpha up-regulates ICAM-1 expression and release in intestinal Myofibroblasts by redox-dependent and -independent mechanisms. J Cell Biochem. 2016;117(2):370–81.
16. Scheller J, Chalaris A, Garbers C, Rose-John S. ADAM17: a molecular switch to control inflammation and tissue regeneration. Trends Immunol. 2011; 32(8):380–7.
17. Kenny PA, Bissell MJ. Targeting TACE-dependent EGFR ligand shedding in breast cancer. J Clin Invest. 2007;117(2):337–45.
18. Vincent B, Checler F. Alpha-secretase in Alzheimer's disease and beyond: mechanistic, regulation and function in the shedding of membrane proteins. Curr Alzheimer Res. 2012;9(2):140–56.
19. Beck Gooz M, Maldonado EN, Dang Y, Amria MY, Higashiyama S, Abboud HE, et al. ADAM17 promotes proliferation of collecting duct kidney epithelial cells through ERK activation and increased glycolysis in polycystic kidney disease. Am J Physiol Renal Physiol. 2014;307(5):F551–9.
20. Lamas JR, Rodriguez-Rodriguez L, Tornero-Esteban P, Villafuertes E, Hoyas J, Abasolo L, et al. Alternative splicing and proteolytic rupture contribute to the generation of soluble IL-6 receptors (sIL-6R) in rheumatoid arthritis. Cytokine. 2013;61(3):720–3.
21. Hanyuda M, Kasama T, Isozaki T, Matsunawa MM, Yajima N, Miyaoka H, et al. Activated leucocytes express and secrete macrophage inflammatory protein-1alpha upon interaction with synovial fibroblasts of rheumatoid arthritis via a beta2-integrin/ICAM-1 mechanism. Rheumatology (Oxford). 2003;42(11):1390–7.
22. Matsunawa M, Isozaki T, Odai T, Yajima N, Takeuchi HT, Negishi M, et al. Increased serum levels of soluble fractalkine (CX3CL1) correlate with disease activity in rheumatoid vasculitis. Arthritis Rheum. 2006;54(11):3408–16.
23. Isozaki T, Rabquer BJ, Ruth JH, Haines GK 3rd, Koch AE. ADAM-10 is overexpressed in rheumatoid arthritis synovial tissue and mediates angiogenesis. Arthritis Rheum. 2013;65(1):98–108.
24. Charbonneau M, Harper K, Grondin F, Pelmus M, McDonald PP, Dubois CM. Hypoxia-inducible factor mediates hypoxic and tumor necrosis factor alpha-induced increases in tumor necrosis factor-alpha converting enzyme/ ADAM17 expression by synovial cells. J Biol Chem. 2007;282(46):33714–24.
25. Ohta S, Harigai M, Tanaka M, Kawaguchi Y, Sugiura T, Takagi K, et al. Tumor necrosis factor-alpha (TNF-alpha) converting enzyme contributes to production of TNF-alpha in synovial tissues from patients with rheumatoid arthritis. J Rheumatol. 2001;28(8):1756–63.
26. Garton KJ, Gough PJ, Blobel CP, Murphy G, Greaves DR, Dempsey PJ, et al. Tumor necrosis factor-alpha-converting enzyme (ADAM17) mediates the cleavage and shedding of fractalkine (CX3CL1). J Biol Chem. 2001;276(41): 37993–8001.
27. Ruth JH, Volin MV, Haines GK 3rd, Woodruff DC, Katschke KJ Jr, Woods JM, et al. Fractalkine, a novel chemokine in rheumatoid arthritis and in rat adjuvant-induced arthritis. Arthritis Rheum. 2001;44(7):1568–81.
28. Umemura M, Isozaki T, Ishii S, Seki S, Oguro N, Miura Y, et al. Reduction of serum ADAM17 level accompanied with decreased cytokines after Abatacept therapy in patients with rheumatoid arthritis. Int J Biomed Sci. 2014;10(4):229–35.
29. Tsakadze NL, Sithu SD, Sen U, English WR, Murphy G, D'Souza SE. Tumor necrosis factor-alpha-converting enzyme (TACE/ADAM-17) mediates the ectodomain cleavage of intercellular adhesion molecule-1 (ICAM-1). J Biol Chem. 2006;281(6):3157–64.
30. Garton KJ, Gough PJ, Philalay J, Wille PT, Blobel CP, Whitehead RH, et al. Stimulated shedding of vascular cell adhesion molecule 1 (VCAM-1) is mediated by tumor necrosis factor-alpha-converting enzyme (ADAM 17). J Biol Chem. 2003;278(39):37459–64.
31. Singh RJ, Mason JC, Lidington EA, Edwards DR, Nuttall RK, Khokha R, et al. Cytokine stimulated vascular cell adhesion molecule-1 (VCAM-1) ectodomain release is regulated by TIMP-3. Cardiovasc Res. 2005;67(1):39–49.

2

IgG Fc galactosylation predicts response to methotrexate in early rheumatoid arthritis

Susanna L. Lundström[1*], Aase H. Hensvold[2,3], Dorothea Rutishauser[1], Lars Klareskog[2,3], A. Jimmy Ytterberg[1,2], Roman A. Zubarev[1*] and Anca I. Catrina[2,3]

Abstract

Background: Methotrexate (MTX) is the standard first-line therapy in rheumatoid arthritis (RA) with variable clinical efficacy that is difficult to predict. The glycosylation status of immunoglobulin G (IgG) is altered in RA and influenced by MTX treatment. We aimed to further investigate if IgG glycosylation in untreated early RA can predict therapeutic response to MTX.

Methods: We used a shotgun proteomic approach to screen for the Fc glycopeptides in the serum of 12 control subjects and 59 untreated patients with early RA prior to and following MTX initiation. MTX treatment response was defined according to the European League Against Rheumatism at a median of 14 weeks (range 13–15) after treatment initiation. Seropositive patients were defined as those testing positive for anticitrullinated protein antibodies and/or rheumatoid factor at baseline ($n = 44$). Data analysis was performed using uni- and multivariate statistics.

Results: We could confirm a low abundance of galactosylated glycans in untreated patients with early RA compared with control subjects that was partially restored by MTX treatment. This was more evident among future nonresponders than among responders to MTX treatment. Results were further validated and confirmed by multivariate statistical analysis of the baseline Fc glycan, proteomic, and clinical data. We found that the ratio between the main agalactosylated (FA2) and main mono- and di-galactosylated Fc glycans (FA2G1 and FA2G2) of IgG1 ranked as the most prominent factor distinguishing responders from nonresponders. A low baseline ratio of FA2/[FA2G1 + FA2G2]-IgG1 was associated with nonresponse (OR 5.3 [1.6–17.0]) and was able to discriminate future nonresponders from responders to MTX therapy with a sensitivity of 70% (95% CI 46–88%) and a specificity of 69% (95% CI 52–83%). For seropositive patients ($n = 44$), this trend was improved with a sensitivity of 73% (95% CI 45–92%) for nonresponse and a specificity of 79% (95% CI 60–92%).

Conclusions: We show that the FA2/[FA2G1 + FA2G2] of IgG1 is a biomarker candidate that is significantly associated with nonresponding patients and has potential value for prediction of MTX clinical response.

Keywords: Immunoglobulin, Glycosylation, Rheumatoid arthritis, Methotrexate, Complement, Biomarker

* Correspondence: susanna.lundstrom@ki.se; roman.zubarev@ki.se
[1]Division of Physiological Chemistry I, Department of Medical Biochemistry and Biophysics, Karolinska Institutet, Scheelesväg 2, SE 17177 Stockholm, Sweden
Full list of author information is available at the end of the article

Background

Rheumatoid arthritis (RA) is an autoimmune disease in which autoantibodies, and especially anticitrullinated protein antibodies (ACPA) and rheumatoid factor (RF), are thought to play an important pathogenic role. Effector functions of antibodies are mediated largely through the fragment crystallizable (Fc) portion, such as phagocytosis; cell cytotoxicity; complement activation; and, more recently, osteoclast activation [1, 2]. In general, these functions are dependent on the glycan structures present on the constant heavy chains of the Fc portion of immunoglobulin G (IgG). The more complex the glycan is (particularly if the glycan contains galactose and sialic acid), the less likely it is for antibodies to have a proinflammatory effect [3–6]. For this reason, it has been suggested that the amount of galactosylated glycans, or the ratio between agalactosylated and galactosylated Fc glycans, is an indicator of inflammation and immune system activation [7]. In RA, agalactosylated and asialylated glycans are prominent, and the presence of these modified glycans often correlates with disease severity and progression [8–10]. Furthermore, ACPA IgGs have a perturbed pattern of Fc glycans compared with the total IgG pool [10–12].

Methotrexate (MTX) is the standard first-line therapy in RA with a varying clinical efficacy that is difficult to predict [13–15]. Several studies have suggested that MTX treatment results in significantly increased numbers of Fc-galactosylated glycans, as demonstrated in several small long-standing RA cohorts [16–18].

The aim of the present study was to investigate IgG Fc glycan structures in untreated early RA and their role as biomarkers for response to MTX treatment, using a sensitive and IgG isotype-specific shotgun proteomic approach. By using this approach, we could simultaneously measure the levels of specific proteins of interest (such as the complement pathway proteins and the IgG1–IgG4 protein isotypes). Via multivariate analysis, we could then investigate how these proteins relate to the observed Fc glycan distribution profile.

Our results indicate a general low abundance of galactosylated glycans in untreated early RA and that this feature is partially restored by MTX treatment. Furthermore, the galactosylation status of the IgG-Fc, and specifically the ratio between the main agalactosylated and mono- and digalactosylated Fc glycans of IgG1, (FA2/[FA2G1 + FA2G2]), was shown to be the best overall biomarker candidate that is predictive of therapeutic response.

Methods

Patients

This study was performed with a cohort of 59 untreated patients with early RA recruited during 1996–2006 at the rheumatology clinic at Karolinska University Hospital, Stockholm, Sweden. The selected cohort is part of the nationwide Epidemiological Investigation of Rheumatoid Arthritis (EIRA) cohort [19, 20], whose demographic characteristics are described in Additional file 1: Table S1. The patients were in the stage of untreated early RA with symptom onset <1 year prior to diagnosis. Serum sample selection was based on availability and to give a representation clinically similar to the larger EIRA cohort. The control subjects were similarly selected from among the healthy control subjects originally included in the EIRA control cohort according to age, sex, and geographical area matched to the RA patient study group. Samples were obtained at baseline and at clinical follow-up, which occurred after a median of 14 weeks (25–75% IQR 13–15). All patients started on MTX, with or without concomitant nonsteroidal anti-inflammatory drugs and/or prednisolone, to a final dose of 10–20 mg/week following local guidelines. Seropositive patients were defined as those testing positive for ACPA and/or RF at baseline ($n = 44$). An overview of recruitment and data collection is presented in Fig. 1. Response to MTX was categorized according to European League Against Rheumatism (EULAR) response criteria [21, 22] at follow-up examinations. Patients with no response to MTX were compared with patients with good and moderate responses to MTX. Additionally, serum samples from 11 healthy individuals who were matched to the patient group by age and sex were analyzed. Ethical approval for this work was obtained from the regional ethical review board (96-174[1996-0419] and 2006-476-31/4), Karolinska Institute, Stockholm, Sweden. An informed consent form (as documented by caregivers in patient records) was given to all participants as specified in the ethical approval and in line with Swedish law. Demographic characteristics of the patients and control subjects are summarized in Table 1.

Sample preparation and analysis

Samples were treated similarly to what has previously been described [23]. Ten micrograms of serum protein were preincubated in 0.3% ProteaseMAX (Promega, Madison, WI, USA) and 3 M urea (30 minutes, 50 °C), followed by bath sonication (for 10 minutes, 20 °C). The samples were diluted three times, and acetonitrile was added to a final concentration of 10% [23]. The proteins were reduced (5 mM dithiothreitol, 30 minutes, 56 °C) and alkylated (14 mM iodoacetamide, 30 minutes in darkness). Trypsin was added at a ratio of 1:50 (enzyme to protein) for overnight digestion at 37 °C. Peptides were desalted using C18 StageTips (Thermo Fisher Scientific, West Palm Beach, FL, USA), dried, and resuspended in 0.2% formic acid and 3% acetonitrile prior to

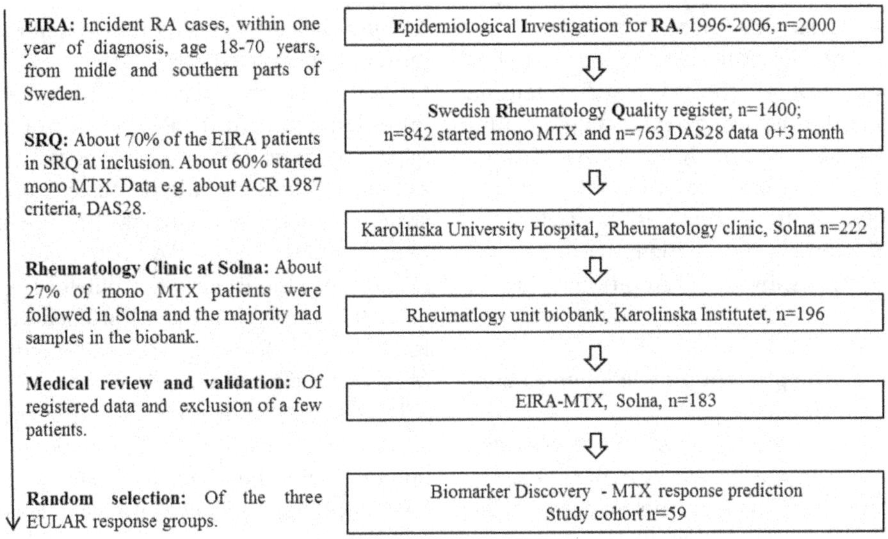

Fig. 1 Overview of study recruitment and data collection. ACR American College of Rheumatology, DAS28 Disease Activity Score in 28 joints, EULAR European League Against Rheumatism, MTX Methotrexate

analysis. Samples were kept at 10 °C, injected into columns in 1-μg aliquots, and analyzed in randomized order using a reversed-phase liquid chromatography system (EASY-nLC) connected to a Q Exactive Orbitrap mass spectrometer (MS; both from Thermo Fisher Scientific). The MS was operating in positive ion mode, and the survey mass spectrum was obtained in the mass-to-charge ratio range of 300–2000 with a nominal resolution of 60,000. Following each survey mass spectrum, the five most abundant precursor ions were selected for and subjected to tandem mass spectrometry (MS/MS) using higher-energy collisional dissociation fragmentation.

Fc glycopeptide identification and quantification

As previously described [11, 23], we screened for 19 different glycoforms N-linked to the tryptic peptides EEQYNSTYR and TKPREEQYNSTYR (IgG1), EEQFNSTFR and TKPREEQFNSTFR (IgG2), as well as EEQFNSTYR/EEQYNSTFR and TKPREEQFNSTYR/TKPREEQYNSTFR (IgG3 and IgG4). Thus, in total, 114 glycopeptides were screened for. Because each glycan substitution site was quantified by two peptides, this corresponds to 57 Fc glycan variants. Quantification was performed in a label-free manner using the Quanti program [24]. Glycopeptide ion abundances were integrated over the respective

Table 1 Characteristics and of patients and healthy control subjects

	Healthy control subjects (*n* = 11)	Early RA				
		All patients (*n* = 59)	GR (*n* = 19)	MR (*n* = 20)	NR (*n* = 20)	*p* Value[a]
Age, years	54 (45–57)	53 (45–62)	49 (41–63)	49 (41–56)	55 (49–65)	0.03
Female sex	73%	72%	68%	65%	80%	0.28
Current smoking	10%	34%	31%	30%	30%	0.52
ACPA- and/or RF-positive	–	75%	74%	75%	75%	0.96
DAS28-ESR	–	5.7 (5.0–6.2)	5.2 (5.0–6.0)	6.0 (5.4–6.4)	5.2 (4.7–6.4)	0.40
HAQ	–	1.3 (0.9–1.6)	1.1 (0.8–1.4)	1.4 (1.0–1.9)	1.3 (0.9–1.6)	0.66
DAS28-ESR follow-up	–	4.5 (2.6–5.1)	2.2 (1.7–2.6)	4.4 (4.0–4.9)	5.4 (4.9–5.8)	<0.0001
MTX duration, weeks	–	14 (13–15)	14 (13–15)	14 (13–15)	14 (14–15)	0.50
Prednisolone	–	25%	31%	30%	15%	0.19

Abbreviations: ACPA Anticitrullinated protein antibodies, *DAS28-ESR* Disease Activity Score in 28 joints based on erythrocyte sedimentation rate, *GR* Good response, *HAQ* Health Assessment Questionnaire, *MR* Moderate response, *MTX* Methotrexate, *NR* No response, *RA* Rheumatoid arthritis, *RF* Rheumatoid factor

All characteristics are from assessments at baseline, except when otherwise stated. Values are of the median (first to third quartiles), except when otherwise indicated. Response was categorized according to European League Against Rheumatism response criteria

[a]Comparison of patients not responding (no European League Against Rheumatism [EULAR] response) and patients responding (EULAR good or moderate response)

chromatographic peaks of monoisotopic ions (<10 ppm deviation from the theoretical mass value) with the charged states described above and within a ±2-minute interval around the expected retention times as determined by human polyclonal IgG standard (Sigma-Aldrich, St. Louis, MO, USA). Glycan abundances were normalized to total content of Fc-glycosylated IgG1 or IgG2 peptides. Extracted ion chromatograms of samples of a patient with RA and a control subject are shown in Additional file 1: Figure S1.

Fc protein isotype and complement protein identification and quantification

Protein identification and quantification were obtained similarly to what has previously been described [11, 23]. Complement pathway proteins were normalized by the logarithmic value of the total intensity of unique peptides for the respective protein. The relative intensity of unique Fc peptides from IgG1, IgG2, IgG3, and IgG4 were used to calculate the IgG isotype distribution. A list of the number of peptides and scores used for identification/quantification of the complement proteins and IgG isotypes is given in Additional file 1: Table S2.

Statistical analysis

Univariate statistical analysis was performed using Student's t test (with equal or unequal variance depending upon the F-test) for interindividual variation and with Student's paired t test for intraindividual variation, respectively. Because the majority of the less significant p values (i.e., 0.05–0.01) are confirmed to be more prominent for nonresponders (interindividually) or good responders (intraindividually), we chose to show the uncorrected values to easily point out these trends. False discovery rate (FDR) correction of p values was performed according to the total number of comparisons ($n = 522$) in the study. p Values <0.02 ($n = 130$) remained significant following the correction. ROC curve analysis was performed using Prism version 5.02 for Windows software (GraphPad Software, La Jolla, CA, USA). Sensitivity and specificity were estimated by 2 × 2 contingency tables using SAS version 9.3 software (SAS Institute, Cary, NC, USA). Principal component analysis (PCA) and orthogonal projections to latent structures discriminant analysis (OPLS-DA) were performed using SIMCA 14.0 (Umetrics, Umeå, Sweden) following mean centering, logarithmic transformation, and univariate scaling. Model performance was reported as cumulative correlation coefficients for the model ($R^2 \times$ [cum]), with predictive performance being based on sevenfold cross-validation calculations (Q^2[cum]) and analysis of variance of cross-validated residuals (CV-ANOVA) p values.

Results

A high agalactosylated/galactosylated Fc glycan ratio is present in untreated early RA

Of the 57 Fc glycopeptides we screened for (based on pure standard IgG), 12 Fc glycans from IgG1 and 7 from IgG2 were profiled directly in the trypsin-digested serum samples (Additional file 1: Table S3). Identified glycan structures are shown in Fig. 2a. When comparing patients with untreated RA with control subjects, it was evident that the Fc glycan profile of RA was significantly ($p < 0.05$) altered: Of the 19 profiled glycans, 12 (8 from IgG1 and 4 from IgG2) were significantly different (Additional file 1: Table S4).

To test the influence that the different Fc glycan sugar types have on the RA patient profile and their potential as biomarkers for response to treatment, the IgG1- and IgG2-Fc glycans were grouped as galactosylated (containing galactose [G]), agalactosylated (lacking galactose [aG]), afucosylated (lacking fucose [aF]), bisected (containing glycan bisection [B]), and sialylated (containing sialic acid [S]). Similarly to what has previously been reported [25, 26], among the Fc glycans, the agalactosylated forms were in general more abundant ($p < 0.05$), whereas the galactosylated forms were less abundant ($p < 0.05$) in patients with early RA as than in healthy control subjects (Fig. 2b and Additional file 1: Table S5). Noteworthy among sialylated and afucosylated glycans (which have been reported as perturbed in RA pathogenesis [27, 28]) is that no significant differences were observed between patients with RA and control subjects. Interestingly, significantly lower abundance of the bisected forms of IgG2 was observed.

MTX partially restores IgG-Fc glycan profiles in early RA

MTX treatment made the early RA Fc glycan profile more similar to that of the control subjects (Additional file 1: Tables S4 and S6). More specifically, we observed in responding patients a significant intraindividual decline in the agalactosylated IgG1 glycans, an increase of the galactosylated glycans particularly in IgG1, and an increase in bisected glycans of IgG2 (Table 2). However, this intraindividual shift was not evident in patients with no response to treatment (Table 2, Additional file 1: Figure S2). Similarly, a significant decline in the ratio between the agalactosylated and galactosylated (aGal/Gal) glycans was observed in the patients responding to MTX but not in the nonresponding patients (Table 2).

We further tested if other structural variations in the Fc glycan would affect the aGal/Gal ratio. The results (Table 2, Additional file 1: Figure S3) indicated a similar trend in all galactosylated species (i.e., independent of other glycan substitution patterns, such as N-acetylglucosamine bisection or fucosylation to the

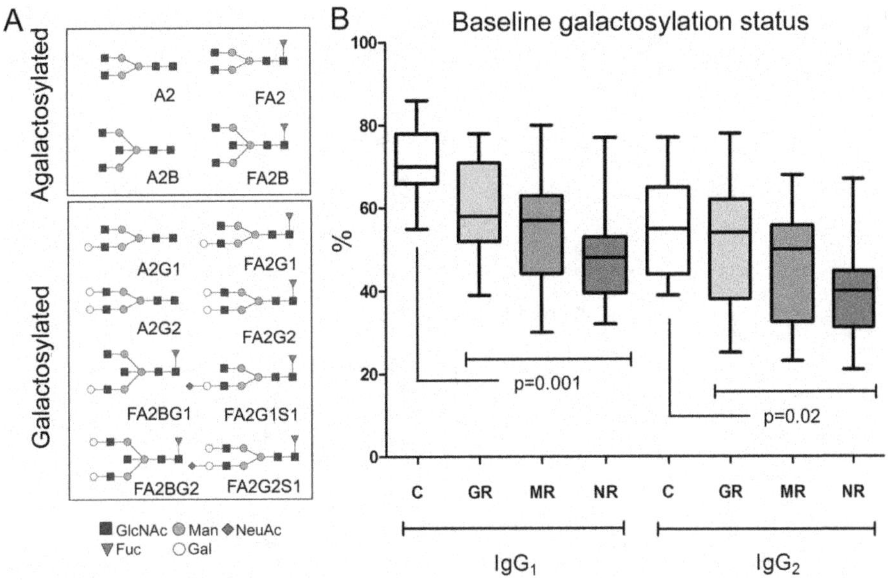

Fig. 2 Distribution of galactosylated immunoglobulin G1 (IgG1)- and IgG2-fragment crystallizable (Fc) glycans. a Quantified glycan structures grouped as agalactosylated, (aGal) and galactosylated (Gal) glycans. Glycan nomenclature is according to Royle et al. [35]. The core oligosaccharide structure comprises a biantennary heptasaccharide moiety (A2). Usually, the first sugar unit (an N-acetylglucosamine) is additionally core-fucosylated (e.g., FA2). The biantennary structure can also be transected by an additional N-acetylglucosamine (FA2B). Furthermore, the outer glucosamine units can be elongated with galactoses (FA2Gn, n = 1 or 2), and the galactoses can be further extended with sialic acids (FA2GnSn, n = 1 or 2). b Distribution of galactosylated IgG1- and IgG2-Fc glycans at baseline in healthy control subjects and in patients with early rheumatoid arthritis (RA). The relative distribution (%) of galactosylated Fc glycans differed significantly ($p < 0.05$) in healthy control subjects compared with patients with early RA and when comparing patients with good response and no response. Collectively, these data demonstrate a changed galactosylation pattern of Fc glycans in RA, with lower proportions of galactosylated glycans than their agalactosylated counterparts. The effect is most pronounced in IgG1. Following false discovery rate correction, $p = 0.001$ remains significant. C Complement protein, MR Moderate response

inner core unit). Similarly, even though IgG2 contained less Fc-galactosylated species than IgG1 in all tested individuals (Fig. 2b), the aGal/Gal ratios correlated between IgG1 and IgG2 relatively well intraindividually (Additional file 1: Figure S3), thus indicating that in patients with RA, both IgG1 and IgG2 contain lower amounts of Fc-galactosylated species than what is normal.

Baseline Fc galactosylation status ranks high in distinguishing responders and nonresponders in a multivariate model

Multivariate statistical modeling was done to find out how well the baseline levels of the Fc glycans would correlate with other variables and reflect the response (or absence thereof) to treatment. Other biomarker candidates included in the analysis were proteins involved in the complement pathways and the IgG1–IgG4 protein isotypes that were present in the proteomic analysis (i.e., acquired simultaneously with the Fc glycans in the analyses of sera by liquid chromatography-tandem mass spectrometry [LC-MS/MS]), as well as patient information obtained from the clinic (i.e., C-reactive protein [CRP] levels, sex, age, smoking history, Disease Activity Score [DAS] and Health Assessment Questionnaire [HAQ] scores). In Fig. 3a, a PCA model ($R^2 = 0.33$, $Q^2 = 0.17$) of the data is presented. It is evident that the majority of the patients with no response to treatment (*dark circles*) cluster in one part of the plot. This clustering indicates that there are features within the model that have a predictive value for future response to treatment. However, there are also patients who did respond to treatment found within this cluster. To distinguish which factors most prominently separated the response to MTX from no response to MTX, an OPLS-DA model of the data was created ($R^2 = 0.28$, $Q^2 = 0.17$, CV-ANOVA p value = 0.01). In Fig. 2b, the features of this model that correlate with 95% confidence with the respective patient group are shown. Particularly, the Fc galactosylation factors are very prominent, with the most robust marker (signified by the top ranking and small error bar) being the ratio between the main agalactosylated and mono- and di-galactosylated Fc glycans of IgG1, (i.e., FA2/[FA2G1 + FA2G2]). In addition to the Fc galactosylation status, several of the complement proteins (complement factors I and H as well as complements 5 and 9) were ranked higher than the inflammatory marker CRP.

Table 2 Immunoglobulin G fragment crystallizable glycan distribution of IgG1 and IgG2 in patients with rheumatoid arthritis prior to and following methotrexate treatment

Type	Isotype	Glycan[a]	Good responders		Moderate responders		Non responders		Intraindividual change			Interindividual differences	
									Prior/following			Prior	Following
			Prior	Following	Prior	Following	Prior	Following	GR	MR	NR	(GR + MR)/NR	(GR + MR)/NR
	IgG1	Σ[Galactosylated glycans][b]	60 ± 12	63 ± 13	54 ± 13	57 ± 13	49 ± 12	47 ± 14	0.004	0.03	0.5	0.02	0.001
		Σ[Agalactosylated glycans][c]	40 ± 12	37 ± 13	46 ± 13	43 ± 13	51 ± 12	53 ± 14	0.004	0.03	0.5	0.02	0.001
		Σ[Afucosylated glycans][d]	4 ± 3	4 ± 3	3 ± 2	4 ± 2	3 ± 1	4 ± 2	0.8	0.4	0.2	0.2	1
		Σ[Bisected glycans][e]	12 ± 4	13 ± 4	12 ± 2	14 ± 3	13 ± 3	14 ± 5	0.2	0.0003	0.3	0.7	1
		Σ[Sialylated glycans][f]	4 ± 4	4 ± 3	3 ± 2	4 ± 3	2 ± 2	3 ± 2	0.5	0.3	0.5	0.1	0.04
	IgG2	Σ[Galactosylated glycans][g]	52 ± 14	54 ± 15	45 ± 13	47 ± 13	40 ± 11	39 ± 11	0.2	0.1	0.7	0.01	0.003
		Σ[Agalactosylated glycans][h]	48 ± 14	46 ± 15	55 ± 13	53 ± 13	60 ± 11	61 ± 11	0.2	0.1	0.7	0.01	0.003
		Σ[Bisected glycans][i]	7 ± 3	8 ± 3	6 ± 2	7 ± 3	7 ± 3	7 ± 3	0.01	0.004	1	0.7	0.5
		Σ[Sialylated glycans][j]	6 ± 5	6 ± 5	5 ± 3	5 ± 4	4 ± 2	4 ± 2	0.5	0.9	0.9	0.02	0.1
aGal/Gal ratio	All IgG1	Log [Σ(Agalactosylated glycans)/Σ(galactosylated glycans)]	−0.18 ± 0.24	−0.25 ± 0.26	−0.08 ± 0.25	−0.14 ± 0.25	0.02 ± 0.21	0.05 ± 0.26	0.003	0.03	0.42	0.03	0.006
	All IgG2	Log [Σ(agalactosylated glycans)/Σ(galactosylated glycans)]	−0.05 ± 0.26	−0.07 ± 0.27	0.09 ± 0.24	0.05 ± 0.24	0.19 ± 0.21	0.20 ± 0.22	0.2	0.05	0.62	0.007	0.006
	Main IgG1	Log[FA2/(FA2G1 + FA2G2)]	−0.17 ± 0.21	−0.24 ± 0.23	−0.07 ± 0.23	−0.13 ± 0.22	0.02 ± 0.20	0.05 ± 0.24	0.001	0.02	0.4	0.02	0.001
	Main IgG2	Log[FA2/(FA2G1 + FA2G2)]	0.02 ± 0.23	−0.05 ± 0.24	0.11 ± 0.23	0.06 ± 0.21	0.20 ± 0.21	0.22 ± 0.20	0.1	0.02	0.6	0.02	0.001
	Bisected IgG1	Log[FA2B/(FA2BG1 + FA2BG2)]	−0.15 ± 0.29	−0.21 ± 0.29	−0.08 ± 0.26	−0.12 ± 0.25	0.06 ± 0.24	0.07 ± 0.26	0.03	0.1	0.7	0.02	0.002
	Bisected IgG2	Log[FA2B/FA2BG1]	0.40 ± 0.35	0.35 ± 0.42	0.68 ± 0.48	0.52 ± 0.46	0.76 ± 0.38	0.70 ± 0.29	0.4	0.03	0.3	0.1	0.02
	Afucosylated IgG1	Log[A2/(A2G1 + A2G2)]	−0.51 ± 0.62	−0.72 ± 0.71	−0.36 ± 0.59	−0.53 ± 0.58	−0.17 ± 0.56	−0.19 ± 0.56	0.02	0.04	0.8	0.1	0.01

Abbreviations: *aGal/Gal* Ratio between agalactosylated and galactosylated glycans, *GR* Good response, *MR* Moderate response, *NR* No response
Patients are grouped according to response to MTX. Figures are given for average values (%) ± SD. *p* Values <0.02 remained significant following false discovery rate correction
[a]Glycan abbreviations are provided in Fig. 2a legend
[b]Σ[IgG1: A2G1, A2G2, FA2G1, FA2BG1, FA2G1S1, FA2G2, FA2BG2, FA2G2S1]
[c]Σ[IgG1: FA2, FA2B, A2 and A2B]
[d]Σ[IgG1: A2, A2B, A2G1, A2G2]
[e]Σ[IgG1: A2B, FA2B, FA2BG1, FA2BG2]
[f]Σ[IgG1: FA2G1S1, FA2G2S1]
[g]Σ[IgG2: FA2G1, FA2BG1, FA2G2, FA2G1S1, FA2G2, FA2G2S1]
[h]Σ[IgG2: FA2, FA2B]
[i]Σ[IgG2: FA2B, FA2BG1]
[j]Σ[IgG2: FA2G1S1, FA2G2S1]

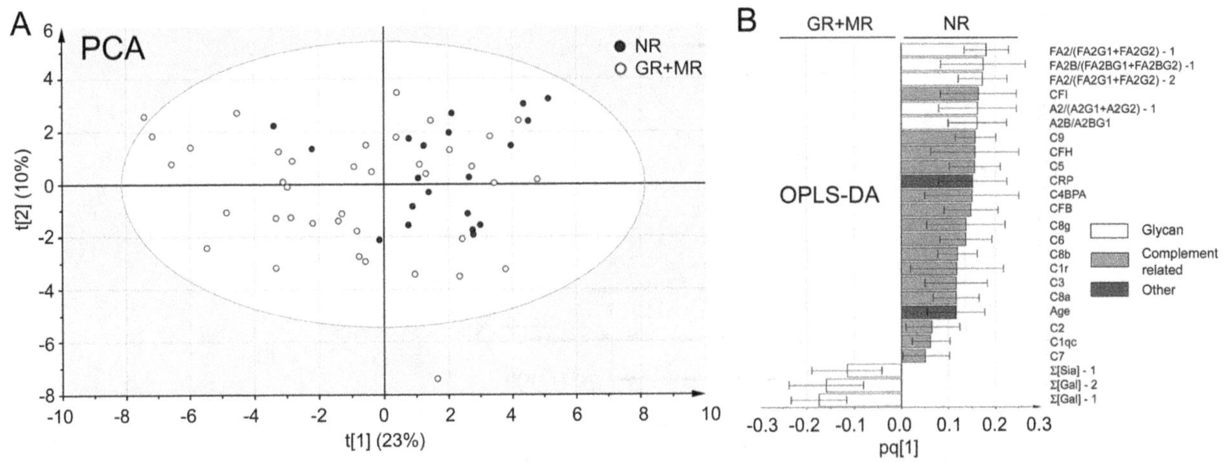

Fig. 3 Multivariate model based on baseline information of the patients prior to methotrexate treatment. a Principal component analysis (PCA) score plot. The majority of patients with no response to treatment (NR, dark circles) cluster together along component 1 (x-axis). This indicates that there are factors at baseline that are characteristic for this patient group within the model. b The orthogonal projections to latent structures discriminant analysis (OPLS-DA) loading plot of the same data reveals which factors these are. The error bars represent the range of each marker's value (with >95% confidence). Features that are positive correlate with no response, features that are negative correlate with response. Shown are only the features correlating with 95% confidence. For details of the complete model, see Additional file 1: Table S7. C Complement protein, CF Complement factor, FA2 Main agalactosylated Fc glycan, FA2G1 Main monogalactosylated Fc glycan, FA2G2 Main digalactosylated Fc glycan, GR Good response, MR Moderate response, NR No response

Baseline FA2/(FA2G1 + FA2G2) of IgG1 can predict response to MTX treatment in early RA

Because uni- and multivariate data analyses indicated that the baseline Fc glycan ratio of FA2/(FA2G1 + FA2G2) of IgG1 was the top candidate for distinguishing between MTX responders and nonresponders, we further investigated this marker's performance in predicting therapeutic response (Table 3). We created a dichotomous biomarker choosing a cutoff (−0.045) of log[FA2/(FA2G1 + FA2G2)] (Fig. 4a) for optimal sensitivity and specificity determined by ROC curve of the model based on all patients (Fig. 4b). FA2/(FA2G1 + FA2G2) of IgG1 was significantly associated with lack of response among all patients (OR 5.3, 95% CI 1.6–17.0, $p = 0.006$). At the cutoff of −0.045, this parameter distinguished responders from nonresponders with a sensitivity of 70% (95% CI 46–88%) and specificity of 69% (95% CI 52–83%) (Table 3).

Noteworthy among seropositive patients (i.e., patients who at baseline were testing positive for ACPA and/or RF, $n = 44$) is that the marker was even more selective (OR 10.5, 95% CI 2.5–45, $p = 0.001$). Responding patients could be predicted with a sensitivity of 73% (95% CI 45–92%) and a specificity of 79% (95% CI 60–92%) according to the −0.045 cutoff (Table 3). ROC curve analysis of seropositive patients generated an AUC of 81 ± 13% compared with the ROC curve model based on all patients (71 ± 14% for all patients) (Fig. 4).

Using logistic regression models, we identified significant association of lack of response with age ($p = 0.03$), whereas other tested variables (DAS score based on erythrocyte sedimentation rate [ESR], CRP levels, HAQ scores, sex, smoking status, use of prednisolone) were not significant predictors. When we included age as a possible predictor in the model, we observed that the FA2/(FA2G1 + FA2G2)-IgG1 biomarker remained a significant predictive factor associated with lack of response (all patients, OR 4.2, 95% CI 1.2–14.1, $p = 0.02$) and seropositive patients (OR 8.8, 95% CI 1.9–41.2, $p = 0.006$), respectively).

Table 3 Predictive value of immunoglobulin G1 $\log_{10}$[FA2/(FA2G2 + FA2G2)] as a response biomarker[a]

Test		Result	NR	GR + MR	Sensitivity (nonresponse) (95% CI)	Specificity (response) (95% CI)	OR (95% CI)
All patients	FA2/(FA2G2 + FA2G2)-IgG1	Positive	14	12	70% (46–88)	69% (52–83)	5.3 (1.6–17.0)
		Negative	6	27			
ACPA+ and/or RF+	FA2/(FA2G2 + FA2G2)-IgG1	Positive	11	6	73% (45–92)	79% (60–92)	10.5 (2.5–45)
		Negative	4	23			

Abbreviations: *ACPA* Anticyclic citrullinated peptide antibody, *FA2* Main agalactosylated, *FA2G1* Main monogalactosylated Fc glycan, *FA2G2* Main digalactosylated Fc, *GR* Good response, *IgG1* Immunoglobulin G1, *MR* Moderate response, *NR* No response, *RF* Rheumatoid factor

[a]Cutoff −0.045

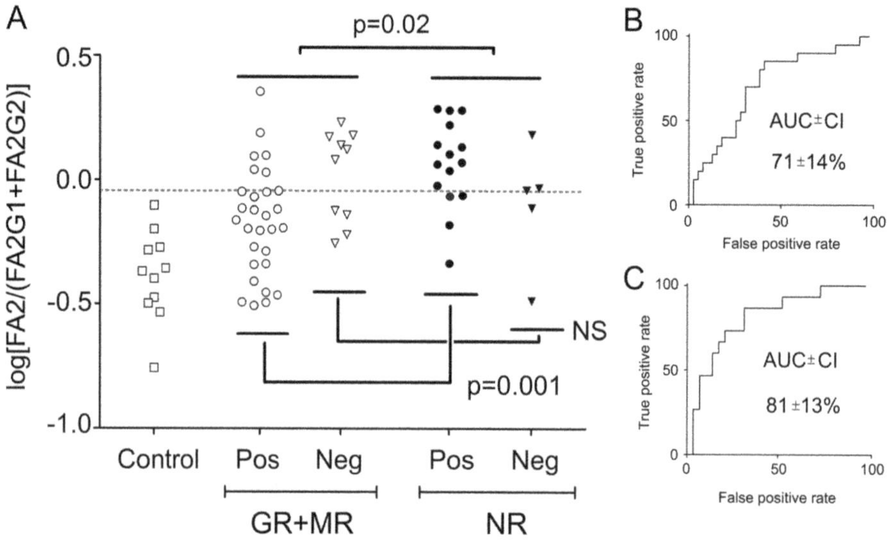

Fig. 4 The log[FA2/(FA2G1 + FA2G2)] value of immunoglobulin G1 (IgG1) as a predictive factor for response. a Good (GR) and moderate responders (MR) compared with patients with no response (NR) to methotrexate treatment. Patients are split into seropositive (Pos) and seronegative (Neg) groups. Cutoff −0.045. b ROC curve for distinguishing the responding and nonresponding patient cohorts. c ROC curve for distinguishing the responding and nonresponding patient cohorts when only seropositive patients were included. Following false discovery rate correction, p = 0.001 remains significant. FA2 Main agalactosylated, FA2G1 Main monogalactosylated Fc glycan, FA2G2 Main digalactosylated Fc, NS Not significant

Discussion

The glycosylation pattern of the IgG-Fc glycans has been associated with inflammation and immune activation in RA [8–10]. We confirm a changed galactosylation pattern of Fc glycans in RA that is partially reversed following MTX treatment [16, 18, 25]. We further show that specific Fc glycans (i.e., the ratio between the most abundant agalactosylated glycan versus the most abundant mono- and di-galactosylated Fc glycans of IgG1 [FA2/{FA2G1 + FA2G2}]) are associated with and have predictive value for MTX response. This result suggests a potential use of this marker in the clinic.

We used a previously validated sensitive proteomic approach [23] that enables quantification of a larger number of Fc glycans and distinguishes different IgG isotypes without any need for IgG enrichment. Given that protein G and protein A columns are based on Fc binding interactions, the regular "high-throughput" IgG enrichment approaches may affect the distribution of which Fc glycans are enriched. In addition, our method has the benefit of acquiring information on the regular proteome during the same analysis. This information can be used as an additional internal validation (as demonstrated by the complement pathway and glycan correlations presented herein). Thus, this approach provides a descriptive and direct measure of the polyclonal IgG-Fc glycan structures combined with the information on the regular proteome status [23]. A disadvantage of not including an IgG enrichment step is that the low abundant Fc glycopeptides, such as the IgG3/IgG4 Fc glycans, are below the limit of quantification. Additionally, owing to the complexity of the sample, the LC-MS/MS analysis time will be longer than the regular high-throughput approaches (1–2 h versus 5–30 minutes).

The altered Fc glycosylation pattern in RA is due mainly to the generally higher abundance of the agalactosylated glycans than that of their galactosylated counterparts. In the present study, we found that this perturbation in the Fc glycan profile occurs not only in IgG1 but also in IgG2 and that MTX treatment partially restores both profiles. Restoration of Fc galactosylation following treatment has been indicated in two previous RA studies [16, 18]. This change is likely a reflection and a marker of an overall decline in ongoing proinflammatory pathological processes following treatment. For example, a decline in IgG-Fc galactosylation has previously been associated with a proinflammatory status and correlates with CRP or ESR levels [9, 10, 12, 16]. Similarly to other reports in the literature, we also found a correlation between IgG1 [FA2/(FA2G1 + FA2G2)] and CRP ($R^2 = 0.3$ both prior to and following treatment). However, in contrast to FA2/(FA2G1 + FA2G2)-IgG1, baseline DAS measured by DAS28-ESR and baseline CRP levels were not significantly associated with response, suggesting that the IgG galactosylation patterns in RA likely reflect complex disease processes beyond inflammation. Furthermore, the DAS correlated only with IgG1 [FA2/(FA2G1 + FA2G2)] following treatment ($R^2 = 0.2$); at baseline, the trend was insignificant ($R^2 = 0.02$).

Of the 59 patients with RA, 15 (6 with good, 6 with moderate, and 3 with no MTX response) were treated with prednisolone. Corticosteroids such as prednisolone have been shown to affect protein glycosylation, particularly sialylation [29–31]. In the present study, we could not see an effect of prednisolone on sialylation levels or galactosylation status. When we excluded the prednisolone-treated patients, log(FA2/(FA2G1 + FA2G2) remained significant ($p < 0.03$).

Because Fc galactosylation status has been linked to both regulation of the lectin complement pathway (via agalactosylated Fc glycans) [3] and the classical complement pathway (via galactosylated Fc glycans) [32, 33], we tested how these proteins (also analyzed in the same sera LC-MS/MS measurements) would correlate with the galactosylation status. It is noteworthy that, in the multivariate model, both proteins that were highest-ranked in distinguishing responding and nonresponding patients and that could be linked to a specific pathway were regulatory proteins of the alternative complement pathway (CFI and CFH). Additionally, the membrane attack complex-forming proteins (C5 and C9) strongly correlated with no response to MTX, suggesting a high level of proinflammatory activity in these patients. Note that both the classical pathway proteins C1qb and C1qc had significantly lower abundance in patients with RA than in control subjects (Additional file 1: Figure S4). This is in line with previous studies that have demonstrated a positive correlation between Fc galactosylation and classical complement pathway activation via C1q binding [32, 33]. It is noteworthy that the protein which showed the best intraindividual correlation with galactosylation status (including control subjects and patients with RA) was the inhibitor of the classical and lectin complement pathways C4bBPα, whose abundance was positively correlated with agalactosylation (Additional file 1: Figure S5).

By investigating the discriminatory value of several different Fc glycans, we found that FA2/(FA2G1 + FA2G2) of IgG1 was the best predictive factor for therapeutic response to MTX. Interestingly, among seropositive (ACPA- and/or RF-positive) patients, this trend was enhanced, suggesting a potential pathogenic relevance of the glycosylation status of RA-associated antibodies similar to what has previously been proposed [2, 11, 12, 34]. However, this observation needs to be confirmed and validated in a larger cohort.

Researchers in one previous study on patients with long-standing RA treated with MTX or anti-tumor necrosis factor drugs tested the use of Fc galactosylation status as a biomarker for predicting MTX response [16]. In that study, the results were negative. Besides the clinical difference between the cohorts (early RA versus long-standing RA, naive versus previous exposure to disease-modifying antirheumatic drugs), another possible explanation for this discrepancy might rely on the differences in analytical techniques. This previous report was limited to the mono-galactosylated glycan abundance (FAG1) from unspecific IgGs [16], whereas in the present study, we found more prominent differences for the di-galactosylated counterpart (FA2G2) than for FA2G1.

Conclusions

In this pilot, we show that the IgG-Fc galactosylation status is changed in untreated patients with early RA, which likely has perturbing effects on activation and regulation of the complement pathways. Furthermore, FA2/(FA2G1 + FA2G2) of IgG1 at baseline is significantly associated with nonresponse and thus is a potential biomarker for MTX clinical response prediction. The overall results, and particularly the specific differences in predicting the MTX response comparing seropositive and seronegative patients, are interesting but need to be validated in larger cohorts.

Additional file

Additional file 1: Table S1. Demographic characteristics of the nationwide EIRA cohort. **Table S2.** Characterized complement pathway proteins and IgG-isotype proteins. **Table S3.** Individual IgG-Fc glycan distribution values in IgG1 and in IgG2 in control subjects, as well as in patients with RA prior to and following MTX treatment. **Table S4.** Significant differences for the 19 characterized glycan species when comparing healthy versus all, good, moderate, and nonresponding patients prior to and following MTX treatment. **Table S5.** IgG1 and IgG2 Fc glycan distributions grouped according to structural features, comparing healthy control subjects and patients with RA prior to and following MTX treatment. **Table S6.** Intra- and interindividual differences in the patients with RA, comparing individual glycan species prior to and following MTX treatment. **Table S7.** Complete list, ranking, and correlation (with response versus no response to MTX) of the features used in the OPLS-DA model shown in Fig. 3b. **Figure S1.** Extracted ion chromatograms of IgG1 and IgG2 Fc glycans quantified in a control subject and a patient with RA. **Figure S2.** Intraindividual changes in galactosylation status on IgG1 and on IgG2 for good and moderate responders and for nonresponders. **Figure S3.** Intraindividual correlation between the aGal/Gal status of glycans with different types of structural features and of IgG1 and IgG2 substituted glycans. **Figure S4.** Significant differences between control subjects and patients with early RA at baseline in the classical pathway initiating complements C1 and C9. **Figure S5.** Intraindividual correlation between the classical and lectin pathway inhibitor C4bBPα versus FA2/(FA2G1 + FA2G2). (DOCX 1180 kb)

Abbreviations

ACPA: Anticitrullinated protein antibodies; aF: Lacking fucose; aG: Lacking galactose; aGal/Gal: Ratio between agalactosylated and galactosylated glycans; B: Bisected glycans; C: Complement protein; CF: Complement factor; CRP: C-reactive protein; CV-ANOVA: Analysis of variance of cross-validated residuals; DAS-ESR: Disease Activity Score based on erythrocyte sedimentation rate; EIRA: Epidemiological Investigation of Rheumatoid Arthritis; EULAR: European League Against Rheumatism; FA2: Main agalactosylated Fc glycan ; FA2G1: Main monogalactosylated Fc glycan; FA2G2: Main digalactosylated Fc glycan; Fc: Fragment crystallizable; FDR: False discovery rate; G: Galactose; GR: Good response; HAQ: Health Assessment Questionnaire; IgG: Immunoglobulin G; MR: Moderate response; MS: Mass spectrometer; MS/MS: Tandem mass spectrometry; LC-MS/MS: Liquid chromatography-tandem mass spectrometry; MTX: Methotrexate;

NR: No response; OPLS-DA: Orthogonal projections to latent structures discriminant analysis; PCA: Principal component analysis; RA: Rheumatoid arthritis; RF: Rheumatoid factor; S: Sialic acid

Acknowledgements

We thank Marie Ståhlberg and Carina Palmberg at the Proteomics Karolinska/Karolinska Institutet core facility, Medical Biochemistry and Biophysics, Karolinska Institutet, for help with sample preparation and LC-MS/MS proteomic analysis.

Funding

This work was supported by research funding from the Innovative Medicine Initiative BTCure Project (115142-2), FP7-HEALTH-2012-INNOVATION-1 Euro--TEAM (305549-2), the Initial Training Networks 7th Framework Programme OSTEOIMMUNE (289150), the Swedish Research Council, and the Swedish Foundation for Strategic Research.

Authors' contributions

SLL, AHH, AJY, RAZ, and AIC made substantial contributions to the study's conception and design. DR, LK, RAZ, and AIC contributed reagents, materials, and analytical tools. SLL, AHH, DR, and AJY analyzed and interpreted data. SLL and AHH drafted the manuscript. DR, LK, AJY, RAZ, and AIC revised the manuscript critically for important intellectual content. All authors read and approved the final manuscript.

Competing interests

The authors declare that they have no competing interests.

Author details

[1]Division of Physiological Chemistry I, Department of Medical Biochemistry and Biophysics, Karolinska Institutet, Scheelesväg 2, SE 17177 Stockholm, Sweden. [2]Rheumatology Unit, Department of Medicine, Karolinska Institutet, Stockholm, Sweden. [3]Rheumatology Unit, Karolinska University Hospital, Stockholm, Sweden.

References

1. Negishi-Koga T, Gober HJ, Sumiya E, Komatsu N, Okamoto K, Sawa S, et al. Immune complexes regulate bone metabolism through FcRγ signalling. Nat Commun. 2015;6:6637.
2. Harre U, Lang SC, Pfeifle R, Rombouts Y, Fruhbeisser S, Amara K, et al. Glycosylation of immunoglobulin G determines osteoclast differentiation and bone loss. Nat Commun. 2015;6:6651.
3. Malhotra R, Wormald MR, Rudd PM, Fischer PB, Dwek RA, Sim RB. Glycosylation changes of IgG associated with rheumatoid arthritis can activate complement via the mannose-binding protein. Nat Med. 1995;1(3):237–43.
4. Anthony RM, Wermeling F, Karlsson MC, Ravetch JV. Identification of a receptor required for the anti-inflammatory activity of IVIG. Proc Natl Acad Sci U S A. 2008;105(50):19571–8.
5. Anthony RM, Wermeling F, Ravetch JV. Novel roles for the IgG Fc glycan. Ann N Y Acad Sci. 2012;1253:170–80.
6. Collin M, Ehlers M. The carbohydrate switch between pathogenic and immunosuppressive antigen-specific antibodies. Exp Dermatol. 2013;22(8):511–4.
7. de Jong SE, Selman MH, Adegnika AA, Amoah AS, van Riet E, Kruize YC, et al. IgG1 Fc N-glycan galactosylation as a biomarker for immune activation. Sci Rep. 2016;6:28207.
8. Rombouts Y, Ewing E, van de Stadt LA, Selman MH, Trouw LA, Deelder AM, et al. Anti-citrullinated protein antibodies acquire a pro-inflammatory Fc glycosylation phenotype prior to the onset of rheumatoid arthritis. Ann Rheum Dis. 2015;74(1):234–41.
9. Collins ES, Galligan MC, Saldova R, Adamczyk B, Abrahams JL, Campbell MP, et al. Glycosylation status of serum in inflammatory arthritis in response to anti-TNF treatment. Rheumatology (Oxford). 2013;52(9):1572–82.
10. Ercan A, Cui J, Chatterton DE, Deane KD, Hazen MM, Brintnell W, et al. Aberrant IgG galactosylation precedes disease onset, correlates with disease activity, and is prevalent in autoantibodies in rheumatoid arthritis. Arthritis Rheum. 2010;62(8):2239–48.
11. Lundstrom SL, Fernandes-Cerqueira C, Ytterberg AJ, Ossipova E, Hensvold AH, Jakobsson PJ, et al. IgG antibodies to cyclic citrullinated peptides exhibit profiles specific in terms of IgG subclasses, Fc-glycans and a Fab-peptide sequence. PLoS One. 2014;9(11):e113924.
12. Scherer HU, van der Woude D, Ioan-Facsinay A, el Bannoudi H, Trouw LA, Wang J, et al. Glycan profiling of anti-citrullinated protein antibodies isolated from human serum and synovial fluid. Arthritis Rheum. 2010;62(6):1620–9.
13. McInnes IB, O'Dell JR. State-of-the-art: rheumatoid arthritis. Ann Rheum Dis. 2010;69(11):1898–906.
14. Smolen JS, Landewé R, Breedveld FC, Buch M, Burmester G, Dougados M, et al. EULAR recommendations for the management of rheumatoid arthritis with synthetic and biological disease-modifying antirheumatic drugs: 2013 update. Ann Rheum Dis. 2014;73(3):492–509.
15. O'Dell JR, Curtis JR, Mikuls TR, Cofield SS, Bridges Jr SL, Ranganath VK, et al. Validation of the methotrexate-first strategy in patients with early, poor-prognosis rheumatoid arthritis: results from a two-year randomized, double-blind trial. Arthritis Rheum. 2013;65(8):1985–94.
16. Ercan A, Cui J, Hazen MM, Batliwalla F, Royle L, Rudd PM, et al. Hypogalactosylation of serum N-glycans fails to predict clinical response to methotrexate and TNF inhibition in rheumatoid arthritis. Arthritis Res Ther. 2012;14(2):R43.
17. Pasek M, Duk M, Podbielska M, Sokolik R, Szechinski J, Lisowska E, et al. Galactosylation of IgG from rheumatoid arthritis (RA) patients – changes during therapy. Glycoconj J. 2006;23(7-8):463–71.
18. Gindzienska-Sieskiewicz E, Radziejewska I, Domyslawska I, Klimiuk PA, Sulik A, Rojewska J, et al. Changes of glycosylation of IgG in rheumatoid arthritis patients treated with methotrexate. Adv Med Sci. 2016;61(2):193–7.
19. Saevarsdottir S, Wedren S, Seddighzadeh M, Bengtsson C, Wesley A, Lindblad S, et al. Patients with early rheumatoid arthritis who smoke are less likely to respond to treatment with methotrexate and tumor necrosis factor inhibitors: observations from the Epidemiological Investigation of Rheumatoid Arthritis and the Swedish Rheumatology Register cohorts. Arthritis Rheum. 2011;63(1):26–36.
20. Hensvold AH, Joshua V, Li W, Larkin M, Qureshi F, Israelsson L, et al. Serum RANKL levels associate with anti- citrullinated protein antibodies in early untreated rheumatoid arthritis and are modulated following methotrexate. Arthritis Res Ther. 2015;17:239.
21. van Gestel AM, Prevoo ML, Hof MA v 't, van Rijswijk MH, van de Putte LB, van Riel PL. Development and validation of the European League Against Rheumatism response criteria for rheumatoid arthritis: comparison with the preliminary American College of Rheumatology and the World Health Organization/International League Against Rheumatism Criteria. Arthritis Rheum. 1996;39(1):34–40.
22. Aletaha D, Landewé R, Karonitsch T, Bathon J, Boers M, Bombardier C, et al. Reporting disease activity in clinical trials of patients with rheumatoid arthritis: EULAR/ACR collaborative recommendations. Arthritis Rheum. 2008;59(10):1371–7.
23. Lundstrom SL, Yang H, Lyutvinskiy Y, Rutishauser D, Herukka SK, Soininen H, et al. Blood plasma IgG Fc glycans are significantly altered in Alzheimer's disease and progressive mild cognitive impairment. J Alzheimers Dis. 2014;38(3):567–79.
24. Lyutvinskiy Y, Yang H, Rutishauser D, Zubarev RA. In silico instrumental response correction improves precision of label-free proteomics and accuracy of proteomics-based predictive models. Mol Cell Proteomics. 2013;12(8):2324–31.
25. Parekh RB, Roitt IM, Isenberg DA, Dwek RA, Ansell BM, Rademacher TW. Galactosylation of IgG associated oligosaccharides: reduction in patients with adult and juvenile onset rheumatoid arthritis and relation to disease activity. Lancet. 1988;1(8592):966–9.
26. Nakagawa H, Hato M, Takegawa Y, Deguchi K, Ito H, Takahata M, et al. Detection of altered N-glycan profiles in whole serum from rheumatoid arthritis patients. J Chromatogr B Analyt Technol Biomed Life Sci. 2007;853(1-2):133–7.

27. Gornik I, Maravic G, Dumic J, Flogel M, Lauc G. Fucosylation of IgG heavy chains is increased in rheumatoid arthritis. Clin Biochem. 1999;32(8):605–8.
28. van de Geijn FE, Wuhrer M, Selman MH, Willemsen SP, de Man YA, Deelder AM, et al. Immunoglobulin G galactosylation and sialylation are associated with pregnancy-induced improvement of rheumatoid arthritis and the postpartum flare: results from a large prospective cohort study. Arthritis Res Ther. 2009;11(6):R193.
29. Rouiller Y, Perilleux A, Marsaut M, Stettler M, Vesin MN, Broly H. Effect of hydrocortisone on the production and glycosylation of an Fc-fusion protein in CHO cell cultures. Biotechnol Prog. 2012;28(3):803–13.
30. Maguire TM, Coughlan CM, Seckl JR, Breen KC. The effect of corticosteroids on serum sialyltransferase enzyme activities in the rat. Biochim Biophys Acta. 1998;1379(1):23–8.
31. Saldova R, Huffman JE, Adamczyk B, Muzinic A, Kattla JJ, Pucic M, et al. Association of medication with the human plasma N-glycome. J Proteome Res. 2012;11(3):1821–31.
32. Boyd PN, Lines AC, Patel AK. The effect of the removal of sialic acid, galactose and total carbohydrate on the functional activity of Campath-1H. Mol Immunol. 1995;32(17-18):1311–8.
33. Hodoniczky J, Zheng YZ, James DC. Control of recombinant monoclonal antibody effector functions by Fc N-glycan remodeling in vitro. Biotechnol Prog. 2005;21(6):1644–52.
34. Banda NK, Wood AK, Takahashi K, Levitt B, Rudd PM, Royle L, et al. Initiation of the alternative pathway of murine complement by immune complexes is dependent on N-glycans in IgG antibodies. Arthritis Rheum. 2008;58(10):3081–9.
35. Royle L, Campbell MP, Radcliffe CM, White DM, Harvey DJ, Abrahams JL, et al. HPLC-based analysis of serum N-glycans on a 96-well plate platform with dedicated database software. Anal Biochem. 2008;376(1):1–12.

3

Use of a baseline risk score to identify the risk of serious infectious events in patients with rheumatoid arthritis during certolizumab pegol treatment

Jeffrey R. Curtis[1*], Kevin Winthrop[2], Cathy O'Brien[3], 'Matladi N. Ndlovu[3], Marc de Longueville[3] and Boulos Haraoui[4]

Abstract

Background: The risk of serious infectious events (SIEs) is increased in patients with rheumatoid arthritis (RA). The aim of this study was to develop an age-adjusted comorbidity index (AACI) to predict, using baseline characteristics, the SIE risk in patients with RA treated with certolizumab pegol (CZP).

Methods: Data of CZP-treated patients with RA were pooled from the RAPID1/RAPID2 randomized controlled trials (RCT CZP) and their open-label extensions (All CZP). Predictors of the first SIE were examined using multivariate Cox models. The AACI was developed by assigning specific weights to patient age and comorbidities on the basis of relative SIE risk. SIE rates were predicted using AACI score and baseline glucocorticoid use, and they were compared with observed rates. The percentage of patients in each SIE risk group achieving low disease activity (LDA)/remission was examined at 1 year of treatment.

Results: Among 1224 RCT CZP patients, 40 reported ≥ 1 SIE (incidence rate [IR] 5.09/100 patient-years [PY]), and 201 of 1506 All CZP patients reported ≥ 1 SIE (IR 3.66/100 PY). Age ≥ 70 years, diabetes mellitus, and chronic obstructive pulmonary disease/asthma made the greatest contributions to AACI score. SIE rates predicted using AACI and glucocorticoid use at baseline showed good agreement with observed SIE rates across low-risk and high-risk groups. At 1 year, more high-risk All CZP patients than low-risk All CZP patients reported SIEs (IR 8.4/100 PY vs. IR 3.4/100 PY). Rates of LDA/remission were similar between groups.

Conclusions: AACI and glucocorticoid use were strong baseline predictors of SIE risk in CZP-treated patients with RA. Predicted SIE risk was not associated with patients' likelihood of clinical response. This SIE risk score may provide a valuable tool for clinicians when considering the risk of infection in individual patients with RA.

Keywords: Certolizumab pegol, Safety, Global risk score, Comorbidity, Serious infection

* Correspondence: jrcurtis@uabmc.edu
[1]University of Alabama at Birmingham, Birmingham, AL, USA
Full list of author information is available at the end of the article

Background

Anti-tumor necrosis factor (anti-TNF) agents are often the first class of biologic drugs prescribed to patients with rheumatoid arthritis (RA), providing an effective therapeutic option that improves clinical, radiographic, and functional outcomes [1]. Owing to their immunomodulatory action, anti-TNFs have been linked to an increased risk of serious infectious events (SIEs), although the strength of this association remains a topic of debate [2–5]. In light of these concerns, biologic registries have been established in several countries to examine the long-term safety of anti-TNFs and to investigate how different patient characteristics affect the risk of serious infection [6–9].

In addition, older age and specific comorbidities that are relatively prevalent in the RA population, such as diabetes mellitus or chronic obstructive pulmonary disease (COPD), have been associated with an increased risk of SIEs during anti-TNF therapy [9–14]. Concomitant treatment with systemic glucocorticoids has also been linked to an increased susceptibility to infection [6, 8, 12, 15]. In clinical practice, physicians have to balance the benefits of the different available treatments against their overall risk, as well as the risks associated with the characteristics of each patient. This often involves the complex task of extrapolating data from study populations to the individual patient level. Infection risk scores, which summarize the relative contributions of various patient characteristics in a single composite measure, may help clinicians to anticipate the potential risk of SIEs in individual patients and make better-informed treatment decisions when balancing the expected therapeutic risks and benefits for an individual patient [11, 16, 17].

Certolizumab pegol (CZP) is a PEGylated, Fc-free anti-TNF approved for the treatment of adult patients with moderate to severe active RA [18–21]. Using baseline patient characteristics, we developed and tested an age-adjusted comorbidity index (AACI) to predict the risk of SIEs in patients with RA at the start of CZP treatment. In addition, we investigated if the predicted SIE risk was associated with the likelihood of clinical response at 1 year of CZP treatment.

Methods

Patient population and study design

To develop an AACI predictive of SIE risk in patients with RA initiating CZP treatment, we pooled baseline data from anti-TNF naive patients with RA who participated in the Rheumatoid Arthritis PreventIon of structural Damage 1 (RAPID1) and RAPID2 randomized controlled trials (RCTs; ClinicalTrials.gov, NCT00152386 and NCT00160602, respectively) and their respective open-label extensions (OLEs; NCT00175877 and NCT00160641, respectively). These pivotal registration studies have been described in detail elsewhere [20–23], and their study design is summarized in Fig. 1.

Oral glucocorticoids (≤10 mg/day prednisone equivalent) were permitted, provided that doses remained stable within 28 days of baseline and throughout the RCTs; doses were allowed to change during the OLEs. Additional details concerning patients' eligibility criteria and permitted medications are reported elsewhere [20, 21].

Definition of serious infectious events and patient groups analyzed

SIEs were classified according to the Medical Dictionary for Regulatory Activities (MedDRA) version 9.0. The definition of SIE encompassed the regulatory definition of serious adverse event (SAE) of infection [24] plus any medical events deemed important by the investigator, regardless of infection severity. All suspected SIEs were subsequently expert-reviewed by an external independent safety steering committee that classified SIEs by the regulatory definition of SAE of infection, with an additional criterion of the need for intravenous antibiotics [25].

For each patient, analyses included the first SIE that occurred after the first dose of CZP and up to 84 days (six times the half-life of CZP) after the last study dose or patient withdrawal; any subsequent SIEs were not included. Two overlapping patient groups were analyzed: (1) patients randomized to CZP in the RCTs (RCT CZP; only SIEs occurring during the RCTs were included) and (2) all patients treated with CZP during the RCTs and/or OLEs, including RCT placebo completers switched to CZP at the start of OLE as well as patients withdrawn from the RCTs at week 16 who reconsented to enter the OLE (All CZP; SIEs occurring during the RCTs or OLEs were included).

Derivation of age-adjusted comorbidity index

An AACI was developed to predict the influence of baseline age and medically treated comorbidities on the risk of SIEs during CZP treatment. The AACI was conceptually similar to the Charlson comorbidity index [26], but it was designed to better reflect the age and specific comorbidity burden of an RA patient population similar to participants in the RAPID1/RAPID2 trials. Age at baseline (<50, ≥ 50 to < 60, ≥ 60 to < 70, and ≥ 70 years) and the most frequent medically treated comorbidities (diabetes mellitus, COPD/asthma, cardiac disorder [including coronary artery disease and heart failure], hypertension, hyperlipidemia, thyroid disorder, osteoporosis, and depression) were considered for inclusion in the AACI. Medically treated comorbidities were identified on the basis of patients' medical histories or medications at baseline.

Using the RCT CZP data, the weight attributed to each baseline covariate in the AACI was derived by including all candidate covariates (described below) in a

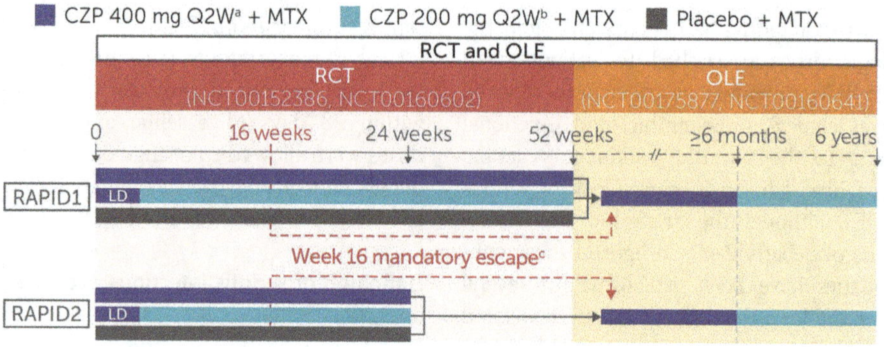

Fig. 1 Rheumatoid Arthritis Prevention of structural Damage 1 (RAPID1) and RAPID2 study design. Patients were randomized 2:2:1 to CZP 400 mg Q2W, CZP 200 mg Q2W, or placebo Q2W, respectively, in combination with MTX. The loading dose (LD) was CZP 400 mg at weeks 0, 2, and 4. [a]Twice the registered CZP dose. [b]Registered CZP dose. [c]At week 16, American College of Rheumatology 20% improvement nonresponders at weeks 12 and 14 were withdrawn from the RCTs; these patients, as well as those who completed the RCTs, were allowed to enter the OLEs, receiving CZP 400 mg Q2W + MTX for ≥ 6 months before being switched to CZP 200 mg Q2W + MTX. *CZP* Certolizumab pegol, *Q2W* Every 2 weeks, *Q4W* Every 4 weeks, *MTX* Methotrexate, *RCT* Randomized controlled trial, *OLE* Open-label extension

multivariate Cox proportional hazards model to estimate the relative risk of SIEs associated with each factor. The same analysis was repeated using the All CZP data. The two HRs obtained for each covariate in the RCT CZP and All CZP analyses were averaged to assign the corresponding weight (HR <1.2, weight = 0; HR ≥ 1.2 and < 1.5, weight = 1; HR ≥ 1.5 and < 2.5, weight = 2; HR ≥ 2.5 and < 3.5, weight = 3). An individual patient's AACI score corresponded to the sum of the weights associated with their age and specific comorbidities (Table 1 and Additional file 1: Table S1).

Evaluation of risk of SIEs

Observed incidence rates (IRs) of SIEs per 100 patient-years (PY) together with 95% CIs were calculated. Time at risk was measured from initiation of CZP up to the occurrence of the first SIE, or the total time at risk was measured for patients without SIEs (up to 84 days after the last study

Table 1 Relative serious infectious event risk associated with baseline age categories and medically treated comorbidities included in age-adjusted comorbidity index

Category		HR (95% CI)		Weight in the AACI[a]
		RCT CZP (*n* = 1224)	All CZP (*n* = 1506)	
Age, years	<50	Reference	Reference	0
	≥50 to < 60	1.29 (0.58–2.87)	1.39 (0.99–1.96)	1
	≥60 to < 70	1.14 (0.44–2.94)	1.40 (0.92–2.12)	1
	≥70	2.18 (0.70–6.84)	2.93 (1.69–5.09)	3
Diabetes mellitus		1.98 (0.59–6.58)	1.61 (0.90–2.89)	2
COPD/asthma		2.67 (0.77–9.27)	1.29 (0.56–2.97)	2
Cardiac disorder		N/C	1.33 (0.52–3.43)	0
Hypertension		1.34 (0.69–2.63)	0.96 (0.70–1.32)	0
Hyperlipidemia		2.39 (0.82–6.93)	1.47 (0.81–2.67)	2
Thyroid disorder		N/C	0.87 (0.42–1.78)	0
Osteoporosis		2.30 (0.98–5.39)	1.16 (0.73–1.86)	2
Depression		1.00 (0.22–4.51)	1.46 (0.75–2.83)	1

Abbreviations: SIE Serious infectious event, *AACI* Age-adjusted comorbidity index, *CZP* Certolizumab pegol, *COPD* Chronic obstructive pulmonary disease, *N/C* Not calculable (no patients with the indicated comorbidity experienced an SIE during the randomized controlled trials), *RCT CZP* Patients randomized to CZP in the RAPID1/RAPID2 randomized controlled trials, *All CZP* All patients treated with CZP during the RAPID1/RAPID2 randomized controlled trials and/or open label extensions

HRs were derived from a Cox proportional hazards model fitted with the indicated age categories and medically treated comorbidities; no other baseline covariates were included

[a]Weight of each category in the AACI was based on the average HR between the RCT CZP and All CZP populations (HR ≥ 1.2 and < 1.5, weight = 1; HR ≥ 1.5 and < 2.5, weight = 2; HR ≥ 2.5 and < 3.5, weight = 3)

dose or patient withdrawal). Placebo-treated patients did not contribute any data to the analysis until they entered the OLE and began treatment with CZP.

To identify all clinically relevant predictors of SIEs, a stepwise Cox proportional hazards model was fitted with AACI categories (0, 1, ≥ 2) and additional baseline covariates: body mass index (BMI; < 20, 20–30, or > 30 kg/m^2), 28-joint Disease Activity Score with C-reactive protein (DAS28[CRP]), disease duration (<2 or ≥ 2 years), Health Assessment Questionnaire Disability Index (HAQ-DI), joint erosion score (computed as log[erosion score] and included as a proxy for disease severity), methotrexate dose (≤15 or > 15 mg/week), and systemic glucocorticoid use (yes or no). Covariates were retained in the Cox model if there was an indication of a link with the occurrence of the first SIE ($p \leq 0.25$); covariates with $p \leq 0.05$ were identified as risk factors. All p values were nominal only. RCT CZP and All CZP patients were then categorized into six different risk groups based on AACI categories (0, 1, ≥ 2) and systemic glucocorticoid use (yes or no).

The Kaplan-Meier estimator was used to analyze the time to first SIE. Predicted SIE rates were based upon each patient's covariate distribution and were obtained at regular time intervals up to the date of the last recorded SIE in RCT CZP (day 301) and up to 2 years in the All CZP group. The ability of the model to discriminate between risk groups was evaluated by calculating the c-index [27]. As a sensitivity analysis, the Rheumatoid Arthritis Observation of Biologic Therapy (the German biologics register) (RABBIT) Risk Score [17] was tested in the All CZP group (*see* Additional file 1: Methods).

Clinical outcomes

For each of the six SIE risk groups in All CZP, the percentage of patients with low disease activity (LDA; DAS28[CRP] ≤ 2.7, Clinical Disease Activity Index [CDAI] ≤ 10, and Simplified Disease Activity Index [SDAI] ≤ 11) and in remission (DAS28[CRP] < 2.3, CDAI ≤ 2.8, and SDAI ≤ 3.3) was evaluated at 1 year of CZP exposure. Missing data were imputed using nonresponder imputation.

Results

Patient population and overall incidence of SIEs

The anti-TNF naive RA population pooled from RAPID1 and RAPID2 comprised 1224 patients in the RCT CZP group, with a total CZP exposure of 798.5 PY and median exposure per patient of 0.5 PY. The All CZP group comprised 1506 patients (including 282 of 311 RCT placebo patients and 1074 of 1224 RCT CZP patients who reconsented to enter the OLEs) with a total CZP exposure of 5778.6 PY and median exposure per patient of 4.8 PY. Demographic characteristics, baseline disease activity, and the prevalence of medically treated comorbidities were similar between the two patient groups (Table 2). Over 50% of patients in each group used systemic glucocorticoids at baseline.

During the RCTs, 40 of 1224 RCT CZP patients reported ≥ 1 SIE (IR 5.09/100 PY [3.64–6.93]). Over the combined RCT and OLE periods, 201 of 1506 All CZP patients reported ≥ 1 SIE (IR 3.66/100 PY [3.17–4.21]). Pneumonia and cellulitis were the most common SIEs (39 and 16 events, respectively, in All CZP). Overall, 15 RCT CZP patients and 69 All CZP patients were withdrawn from the studies because of SIEs.

Contribution of age and comorbidities selected for inclusion in age-adjusted comorbidity index

Age ≥ 70 years was strongly associated with the risk of SIEs, contributing 3 points to the AACI score. Diabetes mellitus and COPD/asthma were also important predictors of SIEs and were assigned a weight of 2 points each (Table 1). Other comorbidities contributing to AACI score were hyperlipidemia, osteoporosis, and depression.

Among all patients, the distribution of AACI scores ranged between 0 and 8, and the observed percentage of patients with SIEs generally increased with AACI score (Additional file 1: Table S1). Most patients (80% in both groups) had AACI scores ≤ 1; only one patient in the All CZP group had an AACI score of 8. Owing to the limited number of patients with high AACI scores, those with AACI scores ≥ 2 were pooled in subsequent analyses.

Identification of baseline risk factors for first SIE

AACI scores ≥ 2 and baseline systemic glucocorticoid use were identified by the Cox model as the main risk factors for the first SIE (Fig. 2). In both RCT CZP and All CZP, an AACI ≥ 2 was associated with an increase in the risk of SIEs compared with AACI of 0 (RCT CZP HR 2.86 [1.23–6.62]; All CZP HR 2.59 [1.79–3.76]), and an AACI of 1 was also associated with increased SIE risk in All CZP (HR 1.42 [1.01–2.01]). Baseline systemic glucocorticoid use was also associated with an increased risk of SIEs in RCT CZP patients (HR 2.33 [1.10–4.95]). The association was weaker in the All CZP group (HR 1.26 [0.95–1.68]). In a sensitivity analysis examining different baseline glucocorticoid doses, the risk of SIEs was similar between glucocorticoid doses > 0–5 mg/day and > 5 mg/day (data not shown).

Baseline DAS28(CRP) and erosion scores did not contribute to SIE risk in the All CZP group, but they showed a modest association in the RCT CZP group. No other covariates tested (BMI, disease duration, HAQ-DI, and MTX dose) showed a detectable association with the risk of SIEs ($p > 0.25$). Replacing DAS28(CRP) in the Cox model with alternative measures of disease activity (CRP, DAS28[erythrocyte sedimentation rate], CDAI, and SDAI)

Table 2 Baseline patient characteristics

		RCT CZP (*n* = 1224)	All CZP (*n* = 1506)
Female sex, *n* (%)		1008 (82.4)	1245 (82.7)
Age, years, *n* (%)	<50	470 (38.4)	580 (38.5)
	≥50 to < 60	440 (35.9)	546 (36.3)
	≥60 to < 70	247 (20.2)	300 (19.9)
	≥70	67 (5.5)	80 (5.3)
Disease duration (years), *n* (%)	<2	261 (21.3)	323 (21.4)
	≥2	963 (78.7)	1183 (78.6)
DAS28(CRP), mean (SD)		6.20 (0.83)	6.20 (0.85)
HAQ-DI, mean (SD)		1.65 (0.60)	1.65 (0.60)
CRP, mg/L, median (IQR)		15.0 (6.0–32.0)	15.0 (6.0–32.0)
Rheumatoid factor, IU/ml, median (IQR)		68.3 (18.9–201.1)	70.0 (19.4–200.0)
mTSS, median (IQR)		20.0 (5.5–54.7)	20.0 (6.0–55.0)
BMI, kg/m^2, *n* (%)	<20	83 (6.8)	104 (6.9)
	20–30	833 (68.1)	1024 (68.0)
	>30	308 (25.2)	378 (25.1)
Glucocorticoid dose, mg/day, *n* (%)	0	518 (42.3)	637 (42.3)
	>0–5	332 (27.1)	402 (26.7)
	>5	374 (30.6)	467 (31.0)
Systemic MTX dose, mg/week, *n* (%)	≤15	1018 (83.2)	1261 (83.7)
	>15	206 (16.8)	245 (16.3)
Medically treated comorbidities, *n* (%)[a]			
Diabetes mellitus		47 (3.8)	53 (3.5)
COPD/asthma		34 (2.8)	38 (2.5)
Cardiac disorder[b]		15 (1.2)	17 (1.1)
Hypertension[c]		387 (31.6)	465 (30.9)
Hyperlipidemia		55 (4.5)	66 (4.4)
Thyroid disorder		55 (4.5)	63 (4.2)
Osteoporosis		92 (7.5)	113 (7.5)
Depression		37 (3.0)	45 (3.0)

Abbreviations: CZP Certolizumab pegol, *RCT* Randomized controlled trial, *DAS28(CRP)* 28-joint Disease Activity Score with C-reactive protein, *CRP* C-reactive protein, *HAQ-DI* Health Assessment Questionnaire Disability Index, *mTSS* Modified total Sharp score, *MTX* Methotrexate, *BMI* Body mass index, *COPD* Chronic obstructive pulmonary disease, *RCT CZP* Patients randomized to CZP in the RAPID1/RAPID2 randomized controlled trials, *All CZP* All patients treated with CZP during the RAPID1/RAPID2 randomized controlled trials and/or open label extensions

[a]Medically treated comorbidities were identified on the basis of patients' medical histories and medications at baseline

[b]Cardiac disorder included coronary artery disease and heart failure

[c]Hypertension included patients with history of cerebrovascular disorder (*n* = 5 in RCT CZP and *n* = 5 in All CZP) and transient ischemic attack (*n* = 4 in RCT CZP and *n* = 5 in All CZP)

produced results similar to those of the main analyses (data not shown).

Use of baseline age-adjusted comorbidity index and systemic glucocorticoids to predict rate of SIEs

In the RCT CZP group, the predicted risk of SIEs was lowest for patients with an AACI of 0 and no systemic glucocorticoid use at baseline, and highest in patients with an AACI ≥ 2 who used systemic glucocorticoids (Fig. 3a). Within the same AACI category, the percentage of patients reporting a first SIE was approximately twofold higher if patients also used systemic glucocorticoids at baseline. The c-index (0.66 [0.33–0.93]) indicated fair discrimination between patient groups.

In the All CZP group, the predicted risk of SIEs was lowest for the patient groups defined by AACI of 0 and highest for patients with AACI ≥ 2, regardless of systemic glucocorticoid use (Fig. 3b). The c-index (0.85 [0.73–0.93]) suggested excellent discrimination between patient groups.

Across the different risk groups, observed SIE rates generally matched model predictions, demonstrating that the prediction model was well-calibrated (Table 3).

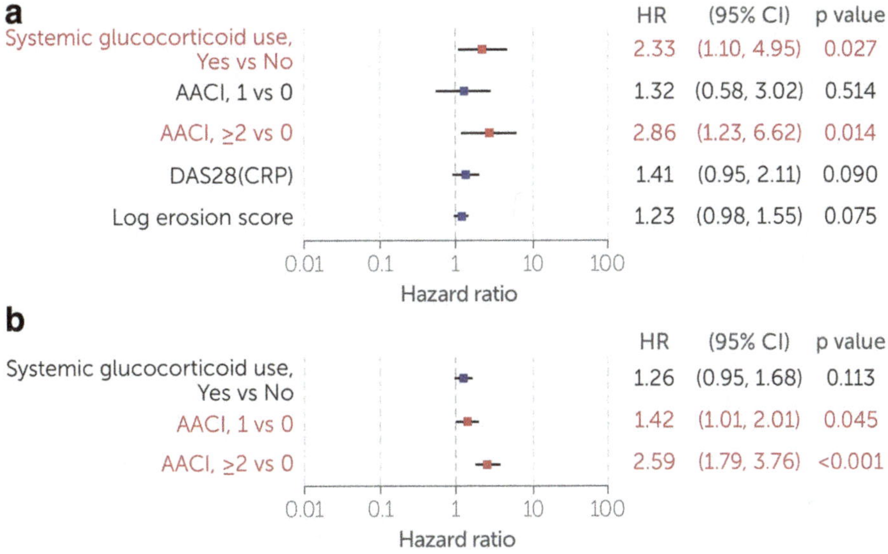

Fig. 2 Multivariate analysis of baseline predictors to the first SIE. **a** RCT CZP group. **b** All CZP group. A Cox proportional hazards model fitted with AACI categories was used to identify baseline covariates linked to SIE risk ($p \leq 0.25$). Baseline covariates identified as risk factors ($p \leq 0.05$) are highlighted in *red*. No other baseline covariates examined (BMI, disease duration, HAQ-DI, and MTX dose) were considered relevant to the outcome ($p > 0.25$). *SIE* Serious infectious event, *RCT* Randomized controlled trial, *CZP* Certolizumab pegol, *AACI* Age-adjusted comorbidity index, *DAS28(CRP)* 28-joint Disease Activity Score with C-reactive protein, *BMI* Body mass index, *HAQ-DI* Health Assessment Questionnaire Disability Index, *MTX* Methotrexate, *RCT CZP* Patients randomized to CZP in the RAPID1/RAPID2 randomized controlled trials, *All CZP* All patients treated with CZP during the RAPID1/RAPID2 randomized controlled trials and/or open label extensions

Consistent with model predictions, the observed IRs of SIEs were higher for patients with AACI ≥ 2 and baseline systemic glucocorticoid use, and lower for patients with AACI of 0 and no baseline systemic glucocorticoid use (Table 4).

As a sensitivity analysis, the RABBIT Risk Score was tested in the All CZP group. On the basis of expected SIE risk, patients were assigned only to the first three deciles of RABBIT Risk Scores published by Zink et al. [17]. Predicted SIE rates were generally comparable to observed rates, with some underestimation of SIE rates in patients with lower RABBIT Risk Scores (Additional file 1: Figure S1).

Observed rates of LDA and remission in different SIE risk groups

We investigated if the predicted SIE risk influenced the achievement of LDA and remission at 1 year of CZP treatment according to DAS28(CRP), CDAI, and SDAI criteria (Fig. 4). In All CZP, the percentage of patients achieving LDA was comparable across the different SIE risk groups, albeit with a numerically higher proportion in the low-risk group (AACI of 0 and no baseline systemic glucocorticoid use). Likewise, the rates of remission did not vary considerably between SIE risk groups.

Discussion

Patients with RA are reported to have an increased susceptibility to infection compared with patients without RA [28]. Although the strength of association between anti-TNFs and the risk of infection remains a topic of debate [2–5], the evidence published so far underscores the need for clinicians to carefully balance the clinical benefits and potential harms of initiating anti-TNF therapy in individual patients.

Using data pooled from the pivotal RAPID1 and RAPID2 RCTs and OLEs [20–23], we derived and tested a new AACI to predict the risk of SIEs during CZP treatment, based on the baseline characteristics of anti-TNF naive patients with moderate to severe active RA and inadequate response to prior disease-modifying antirheumatic drugs. AACI ≥ 2 and systemic glucocorticoid use were identified as the main baseline risk factors for the occurrence of SIEs. With up to 2 years of CZP exposure, predicted SIE rates matched the observed rates, suggesting that the model was well-calibrated for the outcome. Discrimination between different risk groups in the model was fair (RCT CZP) to excellent (All CZP).

As expected, the IRs of SIEs in groups defined as being at high risk were higher than reported previously in a pooled safety analysis of patients with RA in CZP clinical trials (IR 3.7/100 PY [3.3–4.1] [25]). Consistent with previous CZP safety data [25] and registry data [10, 13], the highest incidence of SIEs was seen during the first 6 months of anti-TNF treatment and decreased thereafter.

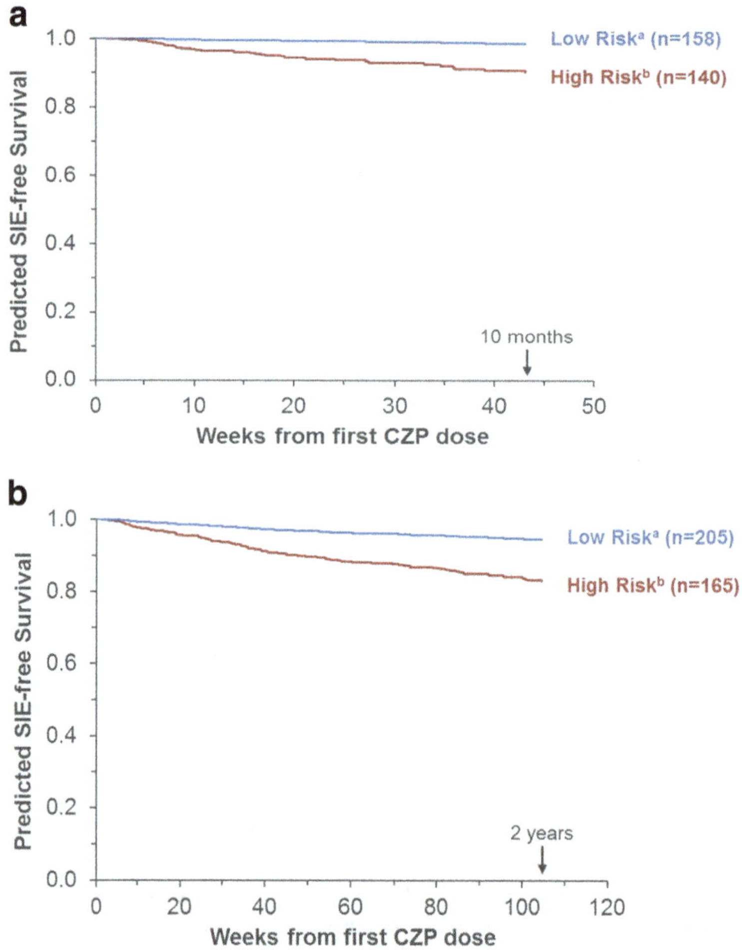

Fig. 3 Predicted time to first SIE, by baseline systemic glucocorticoid use and AACI. **a** RCT CZP. **b** All CZP. Predicted SIE-free survival curves correspond to Kaplan-Meier estimates for the indicated risk groups, based on the covariates selected by the Cox models. The c-indexes were 0.66 (95% CI 0.33–0.93) for the RCT CZP model and 0.85 (95% CI 0.73–0.93) for the All CZP model. [a]Low risk at baseline: AACI of 0, without systemic glucocorticoid use. [b]High risk at baseline: AACI ≥ 2, with systemic glucocorticoid use. *SIE* Serious infectious event, *CZP* Certolizumab pegol, *AACI* Age-adjusted comorbidity index, *RCT CZP* Patients randomized to CZP in the RAPID1/RAPID2 randomized controlled trials, *All CZP* All patients treated with CZP during the RAPID1/RAPID2 randomized controlled trials and/or open label extensions, *CI* Confidence interval

In All CZP, the rates of LDA and remission observed at 1 year were similar across all six risk groups, suggesting that the baseline risk of SIEs was not associated with the likelihood of response to CZP treatment. Indeed, poor prognostic factors for RA progression, such as longer disease duration, greater disability, and erosive disease [29, 30], were not associated with SIE risk when tested in the Cox model.

In line with previous studies [9–14], older age (≥70 years), diabetes mellitus, and COPD/asthma were strongly associated with SIE risk in this RA population, making an important contribution to patients' AACI scores. Consistent with our results, older age and comorbidities also featured in other SIE risk scores in RA, developed using data from biologics registries and administrative databases [11, 16, 17]. In addition, we found that hyperlipidemia, osteoporosis, and depression were associated with an increased risk of SIEs in the RAPID1/RAPID2 patient population. Depression and the use of certain antidepressant medications have previously been associated with an increased risk of some infections [31]. However, it is uncertain whether some of these associations might have a true biologic basis, be driven by the effects of medications used to treat the condition, be a proxy for a shared risk factor (e.g., frailty), or reflect other confounding factors.

The increased risk of infection associated with systemic glucocorticoids is widely recognized [6, 8, 12, 15]. Our data revealed a dose-independent association between baseline systemic glucocorticoid use and SIEs in the RCT CZP group, where doses were required to remain stable throughout the RCTs [20, 21]. By contrast, systemic glucocorticoid doses were allowed to change during the OLEs, which may have minimized our ability to detect a stronger association with SIE

Table 3 Predicted and observed percentages of patients affected by first serious infectious event

Time since first CZP dose	Data						
RCT CZP	Percentage of patients affected by the first SIE[a]	Without systemic glucocorticoid use			With systemic glucocorticoid use		
		AACI = 0 (n = 158)	AACI = 1 (n = 250)	AACI ≥ 2 (n = 110)	AACI = 0 (n = 271)	AACI = 1 (n = 295)	AACI ≥ 2 (n = 140)
3 months	Predicted (95% CI)	0.5 (0.0–1.0)	0.7 (0.1–1.3)	1.4 (0.2–2.7)	1.2 (0.3–2.1)	1.7 (0.6–2.8)	3.8 (1.4–6.1)
	Observed	0.6	1.2	1.8	1.1	2.4	2.9
6 months	Predicted (95% CI)	0.9 (0.1–1.8)	1.2 (0.3–2.2)	2.5 (0.4–4.5)	2.1 (0.6–3.5)	3.0 (1.2–4.7)	6.5 (2.7–10.1)
	Observed	0.6	1.6	2.7	2.2	3.7	5.0
1 year	Predicted (95% CI)[b]	1.5 (0.2–2.8)	1.9 (0.4–3.4)	3.9 (0.7–7.0)	3.3 (1.0–5.5)	4.7 (2.0–7.2)	10.0 (4.3–15.4)
	Observed	0.6	2.0	3.6	3.0	4.1	7.1
All CZP	Percentage of patients affected by the first SIE[a]	Without systemic glucocorticoid use			With systemic glucocorticoid use		
		AACI = 0 (n = 205)	AACI = 1 (n = 302)	AACI ≥ 2 (n = 130)	AACI = 0 (n = 325)	AACI = 1 (n = 379)	AACI ≥ 2 (n = 165)
3 months	Predicted (95% CI)	0.9 (0.4–1.3)	1.2 (0.6–1.8)	2.2 (1.1–3.3)	1.1 (0.6–1.6)	1.5 (0.8–2.2)	2.8 (1.5–4.1)
	Observed	0.5	1.0	1.5	0.9	2.1	3.0
6 months	Predicted (95% CI)	1.6 (0.9–2.3)	2.3 (1.4–3.2)	4.2 (2.5–5.8)	2.1 (1.2–2.9)	2.9 (1.9–3.9)	5.2 (3.3–7.2)
	Observed	2.0	1.3	2.3	2.2	3.7	5.5
1 year	Predicted (95% CI)	3.3 (2.1–4.5)	4.6 (3.2–6.1)	8.3 (5.5–11.0)	4.1 (2.8–5.5)	5.8 (4.1–7.5)	10.4 (7.2–13.4)
	Observed	4.4	2.0	4.6	4.0	7.1	10.9
2 years	Predicted (95% CI)	5.5 (3.6–7.4)	7.7 (5.5–9.9)	13.7 (9.5–17.7)	6.9 (4.8–8.9)	9.6 (7.2–12.0)	16.9 (12.3–21.3)
	Observed	5.9	4.6	13.8	6.8	9.8	12.7

Abbreviations: SIE Serious infectious event, *CZP* Certolizumab pegol, *AACI* Age-adjusted comorbidity index, *RCT CZP* Patients randomized to CZP in the RAPID1/RAPID2 randomized controlled trials, *All CZP* All patients treated with CZP during the RAPID1/RAPID2 randomized controlled trials and/or open label extensions, *CI* Confidence interval

[a]Percentage of patients affected by the first SIE up to the indicated time since the first CZP dose

[b]One-year predicted rates in RCT CZP correspond to 301 days (~10 months) because Kaplan-Meier estimates were not defined beyond the last SIE date

Table 4 Observed incidence of serious infectious events in patients categorized by age-adjusted comorbidity index and baseline systemic glucocorticoid use

Time since first CZP dose	IR/100 PY (95% CI)[a]					
	Without systemic glucocorticoid use			With systemic glucocorticoid use		
	AACI = 0	AACI = 1	AACI ≥ 2	AACI = 0	AACI = 1	AACI ≥ 2
RCT CZP						
Patients, *n*	158	250	110	271	295	140
3 months	2.6 (0.1–14.5)	4.9 (1.0–14.3)	7.8 (1.0–28.2)	4.5 (0.9–13.3)	9.8 (3.9–20.2)	11.9 (3.2–30.5)
6 months	1.4 (0.0–8.0)	3.7 (1.0–9.6)	6.8 (1.4–19.9)	5.1 (1.9–11.1)	8.6 (4.3–15.4)	12.1 (4.9–25.0)
1 year	1.0 (0.0–5.3)	3.2 (1.0–7.4)	6.2 (1.7–15.9)	4.6 (2.0–9.1)	6.2 (3.2–10.9)	12.1 (5.8–22.2)
All CZP						
Patients, *n*	205	302	130	325	379	165
3 months	2.0 (0.1–11.1)	4.1 (0.8–11.9)	6.6 (0.8–23.7)	3.8 (0.8–11.1)	8.7 (3.8–17.1)	12.6 (4.1–29.4)
6 months	4.1 (1.1–10.5)	2.8 (0.8–7.1)	5.1 (1.0–14.8)	4.5 (1.8–9.3)	7.8 (4.3–13.1)	11.7 (5.4–22.2)
1 year	4.8 (2.2–9.1)	2.2 (0.8–4.7)	5.3 (2.0–11.6)	4.3 (2.3–7.4)	8.0 (5.3–11.7)	12.6 (7.5–20.0)
2 years	3.4 (1.8–6.0)	2.7 (1.5–4.5)	8.9 (5.3–14.0)	3.9 (2.5–5.9)	6.0 (4.3–8.3)	8.4 (5.2–12.8)

Abbreviations: SIE Serious infectious event, *CZP* Certolizumab pegol, *IR* Incidence rate, *PY* Patient-years, *AACI* Age-adjusted comorbidity index, *RCT CZP* Patients randomized to CZP in the RAPID1/RAPID2 randomized controlled trials, *All CZP* All patients treated with CZP during the RAPID1/RAPID2 randomized controlled trials and/or open label extensions, *CI* Confidence interval

[a]IR of SIEs observed during the indicated time interval since the first day on CZP

risk in the All CZP group. Furthermore, we cannot discount the possibility that doses taken over the previous 2–3 years may have had a cumulative impact on the risk of SIEs [32]. Despite such limitations, our results suggest potential benefits of avoiding concomitant systemic glucocorticoid use in CZP-treated patients with RA as early as possible, as recommended by the 2015 American College of Rheumatology RA guidelines [33].

High disease activity has been associated with an increased risk of infection [34, 35]. However, in our model, baseline disease activity showed only a modest association with the risk of SIEs. One likely explanation is the fact that all patients enrolled in the RAPID1/RAPID2 RCTs had moderate to high disease activity at baseline. The relatively narrow range of baseline DAS28(CRP) scores in this RA population may have concealed a stronger association with SIE risk.

Several studies have reported that the relative risk of infection decreases over time in patients with RA treated with anti-TNF [13, 25, 36–38]. This has been attributed not only to the depletion of susceptible patients from the study cohorts but also to an improvement in the clinical status of patients, either as a direct result of reduced disease activity or owing to a decline in the use of concomitant glucocorticoids [8]. The model that we developed tested only the effect of baseline patient characteristics. Although AACI, which is a static patient characteristic, was the strongest predictor of SIEs, clinical parameters such as disease activity and physical function (HAQ-DI) may have changed considerably over time as a result of CZP treatment, resulting in weaker prediction of SIE rates for CZP exposures > 2 years.

A limitation of the method used to derive the AACI is the fact that the HRs for each age category and individual comorbidity were averaged across the RCT CZP and All CZP groups in order to assign the respective weighting. Our intention with the AACI was to provide an indication of SIE risk not only in the first year of treatment but also over a longer period of time. Had we used just the RCT period to derive the weightings for each age category and comorbidity, we would have potentially overestimated the risk of SIEs during the OLE. For this reason, the averaging of HRs seemed to be a reasonable approach, albeit at the expense of some predictive accuracy.

Prior epidemiologic work has suggested that although some risk estimation models can be generalized, model performance is optimized when population-specific weights can be derived [11]. As such, the weighting for each risk factor in one population may not be generalizable to a different RA population. For instance, the RABBIT Risk Score performed well in the All CZP group, but SIE rates were underestimated at the lower end of the risk spectrum. One possible explanation is the fact that the RABBIT Risk Score may be better calibrated for real-world patient populations with a higher propensity for SIEs [17]. For example, chronic renal disease and chronic lung disease, which contribute to the RABBIT Risk Score, were less prevalent or absent in our study population. Furthermore, our assumption that there were zero patients with a history of prior SIEs

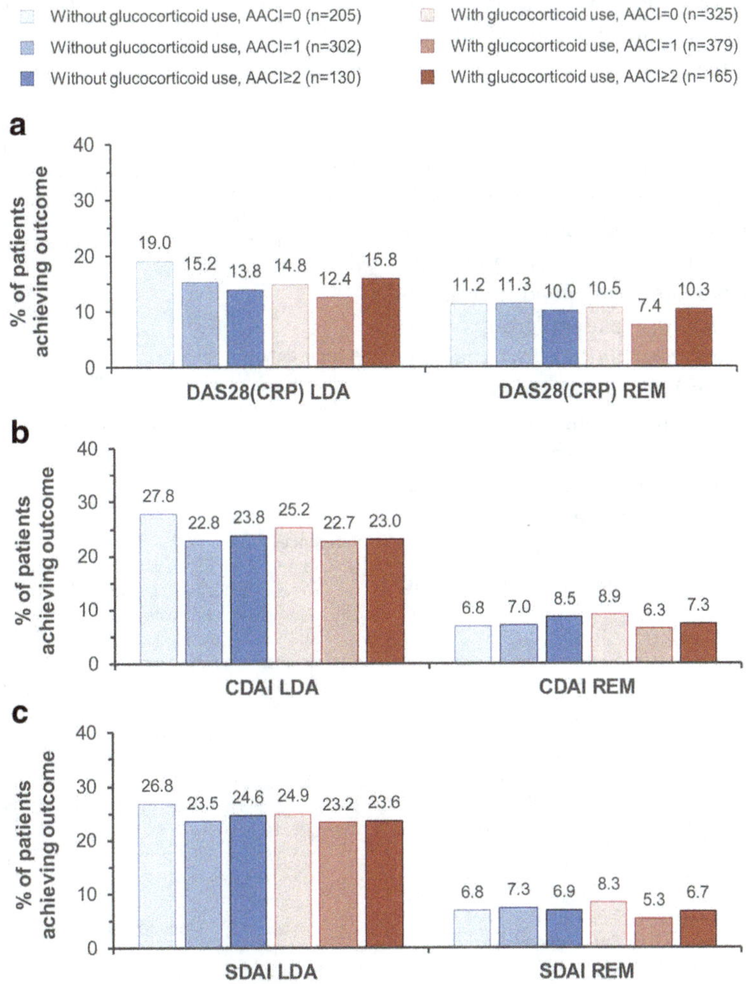

Fig. 4 Observed proportion of All CZP patients achieving LDA and remission at 1 year of treatment. **a** DAS28(CRP). **b** CDAI. **c** SDAI. LDA was defined as DAS28(CRP) ≤ 2.7, CDAI ≤ 10, and SDAI ≤ 11; remission corresponded to DAS28(CRP) < 2.3, CDAI ≤ 2.8, and SDAI ≤ 3.3. Missing data were imputed using nonresponder imputation. *LDA* Low disease activity, *CZP* Certolizumab pegol, *AACI* Age-adjusted comorbidity index, *DAS28(CRP)* 28-joint Disease Activity Score with C-reactive protein, *REM* Remission, *CDAI* Clinical Disease Activity Index, *SDAI* Simplified Disease Activity Index, *All CZP* All patients treated with CZP during the RAPID1/RAPID2 randomized controlled trials and/or open label extensions

may also have contributed to the underestimation of RABBIT Risk Scores.

At initiation of anti-TNF therapy, prescribers need to consider the infection risk in each individual patient, which must take into account the patient's age, comorbidities, concomitant medications, and clinical history. However, most data currently available consist of mean infection rates observed in relatively large, heterogeneous populations. Although group-level infection rates are informative, they are not always relevant at the individual patient level in clinical practice. This is why stratifying patients according to comorbidity burden and other infection risk factors can help clinicians to make more accurate risk-benefit assessments regarding anti-TNF therapy and ultimately make better-informed treatment decisions at the individual-patient level.

However, in clinical practice, prescribers tend to channel higher-risk patients away from anti-TNF therapy, owing to the commonly held view that older patients or those with more severe comorbidities are less likely to benefit clinically from anti-TNF treatment [11, 39, 40]. However, there is published evidence suggesting that responsiveness to treatment and the incremental infection risk associated with anti-TNFs is similar for higher- and lower-risk groups [41, 42]. Consistent with this, our data showed that the rates of LDA and remission at 1 year of CZP treatment were similar across all AACI risk groups. Although the limited placebo exposure did not allow us to quantify the incremental risk associated with CZP, the results of our study are reassuring for patients with higher AACI scores at baseline and may encourage clinicians to avoid concomitant glucocorticoids to reduce the SIE risk. Further research is needed to examine how the disease-modifying effects of CZP treatment, as well as changes in glucocorticoid use, influence the risk of SIEs in a time-dependent manner.

Conclusions

In this population of patients with moderate to severe active RA and no prior anti-TNF use, the rate of SIEs during CZP treatment was predicted with considerable accuracy using a combination of AACI score and baseline systemic glucocorticoid use, with good discrimination between high- and low-risk patient groups. This SIE risk score may provide a valuable tool for clinicians when considering the risk of infection in individual patients with RA. One of the greatest strengths of our analysis was the use of a large, very comprehensive clinical trial database to derive the AACI. However, we should note that the AACI model has not been validated in a different population. It would be valuable to assess how the AACI performs in other RA trials and in real-world settings.

Abbreviations

AACI: Age-adjusted comorbidity index; BMI: Body mass index; CDAI: Clinical Disease Activity Index; CI: Confidence interval; COPD: Chronic obstructive pulmonary disease; CRP: C-reactive protein; CZP: Certolizumab pegol; DAS28(CRP): 28-joint Disease Activity Score with C-reactive protein; HAQ-DI: Health Assessment Questionnaire Disability Index; HR: Hazard ratio; IR: Incidence rate; LD: Loading dose; LDA: Low disease activity; MedDRA: Medical Dictionary for Regulatory Activities; mTSS: Modified total Sharp score; MTX: Methotrexate; OLE: Open-label extension; PY: Patient-years; RA: Rheumatoid arthritis; RABBIT: Rheumatoid Arthritis Observation of Biologic Therapy (the German biologics register); RAPID: Rheumatoid Arthritis Prevention of structural Damage; RCT: Randomized controlled trial; SAE: Serious adverse event; SDAI: Simplified Disease Activity Index; SIE: Serious infectious event; TNF: Tumor necrosis factor

Acknowledgements

The authors thank the patients and their caregivers in addition to the investigators and their teams who contributed to this study. The authors acknowledge Pauline Ralston, MSc, UCB Pharma, Brussels, Belgium, for statistical assistance; and Ricardo Milho, PhD, and Debbie Nixon, DPhil, from Costello Medical, Cambridge, UK, for medical writing and editorial assistance in the preparation of this manuscript for publication based on the authors' input and direction.

Funding

This study was funded by UCB Pharma.

Authors' contributions

JRC, KW, CO'B, 'MNN, MdL, and BH contributed to the conception, design, execution, or analysis and interpretation of the data. The authors read and approved the final manuscript to be published after critically revising it for important intellectual content.

Competing interests

JRC has received research grants and consultant fees from Roche, Genentech, UCB Pharma, Janssen, Corrona, Amgen, Pfizer, Bristol-Myers Squibb, Crescendo, and AbbVie. KW has received consultant fees from UCB Pharma, Pfizer, Bristol-Myers Squibb, Eli Lilly, AbbVie, and Roche. CO'B was an employee of UCB Pharma at the time of this work. 'MNN is an employee of UCB Pharma. MdL is an employee of UCB Pharma. BH has received research grants and consultant fees from Abbott, Amgen, Bristol-Myers Squibb, Janssen, Pfizer, Roche, and UCB Pharma. UCB sponsored the study and the development of the manuscript/publication and reviewed the text to ensure that, from UCB's perspective, the data presented in this article are scientifically, technically, and medically supportable; that they do not contain any information that has the potential to damage the intellectual property of UCB; and that the publication complies with applicable laws, regulations, guidelines, and good industry practice.

Author details

[1]University of Alabama at Birmingham, Birmingham, AL, USA. [2]Oregon Health and Science University, Portland, OR, USA. [3]UCB Pharma, Brussels, Belgium. [4]Department of Medicine, Centre Hospitalier de l'Université de Montréal, Montréal, QC, Canada.

References

1. Nam JL, Ramiro S, Gaujoux-Viala C, Takase K, Leon-Garcia M, Emery P, Gossec L, Landewé R, Smolen JS, Buch MH. Efficacy of biological disease-modifying antirheumatic drugs: a systematic literature review informing the 2013 update of the EULAR recommendations for the management of rheumatoid arthritis. Ann Rheum Dis. 2014;73(3):516–28.
2. Bongartz T, Sutton AJ, Sweeting MJ, Buchan I, Matteson EL, Montori V. Anti-TNF antibody therapy in rheumatoid arthritis and the risk of serious infections and malignancies: systematic review and meta-analysis of rare harmful effects in randomized controlled trials. JAMA. 2006;295(19):2275–85.
3. Leombruno JP, Einarson TR, Keystone EC. The safety of anti-tumour necrosis factor treatments in rheumatoid arthritis: meta and exposure-adjusted pooled analyses of serious adverse events. Ann Rheum Dis. 2009;68(7):1136–45.
4. Singh JA, Cameron C, Noorbaloochi S, Cullis T, Tucker M, Christensen R, Ghogomu ET, Coyle D, Clifford T, Tugwell P, Wells GA. Risk of serious infection in biological treatment of patients with rheumatoid arthritis: a systematic review and meta-analysis. Lancet. 2015;386(9990):258–65.
5. Thompson AE, Rieder SW, Pope JE. Tumor necrosis factor therapy and the risk of serious infection and malignancy in patients with early rheumatoid arthritis: a meta-analysis of randomized controlled trials. Arthritis Rheum. 2011;63(6):1479–85.
6. Greenberg JD, Reed G, Kremer JM, Tindall E, Kavanaugh A, Zheng C, Bishai W, Hochberg MC. Association of methotrexate and tumour necrosis factor antagonists with risk of infectious outcomes including opportunistic infections in the CORRONA registry. Ann Rheum Dis. 2010;69(2):380–6.
7. Listing J, Gerhold K, Zink A. The risk of infections associated with rheumatoid arthritis, with its comorbidity and treatment. Rheumatology. 2013;52(1):53–61.
8. Strangfeld A, Eveslage M, Schneider M, Bergerhausen HJ, Klopsch T, Zink A, Listing J. Treatment benefit or survival of the fittest: what drives the time-dependent decrease in serious infection rates under TNF inhibition and what does this imply for the individual patient? Ann Rheum Dis. 2011;70(11):1914–20.
9. Zink A, Askling J, Dixon WG, Klareskog L, Silman AJ, Symmons DP. European biologicals registers: methodology, selected results and perspectives. Ann Rheum Dis. 2009;68(8):1240–6.
10. Cobo-Ibáñez T, Descalzo MÁ, Loza-Santamaría E, Carmona L, Muñoz-Fernández S. Serious infections in patients with rheumatoid arthritis and other immune-mediated connective tissue diseases exposed to anti-TNF or rituximab: data from the Spanish registry BIOBADASER 2.0. Rheumatol Int. 2014;34(7):953–61.
11. Curtis JR, Xie F, Chen L, Muntner P, Grijalva CG, Spettell C, Fernandes J, McMahan RM, Baddley JW, Saag KG, et al. Use of a disease risk score to compare serious infections associated with anti-tumor necrosis factor therapy among high- versus lower-risk rheumatoid arthritis patients. Arthritis Care Res. 2012;64(10):1480–9.
12. Doran MF, Crowson CS, Pond GR, O'Fallon WM, Gabriel SE. Predictors of infection in rheumatoid arthritis. Arthritis Rheum. 2002;46(9):2294–300.

13. Galloway JB, Hyrich KL, Mercer LK, Dixon WG, Fu B, Ustianowski AP, Watson KD, Lunt M, Symmons DP, Consortium BCC, et al. Anti-TNF therapy is associated with an increased risk of serious infections in patients with rheumatoid arthritis especially in the first 6 months of treatment: updated results from the British Society for Rheumatology Biologics Register with special emphasis on risks in the elderly. Rheumatology. 2011;50(1):124–31.
14. Van Dartel SA, Fransen J, Kievit W, Dutmer EA, Brus HL, Houtman NM, Van De Laar MA, Van Riel PL. Predictors for the 5-year risk of serious infections in patients with rheumatoid arthritis treated with anti-tumour necrosis factor therapy: a cohort study in the Dutch Rheumatoid Arthritis Monitoring (DREAM) registry. Rheumatology. 2013;52(6):1052–7.
15. Haraoui B, Combe B, Champsaur M, Luijtens K, Keystone E. Effects of different steroid doses on adverse events and radiographic progression of certolizumab pegol-treated rheumatoid arthritis patients [abstract]. Ann Rheum Dis. 2013;71 Suppl 3:498.
16. Crowson CS, Hoganson DD, Fitz-Gibbon PD, Matteson EL. Development and validation of a risk score for serious infection in patients with rheumatoid arthritis. Arthritis Rheum. 2012;64(9):2847–55.
17. Zink A, Manger B, Kaufmann J, Eisterhues C, Krause A, Listing J, Strangfeld A. Evaluation of the RABBIT Risk Score for serious infections. Ann Rheum Dis. 2014;73(9):1673–6.
18. Karmiris K, Paintaud G, Noman M, Magdelaine-Beuzelin C, Ferrante M, Degenne D, Claes K, Coopman T, Van Schuerbeek N, Van Assche G, et al. Influence of trough serum levels and immunogenicity on long-term outcome of adalimumab therapy in Crohn's disease. Gastroenterology. 2009;137(5):1628–40.
19. European Medicines Agency (EMA). Annex I: summary of product characteristics (Cimzia). London: EMA; 2013.
20. Keystone E, Heijde D, Mason Jr D, Landewé R, Vollenhoven RV, Combe B, Emery P, Strand V, Mease P, Desai C, et al. Certolizumab pegol plus methotrexate is significantly more effective than placebo plus methotrexate in active rheumatoid arthritis: findings of a fifty-two-week, phase III, multicenter, randomized, double-blind, placebo-controlled, parallel-group study. Arthritis Rheum. 2008;58(11):3319–29.
21. Smolen J, Landewé RB, Mease P, Brzezicki J, Mason D, Luijtens K, van Vollenhoven RF, Kavanaugh A, Schiff M, Burmester GR, et al. Efficacy and safety of certolizumab pegol plus methotrexate in active rheumatoid arthritis: the RAPID 2 study. A randomised controlled trial. Ann Rheum Dis. 2009;68(6):797–804.
22. Keystone E, Landewé R, van Vollenhoven R, Combe B, Strand V, Mease P, Shaughnessy L, Vanlunen B, van der Heijde D. Long-term safety and efficacy of certolizumab pegol in combination with methotrexate in the treatment of rheumatoid arthritis: 5-year results from the RAPID 1 trial and open-label extension. Ann Rheum Dis. 2014;73(12):2094–100.
23. Smolen JS, van Vollenhoven R, Kavanaugh A, Strand V, Vencovsky J, Schiff M, Landewé R, Haraoui B, Arendt C, Mountian I, et al. Certolizumab pegol plus methotrexate 5-year results from the rheumatoid arthritis prevention of structural damage (RAPID) 2 randomized controlled trial and long-term extension in rheumatoid arthritis patients. Arthritis Res Ther. 2015;17:245.
24. U.S. Food and Drug Administration (FDA). Reporting serious problems to the FDA: what is a serious adverse event? Silver Spring, MD: FDA; 2012. https://www.fda.gov/safety/medwatch/howtoreport/ucm053087.htm. Accessed 15 Feb 2017.
25. Bykerk VP, Cush J, Winthrop K, Calabrese L, Lortholary O, de Longueville M, van Vollenhoven R, Mariette X. Update on the safety profile of certolizumab pegol in rheumatoid arthritis: an integrated analysis from clinical trials. Ann Rheum Dis. 2015;74(1):96–103.
26. Charlson ME, Pompei P, Ales KL, MacKenzie CR. A new method of classifying prognostic comorbidity in longitudinal studies: development and validation. J Chronic Dis. 1987;40(5):373–83.
27. Gönen M, Heller G. Concordance probability and discriminatory power in proportional hazards regression. Biometrika. 2005;92(4):965–70.
28. Doran MF, Crowson CS, Pond GR, O'Fallon WM, Gabriel SE. Frequency of infection in patients with rheumatoid arthritis compared with controls: a population-based study. Arthritis Rheum. 2002;46(9):2287–93.
29. Quinn MA, Conaghan PG, O'Connor PJ, Karim Z, Greenstein A, Brown A, Brown C, Fraser A, Jarret S, Emery P. Very early treatment with infliximab in addition to methotrexate in early, poor-prognosis rheumatoid arthritis reduces magnetic resonance imaging evidence of synovitis and damage, with sustained benefit after infliximab withdrawal: results from a twelve-month randomized, double-blind, placebo-controlled trial. Arthritis Rheum. 2005;52(1):27–35.
30. Jayakumar K, Norton S, Dixey J, James D, Gough A, Williams P, Prouse P, Young A. Sustained clinical remission in rheumatoid arthritis: prevalence and prognostic factors in an inception cohort of patients treated with conventional DMARDs. Rheumatology. 2012;51(1):169–75.
31. Rogers MA, Greene MT, Young VB, Saint S, Langa KM, Kao JY, Aronoff DM. Depression, antidepressant medications, and risk of *Clostridium difficile* infection. BMC Med. 2013;11:121.
32. Dixon WG, Abrahamowicz M, Beauchamp ME, Ray DW, Bernatsky S, Suissa S, Sylvestre MP. Immediate and delayed impact of oral glucocorticoid therapy on risk of serious infection in older patients with rheumatoid arthritis: a nested case-control analysis. Ann Rheum Dis. 2012;71(7):1128–33.
33. Singh JA, Saag KG, Bridges Jr SL, Akl EA, Bannuru RR, Sullivan MC, Vaysbrot E, McNaughton C, Osani M, Shmerling RH, et al. 2015 American College of Rheumatology Guideline for the Treatment of Rheumatoid Arthritis. Arthritis Rheumatol. 2016;68(1):1–26.
34. Au K, Reed G, Curtis JR, Kremer JM, Greenberg JD, Strand V, Furst DE. High disease activity is associated with an increased risk of infection in patients with rheumatoid arthritis. Ann Rheum Dis. 2011;70(5):785–91.
35. Emery P, Gallo G, Boyd H, Morgan CL, Currie CJ, Poole CD, Nab HW. Association between disease activity and risk of serious infections in subjects with rheumatoid arthritis treated with etanercept or disease-modifying anti-rheumatic drugs. Clin Exp Rheumatol. 2014;32(5):653–60.
36. Askling J, Fored CM, Brandt L, Baecklund E, Bertilsson L, Feltelius N, Coster L, Geborek P, Jacobsson LT, Lindblad S, et al. Time-dependent increase in risk of hospitalisation with infection among Swedish RA patients treated with TNF antagonists. Ann Rheum Dis. 2007;66(10):1339–44.
37. Curtis JR, Patkar N, Xie A, Martin C, Allison JJ, Saag M, Shatin D, Saag KG. Risk of serious bacterial infections among rheumatoid arthritis patients exposed to tumor necrosis factor α antagonists. Arthritis Rheum. 2007;56(4):1125–33.
38. Klareskog L, Gaubitz M, Rodriguez-Valverde V, Malaise M, Dougados M, Wajdula J. Assessment of long-term safety and efficacy of etanercept in a 5-year extension study in patients with rheumatoid arthritis. Clin Exp Rheumatol. 2011;29(2):238–47.
39. Radner H, Yoshida K, Hmamouchi I, Dougados M, Smolen JS, Solomon DH. Treatment patterns of multimorbid patients with rheumatoid arthritis: results from an international cross-sectional study. J Rheumatol. 2015;42(7):1099–104.
40. Turesson C. Comorbidity in rheumatoid arthritis. Swiss Med Wkly. 2016;146:w14290.
41. Bathon JM, Fleischmann RM, Van der Heijde D, Tesser JR, Peloso PM, Chon Y, White B. Safety and efficacy of etanercept treatment in elderly subjects with rheumatoid arthritis. J Rheumatol. 2006;33(2):234–43.
42. Koller MD, Aletaha D, Funovits J, Pangan A, Baker D, Smolen JS. Response of elderly patients with rheumatoid arthritis to methotrexate or TNF inhibitors compared with younger patients. Rheumatology. 2009;48(12):1575–80.

4

One-year risk of serious infection in patients treated with certolizumab pegol as compared with other TNF inhibitors in a real-world setting: data from a national U.S. rheumatoid arthritis registry

Leslie R. Harrold[1,2*], Heather J. Litman[2], Katherine C. Saunders[2], Kimberly J. Dandreo[2], Bernice Gershenson[1,2], Jeffrey D. Greenberg[3], Robert Low[4], Jeffrey Stark[4], Robert Suruki[5], Srihari Jaganathan[4], Joel M. Kremer[6] and Mohamed Yassine[4]

Abstract

Background: Registry studies provide a valuable source of comparative safety data for tumor necrosis factor inhibitors (TNFi) used in rheumatoid arthritis (RA), but they are subject to channeling bias. Comparing safety outcomes without accounting for channeling bias can lead to inaccurate comparisons between TNFi prescribed at different stages of the disease. In the present study, we examined the incidence of serious infection and other adverse events during certolizumab pegol (CZP) use vs other TNFi in a U.S. RA cohort before and after using a methodological approach to minimize channeling bias.

Methods: Patients with RA enrolled in the Corrona registry, aged ≥ 18 years, initiating CZP or other TNFi (etanercept, adalimumab, golimumab, or infliximab) after May 1, 2009 ($n = 6215$ initiations), were followed for ≤ 12 months. A propensity score (PS) model was used to control for baseline characteristics associated with the probability of receiving CZP vs other TNFi. Incidence rate ratios (IRRs) of serious infectious events (SIEs), malignancies, and cardiovascular events (CVEs) in the CZP group vs other TNFi group were calculated with 95% CIs, before and after PS matching.

Results: Patients were more likely to initiate CZP later in the course of therapy than those initiating other TNFi. CZP initiators ($n = 975$) were older and had longer disease duration, more active disease, and greater disability than other TNFi initiators ($n = 5240$). After PS matching, there were no clinically important differences between CZP ($n = 952$) and other TNFi ($n = 952$). Before PS matching, CZP was associated with a greater incidence of SIEs (IRR 1.53 [95% CI 1.13, 2.05]). The risk of SIEs was not different between groups after PS matching (IRR 1.26 [95% CI 0.84, 1.90]). The 95% CI of the IRRs for malignancies or CVEs included unity, regardless of PS matching, suggesting no difference in risk between CZP and other TNFi.

Conclusions: After using PS matching to minimize channeling bias and compare patients with a similar likelihood of receiving CZP or other TNFi, the 1-year risk of SIEs, malignancies, and CVEs was not distinguishable between the two groups.

Keywords: Rheumatoid arthritis, TNF inhibitors, Serious infection, Malignancy, Cardiovascular events

* Correspondence: lharrold@corrona.org
[1]University of Massachusetts Medical School, Worcester, MA, USA
[2]Pharmacoepidemiology and Outcomes Research, Corrona, 352 Turnpike Road, Suite 325, Southborough, MA 01772, USA
Full list of author information is available at the end of the article

Background

Rheumatoid arthritis (RA) is a chronic autoimmune disease that causes persistent synovial inflammation. When not treated adequately, active RA can lead to progressive joint damage, significant pain, disability, and reduced quality of life [1, 2]. The chronic inflammation inherent to RA has consequences that go beyond the damage to the musculoskeletal system. Compared with the general population, RA is associated with substantial morbidity and premature mortality, which is attributed mainly to serious infection, cardiovascular disease, and certain types of cancer [3–5]. The substantial disease burden of RA underscores the importance of effective therapy.

Tumor necrosis factor inhibitors (TNFi), often the first class of biologic therapy prescribed to patients with RA, have been demonstrated to reduce disease activity and improve clinical, radiographic, and functional outcomes [6]. Effective control of disease activity with TNFi has been linked with a reduced risk of cardiovascular disease [7, 8]. Conversely, the immunosuppressive effect of TNFi has raised concerns over an increased risk of infection [9], although the magnitude of this risk remains a topic of intense debate [10–21]. The impact of TNFi on the incidence of cancer is also unclear [11, 22–25].

Overall, it is difficult to assess the risks associated with TNFi therapy, owing to the influence of patients' demographic characteristics, clinical history, and concomitant immunomodulatory treatments. Furthermore, in clinical practice, drugs with similar therapeutic indications can be prescribed selectively to patients with different baseline prognoses, a phenomenon termed *channeling bias* [26]. Consequently, the line of TNFi therapy may also influence the safety risks observed in clinical practice.

Certolizumab pegol (CZP), a PEGylated, Fc-free TNFi, is approved for the treatment of adult patients with moderate to severe active RA [27]. Currently, there is limited evidence on the safety of CZP compared with other TNFi drugs in the context of U.S. clinical practice. The objective of this prospective, observational cohort study was to examine the 1-year incidence of serious infectious events (SIEs) during CZP use compared with other TNFi drugs (golimumab, etanercept, adalimumab, and infliximab), with and without a methodological approach accounting for channeling bias in patients with moderate to severe RA enrolled in the Consortium of Rheumatology Researchers of North America (Corrona) registry. The 1-year risk of malignancies and cardiovascular events (CVEs) was also assessed, owing to their importance for decision-making in clinical practice.

Methods

Data source

The Corrona registry is an independent, prospective, observational cohort of patients with RA recruited from 169 private and academic practice sites across 40 states in the United States [28]. Data on 43,099 patients with RA had been collected as of June 30, 2016. The Corrona database comprises information from 326,613 patient visits and approximately 145,526.5 patient-years (PY) of total follow-up, with a mean patient follow-up of 4.13 years, and median time between follow-up visits of 4.90 months. Institutional review board (IRB) approvals for this study were obtained from a central IRB (New England IRB) for private practice sites and local IRBs of participating academic sites.

Study population

Data were provided by treating rheumatologists for patients with RA enrolled in the Corrona registry who initiated treatment with CZP or other TNFi (adalimumab, etanercept, golimumab, and infliximab) between May 1, 2009, and March 31, 2016. Patients could have been treated with TNFi before this study, so index drug corresponded to any line of therapy. If patients were treated with more than one TNFi during the study, all TNFi initiations were included in the analysis. The study population comprised patients aged ≥ 18 years with at least one follow-up visit post-drug initiation. All patients provided written informed consent prior to participation.

Adverse events of interest

Physician-reported adverse events (AEs) of interest that occurred from drug initiation up to 90 days following discontinuation/switch of TNFi, or up to 12 months from drug initiation, were included in the analysis. SIEs were the main AE of interest (infections requiring hospitalization and/or intravenous antibiotics); when data were available, information was also provided about the SIE microorganism (opportunistic vs nonopportunistic), malignancies, and CVEs (Table 1).

Other AEs of interest included anaphylaxis/allergic reaction, drug-induced systemic lupus erythematosus, gastrointestinal perforation, hepatic events, progressive multifocal leukoencephalopathy, other neurological events with hospitalization and/or other demyelinating disease, and spontaneous serious bleeding (*see* Additional file 1: Table S1). Corrona has an established system for the validation of physician-reported AEs. Briefly, serious AEs and AEs of special interest are recorded by treating physicians using Targeted Adverse Event questionnaires. These questionnaires, alongside supporting documents appropriate to the event (e.g., hospitalization records, pathology reports), are submitted to Corrona for validation, with a subset triaged for expert adjudication. Previous validation of Corrona's AE reporting has found positive predictive values of 86% for malignancies [29], 96% for CVEs [30], and 71% for SIEs [31].

Table 1 Adverse events of interest

AE category	Physician-reported AEs included in the analysis
SIEs	Infections for which the patient was hospitalized and/or received intravenous antibiotics, which were categorized as follows: joint/bursa, cellulitis/skin, sinusitis, diverticulitis, sepsis, pneumonia, bronchitis, gastroenteritis, meningitis/encephalitis, urinary tract infection, upper respiratory infection, active tuberculosis (latent tuberculosis infection was not included), and other infections
SIE microorganism	Opportunistic infections: coccidioidomycosis, *Cryptococcus*, herpes zoster, histoplasmosis, John Cunningham virus, *Listeria*, *Pneumocystis*, active tuberculosis (latent tuberculosis infection was not included), and other opportunistic infections. Nonopportunistic infections: methicillin-resistant *Staphylococcus aureus* (MRSA), bacterial infection other than MRSA, and other nonopportunistic infections
Malignancies	Nonmelanoma skin cancer, melanoma skin cancer, lymphoma, breast cancer, lung cancer, and other cancers
CVEs	Myocardial infarction, transient ischemic attack, stroke, congestive heart failure with hospitalization, cardiac revascularization procedure, ventricular arrhythmia, cardiac arrest, acute coronary syndrome, unstable angina, hypertension with hospitalization, peripheral arterial thromboembolic event, urgent peripheral arterial revascularization, peripheral ischemia or gangrene (necrosis), and other CVEs

Abbreviations: AE Adverse event, *SIE* Serious infection event, *CVE* Cardiovascular event

Propensity score matching

To control for baseline patient characteristics associated with the likelihood of receiving CZP or an alternative TNFi, a propensity score (PS; i.e., the probability of treatment selection) was calculated for each patient using a logistic regression model that included baseline covariates with $p < 0.1$ for the difference between CZP and other TNFi and thought to be independently associated with treatment on the basis of clinical expertise and prior group consensus. CZP and other TNFi patients were matched by estimated PS from a model including age, sex, disease duration, Clinical Disease Activity Index (CDAI) at drug initiation, and physician-reported line of TNFi therapy. Matching was performed in a 1:1 ratio without replacement, using a maximum tolerated difference (caliper) of 0.01.

Statistical analysis

Patients' comorbidity scores were calculated using a modified version of the Charlson comorbidity index [32] (*see* Additional file 1). All patients had a modified Charlson comorbidity index ≥ 1 because RA is included under connective tissue disease.

Baseline characteristics were compared between CZP and other TNFi patients before and after PS matching. Student's two-sample t tests were used for continuous variables (or Wilcoxon rank-sum tests if variables were skewed), and chi-square tests were used for categorical variables (or Fisher's exact test in the case of small counts). All p values were nominal in nature and should be interpreted in an exploratory manner.

Observed incidence rates (IRs) of AEs of interest were calculated per 100 PY, with 95% CIs calculated using the Poisson distribution assumption. For each AE category, time at risk was measured from drug initiation up to either the occurrence of the first event of interest under that category, 90 days following discontinuation/switch of biologic (censored), or up to 12 months after drug initiation (censored). Incidence rate ratios (IRRs) were calculated in both unmatched and PS-matched comparisons for overall SIEs, malignancies, and CVEs, with CZP as numerator and other TNFi as denominator; 95% CIs were calculated using the exact distribution derived using Stata® version 14.1 software (StataCorp LP, College Station, TX, USA).

Results

Baseline demographics

A total of 5363 patients with RA in the Corrona database met the inclusion criteria and initiated TNFi therapy between May 1, 2009, and March 31, 2016. There were a total of 6215 TNFi initiations comprising 975 CZP initiators and 5240 initiators of other TNFi (adalimumab, etanercept, golimumab, and infliximab). After PS matching, the CZP and other TNFi groups included 952 patients each (Fig. 1).

Among all initiators (before PS matching), on average, patients initiating CZP were older, had longer disease duration, had more active disease based on the CDAI, and had more functional impairment based on the modified Health Assessment Questionnaire than patients in the other TNFi group ($p \leq 0.01$) (Table 2). Race and Medicare insurance status also showed an imbalance between the two groups ($p < 0.001$). Sex, body mass index (BMI), age at RA onset, and the prevalence of comorbidities were balanced between groups (Table 2), as were rheumatoid factor positivity, anticitrullinated protein antibody positivity, smoking status, and blood pressure (not shown). Patients were more likely to initiate CZP later in the course of therapy, with approximately 44.8% of CZP initiators corresponding to third-line therapy or later, compared with 20.1% in the other TNFi group (Table 2). Concomitant disease-modifying antirheumatic drug (DMARD) and prednisone use were similar between the two groups, except for methotrexate (MTX) and other nonbiologic DMARD use, which was more prevalent among other TNFi initiators (Table 2).

After PS matching, there were no clinically relevant baseline differences between the CZP and other TNFi groups; line of TNFi therapy and concomitant medication use were also similar (Table 2).

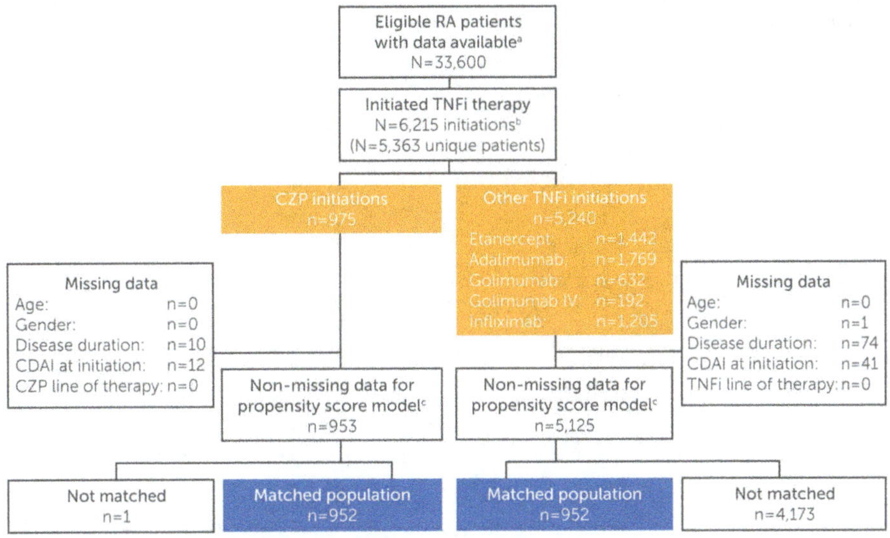

Fig. 1 Patient disposition. Data from May 1, 2009, through March 31, 2016, were available. There were 975 unique CZP patients and 4625 unique other TNFi patients. [a]Eligible patients with RA were ≥ 18 years of age, had at least one follow-up visit post-index drug initiation, and provided written informed consent prior to participation. [b]Initiations refer to the total number of TNFi initiated during the period of observation because patients may have used more than one TNFi during the study (e.g., if one patient switched from etanercept to CZP, both initiations would have been included in the analysis). [c]Propensity scores were calculated using a logistic regression model fitted with the following baseline covariates: age, sex, disease duration, CDAI at initiation, and TNFi line of therapy. *RA* rheumatoid arthritis, *CZP* certolizumab pegol, *TNFi* tumor necrosis factor inhibitor, *IV* intravenous, *CDAI* Clinical Disease Activity Index

Observed incidence of AEs in the unmatched population

Average follow-up for each of the AEs can be calculated as the number of PY at risk divided by the number of patients considered. For instance, with SIEs in the CZP group, the average follow-up time was 820/975 = 0.84 PY (approximately 10 months).

Among all initiators, the IR of SIEs was higher in the CZP group than in the other TNFi group (Table 3). The 95% CI of the corresponding IRR excluded unity (IRR 1.53 [1.13, 2.05]), suggesting that CZP was associated with a greater risk of SIEs than other TNFi (Fig. 2a). By contrast, the IRs of malignancies and CVEs did not differ substantially between CZP and other TNFi (Table 3). The 95% CI of the IRRs for malignancies (IRR 0.86 [0.46, 1.49]) and CVEs (IRR 1.22 [0.67, 2.08]) included unity, suggesting no difference in risk between the two groups (Fig. 2a).

Cellulitis/skin infection, pneumonia, and urinary tract infection were the most frequently reported SIEs. There were no cases of active tuberculosis among CZP initiators, and there were two cases in the other TNFi group (Table 3). Regarding other AEs of interest, rare cases of anaphylaxis/allergic reaction were reported for both CZP (4 events) and other TNFi (14 events). Patients in the other TNFi group also reported gastrointestinal perforation (three events), hepatic events (ten events), other neurological events (four events), and spontaneous serious bleeding (five events) (Table 3).

Observed incidence of AEs in the PS-matched population

In contrast with the unmatched population, the IR of SIEs was similar between CZP and other TNFi after PS matching (Table 4). The 95% CI of the IRR included unity (IRR 1.26 [0.84, 1.90]), suggesting that the risk of SIEs was not different between the PS-matched groups (Fig. 2b). Similar to what was seen in the unmatched population, the IRs of malignancies and CVEs in the CZP and other TNFi groups did not differ substantially after PS matching (Table 4). The 95% CI of the IRRs for malignancies (IRR 0.71 [0.33, 1.47]) and CVEs (IRR 1.01 [0.49, 2.11]) included unity, suggesting no difference in risk between the PS-matched groups (Fig. 2b).

Cellulitis/skin infection, pneumonia, and urinary tract infection were still the most frequent SIEs. The incidence rates of other AEs of interest remained low in the PS-matched groups (Table 4).

Discussion

When initiating TNFi therapy in RA, rheumatologists need to carefully balance the potential clinical benefits of treatment with the anticipated risks in each individual patient in light of their demographic characteristics, clinical history, and concomitant medications. Excepting a recently completed head-to-head randomized controlled trial (RCT) comparing the efficacy and safety of CZP and adalimumab, in which investigators reported no clinically significant differences between the

Table 2 Baseline demographics, disease characteristics, tumor necrosis factor inhibitor line of therapy, and concomitant medications, before and after propensity score matching

	Before PS matching			After PS matching		
	CZP (*n* = 975)	Other TNFi (*n* = 5240)	Nominal *p* value	CZP (*n* = 952)	Other TNFi (*n* = 952)	Nominal *p* value
Demographics						
Age, years, median (IQR)	58 (18.0)	56 (16.5)	< 0.001	58 (17.0)	58 (16.0)	0.48
Female sex, *n* (%)	769 (78.9)	4107 (78.4)	0.74	751 (78.9)	750 (78.8)	0.96
Race, white, *n* (%)	840 (86.2)	4310 (82.3)	< 0.001	820 (86.1)	786 (82.6)	0.03[a]
BMI, kg/m^2, mean (SD)	30.0 (7.3)	30.1 (7.3)	0.49	30.0 (7.3)	30.1 (7.5)	0.68
Insurance[b]						
Medicare, *n* (%)	321 (32.9)	1363 (26.0)	< 0.001	315 (33.1)	293 (30.8)	0.28
Medicaid, *n* (%)	48 (4.9)	327 (6.2)	0.12	48 (5.0)	59 (6.2)	0.32
Private, *n* (%)	712 (73.0)	4034 (77.0)	0.01	700 (73.5)	719 (75.5)	0.32
None, *n* (%)	23 (2.4)	136 (2.6)	0.74	22 (2.3)	14 (1.5)	0.24
Clinical characteristics						
Age at RA onset, years, mean (SD)	46.9 (14.4)	47.4 (13.5)	0.35	47.0 (14.4)	46.7 (13.8)	0.73
Disease duration, years, median (IQR)	9 (12.0)	5 (10.0)	< 0.001	9 (12.0)	8 (12.5)	0.26
CDAI, median (IQR)	19.0 (20.2)	17.0 (19.0)	0.01	19.0 (20.2)	18.5 (20.0)	> 0.99
mHAQ, median (IQR)	0.5 (0.8)	0.4 (0.8)	< 0.001	0.5 (0.8)	0.5 (0.8)	0.89
History of comorbidities						
Diabetes, *n* (%)	75 (7.7)	467 (8.9)	0.22	75 (7.9)	96 (10.1)	0.09
Pulmonary disease,[c] *n* (%)	58 (5.9)	347 (6.6)	0.43	58 (6.1)	64 (6.7)	0.57
Cardiovascular disease,[d] *n* (%)	57 (5.8)	283 (5.4)	0.57	54 (5.7)	57 (6.0)	0.77
Malignancy,[e] *n* (%)	48 (4.9)	225 (4.3)	0.38	46 (4.8)	45 (4.7)	0.91
Serious infection,[f] *n* (%)	64 (6.6)	348 (6.6)	0.93	63 (6.6)	80 (8.4)	0.14
Comorbidity index[g]						
Median score (IQR)	1 (0)	1 (0)	0.60	1 (0)	1 (0)	0.12
Score ≥ 2, *n* (%)	197 (21.1)	1029 (20.3)	0.60	191 (20.9)	216 (23.7)	0.16
Line of TNFi therapy			< 0.001[h]			0.69[h]
First, *n* (%)	253 (25.9)	2594 (49.5)		250 (26.3)	236 (24.8)	
Second, *n* (%)	285 (29.2)	1593 (30.4)		276 (29.0)	290 (30.5)	
Third or later, *n* (%)	437 (44.8)	1053 (20.1)		426 (44.7)	426 (44.7)	
Concomitant DMARD use						
Nonbiologic DMARDs (excluding MTX), *n* (%)	146 (15.0)	819 (15.6)	0.60	143 (15.0)	166 (17.4)	0.15
MTX and other nonbiologic DMARDs, *n* (%)	85 (8.7)	661 (12.6)	< 0.001	84 (8.8)	105 (11.0)	0.11
MTX (excluding other nonbiologic DMARDs), *n* (%)	469 (48.0)	2597 (49.6)	0.40	456 (47.9)	450 (47.3)	0.78
Concomitant prednisone use			0.45[h]			0.26[h]
None, *n* (%)	679 (70.1)	3695 (70.9)		661 (69.9)	658 (69.3)	
< 10 mg/day, *n* (%)	197 (20.4)	982 (18.8)		193 (20.4)	179 (18.9)	
≥ 10 mg/day, *n* (%)	92 (9.5)	538 (10.3)		91 (9.6)	112 (11.8)	

Abbreviations: CZP Certolizumab pegol, *TNFi* Tumor necrosis factor inhibitor, *PS* Propensity score, *BMI* Body mass index, *RA* Rheumatoid arthritis, *CDAI* Clinical Disease Activity Index, *mHAQ*, Modified Health Assessment Questionnaire (disability index), *COPD* Chronic obstructive pulmonary disease, *NMSC* Nonmelanoma skin cancer, *DMARD* Disease-modifying antirheumatic drug, *MTX* Methotrexate

[a]Race was statistically different between the PS-matched groups ($p = 0.03$), but this was not thought to be clinically significant

[b]Insurance categories were not mutually exclusive; therefore, patients could be captured in more than one category

[c]Pulmonary disease included asthma, COPD, and interstitial lung disease/pulmonary fibrosis

[d]Cardiovascular disease included coronary artery disease, myocardial infarction, coronary heart failure requiring hospitalization, acute coronary syndrome, unstable angina, cardiac revascularization procedure, cardiac arrest, ventricular arrhythmia, and other cardiovascular diseases

[e]Malignancy included lung cancer, breast cancer, melanoma skin cancer, and other cancers

[f]Serious infection was defined as any infection for which the patient was hospitalized and/or received intravenous antibiotics

[g]Comorbidity index was a modified version of the Charlson comorbidity index and corresponded to the sum of scores for current and physician-reported prior comorbid conditions, namely myocardial infarction, congestive heart failure, peripheral vascular disease, cerebrovascular disease (captured as stroke or transient ischemic attack), COPD, history of bleeding and/or peptic ulcer, diabetes mellitus, leukemia, lymphoma, solid tumor cancer (excluding nonmelanoma skin cancer [NMSC]), liver disease, and connective tissue disease (including RA, so all patients had a comorbidity index ≥ 1)

[h]*p* Values were based on chi-square tests to ascertain if the overall distribution differed significantly between the CZP and other TNFi groups

Table 3 Rates of adverse events of interest before propensity score matching (all initiators)

	CZP ($n = 975$)			Other TNFi ($n = 5240$)		
	PY at risk[a]	Events[b]	IR/100 PY (95% CI)	PY at risk[a]	Events[b]	IR/100 PY (95% CI)
Serious infectious events	820	59	**7.20 (5.58, 9.29)**	4566	215	**4.71 (4.12, 5.38)**
Joint/bursa	847	2	0.24 (0.06, 0.94)	4660	16	0.34 (0.21, 0.56)
Cellulitis/skin	841	13	1.55 (0.90, 2.66)	4650	36	0.77 (0.56, 1.07)
Sinusitis	847	2	0.24 (0.06, 0.94)	4660	10	0.21 (0.12, 0.40)
Diverticulitis	847	2	0.24 (0.06, 0.94)	4660	10	0.21 (0.12, 0.40)
Sepsis	848	1	0.12 (0.02, 0.84)	4657	16	0.34 (0.21, 0.56)
Pneumonia	842	15	1.78 (1.07, 2.95)	4641	58	1.25 (0.97, 1.62)
Bronchitis	846	5	0.59 (0.25, 1.42)	4660	11	0.24 (0.13, 0.43)
Gastroenteritis	847	4	0.47 (0.18, 1.26)	4659	14	0.30 (0.18. 0.51)
Meningitis/encephalitis	848	0	0 (NC)	4665	2	0.04 (0.01, 0.17)
Urinary tract infection	842	10	1.19 (0.64, 2.21)	4650	29	0.62 (0.43, 0.90)
Upper respiratory infection	848	2	0.24 (0.06, 0.94)	4660	10	0.21 (0.12, 0.40)
Active tuberculosis[c]	848	0	0 (NC)	4664	2	0.04 (0.01, 0.17)
Other	844	9	1.07 (0.55, 2.05)	4649	36	0.77 (0.56, 1.07)
Identified serious infectious organism	839	15	**1.79 (1.08, 2.96)**	4636	65	**1.40 (1.10, 1.79)**
Opportunistic	848	0	0.00 (NC)	4664	2	0.04 (0.01, 0.17)
Nonopportunistic	843	8	0.95 (0.47, 1.90)	4648	30	0.65 (0.45, 0.92)
Unknown	844	7	0.83 (0.40, 1.74)	4648	34	0.73 (0.52, 1.02)
Malignancies	841	15	**1.78 (1.08, 2.96)**	4622	96	**2.08 (1.70, 2.54)**
Lymphoma	848	0	0 (NC)	4664	4	0.09 (0.03, 0.23)
Breast cancer	848	1	0.12 (0.02, 0.84)	4660	9	0.19 (0.10, 0.37)
Lung cancer	848	2	0.24 (0.06, 0.94)	4664	3	0.06 (0.02, 0.20)
Skin cancer – melanoma	848	0	0 (NC)	4662	6	0.13 (0.06, 0.29)
Skin cancer – basal/squamous	845	5	0.59 (0.25, 1.42)	4641	49	1.06 (0.80, 1.40)
Other cancer	844	7	0.83 (0.40, 1.74)	4655	26	0.56 (0.38, 0.82)
Cardiovascular events	840	17	**2.02 (1.26, 3.26)**	4633	77	**1.66 (1.33, 2.08)**
Myocardial infarction	847	3	0.35 (0.11, 1.10)	4661	11	0.24 (0.13, 0.43)
TIA/stroke	846	5	0.59 (0.25, 1.42)	4650	34	0.73 (0.52, 1.02)
Other cardiovascular event[d]	843	10	1.19 (0.64, 2.20)	4649	43	0.93 (0.69, 1.25)
Other AEs of interest						
Anaphylaxis/allergic reaction	845	4	0.47 (0.18, 1.26)	4660	14	0.30 (0.18, 0.51)
Drug-induced SLE	848	0	0 (NC)	4665	0	0 (NC)
Gastrointestinal perforation	848	0	0 (NC)	4663	3	0.06 (0.02, 0.20)
Hepatic event	848	0	0 (NC)	4660	10	0.21 (0.12, 0.40)
Progressive multifocal leukoencephalopathy	848	0	0 (NC)	4665	0	0 (NC)
Other neurological event (with hospitalization) /other demyelinating disease	848	0	0 (NC)	4664	4	0.09 (0.03, 0.23)
Spontaneous serious bleeding	848	0	0 (NC)	4664	5	0.11 (0.04, 0.26)

Abbreviations: AE Adverse events, *PS* Propensity score, *CZP* Certolizumab pegol, *TNFi* Tumor necrosis factor inhibitor, *PY* Patient-years, *IR* Incidence rate, *NC* Not calculable, *CVE* Cardiovascular event, *TIA* Transient ischemic attack, *SLE* Systemic lupus erythematosus

[a]Time at risk was measured from drug initiation up to either the occurrence of the first event of interest under that category, 90 days following discontinuation/switch of TNFi, or up to 12 months after drug initiation

[b]Patients may have experienced more than one AE, so the sum of individual conditions may be greater than the total number of first AEs for the overall categories; however, only the time to the first event was considered to calculate the corresponding IRs

[c]Latent tuberculosis was not included

[d]Included congestive heart failure with hospitalization, cardiac revascularization procedure, ventricular arrhythmia, cardiac arrest, acute coronary syndrome, unstable angina, hypertension with hospitalization, peripheral arterial thromboembolic event, urgent peripheral arterial revascularization, peripheral ischemia or gangrene (necrosis), and other CVEs

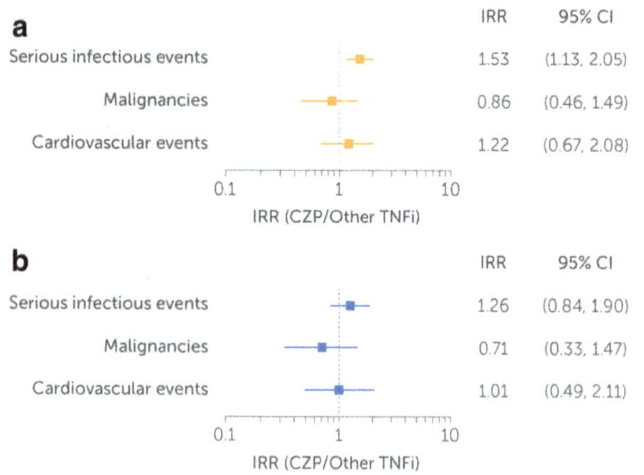

Fig. 2 IRRs of SIEs, malignancies, and CVEs between the CZP and other TNFi groups. **a** Before PS matching (all initiators). **b** After PS matching. IRRs were calculated with the CZP group in the numerator and the other TNFi in the denominator. *IRR* Incidence rate ratio, *SIE* Serious infectious event, *CVE* Cardiovascular event, *CZP* Certolizumab pegol, *TNFi* Tumor necrosis factor inhibitor, *PS* Propensity score

two drugs [33], there is a paucity of head-to-head RCTs comparing the safety of TNFi drugs in RA. Observational studies therefore provide a valuable source of comparative safety data.

Using data from the Corrona registry, we compared the safety of CZP with other TNFi as a group (golimumab, etanercept, adalimumab, and infliximab). As with any registry study, channeling bias can arise from the fact that clinicians prescribe treatment not at random but based on personal clinical experience and their patients' clinical characteristics [26]. To overcome this limitation, we assessed safety outcomes in two cohorts: (1) all patients initiating CZP or other TNFi therapy and (2) the subset of patients matched by PS. In the unmatched population, the rate of SIEs was approximately 50% higher in the CZP group than in the other TNFi group. After using the PS-matched model to minimize channeling bias and resolve clinically significant baseline differences between CZP and other TNFi initiators, the risk of SIEs associated with each group was no longer distinguishable.

The contrasting results in the unmatched and PS-matched cohorts highlight the need to consider baseline patient differences when comparing the risk of AEs between TNFi drugs prescribed at different stages in the course of RA. CZP was prescribed later in the line of therapy than other TNFi. Consequently, patients initiating CZP were, on average, older and had longer disease duration, more active disease, and more functional impairment than patients initiating treatment with other TNFi. This probably explains the higher rate of SIEs in the unmatched CZP group because older age, high disease activity, and disability have previously been identified as risk factors for serious infection in RA [9, 34–38].

Meta-analyses of RCTs have demonstrated that the different TNFi drugs available in RA are equally efficacious at reducing disease activity [18]. Therefore, on the basis of clinical efficacy alone, there has been relative equipoise among rheumatologists regarding which therapy to choose as first and subsequent lines of treatment [39]. However, the safety of TNFi therapy, particularly with regard to infection, continues to be debated. The authors of the first published meta-analysis of serious infection in RA detected an association with TNFi treatment [11], but subsequent meta-analyses performed with greater sample sizes have produced discordant results [14, 15, 17, 18, 20]. Similarly, whereas researchers in some observational studies have reported an association between TNFi and the risk of serious infection [10, 13, 19], others did not find a clear link [12, 16, 21]. In a large meta-analysis of RCTs in which authors compared the safety of all five TNFi drugs across multiple diseases, CZP was associated with higher odds of serious infection than adalimumab, etanercept, and golimumab [40]. However, the diseases and patient populations captured in this meta-analysis differed substantially between drugs, and no correction was made for placebo exposure, which makes the results difficult to interpret. It is known that the background risk of SIEs varies greatly across diseases [37, 41], and even within indications it is strongly dependent on study inclusion criteria and baseline patient characteristics [35]. By contrast, a recent head-to-head clinical trial comparing the efficacy and safety of CZP with adalimumab in patients with RA provided direct evidence of a comparable safety profile for the two drugs, including a similar incidence of serious infection [33].

The IRs of SIEs reported in the present study are consistent with rates observed in other real-world patient populations. For example, in a retrospective study of medical and pharmaceutical data from a large U.S. health insurer, the rate of hospitalized infections among patients with RA with no prior biologic use was 4.6/100 PY, whereas for patients switching to a new biologic at baseline, an IR of 7.0/100 PY was reported [35]. In a retrospective analysis of Medicare claims data for patients with RA treated with prior biologics, the crude IRs of hospitalized infection during TNFi treatment ranged between 14.1/100 PY (golimumab) and 17.0/100 PY (infliximab; the IR for CZP was 14.2/100 PY) [42]. A prospective observational study using data from the British Society for Rheumatology Biologics Register – Rheumatoid Arthritis (BSRBR-RA) reported rates of SIEs ranging from 2.8/100 PY in patients aged < 55 years to 8.3/100 PY in patients aged > 75 years [13].

Regardless of PS matching, there were no important differences in the IRs of malignancies and CVEs between CZP and other TNFi initiators. Interpretation of these results must take into account the infrequent nature of

Table 4 Rates of adverse events of interest after propensity score matching

	CZP ($n = 952$)			Other TNFi ($n = 952$)		
	PY at risk[a]	Events[b]	IR/100 PY (95% CI)	PY at risk[a]	Events[b]	IR/100 PY (95% CI)
Serious infectious events	799	57	**7.13 (5.50, 9.25)**	814	46	**5.65 (4.23, 7.54)**
Joint/bursa	825	2	0.24 (0.06, 0.97)	836	3	0.36 (0.12, 1.11)
Cellulitis/skin	820	13	1.59 (0.92, 2.73)	833	9	1.08 (0.56, 2.08)
Sinusitis	826	2	0.24 (0.06, 0.97)	835	2	0.24 (0.06, 0.96)
Diverticulitis	826	2	0.24 (0.06, 0.97)	835	2	0.24 (0.06, 0.96)
Sepsis	826	1	0.12 (0.02, 0.86)	836	3	0.36 (0.12, 1.11)
Pneumonia	821	15	1.83 (1.10, 3.03)	833	9	1.08 (0.56, 2.08)
Bronchitis	825	5	0.61 (0.25, 1.46)	835	2	0.24 (0.06, 0.96)
Gastroenteritis	825	4	0.48 (0.18, 1.29)	834	5	0.60 (0.25, 1.44)
Meningitis/encephalitis	827	0	0 (NC)	837	1	0.12 (0.02, 0.85)
Urinary tract infection	821	10	1.22 (0.66, 2.26)	834	6	0.72 (0.32, 1.60)
Upper respiratory infection	827	2	0.24 (0.06, 0.97)	835	3	0.36 (0.12, 1.11)
Active tuberculosis[c]	827	0	0 (NC)	837	1	0.12 (0.02, 0.85)
Other	823	7	0.85 (0.41, 1.78)	832	9	1.08 (0.56, 2.08)
Identified serious infection organism	819	14	**1.71 (1.01, 2.89)**	831	14	**1.69 (1.00, 2.85)**
Opportunistic	827	0	0 (NC)	836	2	0.24 (0.06, 0.96)
Nonopportunistic	822	8	0.97 (0.49, 1.95)	835	4	0.48 (0.18, 1.28)
Unknown	824	6	0.73 (0.33, 1.62)	834	8	0.96 (0.48, 1.92)
Malignancies	821	14	**1.71 (1.01, 2.88)**	827	20	**2.42 (1.56, 3.75)**
Lymphoma	827	0	0 (NC)	836	2	0.24 (0.06, 0.96)
Breast cancer	827	1	0.12 (0.02, 0.86)	837	0	0 (NC)
Lung cancer	827	2	0.24 (0.06, 0.97)	837	0	0 (NC)
Skin cancer – melanoma	827	0	0 (NC)	836	2	0.24 (0.06, 0.96)
Skin cancer – basal/squamous	825	4	0.48 (0.18, 1.29)	833	8	0.96 (0.48, 1.92)
Other cancer	823	7	0.85 (0.41, 1.78)	833	8	0.96 (0.48, 1.92)
Cardiovascular events	819	17	**2.08 (1.29, 3.34)**	829	17	**2.05 (1.27, 3.30)**
Myocardial infarction	825	3	0.36 (0.12, 1.13)	837	1	0.12 (0.02, 0.85)
TIA/stroke	824	5	0.61 (0.25, 1.46)	832	10	1.20 (0.65, 2.23)
Other cardiovascular event[d]	822	10	1.22 (0.65, 2.26)	833	9	1.08 (0.56, 2.08)
Other AEs of interest						
Anaphylaxis/allergic reaction	824	4	0.49 (0.18, 1.29)	835	5	0.60 (0.25, 1.44)
Drug-induced SLE	827	0	0 (NC)	837	0	0 (NC)
Gastrointestinal perforation	827	0	0 (NC)	837	1	0.12 (0.02, 0.85)
Hepatic event	827	0	0 (NC)	834	4	0.48 (0.18, 1.28)
Progressive multifocal leukoencephalopathy	827	0	0 (NC)	837	0	0 (NC)
Other neurological event (with hospitalization) /other demyelinating disease	827	0	0 (NC)	837	0	0 (NC)
Spontaneous serious bleeding	827	0	0 (NC)	837	1	0.12 (0.02, 0.85)

Abbreviations: AE Adverse events, *PS* Propensity score, *CZP* Certolizumab pegol, *TNFi* Tumor necrosis factor inhibitor, *PY* Patient-years, *IR* Incidence rate, *NC* Not calculable, *CVE* Cardiovascular event, *TIA* Transient ischemic attack, *SLE* Systemic lupus erythematosus

[a]Time at risk was measured from drug initiation up to either the occurrence of the first event of interest under that category, 90 days following discontinuation/switch of TNFi, or up to 12 months after drug initiation

[b]Patients may have experienced more than one AE, so the sum of individual conditions may be greater than the total number of first AEs for the overall categories; however, only the time to the first event was considered to calculate the corresponding IRs

[c]Latent tuberculosis was not included

[d]Included congestive heart failure with hospitalization, cardiac revascularization procedure, ventricular arrhythmia, cardiac arrest, acute coronary syndrome, unstable angina, hypertension with hospitalization, peripheral arterial thromboembolic event, urgent peripheral arterial revascularization, peripheral ischemia or gangrene (necrosis), and other CVEs

these AEs and the fact that patients in this study were followed for a maximum of 12 months, which may have been too short to detect meaningful risk differences between groups.

Evaluating the impact of TNFi on the risk of cancer in RA is a challenging task. Because most types of cancer occur very rarely, RCTs often lack sufficient power to conclusively assess the risk of malignancy, owing to the short duration of follow-up. Furthermore, patients with RA with a history of cancer tend to be excluded from participation in RCTs [43]. Given the latency of cancer and its potential for reactivation over time, it is important to evaluate the risks of TNFi use in patients with a history of this condition. Approximately 5% of Corrona patients included in our study had a history of prior malignancy. Regardless of PS matching, the IRs of malignancies reported here for CZP and other TNFi initiators were comparable to those previously reported in the BSRBR-RA [43, 44] and the Swedish Biologics Registry [45]. Also consistent with these two registries, nonmelanoma skin cancer was one of the most commonly reported malignancies [46, 47].

Cardiovascular disease is one of the main causes of morbidity and premature mortality in patients with RA [3]. This has been attributed to the direct impact of chronic inflammation on the vascular system and to the secondary effects of physical inactivity [48]. By effectively reducing disease activity, TNFi treatment may help to mitigate the cardiovascular risk associated with RA [7, 8]. In this study, traditional cardiovascular risk factors such as BMI, smoking status, blood pressure, history of cardiovascular disease, and prednisone use were similar at drug initiation between the CZP and other TNFi groups. By contrast, RA disease activity, which is also associated with cardiovascular risk [8, 49, 50], was higher in the CZP group. Nevertheless, the IRs of CVEs we report, which corresponded mainly to myocardial infarction and transient ischemic attack (TIA)/stroke, did not differ substantially between the CZP and other TNFi groups, regardless of PS matching.

A limitation of this study was that patients were followed for a maximum of 12 months after initiation of a particular TNFi. Although SIE rates tend to be highest during the first 6–12 months of TNFi exposure [13, 51], this time frame may not have been sufficient to detect differences in the rates of CVEs or malignancies, owing to the comparative infrequency and longer-term nature of these AEs. Despite this limitation, the rates of malignancy we report were consistent with a recent meta-analysis of observational studies where there were no differences among the five TNFi drugs regarding the overall risk of cancer [52]. Similarly, the rates of myocardial infarction and TIA/stroke were comparable to those previously reported for the Corrona cohort [8]. The rarity of other AEs of interest prevented further analyses; their inclusion in this report was meant to provide a more complete picture of the AEs reported by the study population. Overall, although AEs were assessed over a 1-year period only, the findings of this study are consistent with previously published long-term safety analyses of CZP in RA [53].

A key strength of this study is the fact that we compared safety outcomes for TNFi in U.S. clinical practice using data from a large, nationwide cohort of patients with RA. Because patient characteristics and access to biologic drugs can vary substantially between countries, owing to payer and regulatory differences, it is important to obtain clinical evidence directly relevant to practicing rheumatologists in the United States. It has been demonstrated that patients in Corrona share similar demographic and clinical characteristics with Medicare beneficiaries with claims for rheumatology or RA, suggesting that the results we present may be generalizable to the wider RA population in the United States [54]. Furthermore, we used PS matching to control for baseline patient characteristics that might have influenced the decision to treat with CZP or other TNFi, thereby helping to minimize channeling bias and allowing for a more accurate comparison of the risk of AEs associated with these therapies.

Conclusions

In a PS-matched cohort of patients with moderate to severe RA enrolled in the Corrona registry, there were no differences in the 1-year risk of SIEs, malignancies, and CVEs between patients treated with CZP and those treated with other TNFi.

Abbreviations

AE: Adverse event; BMI: Body mass index; BSRBR-RA: British Society for Rheumatology Biologics Register – Rheumatoid Arthritis; CDAI: Clinical Disease Activity Index; COPD: Chronic obstructive pulmonary disease; Corrona: Consortium of Rheumatology Researchers of North America; CVE: Cardiovascular event; CZP: Certolizumab pegol; DMARD: Disease-modifying antirheumatic drug; IR: Incidence rate; IRB: Institutional review board; IRR: Incidence rate ratio; IV: Intravenous; mHAQ: Modified Health Assessment Questionnaire; MRSA: Methicillin-resistant *Staphylococcus aureus*; MTX: Methotrexate; NC: Not calculable; NMSC: Nonmelanoma skin cancer; PS: Propensity score; PY: Patient-years; RA: Rheumatoid arthritis; RCT: Randomized controlled trial; SIE: Serious infectious event; SLE: Systemic lupus erythematosus; TIA: Transient ischemic attack; TNF: Tumor necrosis factor

Acknowledgements

The authors thank the patients and their caregivers, in addition to the investigators and their teams, who contributed to this study. The authors acknowledge Ricardo Milho, PhD, and Aimée Hall, MPhys, Costello Medical Consulting, Cambridge, UK, for writing and editorial assistance. All costs associated with the development of this article were funded by UCB Pharma.

Funding

This study was sponsored by Corrona, LLC. Corrona, LLC has been supported through contracted subscriptions in the last 2 years by AbbVie, Amgen, Boehringer Ingelheim, Bristol-Myers Squibb, Crescendo, Eli Lilly and

Company, Genentech, Gilead, GSK, Horizon Pharma USA, Janssen, Momenta Pharmaceuticals, Novartis, Pfizer Inc., Roche, Sun-Merck, UCB Pharma, and Valeant. Support for third-party writing assistance for this article, provided by Ricardo Milho, PhD, and Aimée Hall, MPhys, Costello Medical Consulting, Cambridge, UK, was funded by UCB Pharma.

Authors' contributions

LRH, HJL, KCS, KJD, BG, JDG, RL, JS, RS, SJ, JMK, and MY contributed to the conception, design, execution or analysis, and interpretation of the data. All authors approved the final version to be published after critically revising the manuscript/publication for important intellectual content.

Ethics approval and consent to participate

All participating investigators were required to obtain full board approval for conducting noninterventional research involving human subjects with a limited dataset. Sponsor approval and continuing review were obtained through a central institutional review board (IRB) (New England Independent Review Board; NEIRB number 02-021). For academic investigative sites that did not receive a waiver to use the central IRB, full board approval was obtained from the respective governing IRBs, and documentation of approval was submitted to the sponsor prior to initiating any study procedures. The principal investigator or designee at each site inform patients of the purposes of this registry. Patients who express a willingness to consider participation are given a consent form to review. If patients have any questions related to participation in the registry, these are answered by the principal investigator or designee. Patients sign the voluntary consent form. Patients who consent to participate in the registry receive a signed and dated copy of the consent form. Informed consent must be obtained before any assessments are performed.

Competing interests

LRH has received research grants from Pfizer; stock from Corrona, LLC; consulting fees from Roche and Bristol Myers-Squibb; and is an employee of the University of Massachusetts Medical School and Corrona, LLC. HJL is an employee of Corrona, LLC. KCS is an employee of Corrona, LLC. KJD is an employee of Corrona, LLC. BG is an employee of the University of Massachusetts Medical School and Corrona, LLC. JDG is an employee of New York University School of Medicine and Corrona, LLC; has received stock from Corrona, LLC; and has received consulting fees from AstraZeneca, Celgene, Genentech, Biogen Idec Inc., Janssen Pharmaceutical Products, LP, Novartis Pharmaceutical Corporation, and Pfizer. RL is an employee of UCB Pharma. JS is an employee of UCB Pharma. RS is an employee of UCB Pharma. SJ is an employee of UCB Pharma. JMK is an employee of Corrona, LLC, and has received stock from Corrona, LLC; consulting fees from AbbVie, Amgen, Bristol Myers-Squibb, Genentech, GSK, Eli Lilly and Co., Medimmune, Pfizer, and Sanofi; and research grants from AbbVie, Genentech, Eli Lilly and Co., Novartis, and Pfizer. MY is an employee of UCB Pharma.

Author details

[1]University of Massachusetts Medical School, Worcester, MA, USA. [2]Pharmacoepidemiology and Outcomes Research, Corrona, 352 Turnpike Road, Suite 325, Southborough, MA 01772, USA. [3]New York University School of Medicine, New York, NY, USA. [4]UCB Pharma, Smyrna, GA, USA. [5]UCB Pharma, Raleigh, NC, USA. [6]Albany Medical College, Albany, NY, USA.

References

1. Kvien TK. Epidemiology and burden of illness of rheumatoid arthritis. Pharmacoeconomics. 2004;22(2 Suppl 1):1–12.
2. Scott DL, Wolfe F, Huizinga TW. Rheumatoid arthritis. Lancet. 2010; 376(9746):1094–108.
3. Avina-Zubieta JA, Choi HK, Sadatsafavi M, et al. Risk of cardiovascular mortality in patients with rheumatoid arthritis: a meta-analysis of observational studies. Arthritis Rheum. 2008;59(12):1690–7.
4. Doran MF, Crowson CS, Pond GR, et al. Frequency of infection in patients with rheumatoid arthritis compared with controls: a population-based study. Arthritis Rheum. 2002;46(9):2287–93.
5. Naz SM, Symmons DP. Mortality in established rheumatoid arthritis. Best Pract Res Clin Rheumatol. 2007;21(5):871–83.
6. Nam JL, Ramiro S, Gaujoux-Viala C, et al. Efficacy of biological disease-modifying antirheumatic drugs: a systematic literature review informing the 2013 update of the EULAR recommendations for the management of rheumatoid arthritis. Ann Rheum Dis. 2014;73(3):516–28.
7. Barnabe C, Martin BJ, Ghali WA. Systematic review and meta-analysis: anti-tumor necrosis factor α therapy and cardiovascular events in rheumatoid arthritis. Arthritis Care Res (Hoboken). 2011;63(4):522–9.
8. Solomon DH, Reed GW, Kremer JM, et al. Disease activity in rheumatoid arthritis and the risk of cardiovascular events. Arthritis Rheumatol. 2015; 67(6):1449–55.
9. Listing J, Gerhold K, Zink A. The risk of infections associated with rheumatoid arthritis, with its comorbidity and treatment. Rheumatology (Oxford). 2013;52(1):53–61.
10. Askling J, Fored CM, Brandt L, et al. Time-dependent increase in risk of hospitalisation with infection among Swedish RA patients treated with TNF antagonists. Ann Rheum Dis. 2007;66(10):1339–44.
11. Bongartz T, Sutton AJ, Sweeting MJ, et al. Anti-TNF antibody therapy in rheumatoid arthritis and the risk of serious infections and malignancies: systematic review and meta-analysis of rare harmful effects in randomized controlled trials. JAMA. 2006;295(19):2275–85.
12. Dixon WG, Symmons DP, Lunt M, et al. Serious infection following anti-tumor necrosis factor α therapy in patients with rheumatoid arthritis: lessons from interpreting data from observational studies. Arthritis Rheum. 2007;56(9):2896–904.
13. Galloway JB, Hyrich KL, Mercer LK, et al. Anti-TNF therapy is associated with an increased risk of serious infections in patients with rheumatoid arthritis especially in the first 6 months of treatment: updated results from the British Society for Rheumatology Biologics Register with special emphasis on risks in the elderly. Rheumatology (Oxford). 2011;50(1):124–31.
14. Leombruno JP, Einarson TR, Keystone EC. The safety of anti-tumour necrosis factor treatments in rheumatoid arthritis: meta and exposure-adjusted pooled analyses of serious adverse events. Ann Rheum Dis. 2009;68(7):1136–45.
15. Salliot C, Dougados M, Gossec L. Risk of serious infections during rituximab, abatacept and anakinra treatments for rheumatoid arthritis: meta-analyses of randomised placebo-controlled trials. Ann Rheum Dis. 2009;68(1):25–32.
16. Schneeweiss S, Setoguchi S, Weinblatt ME, et al. Anti-tumor necrosis factor α therapy and the risk of serious bacterial infections in elderly patients with rheumatoid arthritis. Arthritis Rheum. 2007;56(6):1754–64.
17. Singh JA, Cameron C, Noorbaloochi S, et al. Risk of serious infection in biological treatment of patients with rheumatoid arthritis: a systematic review and meta-analysis. Lancet. 2015;386(9990):258–65.
18. Singh JA, Hossain A, Tanjong Ghogomu E, et al. Biologics or tofacitinib for rheumatoid arthritis in incomplete responders to methotrexate or other traditional disease-modifying anti-rheumatic drugs: a systematic review and network meta-analysis. Cochrane Database Syst Rev. 2016;5:CD012183.
19. Strangfeld A, Eveslage M, Schneider M, et al. Treatment benefit or survival of the fittest: what drives the time-dependent decrease in serious infection rates under TNF inhibition and what does this imply for the individual patient? Ann Rheum Dis. 2011;70(11):1914–20.
20. Thompson AE, Rieder SW, Pope JE. Tumor necrosis factor therapy and the risk of serious infection and malignancy in patients with early rheumatoid arthritis: a meta-analysis of randomized controlled trials. Arthritis Rheum. 2011;63(6):1479–85.
21. Wolfe F, Caplan L, Michaud K. Treatment for rheumatoid arthritis and the risk of hospitalization for pneumonia: associations with prednisone, disease-modifying antirheumatic drugs, and anti-tumor necrosis factor therapy. Arthritis Rheum. 2006;54(2):628–34.
22. Askling J, Fored CM, Brandt L, et al. Risks of solid cancers in patients with rheumatoid arthritis and after treatment with tumour necrosis factor antagonists. Ann Rheum Dis. 2005;64(10):1421–6.
23. Bongartz T, Warren FC, Mines D, et al. Etanercept therapy in rheumatoid arthritis and the risk of malignancies: a systematic review and individual patient data meta-analysis of randomised controlled trials. Ann Rheum Dis. 2009;68(7):1177–83.
24. Burmester GR, Panaccione R, Gordon KB, et al. Adalimumab: long-term safety in 23 458 patients from global clinical trials in rheumatoid arthritis, juvenile idiopathic arthritis, ankylosing spondylitis, psoriatic arthritis, psoriasis and Crohn's disease. Ann Rheum Dis. 2013;72(4):517–24.

25. Wong AK, Kerkoutian S, Said J, et al. Risk of lymphoma in patients receiving antitumor necrosis factor therapy: a meta-analysis of published randomized controlled studies. Clin Rheumatol. 2012;31(4):631–6.
26. Petri H, Urquhart J. Channeling bias in the interpretation of drug effects. Stat Med. 1991;10(4):577–81.
27. FDA. Cimzia (certolizumab pegol) Prescribing Information; last updated April 2016. Available at: http://www.accessdata.fda.gov/drugsatfda_docs/label/2016/125160s241lbl.pdf. Last accessed: September 2016.
28. Kremer JM. The CORRONA database. Clin Exp Rheumatol. 2005;23(5 Suppl 39): S172–7.
29. Fisher MC, Furer V, Hochberg MC, et al. Malignancy validation in a United States registry of rheumatoid arthritis patients. BMC Musculoskelet Disord. 2012;13:85.
30. Solomon DH, Kremer J, Curtis JR, et al. Explaining the cardiovascular risk associated with rheumatoid arthritis: traditional risk factors versus markers of rheumatoid arthritis severity. Ann Rheum Dis. 2010;69(11):1920–5.
31. Curtis JR, Patkar NM, Jain A, et al. Validity of physician-reported hospitalized infections in a US arthritis registry. Rheumatology (Oxford). 2009;48(10):1269–72.
32. Charlson ME, Pompei P, Ales KL, et al. A new method of classifying prognostic comorbidity in longitudinal studies: development and validation. J Chronic Dis. 1987;40(5):373–83.
33. Smolen JS, Burmester GR, Combe B, et al. Head-to-head comparison of certolizumab pegol versus adalimumab in rheumatoid arthritis: 2-year efficacy and safety results from the randomised EXXELERATE study. Lancet. 2016;388(10061):2763–74.
34. Au K, Reed G, Curtis JR, et al. High disease activity is associated with an increased risk of infection in patients with rheumatoid arthritis. Ann Rheum Dis. 2011;70(5):785–91.
35. Curtis JR, Xie F, Chen L, et al. The comparative risk of serious infections among rheumatoid arthritis patients starting or switching biological agents. Ann Rheum Dis. 2011;70(8):1401–6.
36. Emery P, Gallo G, Boyd H, et al. Association between disease activity and risk of serious infections in subjects with rheumatoid arthritis treated with etanercept or disease-modifying anti-rheumatic drugs. Clin Exp Rheumatol. 2014;32(5):653–60.
37. Grijalva CG, Chen L, Delzell E, et al. Initiation of tumor necrosis factor-α antagonists and the risk of hospitalization for infection in patients with autoimmune diseases. JAMA. 2011;306(21):2331–9.
38. Weaver A, Troum O, Hooper M, et al. Rheumatoid arthritis disease activity and disability affect the risk of serious infection events in RADIUS 1. J Rheumatol. 2013;40(8):1275–81.
39. Singh JA, Saag KG, Bridges Jr SL, et al. 2015 American College of Rheumatology guideline for the treatment of rheumatoid arthritis. Arthritis Rheumatol. 2016;68(1):1–26.
40. Singh JA, Wells GA, Christensen R, et al. Adverse effects of biologics: a network meta-analysis and Cochrane overview. Cochrane Database Syst Rev. 2011;2:CD008794.
41. Burmester GR, Mease P, Dijkmans BA, et al. Adalimumab safety and mortality rates from global clinical trials of six immune-mediated inflammatory diseases. Ann Rheum Dis. 2009;68(12):1863–9.
42. Yun H, Xie F, Delzell E, et al. Comparative risk of hospitalized infection associated with biologic agents in rheumatoid arthritis patients enrolled in Medicare. Arthritis Rheumatol. 2016;68(1):56–66.
43. Silva-Fernández L, Lunt M, Kearsley-Fleet L, et al. The incidence of cancer in patients with rheumatoid arthritis and a prior malignancy who receive TNF inhibitors or rituximab: results from the British Society for Rheumatology Biologics Register-Rheumatoid Arthritis. Rheumatology (Oxford). 2016;55(11): 2033–9.
44. Morgan CL, Emery P, Porter D, et al. Treatment of rheumatoid arthritis with etanercept with reference to disease-modifying anti-rheumatic drugs: long-term safety and survival using prospective, observational data. Rheumatology (Oxford). 2014;53(1):186–94.
45. Askling J, van Vollenhoven RF, Granath F, et al. Cancer risk in patients with rheumatoid arthritis treated with anti-tumor necrosis factor α therapies: does the risk change with the time since start of treatment? Arthritis Rheum. 2009;60(11):3180–9.
46. Mercer LK, Green AC, Galloway JB, et al. The influence of anti-TNF therapy upon incidence of keratinocyte skin cancer in patients with rheumatoid arthritis: longitudinal results from the British Society for Rheumatology Biologics Register. Ann Rheum Dis. 2012;71(6):869–74.
47. Raaschou P, Simard JF, Holmqvist M, et al. Rheumatoid arthritis, anti-tumour necrosis factor therapy, and risk of malignant melanoma: nationwide population based prospective cohort study from Sweden. BMJ. 2013;346:f1939.
48. Turesson C. Comorbidity in rheumatoid arthritis. Swiss Med Wkly. 2016;146: w14290.
49. Del Rincon I, Williams K, Stern MP, et al. Association between carotid atherosclerosis and markers of inflammation in rheumatoid arthritis patients and healthy subjects. Arthritis Rheum. 2003;48(7):1833–40.
50. Myasoedova E, Crowson CS, Kremers HM, et al. Lipid paradox in rheumatoid arthritis: the impact of serum lipid measures and systemic inflammation on the risk of cardiovascular disease. Ann Rheum Dis. 2011;70(3):482–7.
51. Cobo-Ibanez T, Descalzo MA, Loza-Santamaria E, et al. Serious infections in patients with rheumatoid arthritis and other immune-mediated connective tissue diseases exposed to anti-TNF or rituximab: data from the Spanish registry BIOBADASER 2.0. Rheumatol Int. 2014;34(7):953–61.
52. Ramiro S, Gaujoux-Viala C, Nam JL, et al. Safety of synthetic and biological DMARDs: a systematic literature review informing the 2013 update of the EULAR recommendations for management of rheumatoid arthritis. Ann Rheum Dis. 2014;73(3):529–35.
53. Bykerk VP, Cush J, Winthrop K, et al. Update on the safety profile of certolizumab pegol in rheumatoid arthritis: an integrated analysis from clinical trials. Ann Rheum Dis. 2015;74(1):96–103.
54. Curtis JR, Chen L, Bharat A, et al. Linkage of a de-identified United States rheumatoid arthritis registry with administrative data to facilitate comparative effectiveness research. Arthritis Care Res (Hoboken). 2014; 66(12):1790–8.

5

Synovial IL-9 facilitates neutrophil survival, function and differentiation of Th17 cells in rheumatoid arthritis

Kaustav Chowdhury[1], Uma Kumar[2], Soumabha Das[2], Jaydeep Chaudhuri[4], Prabin Kumar[1], Maumita Kanjilal[2], Parashar Ghosh[3], Geetabali Sircar[3], Ravi Kiran Basyal[2], Uma Kanga[1], Santu Bandyopadhaya[4] and Dipendra Kumar Mitra[1*]

Abstract

Background: Role of Th9 cells and interleukin-9 (IL-9) in human autoimmune diseases such as psoriasis and ulcerative colitis has been explored only very recently. However, their involvement in human rheumatoid arthritis (RA) is not conclusive. Pathogenesis of RA is complex and involves various T cell subsets and neutrophils. Here, we aimed at understanding the impact of IL-9 on infiltrating immune cells and their eventual role in synovial inflammation in RA.

Methods: In vitro stimulation of T cells was performed by engagement of anti-CD3 and anti-CD28 monoclonal antibodies. Flow cytometry was employed for measuring intracellular cytokine, RORγt in T cells, evaluating apoptosis of neutrophils. ELISA was used for measuring soluble cytokine, Western blot analysis and confocal microscopy were used for STAT3 phosphorylation and nuclear translocation.

Results: We demonstrated synovial enrichment of Th9 cells and their positive correlation with disease activity (DAS28-ESR) in RA. Synovial IL-9 prolonged the survival of neutrophils, increased their matrix metalloprotienase-9 production and facilitated Th17 cell differentiation evidenced by induction of transcription factor RORγt and STAT3 phosphorylation. IL-9 also augmented the function of IFN-γ + and TNF-α + synovial T cells.

Conclusions: We provide evidences for critical role of IL-9 in disease pathogenesis and propose that targeting IL-9 may be an effective strategy to ameliorate synovial inflammation in RA. Inhibiting IL-9 may have wider impact on the production of pathogenic cytokines involved in autoimmune diseases including RA and may offer better control over the disease.

Keywords: Rheumatoid arthritis, Interleukin-9, Neutrophils, Th17 cells

Background

Helper T ($CD4^+$) cells preferentially producing interleukin (IL)-9 have recently been described as distinct Th9 cells and implicated in several inflammatory conditions such as infectious, neoplastic and autoimmune diseases [1–4]. Contribution of these cells in the pathogenesis of autoimmunity has been demonstrated in animal studies of colitis [5, 6], uveitis [7], and experimental autoimmune encephalomyelitis (EAE) [8–10]. However, reports on their presence or enrichment at the pathologic sites and impact on the local inflammatory cascade in human autoimmune diseases are limited, except in psoriasis [11], systemic lupus erythematosus [12], and colitis [6].Very recently, Th9 cells have been identified in rheumatoid arthritis (RA) peripheral blood and synovial tissues and fluid, but their precise role in RA pathology is not depicted conclusively [13, 14]. Therefore, investigating Th9 cells in RA seems to be important in determining the local immune response. Therefore, we hypothesized that Th9/IL-9-producing cells would be abundant in RA synovial fluid (SF). This study is an attempt to determine

* Correspondence: salilmitra2@gmail.com
[1]Department of Transplant Immunology and Immunogenetics, All India Institute of Medical Sciences (AIIMS), Room No-75, New Delhi 110029, India
Full list of author information is available at the end of the article

the status of Th9 cells at the disease site of RA patients and their involvement in disease progression.

Pathogenesis of RA involves a complex inflammatory cascade mediated by massive influx of various effector immune cells, their activation leading to copious production of tissue-damaging proteases like matrix metalloproteinases (MMPs) [15], and collagenase. Cellular infiltrates in RA joints majorly constitute neutrophils and lymphocytes (T and B) [16–19]. Neutrophils and various T cell subsets producing distinct pro-inflammatory cytokines have been demonstrated as key effector cells augmenting the local inflammatory response during active disease. Synovial neutrophils are activated by diverse cytokines derived from infiltrating T cells and macrophages [20–22]. Involvement of Th1 and Th17 cells in RA has been demonstrated earlier [23–27]. Among diverse cytokines present in SF of RA joints, interferon gamma (IFN-γ), tumor necrosis alpha (TNF-α), and IL-17 are believed to be critical mediators of inflammation in RA. IL-17 and TNF-α have been documented to activate the neutrophils to produce MMPs [28, 29] which are responsible for joint destruction. Most recent findings implicate Th17 cell as an important effector in pathogenic process of RA [30]. Elucidating functional hierarchy of distinct effector T cells producing key pathogenic cytokine(s) is critical and may provide novel opportunity for modulating inflammation in RA and disease remission.

Recent evidence suggests the role of Th9 cells in psoriatic skin lesions [7] in enhancing other T cell subsets producing effector cytokines like IFN-γ, IL-17. However, Th9 cells and their role in RA still remain unclear. Therefore, in this study we asked following questions: (i) Do Th9 cells exist in RA-affected synovial milieu in patients as a distinct in vivo T cell subset? (ii) If so, do they exert a hierarchic influence on other inflammatory immune cells accumulated in pathologic sites of RA? (iii) Does synovial IL-9 augment the function of infiltrating T cells and neutrophils thereby potentiating the inflammatory cascade in RA?

Here, we show the enrichment of Th9/IL-9+ cells as a distinct inflammatory T cell subset in the SF of active RA patients. Our study demonstrates that (i) Th9 cells are enriched in SF, (ii) SF IL-9 drives the inflammatory cascade by inhibiting apoptosis of neutrophils and production of MMP-9 and (iii) augments the differentiation of Th17 cells in RA-affected synovia. We reveal a hitherto unknown mechanism by which Th9/IL-9 cells may perpetuate synovial inflammation in RA to the best of our current knowledge.

Methods

Study subjects

This study was conducted in treatment-naïve active RA patients, fulfilling the 1987 American College of Rheumatology (ACR) criteria [31]. All RA patients disease activity was measured with 28-joint disease activity score (DAS-28), which is based on the number of tender/swollen joints and the erythrocyte sedimentation rate (ESR). All RA patients had DAS-28 ESR > 5. Out of 28 patients, 20 were female and 8 were male (Additional file 1: Table S1). Fifteen healthy controls (HCs) and 10 osteoarthritis (OA) patients with median age 38.6 ± 8.9 and 43.5 ± 2.98 years respectively were enrolled in this study. The female:male ratios of HC and OA groups were 9:6 and 5:5 respectively. HCs were free from any rheumatologic disorders, acute or chronic ailments such as infections, diabetes mellitus or any other endocrine disorders, liver or renal abnormalities. These were confirmed by clinical as well as appropriate laboratory investigations including radiography, complete blood count (CBC), and serology for HIV and hepatitis, relevant endocrine, renal and hepatic assays. OA patients were diagnosed according to ACR classic clinical criteria (inclusion) supplemented with radiographic evaluation, ESR (<40 mm/hour), white cell count of the synovial aspirate (<1000/μl), rheumatoid factor (RF) titer (<1:40). All of our OA patients presented with involvement of knee joints. This is an ex vivo basic experimental study and it is approved by the institutional ethics committee (All India Institute of Medical Sciences, New Delhi, India, letter no: SH/10/11/TII). All blood and SF samples were collected from RA and OA patients after taking duly signed written consent form.

Cell preparation and enumeration of T cell frequency

Peripheral blood and SF fluid mononuclear cells (PBMCs and SFMCs) were isolated by Ficol hypaque (Lymphoprep, Axis-Shield, Oslo, Norway) density gradient centrifugation. Cell viability was checked by 0.1% trypan blue dye exclusion test and found to be > 95% viable. Cells were suspended in media RPMI-1640 (Caisson Laboratories, Smithfield, UT USA) supplemented with L-Glutamine, HEPES (Sigma-Aldrich, St. Louis, MO, USA), antibiotics (Biological Industries, Kibbutz Beit-Haemek, Israel) and 10% heat inactivated fetal calf serum (FCS, Biological Industries). PBMCs/SFMCs were stimulated with plate-bound anti-CD3 (Clone: UCHIT, BD Pharmingen, San Jose, CA, USA; 5ug/ml) and anti-CD28 (clone: CD28.6 eBiosciences, San Diego, CA, USA, 2.5ug/ml) for 48 hours in humidified 5% CO_2 incubator at 37 °C. In some experiments evaluating reagents rIL-9 (20 ng/ml; Abcam, Cambridge, MA, USA), SF (1:9 ratio SF:media), anti-IL-9 monoclonal antibody (10 μg/ml, Abcam) were added in the cell culture to block endogenous IL-9 present in RA SF. Golgi transport inhibitor monensin was added during last 6 hours of culture. For surface staining, cells were washed with phosphate-buffered saline (PBS) and incubated with CD4 phycoerythrin tandem conjugate with cyanine (PE-Cy5) (BD Pharmingen) for 15 minutes on ice. Intracellular cytokine staining for IL-9, IFN-γ, TNF-α, and IL-17A was done after fixation and a permeabilization process using dye-conjugated monoclonal antibodies Anti-IL-9 PE, (BioLegend, San Diego, CA, USA), anti-IFN-γ fluorescein isothiocyanate (FITC), anti-TNF-α PE (BD Pharmingen), anti-IL-17A FITC (eBiosciences). For Th17 cell transcription factor analysis in HC and RA patients, isolated PBMCs and SFMCs were isolated, washed and surface-stained for CD4 (anti-CD4 PECy5, BD Pharmingen) and after fixation and permeabilization, cells were further incubated with anti-retineic-acid-receptor-related orphan nuclear receptor gamma t (RORγt) PE antibody (eBiosciences) for 30 minutes in dark. Data was acquired in FACS caliber (BD, Franklin Lakes, NJ, USA) and analyzed using FlowJo (Tree Star, Ashland, OR, USA).

Neutrophil isolation and apoptosis

To study the neutrophil apoptosis in the presence of the SF of RA patients, neutrophils were enriched from healthy donor by density gradient centrifugation on polymorphoprep as per the manufacturer's protocol (Axis-Shield PoC AS) [32]. After lysis of red blood cells (RBCs) neutrophils were washed with PBS (pH 7.4) and suspended in media RPMI-1640 (as described in the previous section). Purity and viability (>95%) of enriched neutrophils were assessed using Leishman staining and the trypan blue dye exclusion method. Neutrophils were identified in FACS by using CD15 as a neutrophil identifying marker [33]. To observe the effect of IL-9 on neutrophil survival, neutrophils (isolated freshly from healthy donor peripheral blood) were cultured in the presence and absence of rIL-9 (20 ng/ml, eBioscience), in media for 12 hours at 37 °C. Neutrophils were harvested, washed twice with PBS, and incubated with anti-CD15 PE and anti-annexin V FITC antibody (BD Pharmingen) for 15 minutes on ice. To determine the effect of endogenous IL-9 on neutrophil survival, neutrophils from RA SF (1×10^6) were cultured in the presence of rIL-9, autologous SF (100 µl SF of active RA patient in 400 µl RPMI-1640) and anti-IL-9 antibody (10 µg/ml; Abcam). Cells were harvested after 12 hours and washed twice with PBS. Cells were subjected to FACS-based staining for CD15 and annexin V and acquired by FACSCalibur (BD). Data analysis was done with FlowJo X (Tree Star).

Neutrophils activation and IL-9 receptor expression

To study the neutrophil activation and function, freshly isolated healthy neutrophils (1×10^6) were stimulated with rIL-9 (eBioscience), lipopolysaccharide (LPS) (5 ng/ml, Sigma-Aldrich) and LPS plus rIL-9 for 12 hours. Cells were then incubated with anti-CD69 PE antibody (BD Pharmingen) and anti-IL-9 receptor (anti-CD129) PE antibody (BioLegend) on ice for 15 minutes on ice.

MMP-9 production by neutrophils

To determine the matrix metalloproteinase-9 (MMP-9) production by neutrophils, isolated neutrophils (1×10^6) from healthy controls were stimulated either with RA SF (cell-free SF, DAS-28 score > 5, 1:9 ratio SF:media), rIL-9 (20 ng/ml) or anti-IL-9 blocking antibody (10 µg/ml, Abcam) for 12 hours and monesin was added (as a golgi transport inhibitor, Sigma-Aldrich) during last 6 hours of culture. Neutrophils were fixed with 2% formaldehyde, permeabilized and incubated with rabbit anti-human anti-MMP-9 primary antibody (1:250 dilution, Santa Cruz Biotechnology, Dallas, TX, USA) for 30 minutes at room temperature followed by secondary anti-rabbit IgG FITC (dilution 1:100; Abcam) for another 30 minutes at room temperature. Stained samples were acquired by FACSCalibur (BD) and analyzed with Flow Jo (Tree Star).

Western blot for MCL-1 and STAT3 phosphorylation

Neutrophils were enriched from SF of RA patients and cultured (2×10^6) as mentioned above in apoptosis assay. After 12 hours of culture, cells were harvested and were lysed in lysis buffer [protenase inhibitor cocktail (BD Pharmingen) and phosphoSTOP (Sigma-Aldrich) present in lysis buffer along with radioimmunoprecipitation assay buffer (RIPA, Cell Signaling Technology, Danvers, MA, USA)]. After extracting proteins from each culture condition (media, SF, rIL-9, anti-IL-9), concentration was measured with protein estimation kit (Bio-Rad, Hercules, CA, USA). Each protein sample (50 µg) was subjected to SDS-polyacrylamide gel electrophoresis (PAGE). Proteins were transferred to polyvinylidene difluoride membranes (PVDF, EMD Millipore, Billerica, MA, USA) and western blot was performed using anti-induced myeloid leukemia cell differentiation protein [anti-induced myeloid leukemia cell differentiation protein (MCL-1) monoclonal antibody, 1:500 dilution, Santa Cruz Biotechnology, Dallas, TX, USA]. Beta-actin (anti-β-actin, 1:500 dilutions, Santa Cruz Biotechnology) was used as loading control. Detection of specific protein was done by Luminata Forte HRP substrate (EMD Millipore). To determine signal transducer and activator of transcription 3 (STAT3) phosphorylation in CD4+ T cells, freshly isolated PBMCs (2×10^6) from healthy individuals were enriched for CD4+ T cells with the help of magnetic enrichment kit (Miltenyi Biotec, San Diego, CA, USA). Enriched CD4+ cells (98% purity, viability was 97.8% with trypan blue dye exclusion method) were cultured in presence of rIL-9 (20 ng/ml, eBiosciences), SF of RA patient (DAS28-ESR > 5 +, 100 µl SF in 500 µl RPMI1640) and anti-IL-9 polyclonal goat antibody (20 Abcam) for 12 hours. Cells were harvested and cell lysate was prepared in lysis buffer (mentioned above). After extracting proteins from each culture condition (media, anti-CD3/28, rIL-9, RA SF) protein concentration was measured with protein estimation kit (Bio-Rad). Each protein sample (50 µg) was subjected to

SDS-PAGE. Proteins were transferred to polyvinylidenedifluoride membranes (PVDF, EMD Millipore) and western blot was performed anti-phospho STAT3 (Tyr705, 1:1000 dilution, Cell Signaling Technology) antibody. Detection of specific protein was done by Luminata Forte HRP substrate (EMD Millipore).

Detection of STAT3 co-localization by confocal microscopy

To determine the STAT3 phosphorylation and cellular localization, freshly isolated PBMCs (2×10^6) from healthy subjects were stimulated as per same culture conditions mentioned above for STAT3 western blot. Cells were harvested after 12 hours and washed twice with PBS. Surface staining was done with anti CD4 FITC (BD Pharmingen) incubation on ice for 15 minutes. After fixing and permealization, cells were incubated in dark with DAPI-conjugated Prolong Gold anti-fade reagent as per the manufacturer's protocol (Invitrogen, Waltham, MA, USA) and anti-phopho-STAT3 APC antibody (Tyr705, 1:300 dilution, Lifespan Biosciences, Seattle, WA, USA) at room temperature for 30 minutes. Cells were then observed under a Plan Apo VC 60X/1.40 oil objective on an inverted Eclipse Ti Nikon microscope equipped with a QImaging-Rolera EMC^2 camera to capture image (Nikon, Tokyo, Japan).

Cytokine ELISA

Levels of soluble IL-9 and MMP-9 were assessed in plasma (HC, OA, RA) and SF (RA and OA) by ELISA kit IL-9 (Abcam) and MMP-9 (eBioscience) respectively, as per the manufacturer's protocol.

Statistical analysis

Statistical analysis was done with GraphPad prism5 software (La Jolla, CA, USA) by using Student's t test for unpaired samples. One-way ANOVA, Dunnett's multiple comparison tests was used for statistical significance evaluation in cytokine production study in different conditions. The data were presented as mean ± SEM and values $p < 0.05$ was considered significant.

Results

Enrichment of Th9 cells in the RA SF correlates with disease activity score (DAS28-ESR)

We aimed to enumerate the frequency of IL-9-producing CD4+ T cells in peripheral blood (PBL) and SF of RA patients by flow cytometry. Frequency of Th9 cells was elevated in the PBL of RA patients compared to HC and OA patients. However, it was not significantly higher in the PBL of OA patients compared to HC. Interestingly, frequency of Th9 cells was markedly higher in RA SF relative to their autologous PBL as well as to their disease control group OA SF, suggesting their enrichment at the pathologic site (RA SF, Fig. 1a and b). Th9 cell frequency of both PBL ($r = 0.45$; $p = 0.02$) and SF ($r = 0.79$; $p = 0.0001$) correlated with DAS-28-ESR disease activity score of the patients (Fig. 1c). Soluble level of IL-9 was also significantly elevated in RA PBL and SF compared to OA PBL and SF (Fig. 1d).

Synovial IL-9 of RA patients inhibits apoptosis of neutrophils

We investigated the impact of endogenous IL-9 of RA SF on the survival and activation of synovial neutrophils, the most abundant cells infiltrating in the RA joints [34]. Addition of recombinant IL-9 (rIL-9) significantly reduced the apoptosis of healthy neutrophils in vitro as measured by the annexin V staining (Fig. 2a). To understand it is in vivo relevance, we measured the spontaneous apoptosis of RA SF derived neutrophils in presence and absence of SF. RA SF, and rIL-9 significantly reduced, while blocking IL-9, increased the spontaneous apoptosis of neutrophil (Fig. 2b and Additional file 2: Figure S1). rIL-9 increased the expression of anti-apoptotic protein, MCL-1 (a BCL-2 homolog) in RA SF-derived neutrophils. Addition of RA SF increased the expression of MCL-1, even higher than rIL-9 alone. Moreover, blocking endogenous IL-9 in SF reduced the expression of MCL-1 (Fig. 2c, d). Therefore, we concluded that IL-9 present in the SF of RA patients inhibits the apoptosis and might allow them to cause prolonged tissue damage.

IL-9 activates neutrophils and enhances their matrix metalloproteinase production

Enhanced survival of neutrophils prompted us to investigate the impact of IL-9 on their activation status. rIL-9 could induce IL-9 receptor [CD129/interleukin 9 receptor (IL-9R)] on neutrophils. However, LPS activated healthy neutrophils expressed higher levels of IL-9 receptor, suggesting activation dependence of its expression (Fig. 3a). Similarly, IL-9 receptor was higher on RA SF-derived neutrophils compared to their autologous PBL-derived neutrophils (Fig. 3b). rIL-9 also induced surface expression of CD69, this suggests IL-9 can activate neutrophils (Fig. 3c). MMP-9 is a protease involved in the pathogenesis of RA [35]. Endogenous IL-9 present in the SF of RA patients and rIL-9 both enhanced MMP-9 production by neutrophils derived from healthy individuals. Whereas blocking endogenous IL-9 with anti-IL-9 antibody in RA SF decreased the production of MMP-9 in neutrophils (Fig. 3d). Moreover, the soluble level of MMP-9 was also significantly higher in RA (SF and plasma) than in OA (SF and plasma, Fig. 3e).

IL-9 potentiates functional differentiation of Th17 cells

Increased frequency of synovial Th9 cells and its correlation with the disease activity score (DAS28-ESR) prompted us to investigate the impact of IL-9 on differentiation of Th17 cells. rIL-9 increased the number of IL-

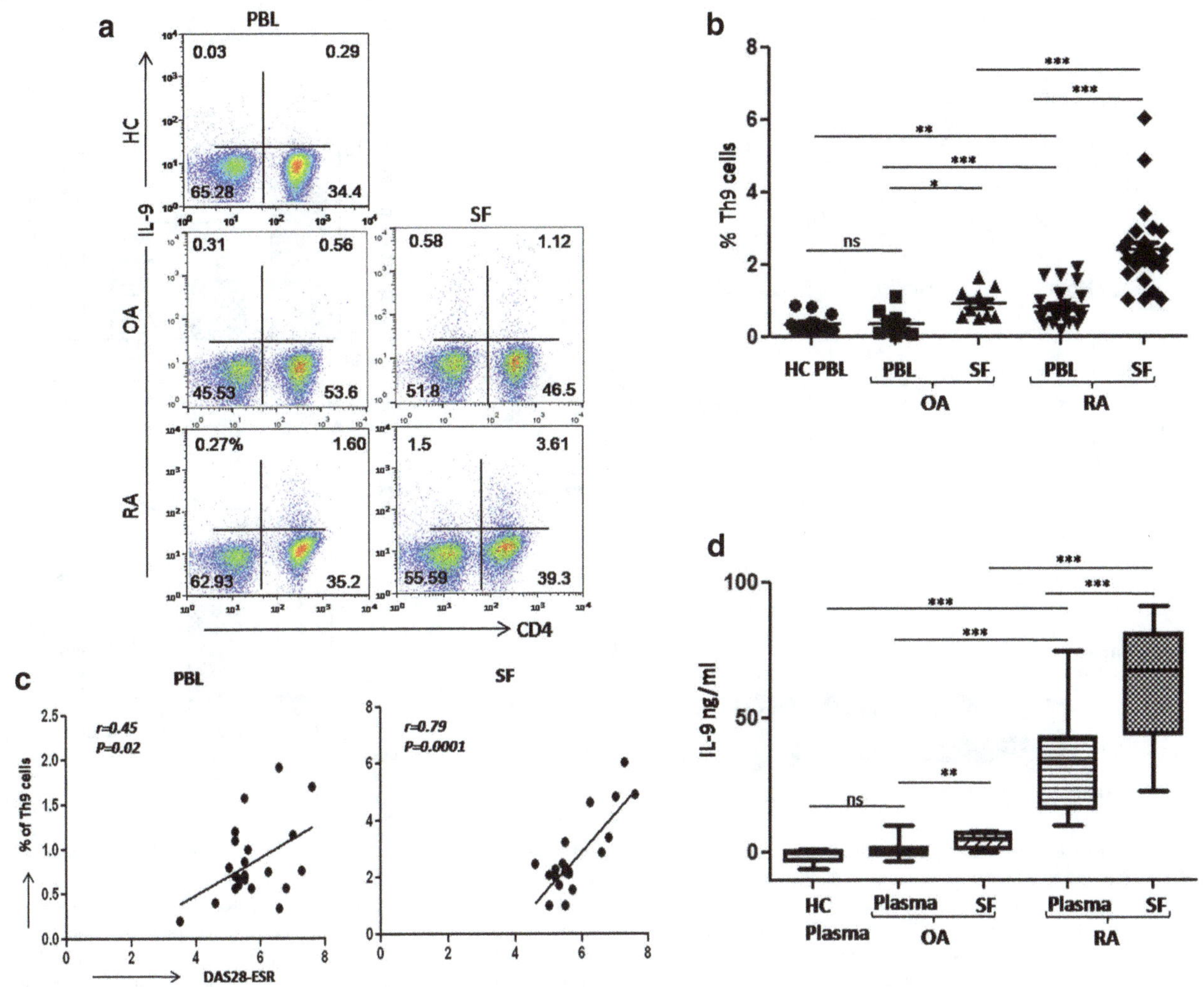

Fig. 1 Th9 cell frequency is higher in SF of RA patients. **a** Representative FACS plots show Th9 cell frequency in PBL (HC, OA, and RA) and SF (OA and RA). **b** Cumulative scatter plot shows frequency of Th9 cells in of RA (PBL and SF; n = 28), OA (PBL and SF; n = 10), HC (PBL; n = 15), significant enrichment of Th9 cells in SF of RA patients. **c** Significantly higher DAS28-ESR correlation with Th9 cell frequency in RA SF ($r = 0.79$, $p = 0.0001$) and RA PBL ($r = 0.45$, $p = 0.02$, n = 28). **d** IL-9 ELISA performed in plasma (HC; n = 15, OA; n = 10, RA; n = 20) and RA SF (n = 20), shows higher levels of soluble IL-9 in RA SF 9pt?>compared to autologous RA plasma (mean ± SEM, $^{*}p < 0.05$, $^{**}p < 0.005$, $^{***}p < 0.0001$). *DAS28* disease activity score of 28 joints, *ESR* erythrocyte sedimentation rate, *IL* interleukin, *OA* osteoarthritis, *PBL* peripheral blood, *RA* rheumatoid arthritis, *SF* synovial fluid, *Th* T helper

17A+ CD4+ T cells in healthy PBMCs stimulated in vitro with TCR engagement especially in memory (CD45RA-) T cells (Fig. 4a, b). This hints toward an IL-9-dependent Th17 differentiation of memory T cells in the synovium of RA patients. We further looked for Th17 differentiation-related transcription factor, Retinoic acid-related orphan receptor γt (RORγt) in presence of endogenous and synthetic IL-9. To this end, we have observed substantial increase in the number of RORγt^{+} T cells in the presence of both rIL-9 and RA SF (Fig. 4c). This is further substantiated by the presence of a higher number of RORγt^{+} T cells (gated on CD4+ cells) in RA SF compared to RA PBL (Fig. 4d). All together, these findings suggest that endogenously produced IL-9 present in RA SF can potentiate differentiation of Th17 cells.

Synovial IL-9 potentiates T cells present in the RA-affected joints

To observe if IL-9 can differentiate IFN-γ^{+}, TNF-α^{+}, and IL-17A^{+} effector T cells, we studied the effect of rIL-9 and RA SF on their frequency in SF of RA patients. The frequency of Th17 cells was significantly higher in the peripheral blood of RA patients compared to that of HC and OA patients (Fig. 5a, b). Th17 cells were even more abundant in the RA SF compared to OA SF, indicating their possible enrichment in the pathogenic milieu (Fig. 5b).To validate this further we stimulated T cells from RA SF in presence of rIL-9 and RA SF. T cells obtained from RA SF showed significantly higher frequency of IFN-γ^{+}, TNF-α^{+}, and IL-17A^{+} cells in presence of rIL-9 and RA SF. Moreover, neutralizing IL-9 of

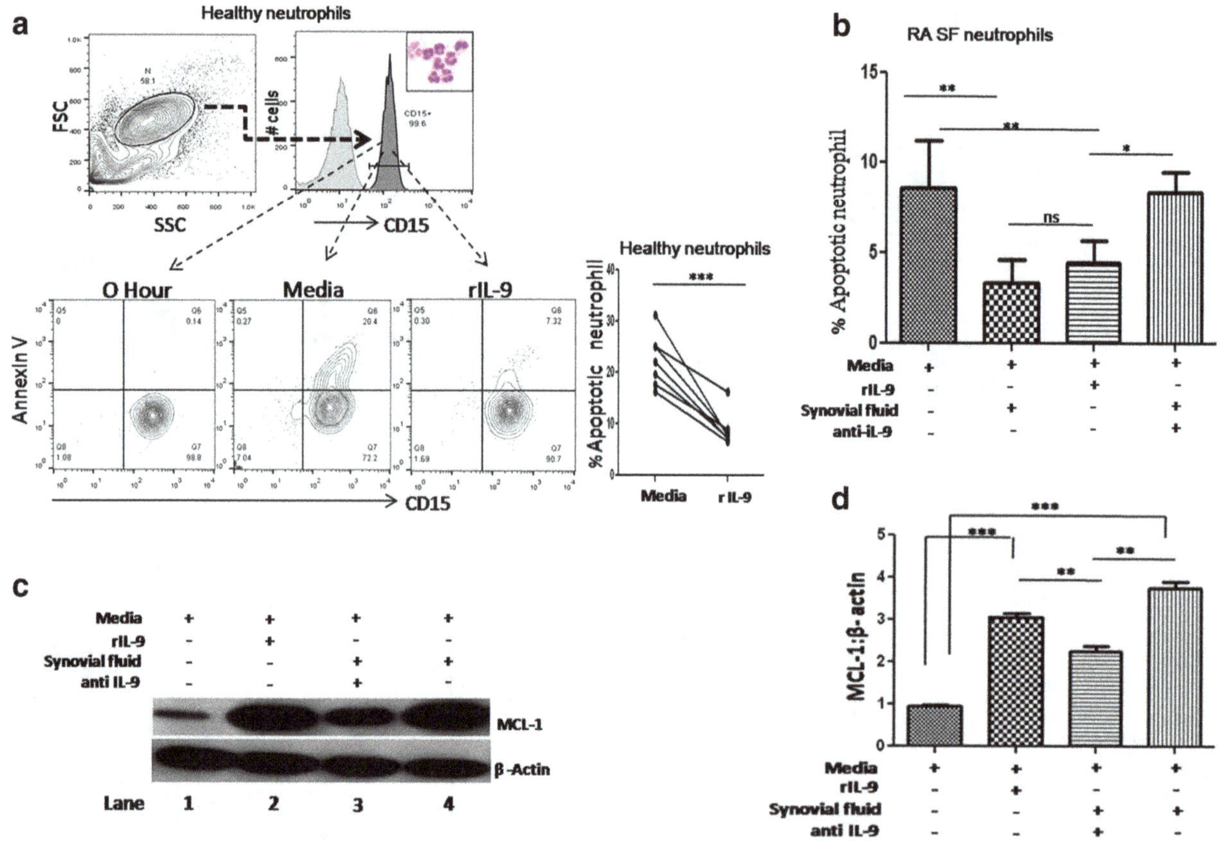

Fig. 2 IL-9 provides survival to RA SF neutrophils. **a** FACS plots show reduced annexin V on CD15-gated neutrophils (*upper panel*, Leishman's stain image of neutrophils in inset) in presence of rIL-9 and cumulative data is shown in line graph (*lower right panel*, n = 7). **b** Cumulative bar graph shows reduction in apoptosis of RA SF-derived neutrophils in the presence of RA SF and rIL-9, addition of anti-IL9 antibody in RA SF increased apoptosis (n = 8, mean ± SEM; $p < 0.006$). **c** Western blot image shows MCL-1 expression in SF-derived neutrophils under different conditions (media, rIL-9, anti-IL-9, RA SF). MCL-1 increases with rIL-9 (*lane 2*), RA SF (*lane 4*) and reduces upon blocking of endogenous IL-9 present in RA SF (*lane no 3*). Data are representative of two different experiments performed. **d** Relative (MCL-1/β-actin) densitometry bar graph of the experiment (n = 3, mean ± SEM, unpaired *t* test, $^*p < 0.05$, $^{**}p < 0.001$, $^{***}p < 0.0001$). *IL* interleukin, *IL-9R* interleukin 9 receptor, *MCL-1* induced myeloid leukemia cell differentiation protein, *RA* rheumatoid arthritis, *SF* synovial fluid, *Th* T helper

SF by blocking antibody significantly reduced their frequencies (Fig. 5c). Interestingly, both the basal and IL-9-induced frequencies of these cytokine-producing T cells were much higher in the SF of RA patients relative to their peripheral compartment (data not shown). This suggests IL-9 mediated potentiation of inflammatory cytokine-producing T cells. This is further supported by higher expression of IL-9 receptors on these effector T cells, both in peripheral and SF (data not shown).

IL-9 of SF of RA patients induces STAT3 phosphorylation and nuclear translocation

To delineate the signaling pathway responsible for Th17 cell differentiation, we studied STAT3 phosphorylation of healthy donor-derived CD4+ T cells enriched by magnetic sorting in the presence of both recombinant and endogenous IL-9 produced in SF of RA patients. rIL-9 and SF of RA patients could phosphorylate the STAT3 and anti-IL-9 addition in RA SF abrogated the same, suggesting that IL-9 of SF indeed triggers STAT3 phosphorylation, a key transcription factor toward Th17 differentiation (Fig. 6a, b). This is further confirmed by confocal microscopy, showing STAT3 phosphorylation and its nuclear translocation in the presence of IL-9 (Fig. 6c). Taken together, our results suggest IL-9 mediated triggering of the signaling event in leading to Th17 cells differentiation in RA.

Discussion

Effector T lymphocytes producing various cytokines like IFN-γ, TNF-α, and IL-17 are involved in the pathogenesis of RA [36]. However, the role of Th9 cells in RA has not been studied conclusively so far. Th9 cells were identified as discrete functional T cell subset and initially observed in various Th2-associated immunopathologic conditions such as parasitic infestation and more elaborately studied in allergic asthma, both in mice as well as human [37, 38]. Their differentiation from naïve T cells under the influence

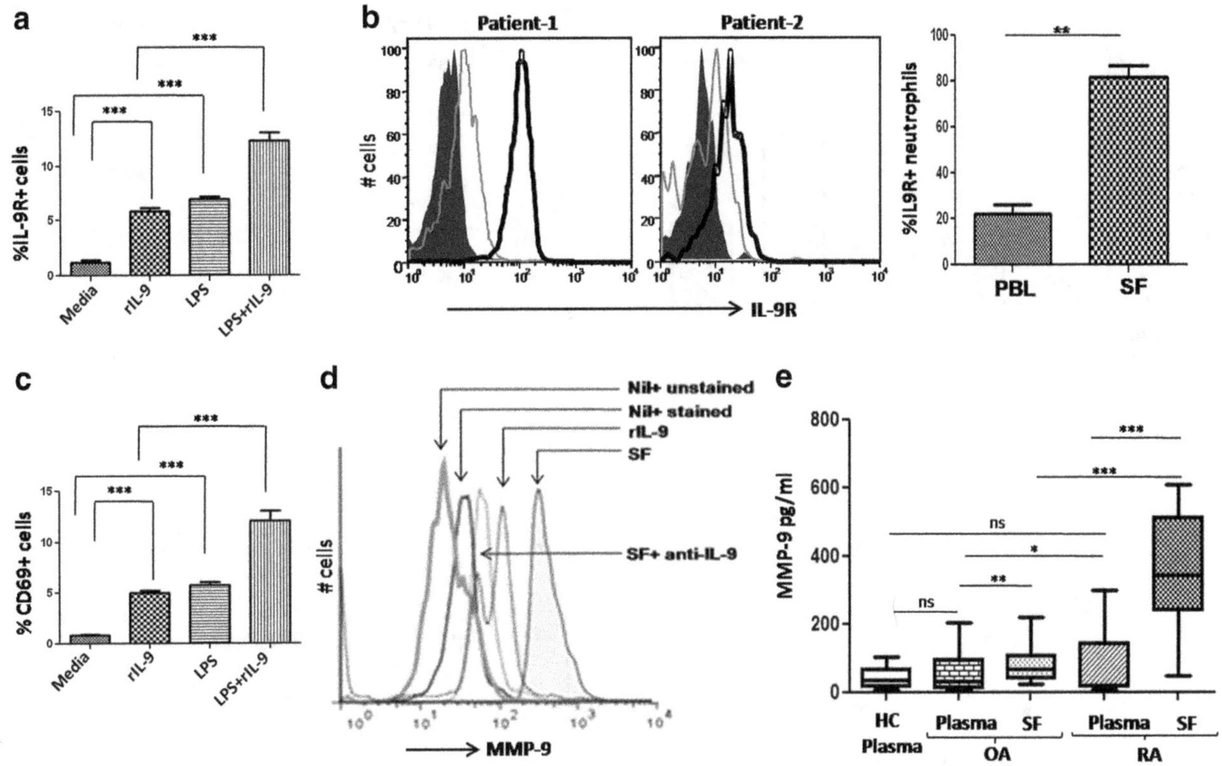

Fig. 3 Effect of IL-9 on neutrophil activation and IL-9R expression. **a** Cumulative bar graph shows IL-9R on neutrophils under different stimulation (rIL-9, LPS, LPS + rIL-9, n = 6, mean ± SEM). **b** Histogram plot shows higher expression of IL-9R on SF-derived (*dark open line*) neutrophils than PBL neutrophils of RA patients (*light open line*, *dark area* is control isotype), cumulative bar graph shows IL-9 receptor expression on neutrophils of RA patients; PBL and SF, n = 7).**c** CD69 expression on neutrophils under different culture conditions (rIL-9, LPS, LPS + rIL-9, n = 6, mean ± SEM). **d** One representative FACS histogram plot of six individual experiments shows intracellular MMP-9 in the presence of rIL-9 (*light open line*), SF (*dark open line*, untreated in *dark shaded area*). **e** Soluble MMP-9 level in plasma (HC; n = 15, OA; n = 10, RA; n = 17) and SF (OA; n = 10, RA; n = 17, unpaired *t* test, mean ± SEM $*p < 0.05$, $**p < 0.001$, $***p < 0.0001$). *HC* healthy control, *IL-9R* interleukin 9 receptor, *LPS* lipopolysaccharide, *MMP-9* matrix metalloproteinase-9, *OA* osteoarthritis, *RA* rheumatoid arthritis, *SF* synovial fluid

of TGF-β and IL-4 was marked by signature transcription factor PU.1 and copious production of IL-9 [39]. Until the recent past, it was thought that these cells belong to the Th2-associated lineage. Several recent animal studies indicate the role of these unique T cell subsets in promoting various autoimmune conditions mediated by pro-inflammatory cytokines like IFN-γ, IL-17. In EAE, Th9 cells have been observed in the lesion sites and IL-9 aggravated the disease severity in EAE [10]. Likewise, in colitis and myasthenia gravis IL-9 has been demonstrated to potentiate the inflammatory pathologies [5, 6, 40]. These results based on animal models indicate a critical role of Th9 cells in the pathogenesis of autoimmune diseases. However, similar reports on IL-9, particularly Th9 cells in human autoimmune conditions are limited, except a few notable very recent studies in psoriasis, colitis, and RA [5, 6, 11, 13]. Schlapbach et al. demonstrated the presence of discrete Th9 cells in the skin, of psoriasis patients, an autoimmune skin proliferative pathology involving various T effector cells. The cells could augment the inflammatory cytokine production by other T cells. Recently, Gerlach et al. identified PU.1 expressing Th9 cell in the lamina propria of ulcerative colitis patients. Ciccia et al. reported that Th9 cells are enriched in synovium of RA patients. These reports not only substantiate the presence of Th9 cells in the pathologic sites, but also suggest their crucial role in autoimmune disease in human.

RA is an autoimmune pathology affecting joints and involves Th1-associated cytokines such as IFN-γ, TNF-α, and Th17-secreted IL-17, etc. In fact, anti-TNF-α therapy in RA patients validates that indeed inflammatory cytokines are involved in the pathogenesis of RA [41]. Here, we show enrichment of Th9 cells in the SF of RA patients, which correlates with disease severity based on DAS-28 ESR scores. Moreover, we demonstrate that rIL-9 as such, but importantly, endogenously produced IL-9 in SF potentiates the differentiation of Th17 cells, as evidenced by (i) expression of signature transcription factor RORγt and increase in IL-17 producers in the SF of RA, (ii) blocking IL-9 present in SF of RA patients abrogates such effects in our experiments. We report similar impact of synovial IL-9 of RA patients on the effector T

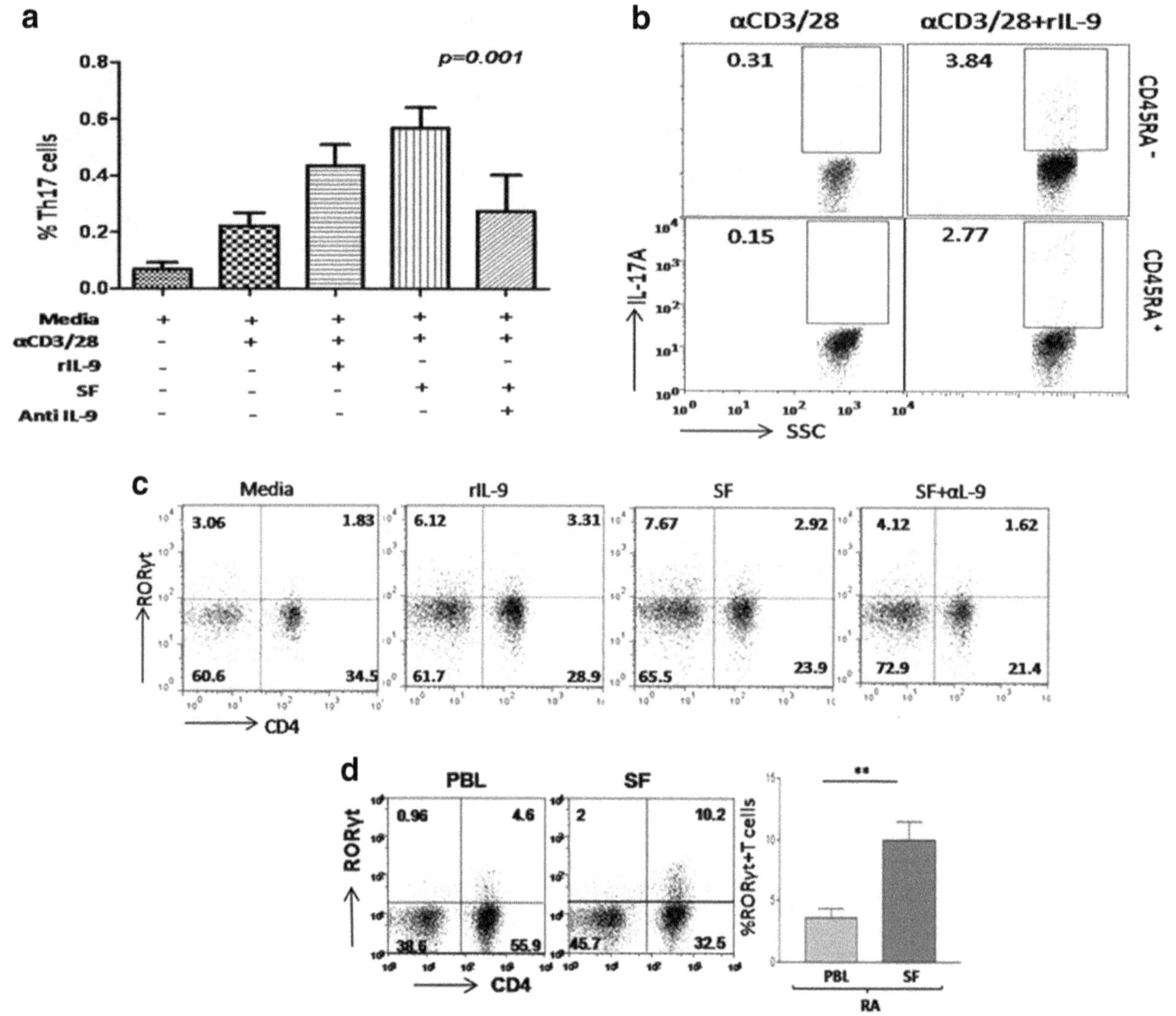

Fig. 4 IL-9 promotes differentiation of Th17 cells. **a** Bar graph shows rIL-9, RA SF can increase level of IL-17A in CD4+ (Th17) cells from healthy donor, decreased upon blocking with anti-IL-9 in RA SF (n = 6, one-way ANOVA analysis with Dunnett's multiple comparison test is applied for statistical significance, $*p < 0.05$). **b** Representative FACS dot plots show frequency of IL-17A^{+} cells in both naïve (CD4 + CD45RA^{+}) and memory (CD4 + CD45RA^{-}) T cell compartment (n = 3). **c** FACS plots show frequency of RORγt + T cells in healthy PBMCs in presence of rIL-9, RA SF, anti-(CD3 + 28). Addition of IL-9 blocking antibody in RA SF reduced the expression of RORγt (n = 5). **d** FACS plots show RORγt^{+}CD4^{+} T cells in RA PBL and RA SF, cumulative bar graph shows RORγt^{+}CD4^{+} T cells in RA PBL and SF (n = 10, unpaired *t* test, mean ± SEM, $**p < 0.005$). *IL* interleukin, *IL-9R* interleukin 9 receptor, *PBL* peripheral blood, *RA* rheumatoid arthritis, *RORγt* retineic-acid-receptor-related orphan nuclear receptor gamma t, *SF* synovial fluid, *Th* T helper

cells producing TNF-α, which is critically involved in the pathogenesis of RA [41].

In the present study, we evaluated the impact of locally enriched IL-9 in RA, and showed that SF IL-9 enhances the survival and activation of neutrophils, evidenced by reduced annexin V expression with concomitant increase of survival protein, MCL-1, and MMP-9 production. Interestingly, MCL-1 upregulation is more pronounced with autologous SF than rIL-9 indicates that other factors including IL-9 may be responsible for delayed apoptosis of neutrophils from RA SF. We demonstrate the potentiating influence of synovial IL-9 on the IL-17+ CD4 T cells derived from RA affected joints, evidenced by their increased production of IL-17(Fig. 5c), upregulation of Th17 related transcription factor expression RORγt (Fig. 4c) and phosphorylation of STAT3 with nuclear translocation (Fig. 6a, c). This is accordance with Elyaman et al., showing IL-9 induces differentiation of Th17 cells in mice [42]. In similar line recently Kundu-Raychaudhuri et al. described IL-9 as a local growth factor for T cells present in RA SF [14]. Therefore, we conclude that enrichment of Th9 cells (and IL-9) in SF facilitates two critical cellular elements involved in augmenting the joint inflammation. Here, we reveal a hitherto unknown interaction between

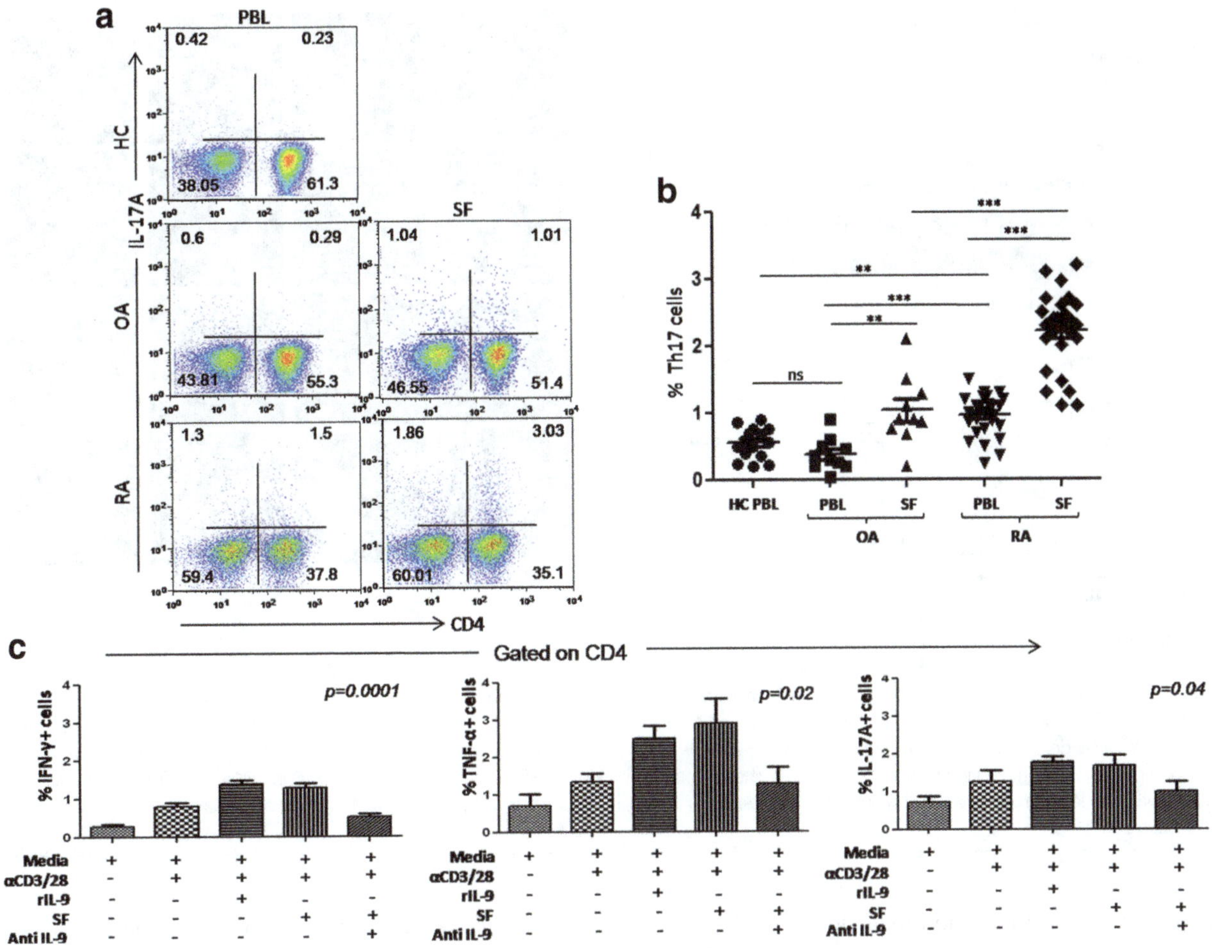

Fig. 5 IL-9 induced differentiation of Th17 and other effector T cells. **a** Representative FACS plots show Th17 cell frequency in PBL (HC, OA, RA) and SF (OA and RA).**b** Cumulative scatter plot shows frequency of Th17 (CD4 + IL-17A+) in RA (PBL and SF, n = 26), OA (PBL and SF, n = 7), HC PBL (n = 12). **c** Cumulative bar graphs show IFN-γ + ($p = 0.0001$) and TNF-α + ($p = 0.02$), IL-17A+ ($p = 0.04$) CD4+ cells were significantly higher in the presence of rIL-9 or RA SF, blocking IL-9 abrogated the same (n = 6, one-way ANOVA analysis with Dunnett's multiple comparison test is applied for statistical significance, $*p < 0.05$). *HC* healthy control, *IL-9R* interleukin 9 receptor, *IFN-γ* interferon gamma, *OA* osteoarthritis, *RA* rheumatoid arthritis, *SF* synovial fluid, *Th* T helper

Th9 cells and neutrophils, which augments joint inflammation in RA. This mechanism may contribute to autoimmune diseases in general, thus necessitating further studies in other autoimmune diseases, particularly where Th9 cells are already reported. Previously, Martin et al. reported that activated neutrophils could recruit Th17 cells, which facilitate neutrophilic infiltration driven by chemokine-receptor interaction in autoimmune diseases such as Crohn's disease and RA [33]. We demonstrate that enriched Th9 cells or IL-9 in SF of RA patients can augment neutrophils activation, survival, and Th17 cell differentiation. This is supported by recent findings of Patricia et al. showing that IL-17 activated neutrophils to kill the *Aspergillus fumigatus* in fungal keratitis [43]. We propose, that enriched Th9 cells possibly trigger and aggravate the synovial inflammation by augmenting Th17 cells and neutrophil survival and activation, thus setting the vicious circuit of their mutual enrichment and activation in the pathologic site of RA. Th9 cells (or IL-9) may be a proximal event in the inflammatory cascade of RA and probable hierarchy of IL-9 may be due to its enhancing impact of synovial T cell function and IL-17 production. Among diverse cytokines present in the SF of RA, possible hierarchy of any of them, particularly newly identified IL-9 may be important in terms of controlling the cascade of inflammation. We have also observed upregulation of rIL-9 receptor expression on IFN-γ, TNF-α, IL-17-producing CD4+ T cells from SF of RA patients (data not shown). Even rIL-9 promoted proliferation of these cytokine-producing cells from RA SF (data not shown). Moreover, enrichment of Th9 cells in the SF may be favored by various IL-1 family cytokines, abundantly present in the affected joints of RA patients [44, 45]. Novel aspects of our study are (i) functionally distinct Th9 cells are enriched in the affected joints of RA patients, (ii) endogenously produced synovial IL-9 prolongs neutrophil

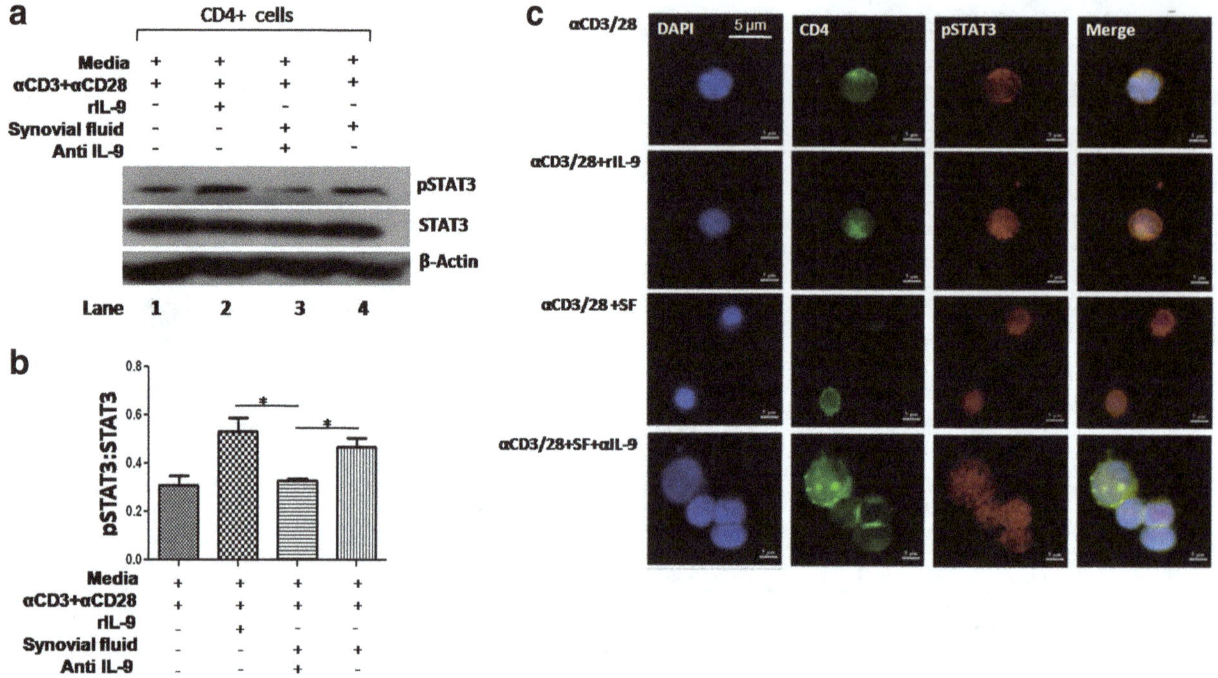

Fig. 6 IL-9 induces transcription factor for Th17 cells. **a** Representative western blot image shows phosphorylation of STAT3 (pSTAT3) in the presence of rIL-9 and SF. pSTAT3 was enhanced with rIL-9 and SF (*lane 2 and 4*) and in presence of anti-IL-9 antibody in SF reduced pSTAT3 (*lane 3*, n = 2). **b** Bar graph shows cumulative densitometry of pSTAT3 (pSTAT3:STAT3, β-actin as loading control, n = 5, unpaired *t* test, mean ± SEM, **p* < 0.05).**c** Representative confocal micrograph from two independent experiments, shows phosphorylation of pSTAT3 (*red*), nucleus (DAPI, *blue*) in CD4+ T cells (*green*) and nuclear translocation (merged image in *violet*). *IL-9R* interleukin 9 receptor, *SF* synovial fluid, *STAT3* signal transducer and activator of transcription 3, *α IL-9* anti-interleukin 9

survival, their activation, and production of MMPs to perpetuate the inflammation of the affected joints of RA, (iii) IL-9 also potentiates inflammatory cytokine producing T helper cells like Th1, Th17, and TNF-α producer (iv) synovial enrichment of Th9 cells correlates with disease severity. The importance of our finding not only lies in elucidating the Th9-mediated mechanism of inflammation in RA, but also in possible therapeutic translation, given its centrality in augmenting different arms of inflammation involving different cell lineages. Last but not the least, is the positive correlation between Th9 cells and the disease activity in RA (DAS28-ESR). This may be utilized as a disease-monitoring signature for clinical management of autoimmune diseases.

Conclusions

Overall, our findings demonstrate the relevance of Th9 cells and IL-9 in the pathogenesis of RA in human. Our results bear several translational implications in the clinical management of RA patients. First, the frequency of Th9 cells, particularly in the SF, may serve as a signature biomarker of disease severity and help monitoring patients and therapeutic response. Second, neutralizing IL-9, especially in the affected joints may inhibit the inflammatory process by suppressing the infiltrating neutrophils (survival and activation) and effector T cells (cytokine production). Third, plausible hierarchy of Th9 cells may even have wider impact on the production of pathogenic cytokines involved in autoimmune diseases including RA and may offer better control over the disease. Therefore, targeting IL-9 may be useful for treating RA patients.

Additional files

Additional file 1: Table S1. Demographic and clinical characteristics of RA patients (n = 28). (DOCX 12 kb)

Additional file 2: Figure S1. Identification and survival of synovial fluid neutrophils in presence of IL-9. Representative gating strategy for FACS plots are showing neutrophils from RA SF. Isolated neutrophils from RA SF were identified with positive staining for CD15 (*dark area* of FACS histogram, *light-shaded area* is isotype control, *right upper panel* FACS plot shows apoptosis of RA SF neutrophils at 0 hour). Apoptosis of neutrophils was measured with Annexin V staining in different culture conditions (media, SF, rIL-9 and anti-IL-9, FACS *dot plots* of *lower panel*). (TIF 360 kb)

Abbreviations

ACR: American College of Rheumatology; ANOVA: Analysis of variance; DAS28: Disease activity score of 28 joints; ELISA: Enzyme-linked immunosorbent assay; ESR: Erythrocyte sedimentation rate; FITC: Fluorescein isothiocyanate; HC: Healthy control; IFN-γ: Interferon gamma; IL: Interleukin; IL-17: Interleukin 17, IL-9R, Interleukin 9 receptor; LPS: Lipopolysaccharide; MCL-1: Induced myeloid leukemia cell differentiation protein; MMP-9: Matrix metalloproteinase-9; OA: Osteoarthritis; PBL: Peripheral blood; PBMC: Peripheral blood mononuclear cell; PBS: Phosphate-buffered saline;

PE: Phycoerythrin; PE-Cy5: Phycoerythrin tandem conjugate with cyanine; RA: Rheumatoid arthritis; RIPA: Radioimmunoprecipitation assay; RORγt: Retineic-acid-receptor-related orphan nuclear receptor gamma t; SF: Synovial fluid; SFMC: Synovial fluid mononuclear cell; STAT3: Signal transducer and activator of transcription 3; Th: T helper; TNF-α: Tumor necrosis factor alpha; α IL-9: Anti-interleukin 9

Acknowledgements
The authors thank all the patients and healthy subjects who participated in this study. The authors are also thankful to Drs. Ankit Saxena, Anupam Mitra, Ambak Rai, and Amar Singh for critical suggestions. The authors thankfully acknowledge the support of Ms. Manju Namdeo, Ms. Soumi Sadhu, and Mr. Abhinav Saurabh for helpful discussions. This work was funded by the Department of Science and Technology, Ministry of Science and Technology, Government of India (Grant No. SR/SO/SH-0159/2010).

Funding
The work was supported by the Department of Science and Technology, Government of India, (SR/SO/SH-0159/2010).

Authors' contributions
DKM along with KC conceptualized, designed experiments and wrote the manuscript. UK, SD, PG, and GS diagnosed and treated the recruited subjects, provided clinical details and specimens for the study. KC and PK performed experiments and data analysis. UK contributed in data analysis and manuscript editing. SB and JC helped in western blot studies with their expertise. All authors read and approved the final manuscript.

Competing interests
All authors declare that they do not have any competing interests.

Author details
[1]Department of Transplant Immunology and Immunogenetics, All India Institute of Medical Sciences (AIIMS), Room No-75, New Delhi 110029, India. [2]Department of Medicine, All India Institute of Medical Sciences (AIIMS), New Delhi, India. [3]Rheumatology Center, Institute of Post Graduate Medical Education and Research (IPGMER), Kolkata, India. [4]Indian Institute of Chemical Biology, Council of Scientific and Industrial Research (CSIR), Kolkata, India.

References

1. Pang N, Zhang F, Ma X, Zhang Z, Zhao H, Xin Y, Wang S, Zhu Y, Wen H, Ding J. Th9/IL-9 profile in human echinococcosis: their involvement in immune response during infection by Echinococcus granulosus. Mediators Inflamm. 2014;2014:781649.
2. Ye ZJ, Yuan M, Zhou Q, Du RH, Yang WB, Xiong XZ, Zhang JC, Wu C, Qin SM, Shi HZ. Differentiation and recruitment of Th9 cells stimulated by pleural mesothelial cells in human Mycobacterium tuberculosis infection. PLoS One. 2012;7(2):e31710.
3. Lu Y, Hong S, Li H, Park J, Hong B, Wang L, Zheng Y, Liu Z, Xu J, He J, Yang J, et al. Th9 cells promote antitumor immune responses in vivo. J Clin Invest. 2012;122(11):1558–8238.
4. Deng Y, Wang Z, Chang C, Lu L, Lau CS, Lu Q. Th9 cells and IL-9 in autoimmune disorders: Pathogenesis and therapeutic potentials. Hum Immunol. 2017;78(2):120–28.
5. Nalleweg N, Chiriac MT, Podstawa E, Lehmann C, Rau TT, Atreya R, Krauss E, Hundorfean G, Fichtner-Feigl S, Hartmann A, et al. IL-9 and its receptor are predominantly involved in the pathogenesis of UC. Gut. 2015;64(5):743–55.
6. Gerlach K, Hwang Y, Nikolaev A, Atreya R, Dornhoff H, Steiner S, Lehr HA, Wirtz S, Vieth M, Waisman A, et al. TH9 cells that express the transcription factor PU.1 drive T cell-mediated colitis via IL-9 receptor signaling in intestinal epithelial cells. Nat Immunol. 2014;15(7):676–86.
7. Xu H, Rizzo LV, Silver PB, Caspi RR. Uveitogenicity is associated with a Th1-like lymphokine profile: cytokine-dependent modulation of early and committed effector T cells in experimental autoimmune uveitis. Cell Immunol. 1997;178(1):69–78.
8. Li H, Nourbakhsh B, Ciric B, Zhang GX, Rostami A. Neutralization of IL-9 ameliorates experimental autoimmune encephalomyelitis by decreasing the effector T cell population. J Immunol. 2010;185(7):4095–100.
9. Li H, Nourbakhsh B, Cullimore M, Zhang GX, Rostami A. IL-9 is important for T-cell activation and differentiation in autoimmune inflammation of the central nervous system. Eur J Immunol. 2011;41(8):2197–206.
10. Jager A, Dardalhon V, Sobel RA, Bettelli E, Kuchroo VK. Th1, Th17, and Th9 effector cells induce experimental autoimmune encephalomyelitis with different pathological phenotypes. J Immunol. 2009;183(11):7169–77.
11. Schlapbach C, Gehad AYC, Watanabe R, Guenova E, Teague JE, Campbell L, Yawalkar N, Kupper TS, Clark RA. Human TH9 cells are skin-tropic and have autocrine and paracrine proinflammatory capacity. Sci Transl Med. 2014;6:219ra8.
12. Ouyang H, Shi Y, Liu Z, Feng S, Li L, Su N, Lu Y, Kong S. Increased interleukin9 and CD4 + IL-9+ T cells in patients with systemic lupus erythematosus. Mol Med Rep. 2013;7(3):1031–7.
13. Ciccia F, Guggino G, Rizzo A, Manzo A, Vitolo B, La Manna MP, Giardina G, Sireci G, Dieli F, Montecucco CM, et al. Potential involvement of IL-9 and Th9 cells in the pathogenesis of rheumatoid arthritis. Rheumatology (Oxford). 2015;54(12):2264–72.
14. Kundu-Raychaudhuri S, Abria C, Raychaudhuri SP. IL-9, a local growth factor for synovial T cells in inflammatory arthritis. Cytokine. 2016;79:45–51.
15. Zhou M, Qin S, Chu Y, Wang F, Chen L, Lu Y. Immunolocalization of MMP-2 and MMP-9 in human rheumatoid synovium. Int J Clin Exp Pathol. 2014;7(6):3048–56.
16. Lundy SK, Sarkar S, Tesmer LA, Fox DA. Cells of the synovium in rheumatoid arthritis. T lymphocytes Arthritis Res Ther. 2007;9(1):202.
17. Zhang X, Burch E, Cai L, So E, Hubbard F, Matteson EL, Strome SE. CD40 mediates downregulation of CD32B on specific memory B cell populations in rheumatoid arthritis. J Immunol. 2013;190(12):6015–22.
18. Doorenspleet ME, Klarenbeek PI, de Hair MJH, van Schaik BDC, Esveldt REE, van Kampen AHC, Gerlag DM, Musters A, Baas F, Tak PP, de Vries N, et al. Rheumatoid arthritis synovial tissue harbours dominant B-cell and plasma-cell clones associated with autoreactivity. Ann Rheum Dis. 2014;73(4):756–2.
19. Bluml S, McKeever K, Ettinger R, Smolen J, Herbst R. B-cell targeted therapeutics in clinical development. Arthritis Res Ther. 2013;15 Suppl 1:S4.
20. Wright HL, Moots RJ, Edwards SW. The multifactorial role of neutrophils in rheumatoid arthritis. Nat Rev Rheumatol. 2014;10:593–601.
21. Edwards SW, Hallett MB. Seeing the wood for the trees: the forgotten role of neutrophils in rheumatoid arthritis. Immunol Today. 1997;18(7):320–4.
22. Mur E, Zabernigg A, Hilbe W, Eisterer W, Halder W, Thaler J. Oxidative burst of neutrophils in patients with rheumatoid arthritis: influence of various cytokines and medication. Clin Exp Rheumatol. 1997;15(3):233–7.
23. Yamada H, Nakashima Y, Okazaki K, Mawatari T, Fukushi JI, Oyamada A, Fujimura K, Iwamoto Y, Yoshikai Y. Preferential accumulation of activated Th1 cells not only in rheumatoid arthritis but also in osteoarthritis joints. J Rheumatol. 2011;38(8):1569–75.
24. Li S, Niu X, Xi Y, Deng S, Li C, Zhao Q, Chen G. T cell vaccination inhibits Th1/Th17/Tfh frequencies and production of autoantibodies in collagen-induced arthritis. Clin Dev Immunol. 2013;2013:967301.
25. Shahrara S, Huang Q, Mandelin 2nd AM, Pope RM. TH-17 cells in rheumatoid arthritis. Arthritis Res Ther. 2008;10(4):R93.
26. van Hamburg JP, Asmawidjaja PS, Davelaar N, Mus AMC, Colin EM, Hazes JMW, Dolhain RJEM, Lubberts E. Th17 cells, but not Th1 cells, from patients with early rheumatoid arthritis are potent inducers of matrix metalloproteinases and proinflammatory cytokines upon synovial fibroblast interaction, including autocrine interleukin-17A production. Arthritis Rheum. 2011;63(1):73–83.
27. Chiang EY, Kolumam GA, Yu X, Francesco M, Ivelja S, Peng I, Gribling P, Shu J, Lee WP, Refino CJ, Balazs M, et al. Targeted depletion of lymphotoxin-alpha-expressing TH1 and TH17 cells inhibits autoimmune disease. Nat Med. 2009;15(7):766–73.
28. Li G, Zhang Y, Qian Y, Zhang H, Guo S, Sunagawa M, Hisamitsu T, Liu Y. Interleukin-17A promotes rheumatoid arthritis synoviocytes migration and invasion under hypoxia by increasing MMP2 and MMP9 expression through NF-kappaB/HIF-1alpha pathway. Mol Immunol. 2013;53(3):227–36.
29. Li G, Zhang Y, Qian Y, Zhang H, Guo S, Sunagawa M, Hisamitsu T, Liu Y. Interleukin-17A promotes rheumatoid arthritis synoviocytes migration and invasion under hypoxia by increasing MMP2 and MMP9 expression through NF-kappaB/HIF-1alpha pathway. J Leukoc Biol. 2006;79(1):214–22.
30. Roeleveld DM, van Nieuwenhuijze AE, van den Berg WB, Koenders MI. The Th17 pathway as a therapeutic target in rheumatoid arthritis and other autoimmune and inflammatory disorders. Bio Drugs. 2013;27(5):439–52.

31. Arnett FC, Edworthy SM, Bloch DA, McShane DJ, Fries JF, Cooper NS, Healey LA, Kaplan SR, Liang MH, Luthra HS, et al. The American Rheumatism Association 1987 revised criteria for the classification of rheumatoid arthritis. Arthritis Rheum. 1988;31(3):315–24.
32. Zhu X, Xiao L, Huo R, Zhang J, Lin J, Xie J, Sun S, He Y, Sun Y, Zhou Z, Shen B, et al. Cyr61 is involved in neutrophil infiltration in joints by inducing IL-8 production by fibroblast-like synoviocytes in rheumatoid arthritis. Arthritis Res Ther. 2013;15(6):R187.
33. Pelletier M, Maggi L, Micheletti A, Lazzeri E, Tamassia N, Costantini C, Cosmi L, Lunardi C, Annunziato F, Romagnani S, Cassatella MA, et al. Evidence for a cross-talk between human neutrophils and Th17 cells. Blood. 2010;115(2):335–43.
34. Wright HL, Moots RJ, Bucknall RC, Edwards SW. Neutrophil function in inflammation and inflammatory diseases. Rheumatology (Oxford). 2010; 49(9):1618–31.
35. Gruber BL, Sorbi D, French DL, Marchese MJ, Nuovo GJ, Kew RR, Arbeit LA. Markedly elevated serum MMP-9 (gelatinase B) levels in rheumatoid arthritis: a potentially useful laboratory marker. Clin Immunol Immunopathol. 1996;78(2):161–71.
36. McInnes IB, Schett G. Cytokines in the pathogenesis of rheumatoid arthritis. Nat Rev Immunol. 2007;7(6):429–42.
37. Xing J, Wu Y, Ni B. Th9: a new player in asthma pathogenesis? J Asthma. 2011;48(2):115–25.
38. Soroosh P, Doherty TA. Th9 and allergic disease. Immunology. 2009; 127(4):450–8.
39. Chang HC, Sehra S, Goswami R, Yao W, Yu Q, Stritesky GL, Jabeen R, McKinley C, Ahyi AN, Han L, Nguyen ET, et al. The transcription factor PU.1 is required for the development of IL-9-producing T cells and allergic inflammation. Nat Immunol. 2010;11(6):527–34.
40. Yao X, Kong Q, Xie X, Wang J, Li N, Liu Y, Sun B, Li Y, Wang G, Li W, Qu S, et al. Neutralization of interleukin-9 ameliorates symptoms of experimental autoimmune myasthenia gravis in rats by decreasing effector T cells and altering humoral responses. Immunology. 2014;143(3):396–405.
41. Meroni PL, Valesini G. Tumour necrosis factor alpha antagonists in the treatment of rheumatoid arthritis: an immunological perspective. Bio Drugs. 2014;Suppl 1:S5–13.
42. Elyaman W, Bradshaw EM, Uyttenhove C, Uyttenhove C, Dardalhon V, Awasthi A, Imitola J, Bettelli E, Oukka M, van Snick J, Renauld JC, Kuchroo VK, Khoury SJ. IL-9 induces differentiation of TH17 cells and enhances function of FoxP3+ natural regulatory T cells. Proc Natl Acad Sci U S A. 2009;106(31):12885–90.
43. Taylor PR, Roy S, Leal Jr SM, Sun Y, Howell SJ, Cobb BA, Li X, Pearlman E. Activation of neutrophils by autocrine IL-17A-IL-17RC interactions during fungal infection is regulated by IL-6, IL-23, RORgammat and dectin-2. Nat Immunol. 2014;15(2):143–51.
44. Kay J, Calabrese L. The role of interleukin-1 in the pathogenesis of rheumatoid arthritis. Rheumatology (Oxford). 2004;43 Suppl 3:iii2–9.
45. Kaplan MH. Th9 cells: differentiation and disease. Immunol Rev. 2013;252(1):104–15.

6

Sirukumab in rheumatoid arthritis refractory to sulfasalazine or methotrexate: a randomized phase 3 safety and efficacy study in Japanese patients

Tsutomu Takeuchi[1], Hisashi Yamanaka[2], Masayoshi Harigai[2], Ryo Tamamura[3], Yuichi Kato[3], Yoshifumi Ukyo[3], Toshikazu Nakano[3], Benjamin Hsu[4*] and Yoshiya Tanaka[5]

Abstract

Background: Sirukumab, a high-affinity human monoclonal antibody that selectively binds to interleukin-6, has demonstrated efficacy in the treatment of rheumatoid arthritis (RA) in global phase 1 and phase 2 studies. The present study evaluated the safety and efficacy of sirukumab, as monotherapy in Japanese patients with RA refractory to methotrexate or sulfasalazine.

Methods: In this phase 3, double-blind study, 122 patients (age ≥ 20 years) were randomized (1:1, 61 patients in each arm) to sirukumab administered subcutaneously: 50 mg once every 4 weeks (q4w) or 100 mg once every 2 weeks (q2w) through 52 weeks. Disease-modifying anti-rheumatic drugs were allowed after 24 weeks. Safety was assessed and efficacy was evaluated using American College of Rheumatology (ACR) responses, Disease Activity Score C-reactive protein (DAS28-CRP) and Health Assessment Questionnaire-Disability Index (HAQ-DI).

Results: Amongst the 122 randomized patients, 99 (81.1%) patients completed the study. Adverse events (AEs) were reported in 114/122 (93.4%) patients and serious AEs were reported in 9/122 (7.4%) patients. No deaths, major cardiovascular AEs, serious gastrointestinal perforations or tuberculosis cases were reported during this study period. Grade 3 hematologic abnormalities (neutropenia and leukopenia) were reported in seven patients and no grade 4 abnormalities were observed. ACR20 responses were observed within 2 weeks, achieved in 47/61 (77.0%, 50 mg q4w) patients and 44/61 (72.1%, 100 mg q2w) patients at week 16 and maintained through week 52. ACR50/70, DAS28-CRP and HAQ-DI responses were also maintained through week 52 in both groups.

Conclusions: Safety findings were comparable between the two treatment groups. The 52-week administration of sirukumab at 50 mg q4w and 100 mg q2w was generally tolerable and with measurable efficacy in Japanese patients with RA refractory to methotrexate and sulfasalazine.

Keywords: Biologicals, Disease-modifying anti-rheumatic drugs, Interleukin-6, Rheumatoid arthritis, Sirukumab

* Correspondence: bhsu@its.jnj.com
[4]Janssen Research & Development, LLC, Spring House, PA, USA
Full list of author information is available at the end of the article

Background

Newer treatment options have been introduced for rheumatoid arthritis (RA) in the past decades and anti-tumor necrosis factor (TNF) alpha agents have been well established as the first-line biologic agent of choice [1]. Although these agents have been used successfully in patients who had failed methotrexate (MTX) therapy, unresponsiveness and tolerability concerns have limited their use. Therefore, there exists an unmet need for newer therapeutic options that will safely alleviate the signs and symptoms of RA in patients who are nonresponsive to anti-TNF agents [2].

Interleukin (IL)-6, a key player in the development of RA, is found at elevated levels in the serum and synovial fluid of RA patients [3]. Currently, tocilizumab and sarilumab, humanized antibodies targeting the IL-6 receptor, are the only approved anti-IL-6 therapy for RA [4–6]. Sirukumab, an anti-IL-6 monoclonal antibody, binds selectively to IL-6 ligand with high affinity. In a phase 1 study, sirukumab demonstrated an acceptable safety and pharmacokinetic profile when administered intravenously (0.3–10 mg/kg) [7]. In a proof-of-concept phase 2 study, sirukumab administered subcutaneously (100 mg once in every 2 weeks) in combination with MTX demonstrated marked improvement (American College of Rheumatology 50 response [ACR50, ≥50% improvement] in 26.7% of patients at week 12) in patients with RA [8].

Patients with moderate to severe active RA refractory to MTX or sulfasalazine (SSZ) have a high unmet need and require strong immunomodulatory therapy to prevent further disease damage and morbidity. Additionally, optional therapies are needed in patients unable to tolerate disease-modifying anti-rheumatic drugs (DMARDs) such as MTX or SSZ due to toxicities such as liver functional failure [9, 10]. In a global phase 3 study (SIRROUND-D) conducted in active RA patients refractory to DMARDs (including MTX or SSZ), sirukumab showed significant improvements in RA symptoms along with inhibition of structural damage progression and improvements in quality of life [11]. Similar results were observed in another global 52-week phase 3 study in patients refractory or intolerant to anti-TNF therapies and other biological treatments (SIRROUND-T) [12]. Thus, sirukumab has demonstrated promise as a clinically efficacious therapy for RA treatment [13].

The current double-blind, randomized, phase 3 study was planned to evaluate the safety and efficacy of sirukumab monotherapy in Japanese patients with RA refractory to MTX or SSZ treatment. This is the first study to evaluate the benefits of sirukumab monotherapy in Japanese patients with active RA refractory to MTX or SSZ.

Methods

Patients

Japanese patients, age ≥ 20 years, diagnosed with RA (according to the revised 1987 criteria of the American Rheumatism Association) for ≥3 months before screening and unresponsive to MTX or SSZ, alone or in combination with other conventional synthetic disease -modifying anti-rheumatic drugs (csDMARDs), were enrolled. Patients with moderate to severely active RA with at least 6 of 68 tender joints and 6 of 66 swollen joints; positive for either rheumatoid factor or anti-cyclic citrullinated peptide or with baseline radiographic erosion; CRP level ≥ 0.8 mg/dl; and if using oral corticosteroids on a stable dose equivalent to ≤ 10 mg/day of prednisolone or on a stable dose of nonsteroidal anti-inflammatory drugs (NSAIDs) or analgesics for 2 weeks before first administration of sirukumab were included.

Patients with prior intolerance or inadequate response to biologic (b)DMARDs such as anti-TNF therapy or tocilizumab within 3 months of therapy, rituximab (other B-cell depleting therapy) within 7 months of therapy or prior sirukumab use were excluded from the study. Previous treatment with bDMARDs with discontinuation for other reasons (e.g., accessibility, inconvenience) was permitted. Other exclusion criteria were: patients who had received corticosteroids via intraarticular, intramuscular or intravenous route within 4 weeks prior to the first sirukumab administration; leflunomide in the past 24 months without any drug elimination procedure; cyclosporine A, azathioprine, tacrolimus, mycophenolate mofetil, oral or parenteral gold, or D-penicillamine within 4 weeks of sirukumab administration; and patients with uncontrolled or severe inflammatory disorders other than RA, hypersensitivity or intolerance to sirukumab, severe infections requiring hospitalization and chronic or recurring infectious disease.

The study protocol was approved by the institutional review board (Keio University Hospital) of the lead investigator (TT) and by the institutional review boards of each of the 20 other participating study sites. The study was conducted in accordance with the Declaration of Helsinki consistent with Good Clinical Practices and applicable regulatory requirements. All participants provided written informed consent.

Study design, randomization and blinding

This phase 3, randomized, double-blind study, was conducted across 21 sites in Japan from October 2012 to March 2015. The study comprised three phases: screening phase (6 weeks), double-blind treatment phase (52 weeks) and posttreatment safety follow-up phase (16 weeks). After screening, the patients were randomized 1:1 to either sirukumab 50 mg every 4 weeks (50 mg q4w group) or sirukumab 100 mg every 2 weeks (100 mg q2w group) administered subcutaneously through week 52. Due to ethical considerations, a placebo group was not included. The two dose regimens were efficacious in the phase 2 study and were being evaluated in this and several phase 3 studies for a possible dose response. Placebo was administered at week 2 and thereafter every 4 weeks through week 52 to the 50 mg q4w group to maintain treatment blinding. Sirukumab (50 mg/1 ml or 100 mg/1 ml) or its placebo was supplied in a 1-ml prefilled syringe. The randomization was performed using a computer-generated randomization schedule and implemented using an interactive voice or web response system. Both patients and investigators were blinded until the safety follow-up was completed and the database finalized. Adjustment in NSAID or analgesic dosage was disallowed 2 weeks prior to first drug administration until week 16 of treatment. Patients with < 20% improvement in swollen or tender joints were allowed to initiate or adjust corticosteroid dosages at the investigator's discretion from week 16 onward. Patients using csDMARDs at enrollment had to discontinue use 4 weeks prior to randomization and concomitant csDMARDS were not allowed until 24 weeks of sirukumab administration. From week 24 through week 52, patients with < 20% improvement from baseline in swollen and tender joints were allowed to take csDMARDs based on the investigator's discretion (Fig. 1).

Safety assessments

Safety (primary objective) was assessed by monitoring AEs, clinical laboratory tests, physical examinations, vital signs and chest X-ray scans for tuberculosis detection. The toxicity grade of clinical laboratory parameters was assessed by Common Terminology Criteria for Adverse Events (CTCAE) grading. The AEs were recorded by the patient's voluntary reporting or their interview in an indirect manner at every visit. All serious AEs (SAEs), serious cardiovascular events, malignancies, infections such as tuberculosis, gastrointestinal perforations and clinical laboratory parameter abnormalities (hematologic, hepatobiliary and lipids) were monitored. Blood samples for clinical laboratory assessments were collected at baseline and weeks 2, 4, 6, 8, 12, 16, 18, 20, 24, 36, 44 and 52.

Efficacy assessments

Efficacy variables included ACR responses and the Disease Activity Score using DAS28-CRP (responder, DAS28-CRP ≤ 3.2 to 5.1 at visit with 0.6 to > 1.2 improvement from baseline; remission, DAS28-CRP < 2.6). Major clinical response was achieved if the ACR70 response was sustained for 6 months. Improvements in disease activity were assessed by Simplified Disease Activity Index (SDAI) and Clinical Disease Activity Index (CDAI) responses. Treatment failures included patients who started treatment with csDMARDs, systemic immunosuppressives (e.g., leflunomide) and/or bDMARDs or required additional treatment or increased dose of oral corticosteroids, intravenous/intramuscular administration of corticosteroids, or discontinued sirukumab for any reason through week 52.

Additionally, physical function was assessed by the Health Assessment Questionnaire-Disability Index (HAQ-DI). Efficacy variables were assessed every 2 weeks from week 0

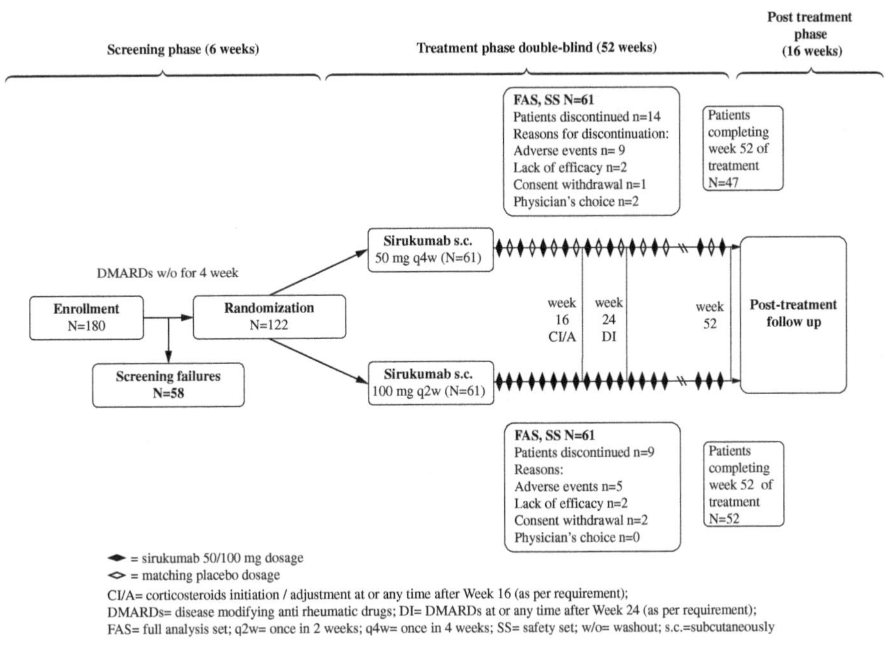

Fig. 1 Study design and patient disposition

to 8, and thereafter every 4 weeks through week 52. Efficacy was also assessed up to 16 weeks in the posttreatment follow-up phase to analyze the effect of concomitant medication.

Immunogenicity assessment

Immunogenicity was assessed from blood samples using a validated drug-tolerant enzyme immunoassay (EIA) at weeks 0, 24 and 52 and final safety follow-up visit (week 68).

Statistical analysis

As per the Japanese regulatory authorities, ≥ 100 patients are recommended to be exposed to the study drug for 1 year to obtain the necessary safety data. Considering the number of Japanese patients in the other global studies of sirukumab, ≥ 40 patients per treatment group were required in this study. Additionally, assuming that about 70% of patients would complete 1 year of treatment as in a study of similar design [14], a minimum enrollment of 120 patients (60 per treatment group) was required.

The safety analysis set included patients who received ≥ 1 dose of sirukumab. The efficacy full analysis set included all patients randomized to the study. Data imputation by the nonresponder imputation (NRI) or the last observation carried forward (LOCF) method was used for categorical and continuous efficacy parameters, respectively. The treatment failure rule was applied to data for posttreatment efficacy analysis. No comparative statistical tests were performed. Descriptive statistics were provided for safety and efficacy parameters (mean and median values of data are provided based on parameter and data distribution).

Results

Patient disposition and characteristics

Of the 180 patients enrolled, 122 patients (50 mg q4w group, N = 61; 100 mg q2w group, N = 61) were randomized, treated and included in the safety and efficacy analysis. Among these, 99 (81.1%) patients completed the study, with the most common reason for study discontinuation being AEs (50 mg q4w group, 9/61 (14.8%) patients; 100 mg q2w group, 5/61 (8.2%) patients) (Fig. 1, Table 2); however, there was no specific trend in these AEs.

The baseline characteristics and demographics between both treatment groups were well balanced. The majority of patients were women (90/122 (73.8%)) with mean (SD) age of 55.1 (11.41) years and body mass index (BMI) 22.3 (3.58) kg/m^2, and the median (range) duration of RA was 5.77 (0.4–41.0) years (Table 1). The baseline RA characteristics for ACR components were

Table 1 Patient demographics and baseline characteristics (efficacy full analysis set)

Characteristic	Sirukumab 50 mg q4w (N = 61)	Sirukumab 100 mg q2w (N = 61)	All (N = 122)
Sex (women), n (%)	47.0 (77.0)	43.0 (70.5)	90 (73.8)
Age (years), mean (SD)	55.4 (10.70)	54.7 (12.16)	55.1 (11.41)
Weight (kg), mean (SD)	55.0 (12.23)	56.8 (9.71)	55.9 (11.03)
Height (cm), mean (SD)	157.9 (7.90)	158.4 (7.80)	158.1 (7.82)
BMI (kg/m^2), mean (SD)	22.0 (3.98)	22.6 (3.13)	22.3 (3.58)
Disease duration (years), median (range)	5.0 (0.4–41.0)	6.3 (0.4–30.0)	5.8 (0.4–41.0)
Swollen joints (number 0–66), median (range)	11.0 (6.0–22.0)	11.0 (5.0–32.0)	11.0 (5.0–32.0)
Tender joints (number 0–68), median (range)	14.0 (6.0–56.0)	15.0 (5.0–48.0)	14.0 (5.0–56.0)
Patient's assessment of pain (VAS; 0–10 cm), median (range)	7.4 (0.7–10.0)	7.4 (0.5–10.0)	7.4 (0.5–10.0)
Patient's global assessment of disease activity (VAS; 0–10 cm), median (range)	7.6 (0.6–10.0)	7.1 (0.6–10.0)	7.5 (0.6–10.0)
Physician's global assessment of disease activity (VAS; 0–10 cm), median (range)	6.5 (2.6–10.0)	6.9 (2.0–10.0)	6.6 (2.0–10.0)
HAQ-DI score (0–3), median (range)	1.4 (0.00–2.75)	1.1 (0.00–2.75)	1.3 (0.00–2.75)
CRP (mg/dl), median (range)	2.7 (0.20– 9.20)	2.5 (0.31–16.60)	2.6 (0.20–16.60)
DAS28-CRP score, median (range)	5.6 (5.14–6.11)	5.9 (4.88–6.57)	5.7 (4.93–6.29)
SDAI score, median (range)	33.2 (28.42–40.38)	38.2 (26.83–52.20)	34.7 (27.70–42.48)
CDAI score, median (range)	30.9 (24.90–37.80)	33.5 (24.20–47.40)	31.8 (24.60–38.80)
Rheumatoid factor-positive, n (%)	48 (78.7)	44 (72.1)	92 (75.4)
Anti-CCP antibody positive, n (%)	55 (90.2)	51 (83.6)	106 (86.9)

BMI body mass index, *CCP* cyclic citrullinated peptide, *CDAI* Clinical Disease Activity Index, *CRP* C-reactive protein, *HAQ-DI* Health Assessment Questionnaire-Disability Index, *q4w* once in 4 weeks, *q2w* once in 2 weeks, *SDAI* Simplified Disease Activity Index, *SD* standard deviation, *VAS* visual analog scale

also balanced with median (range) CRP levels being 2.6 (0.2–16.6) mg/dl. The proportions of patients exposed to prior treatments include ≥ 1 DMARD 100%, ≥ 2 DMARDs 60.7%, MTX 97.5%, SSZ 36.1% and biologics other than sirukumab 19.7% (14 patients (23.0%) in 50 mg q4w group and 10 patients (16.4%) in 100 mg q2w group). The study excluded patients with previous intolerance or inadequate response to tumor necrosis factor (TNF) inhibitor or tocilizumab (anti-IL-6 receptor) therapy and use of B-cell depleting therapy within the previous 7 months. The median sirukumab treatment duration and treatment administrations were 52.14 weeks and 27, respectively. Only three patients (2/61 patients in 50 mg q4w group and 1/61 patient in 100 mg q2w group) initiated DMARDs for minimal improvement in swollen and tender joints at or any time after week 24.

Safety

Adverse events

Of the 122 patients in the safety set, 114 (93.4%) patients experienced ≥ 1 AE and this was comparable between the two treatment groups (50 mg q4w group, 56/61 (91.8%) patients; 100 mg q2w group, 58/61 (95.1%) patients). The most common AEs were nasopharyngitis, injection-site erythema and injection-site swelling (Table 2). Among AEs of special interest, infections were observed in 77/122 (63.1%) patients and injection-site reactions were observed in 47/122 (38.5%) patients.

Serious adverse events

Overall, 9/122 (7.4%) patients had ≥ 1 SAE (50 mg q4w group, 4/61 (6.6%) patients; 100 mg q2w group, 5/61 (8.2%) patients) (Table 2). Serious infections of sinusitis and hepatitis E (one patient each in 100 mg q2w group, 2/61 (3.3%)) and osteomyelitis (50 mg q4w group, 1/61 (1.6%) patient) were observed. Gastrointestinal disorders occurred in one patient each in both groups. Comminuted fracture and schizophrenia (one patient each) were reported in the 50 mg q4w group whereas endometriosis with borderline serous ovary tumor and intervertebral disc protrusion (one patient each) was reported in the 100 mg q2w group. No major cardiovascular events, tuberculosis or gastrointestinal perforations were observed (Table 2). After completion of the posttreatment follow-up period, one patient reported myocardial infarction but the patient recovered from the event. No deaths were observed during the 52-week study treatment.

Hematology and clinical laboratory values

Patients who had grade 0 hematology laboratory values at baseline reported shifts to grade 3 events through week 52 with respect to decreased neutrophils (50 mg q4w group, 3/61 patients; 100 mg q2w group, 2/61 patients) and decreased leukocytes (100 mg q2w group, 2/61 patients) (Table 3). A grade 4 event of decreased platelets (100 mg q2w group, 1/61 patient) was also reported but was considered a technical error, and no events of associated bleeding were reported. Occurrence of severe infection was not observed in patients with grade 3 neutropenia.

Hepatobiliary parameters (aspartate transaminase (AST), alanine transaminase (ALT) and bilirubin) that were grade 0 at baseline did not demonstrate grade 3 or 4 shifts through week 52. Few events of grade 2 shifts (0 at baseline) in ALT (n = 3) and AST (n = 1) were observed, which returned to normal at week 52. In all, seven patients had a grade 2 shift in bilirubin but without any associated increases in ALT or AST. The majority of lipid abnormalities (increased serum triglyceride and cholesterol) were grade 1 or 2 in severity. A grade 3 serum triglyceride increase was observed in two patients (1.7%) and the values remained high even at week 52 (Table 3). Overall, there was no dose-dependent effect on the safety profile of sirukumab with respect to clinical laboratory parameters.

Efficacy

The ACR20/50/70 responses at week 16 were achieved in 77.0%, 47.5% and 26.2% of patients in the 50 mg q4w group and in 72.1%, 57.4% and 32.8% of patients in the 100 mg q2w group, and were maintained through week 52 (Table 4). ACR50/70 responses in the 100 mg q2w group were numerically higher versus the 50 mg q4w group. Major clinical response was achieved by 23/122 (18.9%) patients (50 mg q4w group, 8/61 (13.1%) patients; 100 mg q2w group, 15/61 (24.6%) patients). Overall, subgroup analysis demonstrated that demographics, baseline disease characteristics and medication use did not have any effect on achieving ACR20 at week 16. ACR20 in patients with prior biologic use was 10/17 (58.8%) patients in the 50 mg q4w group and 11/13 (84.6%) patients in the 100 mg q2w group at week 52.

Improvements in HAQ-DI were observed early in the study (50 mg q4w group, week 2; 100 mg q2w group, week 4). The HAQ-DI response (decrease in score ≥ 0.22) was observed in 75.4% patients (50 mg q4w group) and 67.2% patients (100 mg q2w group) at week 16 and the response rates were maintained through week 52 (Table 4). The CRP concentration was almost undetectable from week 16 through week 52. The maximum DAS28-CRP responders were observed at week 4 (58/61 (95.1%) patients in each group), which decreased slightly to 45/61 (73.8%) responders in the 50 mg q4w group and 50/61 (81.9%) responders in the 100 mg q2w group at week 52 (Table 4). The percentage of patients achieving DAS28-CRP remission (< 2.6) increased over time and maximum remission rates were achieved at week 24 (50 mg q4w group, 30/61 (49.2%) patients; 100 mg q2w group, 36/61 (59.0%) patients) and were generally

Table 2 Summary of adverse events through week 52 (safety analysis set)

	Sirukumab 50 mg q4w (*N* = 61)	Sirukumab 100 mg q2w (*N* = 61)	All (*N* = 122)
AEs	56 (91.8)	58 (95.1)	114 (93.4)
Serious AEs	4 (6.6)	5 (8.2)	9 (7.4)
AEs in ≥ 10% patients			
Infections and infestations	39 (63.9)	38 (62.3)	77 (63.1)
Nasopharyngitis	27 (44.3)	27 (44.3)	54 (44.3)
Pharyngitis	6 (9.8)	7 (11.5)	13 (10.7)
General disorders and administration site conditions	26 (42.6)	27 (44.3)	53 (43.4)
Injection-site erythema	19 (31.1)	20 (32.8)	39 (32.0)
Injection-site swelling	10 (16.4)	12 (19.7)	22 (18.0)
Injection-site pruritus	7 (11.5)	13 (21.3)	20 (16.4)
Investigations	28 (45.9)	21 (34.4)	49 (40.2)
Alanine aminotransferase increased	10 (16.4)	10 (16.4)	20 (16.4)
Aspartate aminotransferase increased	9 (14.8)	11 (18.0)	20 (16.4)
White blood cell count decreased	7 (11.5)	7 (11.5)	14 (11.5)
Platelet count decreased	9 (14.8)	3 (4.9)	12 (9.8)
Neutrophil count decreased	7 (11.5)	4 (6.6)	11 (9.0)
Skin and subcutaneous tissue disorders	15 (24.6)	25 (41.0)	40 (32.8)
Eczema	7 (11.5)	7 (11.5)	14 (11.5)
Vascular disorders	5 (8.2)	7 (11.5)	12 (9.8)
Hypertension	5 (8.2)	7 (11.5)	12 (9.8)
Serious AEs			
Infections and infestations	1 (1.6)	2 (3.3)	3 (2.5)
Acute sinusitis	0	1 (1.6)	1 (0.8)
Hepatitis E	0	1 (1.6)	1 (0.8)
Osteomyelitis	1 (1.6)	0	1 (0.8)
Gastrointestinal disorders	1 (1.6)	1 (1.6)	2 (1.6)
Gastroesophageal reflux disease	0	1 (1.6)	1 (0.8)
Large intestine polyp	1 (1.6)	0	1 (0.8)
Injury, poisoning and procedural complications			
Comminuted fracture	1 (1.6)	0	1 (0.8)
Musculoskeletal and connective tissue disorders			
Intervertebral disc protrusion	0	1 (1.6)	1 (0.8)
Neoplasms benign, malignant and unspecified			
Borderline serous tumor of ovary	0	1 (1.6)	1 (0.8)
Psychiatric disorders			
Schizophrenia	1 (1.6)	0	1 (0.8)
Reproductive system and breast disorders			
Endometriosis	0	1 (1.6)	1 (0.8)

Data presented as n (%)
AE adverse event, *q2w* once in 2 weeks, *q4w* once in 4 weeks

maintained at week 52 (50 mg q4w group, 29/61 (47.5%) patients; 100 mg q2w group, 32/61 (52.5%) patients) (Table 4). In patients with prior bDMARD use, the DAS28-CRP remission rates at week 52 were 41.2% (7/17) patients in the 50 mg q4w group and 76.9% (10/13) patients in the 100 mg q2w group. The SDAI and CDAI assessments showed an improvement at week 16, which was consistent until week 52 (Table 4).

Table 3 Summary of safety events related to blood parameters and hematology: shift from CTCAE grade 0 at baseline through week 52 (safety analysis set)

Parameter	Total (*N*)	Grade 0 at baseline	Grade 0	Grade 1	Grade 2	Grade 3	Grade 4
Neutrophils decreased							
Sirukumab 50 mg q4w	61	61 (100.0)	33 (54.1)	17 (27.9)	8 (13.1)	3 (4.9)	0
Sirukumab 100 mg q2w	61	61 (100.0)	34 (55.7)	14 (23.0)	11 (18.0)	2 (3.3)	0
Platelets decreased							
Sirukumab 50 mg q4w	61	61 (100.0)	44 (72.1)	17 (27.9)	0	0	0
Sirukumab 100 mg q2w	61	61 (100.0)	54 (88.5)	6 (9.8)	0	0	1 (1.6)[a]
Leukocytes decreased							
Sirukumab 50 mg q4w	61	61 (100.0)	34 (55.7)	21 (34.4)	6 (9.8)	0	0
Sirukumab 100 mg q2w	61	61 (100.0)	42 (68.9)	11 (18.0)	6 (9.8)	2 (3.3)	0
Lymphocytes decreased							
Sirukumab 50 mg q4w	61	58 (95.1)	51 (83.6)	3 (4.9)	4 (6.6)	0	0
Sirukumab 100 mg q2w	61	58 (95.1)	50 (82.0)	1 (1.6)	7 (11.5)	0	0
Alanine aminotransferase increased							
Sirukumab 50 mg q4w	61	58 (95.1)	30 (49.2)	26 (42.6)	2(3.3)	0	0
Sirukumab 100 mg q2w	61	56 (91.8)	31 (50.8)	24 (39.3)	1 (1.6)	0	0
Aspartate aminotransferase increased							
Sirukumab 50 mg q4w	61	59 (96.7)	33 (54.1)	25 (41.0)	1 (1.6)	0	0
Sirukumab 100 mg q2w	61	55 (90.2)	32 (52.5)	23 (37.7)	0	0	0
Bilirubin increased							
Sirukumab 50 mg q4w	61	61 (100.0)	48 (78.7)	10 (16.4)	3 (4.9)	0	0
Sirukumab 100 mg q2w	61	61 (100.0)	47 (77.0)	10 (16.4)	4 (6.6)	0	0
Cholesterol increased							
Sirukumab 50 mg q4w	59	59 (100.0)	51 (83.6)	5 (8.2)	3 (4.9)	0	0
Sirukumab 100 mg q2w	60	60 (100.0)	54 (88.5)	5 (8.2)	1 (1.6)	0	0
Triglycerides increased							
Sirukumab 50 mg q4w	59	55 (93.2)	34 (55.7)	20 (32.8)	0	1 (1.6)	0
Sirukumab 100 mg q2w	60	54 (90.0)	33 (54.1)	20 (32.8)	0	1 (1.6)	0

Data presented as n **(%) unless stated otherwise**
CTCAE **Common Terminology Criteria For Adverse Events, *q4w* once in 4 weeks, *q2w* once in 2 weeks**
[a]Erroneously reported

Table 4 Summary of efficacy parameters through week 52 (efficacy full analysis set[a])

Efficacy parameter	Sirukumab 50 mg q4w (*N* = 61)	Sirukumab 100 mg q2w (*N* = 61)
ACR20 response, *n* (%)		
Week 16	47 (77.0)	44 (72.1)
Week 24	45 (73.8)	50 (82.0)
Week 52	39 (63.9)	46 (75.4)
ACR50 response, *n* (%)		
Week 16	29 (47.5)	35 (57.4)
Week 24	30 (49.2)	39 (63.9)
Week 52	29 (47.5)	35 (57.4)
ACR70 response, *n* (%)		
Week 16	16 (26.2)	20 (32.8)
Week 24	15 (24.6)	22 (36.1)
Week 52	20 (32.8)	24 (39.3)
HAQ-DI		
Week 16 median decrease from baseline, %	41.2	51.5
Week 52 median decrease from baseline, %	44.5	70.0
CRP levels (mg/dl), mean (SD)		
Week 16	0.02 (0.05)	0.02 (0.02)
Week 52	0.02 (0.06)	0.02 (0.02)
DAS28-CRP response		
Week 16 responders, *n* (%)	55 (90.2)	59 (96.7)
Week 52 responders, *n* (%)	45 (73.8)	50 (82.0)
DAS28-CRP remission		
Week 16 remitters, *n* (%)	28 (45.9)	30 (49.2)
Week 52 remitters, *n* (%)	29 (47.5)	32 (52.5)
SDAI		
Week 16 change from baseline, mean (SD)	−22.4 (12.44)	−25.9 (13.99)
Week 52 change from baseline, mean (SD)	−23.3 (14.02)	−28.5 (15.94)
CDAI		
Week 16 change from baseline, mean (SD)	−19.4 (12.14)	−22.7 (13.23)
Week 52 change from baseline, mean (SD)	−20.4 (13.83)	−25.3 (15.26)
HAQ-DI response		
Week 16 responders, *n* (%)	46 (75.4)	41 (67.2)
Week 52 responders, *n* (%)	44 (72.1)	41 (67.2)

ACR20/50/70 American College of Rheumatology 20/50/70 response, *CDAI* Clinical Disease Activity Index, *CRP* C-reactive protein, *DAS28* Disease Activity Score 28, *HAQ-DI* Health Assessment Questionnaire-Disability Index, *SD* standard deviation, *SDAI* Simplified Disease Activity Index, *q4w* once in 4 weeks, *q2w* once in 2 weeks

[a]Data imputation was nonresponder imputation for categorical parameters and last observation carried forward for noncategorical parameters

Efficacy assessments post sirukumab administration

DMARDs were initiated after the last sirukumab dose at week 52, except in three patients (50 mg q4w group, 2/61 patients; 100 mg q2w group, 1/61 patient) who received DMARDs on or post week 24 (< 20% improvement in swollen and tender joint counts). Proportions of patients with ACR20 and ACR50 response at week 16 post sirukumab treatment were generally similar as compared with week 52 (end of treatment) regardless of DMARDs added (Table 5). In patients using concomitant MTX or corticosteroids (oral or intramuscular), the mean DAS28-CRP was ≤ 2.6 for the 100 mg q2w group at week 52 (Table 5).

Immunogenicity

Only patients in the 50 mg q4w group (6/61 patients) were positive for antibodies against sirukumab through week 68. In two of these patients, immunogenicity was associated with injection-site reactions. No patients were positive for neutralizing antibodies.

Discussion

A 52-week exposure to sirukumab monotherapy (50 mg q4w and 100 mg q2w) was generally tolerable in Japanese patients with active RA who were nonresponders to MTX or SSZ. A retention rate of 81.1% suggests that sirukumab was tolerable, safe and efficacious over 52 weeks of therapy.

Infections related to the immunosuppression were the most commonly observed AEs in anti-IL-6 therapies. The phase 2 trials of sirukumab (100 mg q2w for 24 weeks, 36.7% of patients), sarilumab (200 mg q2w for 12 weeks, 23.5% of patients), tocilizumab (8 mg/kg infusion q4w for 24 weeks, 32.0% of patients) and olokizumab (120 mg q2w for 12 weeks, 27.3% of patients) reported comparable AEs of infections [6, 8, 15, 16]. In all studies, MTX was administered with IL-6 inhibitor, except for the olokizumab study. A phase 2b study in RA patients also reported 12 serious infections (of 28 SAEs) in clazakizumab-treated patients (with or without MTX) [17]. Further, the proportion of patients reporting injection-site reactions was comparable between both treatment groups (50 mg q4w group, 23/61 patients; 100 mg q2w group, 24/61 patients). An association between injection-site reaction and anti-sirukumab antibodies was reported in two patients (50 mg q4w group). Overall, the incidences of ≥ 1 AEs, infections and injection-site reactions were higher in this phase 3 study as compared to observations from a shorter 38-week, phase 2 study (100 mg q2w group: ≥ 1 AEs, 86.7%; infections, 36.7%; injection-site reaction, 16.7%) and two 52-week global phase 3 studies: SIRROUND-D (100 mg q2w group: ≥ 1 AEs, 80.2%; injection-site reactions, 16.3%) and SIRROUND-T (100 mg q2w group: ≥ 1 AEs, 81.0%; injection-site

Table 5 Summary of ACR20 and ACR50 responses and DAS28-CRP based on concomitant medication at and after week 52 (efficacy full analysis set)

Efficacy parameter	Sirukumab 50 mg q4w	Sirukumab 100 mg q2w
ACR20 response		
Methotrexate		
Week 52[a]	29/44 (65.9)	34/42 (81.0)
Week 52[b]	29/36 (80.6)	34/38 (89.5)
Week 16, posttreatment phase[b]	32/36 (88.9)	32/38 (84.2)
DMARDs (including methotrexate)		
Week 52[a]	31/49 (63.3)	34/44 (77.3)
Week 52[b]	31/38 (81.6)	34/38 (89.5)
Week 16, posttreatment phase[b]	33/38 (86.8)	32/38 (84.2)
Corticosteroid (oral)		
Week 52[a]	2/7 (28.6)	8/11 (72.7)
Week 52[b]	2/3 (66.7)	8/9 (88.9)
Week 16, posttreatment phase[b]	3/3 (100.0)	9/9 (100.0)
Corticosteroid (oral, intramuscular)		
Week 52[a]	4/11 (36.4)	11/15 (73.3)
Week 52[b]	4/6 (66.7)	11/12 (91.7)
Week 16, posttreatment phase[b]	5/6 (83.3)	12/12 (100.0)
No DMARD and corticosteroid		
Week 52[a]	7/11 (63.6)	8/12 (66.7)
Week 52[b]	8/8 (100.0)	8/10 (80.0)
Week 16, posttreatment phase[b]	8/8 (100.0)	8/10 (80.0)
ACR50 response		
Methotrexate		
Week 52[a]	21/44 (47.7)	24/42 (57.1)
Week 52[b]	21/36 (58.3)	24/38 (63.2)
Week 16, posttreatment phase[b]	23/36 (63.9)	27/38 (71.1)
DMARDs (including methotrexate)		
Week 52[a]	22/49 (44.9)	24/44 (54.5)
Week 52[b]	22/38 (57.9)	24/38 (63.2)
Week 16, posttreatment phase[b]	23/38 (60.5)	27/38 (71.1)
Corticosteroid (oral)		
Week 52[a]	0/7 (0)	6/11 (54.5)
Week 52[b]	0/3 (0)	6/9 (66.7)
Week 16, posttreatment phase[b]	1/3 (33.3)	8/9 (88.9)
Corticosteroid (oral, intramuscular)		
Week 52[a]	1/11 (9.1)	9/15 (60.0)
Week 52[b]	1/6 (16.7)	9/12 (75.0)
Week 16, posttreatment phase[b]	2/6 (33.3)	11/12 (91.7)
No DMARD and corticosteroid		
Week 52[a]	7/11 (63.6)	8/12 (66.7)
Week 52[b]	7/8 (87.5)	8/10 (80.0)
Week 16, posttreatment phase[b]	7/8 (87.5)	8/10 (80.0)

Table 5 Summary of ACR20 and ACR50 responses and DAS28-CRP based on concomitant medication at and after week 52 (efficacy full analysis set) *(Continued)*

Efficacy parameter	Sirukumab 50 mg q4w	Sirukumab 100 mg q2w
DAS28-CRP score		
All, *n*	61	61
Week 52,[b] *n*	47	52
Mean (SD)	2.4 (1.07)	2.3 (1.03)
Week 16, posttreatment phase, *n*[b]	61	60
Mean (SD)	2.5 (1.17)	2.4 (1.19)
Methotrexate, *n*	44	42
Week 52, *n*[b]	36	38
Mean (SD)	2.5 (1.09)	2.5 (0.94)
Week 16, posttreatment phase, *n*[b]	44	41
Mean (SD)	2.5 (1.10)	2.6 (1.18)
Corticosteroid (oral, intramuscular), *n*	11	15
Week 52, *n*[b]	6	12
Mean (SD)	3.0 (1.69)	1.9 (0.97)
Week 16, posttreatment phase, *n*[b]	11	15
Mean (SD)	3.0 (1.59)	2.1 (0.89)

Data presented as *n/N* (%)
[a]Data imputation was nonresponder imputation for categorical parameters and last observation carried forward for noncategorical parameters
[b]Week 52 and week 16, posttreatment phase: values were as observed
ACR20/50/70 American College of Rheumatology 20/50/70 response, *DMARD* Disease-modifying anti-rheumatic drug, *n* number of patients, *N* total number of patients, *q4w* once in 4 weeks, *q2w* once in 2 weeks, *SD* standard deviation

reactions, 25.0%) [8, 11, 12]. Discontinuations due to AEs in this study were primarily due to infections and infestations (4/122 patients) and the proportion of patients discontinuing treatment due to AEs was lower (3.3%) as compared with the SIRROUND-D (7.8%) and SIRROUND-T (10.1%) studies [11, 12].

The proportion of patients with ≥ 1 SAE was low (7.4%) and comparable with other anti-IL-6 therapy studies of similar treatment duration [4, 6, 16]. The SAEs observed in the earlier phase 2 sirukumab study were similar in profile and frequency to those in this study, suggesting that 52-week sirukumab administration did not significantly affect patient proportions with SAEs. Also, the proportion of patients with SAEs was lower as compared with the rates reported in SIRROUND-D (10.4%) and SIRROUND-T (13.7%) [11, 12]. Overall, three SAEs related to infections (acute sinusitis, hepatitis E and osteomyelitis in one patient each) were reported during the study (50 mg q4w group, 1 SAE; 100 mg q2w group, 2 SAEs). No deaths were reported in this study, although an imbalance in deaths and malignancy has been reported in the sirukumab group as compared with the placebo group in the global SIRROUND-D and SIRROUND-T studies [11, 12]. Incidences of major cardiovascular events, gastrointestinal perforations or tuberculosis have also been reported in these global studies; however, these were absent in the current study [11, 12]. Hematological abnormalities, a common feature noted in all anti-IL-6 therapy studies, were also observed in the current study but no grade 4 events were reported. No patients developed neutralizing antibodies to sirukumab.

Improvements in signs and symptoms of RA based on ACR20/50/70 responses, DAS28-CRP response and HAQ-DI score occurred as early as 2 weeks of treatment with sirukumab and were maintained or improved through week 52. These improvements were numerically greater in the100 mg q2w group versus the 50 mg q4w group. In this 52-week study, the proportion of patients achieving ACR20 responses at week 16 (100 mg q2w group, 72.1% patients) was consistent with the phase 2 study (100 mg q2w group, 63.3%) [8]. Efficacy in the phase 2 studies of sirukumab with respect to ACR20 was similar to those for sarilumab, olokizumab and clazakizumab [4, 6, 8, 15, 16, 18]. However, the ACR70 response at week 52 with both doses (50 mg q4w group, 32.8% patients; 100 mg q2w group, 39.3% patients) was reported in a higher percentage of patients as compared with the SIRROUND-D study (52 weeks; 50 mg q4w group, 16.5%; 100 mg q2w group, 18.5%) and the SIRROUND-T study (24 weeks; 50 mg q4w group, 9%; 100 mg q2w group, 10%) [11, 12]. Similarly, a higher percentage of patients achieved DAS28-CRP remission in the current study at week 52 (50 mg q4w group, 47.5%; 100 mg q2w group, 52.5%) as compared with the phase 2 study (24 weeks; 50 mg q4w group, 13.3%; 100 mg q2w group, 20.0%), the SIRROUND-D study (24 weeks; 50 mg q4w group, 26.0%; 100 mg q2w group, 25.5%) and the SIRROUND-T study (24 weeks; 50 mg q4w group, 19.0%; 100 mg q2w group, 22.0%) [8, 11, 12]. The suppression of inflammation as reflected by the consistently low levels of CRP (0.02 mg/dl from week 16 to 52) may confirm the ability of sirukumab to block IL-6 signaling during the span of the dosing interval [19]. Improvements in CDAI were also consistent with changes in other measures of disease activity (ACR and DAS28-CRP) and maximum improvement was observed at week 52. Concomitant MTX was started post week 52 in most of the patients and demonstrated maintenance of efficacy until week 16 post treatment in both treatment groups. In addition, some patients maintained ACR50 response without concomitant DMARDs and corticosteroids during the posttreatment phase. Overall, the efficacy profile of sirukumab monotherapy over a 52-week period in Japanese patients with active RA support findings from the global SIRROUND-D and SIRROUND-T studies [11, 12]. The current data in combination with previous randomized controlled trials of sirukumab suggest a potential role for sirukumab in RA therapy.

Limitations of this study include the low number of patients and lack of efficacy endpoints. The absence of a placebo control is a limitation for this study with respect to the absolute efficacy achieved but consistent improvement was observed in both sirukumab-treated groups in terms of the clinical signs and symptoms of RA. Generalizability and extrapolation of these results to routine clinical practice should be made within the context that the patients discontinued csDMARDs before study participation, in contrast to the recommended treatment modality that includes continued use of DMARDs for greater efficacy in patients with active RA [14, 20].

Conclusions

Sirukumab monotherapy at both doses (50 mg q4w and 100 mg q2w) was generally tolerable and the safety profile was dosage independent in Japanese patients with RA refractory to MTX and SSZ in this 52-week study. Thus, sirukumab monotherapy has the potential to be a new viable treatment option for RA refractory to conventional synthetic or biologic DMARDs.

Acknowledgements

Sonia Philipose, PhD and Priya Ganpathy, MPharm, ISMPP CMPP™ (both SIRO Clinpharm Pvt. Ltd, Thane, India) provided writing assistance and Akino Tanaka (Janssen Pharmaceutical K.K.) provided additional editorial support for this manuscript. The authors thank Dr Takayuki Ota and Dr Miyo Ota (both The Scripps Research Institute, Department of Immunology and Microbiology) for their contributions to this study. The authors also thank the study participants, without whom this study would never have been accomplished, and the investigators for their participation in this study.

Funding

This study was sponsored by Janssen Pharmaceutical K.K., Japan and Glaxo SmithKline.

Authors' contributions

TT, YT, MH and HY were involved in study design and data interpretation. BH, TN, RT and YK had primary roles in the study design, analyses and data interpretation. YU was the project statistician. All authors contributed to the data interpretation for the results. All authors met the ICMJE criteria and all those who fulfilled those criteria are listed as authors. All authors had access to the study data, provided direction and comments on the manuscript, made the final decision about where to publish these data and approved submission to the journal. All authors read and approved the final manuscript.

Competing interests

TT has received research grants from Astellas Pharma, Bristol-Myers K.K., Chugai Pharmaceutical Co. Ltd, Daiichi Sankyo Co. Ltd, Eisai Co. Ltd, Mitsubishi Tanabe Pharma Co., Pfizer Japan Inc., Santen Pharmaceutical Co. Ltd, Takeda Pharmaceutical Co. Ltd, Teijin Pharma Ltd, AbbVie GK, Asahi Kasei Pharma Corp., Taisho Toyama Pharmaceutical Co. Ltd and SymBio Pharmaceuticals Ltd; has received consulting fees from Astra Zeneca K.K., Eli Lilly Japan K.K., Novartis Pharma K.K., Mitsubishi Tanabe Pharma Co., Asahi Kasei Medical K.K., AbbVie GK, Daiichi Sankyo Co. Ltd, Bristol-Myers K.K. and Nippon Kayaku Co. Ltd; and has received speaking fees from AbbVie GK, Bristol-Myers K.K., Chugai Pharmaceutical Co. Ltd,

Eisai Co. Ltd, Janssen Pharmaceutical K.K., Mitsubishi Tanabe Pharma Co., Pfizer Japan Inc., Takeda Pharmaceutical Co. Ltd, Astellas Pharma, Daiichi Sankyo Co. Ltd, Celtrion and Nippon Kayaku Co. Ltd.
HY has received research grants from AbbVie, Asahi Kasei, Astellas, AstraZeneca, Bristol-Myers Squibb, Chugai, Daiichi Sankyo, Eisai, GlaxoSmithKline, Janssen Pharmaceutical Product, L.P., Mitsubishi Tanabe, MSD, Nippon Kayaku, Pfizer Inc., Santen, Taisho Toyama, Takeda and Teijin; has received consulting fees from AbbVie, Astellas, AstraZeneca, Bristol-Myers Squibb, Chugai, Daiichi Sankyo, Eisai, Mitsubishi Tanabe, Nippon Kayaku, Pfizer Inc., Takeda and Teijin; and has served on a speakers' bureau for AbbVie, Astellas, Bristol-Myers Squibb, Chugai, Eisai, Mitsubishi Tanabe, Pfizer Inc., Takeda and Teijin.
MH has received research grants from AbbVie Japan, Astellas Pharma, Bristol-Myers Squibb, Chugai Pharmaceutical, Eisai, Mitsubishi Tanabe Pharma, Ono Pharmaceuticals, Santen Pharmaceutical, Takeda Pharmaceutical, UCB Japan and Teijin Pharma; and has received consulting fees from AbbVie Japan, Janssen Pharma, Chugai Pharmaceutical, Teijin Pharma, Eli Lilly Japan and Zenyaku Kogyo.
YT has received research grants from Mitsubishi-Tanabe, Takeda, Daiichi-Sankyo, Chugai, Bristol-Myers, MSD, Astellas, Abbvie and Eisai; and has received consulting fees from Abbvie, Chugai, Daiichi-Sankyo, Bristol-Myers, Mitsubishi-Tanabe, Astellas, Takeda, Pfizer, Teijin, Asahi Kasei, YL Biologics, Sanofi, Janssen, Eli Lilly and GlaxoSmithKline.
RT, YK, YU and TN are employees of Janssen Pharmaceutical K.K.
BH is an employee and stockholder of Johnson & Johnson.

Author details

[1]Keio University School of Medicine, Shinjuku-ku, Tokyo, Japan. [2]Tokyo Women's Medical University, Shinjuku-ku, Tokyo, Japan. [3]Janssen Pharmaceutical K.K., Chiyoda-ku, Tokyo, Japan. [4]Janssen Research & Development, LLC, Spring House, PA, USA. [5]University of Occupational & Environmental Health Japan, Kitakyushu, Japan.

References

1. Taylor PC, Feldmann M. Anti-TNF biologic agents: still the therapy of choice for rheumatoid arthritis. Nat Rev Rheumatol. 2009;5(10):578–82.
2. Mewar D, Wilson AG. Treatment of rheumatoid arthritis with tumour necrosis factor inhibitors. Br J Pharmacol. 2011;162(4):785–91.
3. Hirano T, Matsuda T, Turner M, Miyasaka N, Buchan G, Tang B, et al. Excessive production of interleukin 6/B cell stimulatory factor-2 in rheumatoid arthritis. Eur J Immunol. 1988;18(11):1797–802.
4. Maini RN, Taylor PC, Szechinski J, Pavelka K, Broll J, Balint G, et al. Double-blind randomized controlled clinical trial of the interleukin-6 receptor antagonist, tocilizumab, in European patients with rheumatoid arthritis who had an incomplete response to methotrexate. Arthritis Rheum. 2006;54(9): 2817–29. https://doi.org/10.1002/art.22033
5. Nishimoto N, Miyasaka N, Yamamoto K, Kawai S, Takeuchi T, Azuma J. Long-term safety and efficacy of tocilizumab, an anti-IL-6 receptor monoclonal antibody, in monotherapy, in patients with rheumatoid arthritis (the STREAM study): evidence of safety and efficacy in a 5-year extension study. Ann Rheum Dis. 2009;68(10):1580–4.
6. Smolen JS, Beaulieu A, Rubbert-Roth A, Ramos-Remus C, Rovensky J, Alecock E, et al. Effect of interleukin-6 receptor inhibition with tocilizumab in patients with rheumatoid arthritis (OPTION study): a double-blind, placebo-controlled, randomised trial. Lancet. 2008;371(9617):987–97.
7. Xu Z, Bouman-Thio E, Comisar C, Frederick B, Van Hartingsveldt B, Marini JC, et al. Pharmacokinetics, pharmacodynamics and safety of a human anti-IL-6 monoclonal antibody (sirukumab) in healthy subjects in a first-in-human study. Br J Clin Pharmacol. 2011;72(2):270–81.
8. Smolen JS, Weinblatt ME, Sheng S, Zhuang Y, Hsu B. Sirukumab, a human anti-interleukin-6 monoclonal antibody: a randomised, 2-part (proof-of-concept and dose-finding), phase II study in patients with active rheumatoid arthritis despite methotrexate therapy. Ann Rheum Dis. 2014;73(9):1616–25.
9. Kremer JM, Alarcon GS, Lightfoot RW Jr, Willkens RF, Furst DE, Williams HJ, et al. Methotrexate for rheumatoid arthritis. Suggested guidelines for monitoring liver toxicity. American College of Rheumatology. Arthritis Rheum. 1994;37(3):316–28.
10. Schmajuk G, Miao Y, Yazdany J, Boscardin WJ, Daikh DI, Steinman MA. Identification of risk factors for elevated transaminases in methotrexate users through an electronic health record. Arthritis Care Res (Hoboken). 2014;66(8):1159–66.
11. Takeuchi T, Thorne C, Karpouzas G, Sheng S, Xu W, Rao R, et al. Sirukumab for rheumatoid arthritis: the phase III SIRROUND-D study. Ann Rheum Dis. 2017;76(12):2001–08.
12. Aletaha D, Bingham CO 3rd, Tanaka Y, Agarwal P, Kurrasch R, Tak PP, et al. Efficacy and safety of sirukumab in patients with active rheumatoid arthritis refractory to anti-TNF therapy (SIRROUND-T): a randomised, double-blind, placebo-controlled, parallel-group, multinational, phase 3 study. Lancet. 2017;389(10075):1206–17.
13. Pelechas E, Voulgari PV, Drosos AA. Sirukumab: a promising therapy for rheumatoid arthritis. Expert Opin Biol Ther. 2017;17(6):755–63.
14. Takeuchi T, Harigai M, Tanaka Y, Yamanaka H, Ishiguro N, Yamamoto K, et al. Golimumab monotherapy in Japanese patients with active rheumatoid arthritis despite prior treatment with disease-modifying antirheumatic drugs: results of the phase 2/3, multicentre, randomised, double-blind, placebo-controlled GO-MONO study through 24 weeks. Ann Rheum Dis. 2013;72(9):1488–95.
15. Genovese MC, Fleischmann R, Furst D, Janssen N, Carter J, Dasgupta B, et al. Efficacy and safety of olokizumab in patients with rheumatoid arthritis with an inadequate response to TNF inhibitor therapy: outcomes of a randomised phase IIb study. Ann Rheum Dis. 2014;73(9):1607–15.
16. Huizinga TW, Fleischmann RM, Jasson M, Radin AR, van Adelsberg J, Fiore S, et al. Sarilumab, a fully human monoclonal antibody against IL-6Rα in patients with rheumatoid arthritis and an inadequate response to methotrexate: efficacy and safety results from the randomised SARIL-RA-MOBILITY Part A trial. Ann Rheum Dis. 2014;73(9):1626–34.
17. Weinblatt ME, Mease P, Mysler E, Takeuchi T, Drescher E, Berman A, et al. The efficacy and safety of subcutaneous clazakizumab in patients with moderate-to-severe rheumatoid arthritis and an inadequate response to methotrexate: results from a multinational, phase IIb, randomized, double-blind, placebo/active-controlled, dose-ranging study. Arthritis Rheumatol. 2015;67(10):2591–600.
18. Mease P, Strand V, Shalamberidze L, Dimic A, Raskina T, Xu L-A, et al. A phase II, double-blind, randomised, placebo-controlled study of BMS945429 (ALD518) in patients with rheumatoid arthritis with an inadequate response to methotrexate. Ann Rheum Dis. 2012;71(7):1183–89.
19. Burmester GR, Rubbert-Roth A, Cantagrel A, Hall S, Leszczynski P, Feldman D, et al. A randomised, double-blind, parallel-group study of the safety and efficacy of subcutaneous tocilizumab versus intravenous tocilizumab in combination with traditional disease-modifying antirheumatic drugs in patients with moderate to severe rheumatoid arthritis (SUMMACTA study). Ann Rheum Dis. 2014;73(1):69–74.
20. Ogata A, Tanimura K, Sugimoto T, Inoue H, Urata Y, Matsubara T, et al. Phase III study of the efficacy and safety of subcutaneous versus intravenous tocilizumab monotherapy in patients with rheumatoid arthritis. Arthritis Care Res. 2014;66(3):344–54.

7

Calgizzarin (S100A11): a novel inflammatory mediator associated with disease activity of rheumatoid arthritis

Lucie Andrés Cerezo[1,2*†], Barbora Šumová[1,2†], Klára Prajzlerová[1,2], David Veigl[3], Dres Damgaard[4], Claus Henrik Nielsen[4], Karel Pavelka[1,2], Jiří Vencovský[1,2] and Ladislav Šenolt[1,2*]

Abstract

Background: Calgizzarin (S100A11) is a member of the S100 protein family that acts in different tumors by regulating a number of biologic functions. Recent data suggest its association with low-grade inflammation in osteoarthritis (OA). The aim of our study is to compare S100A11 expression in the synovial tissues, synovial fluid and serum of patients with rheumatoid arthritis (RA) and osteoarthritis (OA) and to characterize the potential association between S100A11 and disease activity.

Methods: S100A11 protein expression was detected in synovial tissue from patients with RA ($n = 6$) and patients with OA ($n = 6$) by immunohistochemistry and immunofluorescence. Serum and synovial fluid S100A11 levels were measured by ELISA in patients with RA ($n = 40$) and patients with OA ($n = 34$). Disease activity scores in 28 joints based on C-reactive protein (DAS28-CRP) were used to assess disease activity. Cytokine content in peripheral blood mononuclear cells (PBMCs), synovial fibroblasts (SFs) and synovial fluid was analysed by ELISA, western blotting or cytometric bead array.

Results: S100A11 expression was significantly up-regulated in the synovial lining and sublining layers ($p < 0.01$) and vessels ($p < 0.05$) of patients with RA compared to patients with OA, and was associated with fibroblasts and T cells. S100A11 was significantly increased in synovial fluid ($p < 0.0001$) but not in serum ($p = 0.158$) from patients with RA compared to patients with OA when adjusted for age and sex. Synovial fluid S100A11 correlated with DAS28 ($r = 0.350$, $p = 0.027$), serum CRP ($r = 0.463$, $p = 0.003$), synovial fluid leukocyte count ($r = 0.677$, $p < 0.001$), anti-cyclic citrullinated peptide antibodies (anti-CCP) ($r = 0.424$, $p = 0.006$) and IL-6 ($r = 0.578$, $p = 0.002$) and IL-8 ($r = 0.740$, $p < 0.001$) in synovial fluid from patients with RA. PBMCs and SFs isolated from patients with RA synthesized and spontaneously secreted higher levels of S100A11 in comparison with PBMCs and SFs from patients with OA ($p = 0.011$ and 0.03, respectively). S100A11 stimulated the production of the pro-inflammatory cytokine IL-6 by PBMCs ($p < 0.05$) and SFs ($p < 0.01$).

Conclusions: Our data provide the first evidence of S100A11 up-regulation and its association with inflammation and disease activity in patients with RA.

Keywords: Calgizzarin, S100 proteins, Rheumatoid arthritis, Inflammation, Disease activity

* Correspondence: lucie.andres.cerezo@gmail.com; senolt@revma.cz
†Equal contributors
[1]Institute of Rheumatology, Na Slupi 4, 12850 Prague, Czech Republic
Full list of author information is available at the end of the article

Background

Rheumatoid arthritis (RA) is a chronic systemic autoimmune disease with predominant musculoskeletal manifestations. The hallmark of this condition is persistent synovial inflammation leading to irreversible structural damage and joint failure. Despite intensive research, the exact cause of RA remains elusive. It is well-established that activated immune cells and synovial fibroblasts producing inflammatory factors play a central role in the pathophysiologic mechanisms of RA [1]. Nevertheless, clarifying the roles of cytokines within a complex regulatory network in RA remains a key challenge.

S100A11 (also known as S100C or calgizzarin) is a less well-known member of the large calcium-binding S100 protein family [2] that has been proposed to play specific biologic roles in the processes of endocytosis and exocytosis [3–5], enzyme activity regulation [6], cell growth [7], apoptosis [8] and low-grade inflammation [9]. S100A11 is expressed at different levels in various tissues [10] and is localized in the nucleus, cytoplasm and cell periphery [11–13]. S100A11 is associated with the oncogenesis of many different types of tumour and has been identified as a tumour suppressor in some cancers and as a tumour promoter in other cancers [14]. S100A11 has been found to play an ambivalent role in growth regulation [11, 15] and acts via receptor for advanced glycation end-products (RAGE)-dependent signalling in human keratinocytes [11]. Moreover, S100A11 has been shown to regulate the stability of the cell cycle regulator, cyclin-dependent kinase inhibitor (1p21CIP1/WAF1) in human keratinocytes [16].

Increased S100A11 expression was recently demonstrated in human articular cartilage in patients with osteoarthritis (OA) [17, 18]. S100A11 expression and release from chondrocytes were induced by the pro-inflammatory cytokines interleukin-1β (IL-1β) and tumour necrosis factor-α (TNF-α) and the chemokine CXCL8 [9, 18]. Moreover, extracellular S100A11 was shown to act via RAGE-dependent signalling to activate the p38 mitogen-activated protein kinase (MAPK) pathway and accelerate chondrocyte hypertrophy and matrix catabolism [18]. In addition, S100A11 and several other S100 proteins are up-regulated in the early preclinical phase (before signs of arthritis are present) of adjuvant arthritis [19].

Therefore, the aim of our study was to assess local and systemic S100A11 expression in patients with RA and OA and to investigate the relationship among S100A11, inflammation and RA disease activity.

Methods

Patients

We included 40 patients with active RA (27 female and 13 male, mean age ± SD 54.90 ± 14.25) and 34 patients with knee OA (25 female and 9 male, mean age ± SD 65.20 ± 10.41); see Table 1 for patient characteristics.

Table 1 Characteristics of patients with rheumatoid arthritis (RA) and osteoarthritis (OA)

Characteristics	RA (*n* = 40)	OA (*n* = 34)
Gender (female/male)	27/13	25/9
Age (years)	54.90 ± 14.25	65.21 ± 10.41
CRP (mg/l)	27.88 ± 31.80	4.11 ± 4.30
Disease duration (years)	6.72 ± 8.58	5.57 ± 7.41
Drugs (DMARDs/GCs)	37/26	-
Biological therapy	8[a]	-
DAS28	4.39 ± 1.19	-
RF positivity, *n* (%)	31 (72%)	-
Anti-CCP positivity, *n* (%)	26 (60%)	-

Data are expressed as the mean (± SD) unless stated otherwise. [a]Out of 8 patients, 5 were treated with anti-TNF therapy, 1 with tocilizumab, 1 with rituximab and 1 with anti-IL-17 therapy. *Anti-CCP* anti-cyclic citrullinated peptide antibody, *BMI* body mass index, *CRP* C-reactive protein, *DAS28* disease activity score in 28 joints, *DMARDs* disease-modifying antirheumatic drugs, *GCs* glucocorticoids, *MTX* methotrexate, *RF* rheumatoid factor, *SJC* swollen joints count

Patients with active RA met the American College of Rheumatology criteria for the diagnosis of RA [20]. This study had approval from the Ethics Board of the Institute of Rheumatology, and all subjects provided informed written consent to participate in it.

Laboratory measurements

Paired samples of peripheral blood and synovial fluid were collected at the time of clinically indicated knee arthrocentesis, immediately processed, and stored at -80 °C until use. Prior to analysis, the synovial fluid samples were treated with hyaluronidase (Hylase Dessau; Riemser Arzneimittel, Greifswald, Germany) for 30 minutes at 37 °C. The clinical assessments were performed using the disease activity score in 28 joints based on C-reactive protein (DAS29-CRP). CRP was measured in serum by turbidimetry using an Olympus Biochemical Analyzer (Olympus CO Ltd., Tokyo, Japan). Serum anti-cyclic citrullinated peptide antibody (anti-CCP) and IgM rheumatoid factor (IgM-RF) levels were determined using standard ELISA kits (Test Line s.r.o., Czech Republic).

Measurement of S100A11 and cytokines

Serum and synovial fluid S100A11 levels were measured using a commercially available ELISA kit, according to the manufacturer's protocol (BioVendor, Brno, Czech Republic). The detection limit of the assay is 0.01 ng/ml. The protein levels of the following cytokines in the cell culture supernatants were analysed using the indicated ELISA kits, according to the manufacturers' protocols: TNF-α and IL-6 (Ray Biotech, Norcross, GA, USA) and IL-1β and monocyte chemotactic protein 1 (MCP-1) (R&D Systems, Wiesbaden-Nordenstadt, Germany). The analyses were performed using a SUNRISE ELISA reader (Tecan, Salzburg, Austria) at 450 nm.

The BD Cytometric Bead Array Human Inflammatory Cytokine Kit II (Catalogue number 551811, BD Biosciences, Franklin Lakes, NJ, USA) was used to measure IL-1β, IL-6, IL-8, IL-10 and TNF-α in 5 µl synovial fluid diluted in 20 µl PBS as described in a previous study [21], which included 26 of the patients with RA and 21 of the patients with OA examined in the present study.

Cell isolation, cell cultures and stimulation experiments

Peripheral blood mononuclear cells (PBMCs) were purified using standard Ficoll-Paque density gradient centrifugation. The PBMCs were seeded in 6-well culture plates at a density of 1.0×10^6 cells (to study spontaneous release of S100A11) or 5.0×10^5 cells (for stimulation experiments) per 1 ml of Advanced RPMI-1640 culture medium (Invitrogen, Carlsbad, CA, USA) and were incubated in a humidified atmosphere for 30 minutes at 37 °C with 5% CO_2. For S100A11 analysis, cells from patients with RA ($n = 9$) and OA ($n = 9$) were incubated for 24 h without treatment. The cell culture supernatants were collected and stored at -80 °C.

Synovial fibroblasts (SFs) were isolated from biopsies from patients with RA ($n = 6$) and patients with OA ($n = 6$), which were obtained during surgery as previously described [22]. SFs (passages 4–6) were seeded at a density of 1.0×10^5 cells/per well in 6-well culture plates in 1 ml of DMEM without serum. After the cells were incubated for 24 h without treatment, their supernatants were collected and stored at -80 °C.

PBMCs (n = 8) and SFs (n = 8) from patients with RA (both obtained as described previously) were treated with recombinant TNF-α (10 ng/ml), IL1-β (10 ng/ml), IL-6 (10 ng/ml) (all from R&D Systems, Minneapolis, MN, USA), lipopolysaccharide (LPS) (10 ng/ml) (Sigma-Aldrich, St Louis, MO, USA), polyinosinic:polycytidylic acid (Poly (I:C)) (20 µg/ml) (Invivogen, San Diego, CA, USA) or different concentrations (100–1000 ng/ml) of recombinant S100A11 protein (Biovendor, Brno, Czech Republic). The doses of recombinant S100A11 were selected based on the concentration range detected in the serum and synovial fluid of patients with RA. After the cells were incubated for 24 h, their supernatants were collected and stored at -80 °C.

Immunohistochemical assessment

Samples from synovial biopsies were obtained from patients with RA (four female and two male, mean age ± SD 54.83 ± 9.41 years) from one hip joint, two knee joints, two elbow joints and one hand joint and from six patients with OA (three female and three male, mean age ± SD 66.00 ± 7.77 years) from four knee joints and two hip joints during joint surgery; the samples comprised 5-mm-thick paraffin-embedded sections. The sections were deparaffinised and rehydrated, and endogenous peroxidase activity and background binding were inhibited using 3% hydrogen peroxide in methanol and 1% bovine serum, respectively. Synovial tissue sections were processed for antigen retrieval and immunohistochemical assessment as described elsewhere [23]. The slides were immunoprobed with polyclonal rabbit S100A11 antibodies (ProteinTech, Chicago, IL, USA) in a dilution of 1:20. Blinded, semiquantitative evaluation was performed using a BX53 microscope and DP80 Digital Microscope Camera and CellSens Standard Software (Olympus, Philadelphia, PA, USA). Eight to ten random and non-overlapping fields of synovial tissue were analysed, and S100A11 staining intensity was scored according to a 4-point scale, in which a score of 0 represented negative staining, and scores of 1–3 represented weak, moderate and strong staining intensity, respectively.

Immunofluorescence

For the double-staining experiments, formalin-fixed, paraffin-embedded synovial sections from patients with RA ($n = 4$) were incubated with primary antibodies against S100A11 (diluted 1:100; Abcam, Cambridge, UK), CD68 (diluted 1:100; Abcam, Cambridge, UK), CD3 (diluted 1:100; Abcam, Cambridge, UK), vimentin (diluted 1:50; Sigma-Aldrich, St. Louis, MO, USA), and CD20 (diluted 1:50; Abcam, Cambridge, UK) before being incubated with secondary antibodies coupled to Alexa 488 or Alexa 647 (diluted 1:200) (Abcam, Cambridge, UK). The samples were then analysed using a BX53 microscope with a DP80 Digital Microscope Camera and CellSens Standard Software (Olympus, Philadelphia, PA, USA). S100A11 positivity in different cell populations was quantified in six randomly selected high-power fields per patient by two experienced researchers in a blinded manner and expressed as percentage of S100A11-positive cells.

Western blot analysis

PBMCs and synovial fibroblasts were homogenized and lysed in radioimmunoprecipitation assay (RIPA) buffer (Thermo Fisher, Waltham, MA, USA). Proteins were separated by tricine sodium dodecyl sulfate-polyacrylamide gel electrophoresis and transferred to polyvinylidene difluoride membranes (Biorad Hercules, CA, USA), which were incubated with antibodies against S100A11 (1:100) (Abcam, Cambridge, UK) overnight at 4 °C. Horseradish-peroxidase-conjugated antibodies (1:2000) (Dako, Glostrup, Denmark) were used as secondary antibodies. Beta-actin antibodies (1:5000) (Abcam, Cambridge, UK) were used as loading controls. The ECL™ Prime Western Blotting System (Sigma-Aldrich, St. Louis, MO, USA) was used for protein visualization. The signals were recorded by an Azure Biosystems c300 imaging system (Azure Biosystems, Dublin, CA, USA).

Statistical analysis

The Kolmogorov-Smirnov test of normality was used for all variables. S100A11 in serum and synovial fluid were expressed as median (range). Differences in S100A11 levels between the two groups were analysed using the Mann-Whitney *U* test. Analyses of differences between the groups were further adjusted for confounders (sex and age) using a generalized linear model. The relationships between non-normally distributed variables were determined by calculating the Spearman correlation coefficient. Differences in synovial tissue or PBMC S100A11 expression levels between patients with RA and OA were determined using the Mann-Whitney *U* test. The unpaired *t* test was used for analysis of protein synthesis. Data are expressed as the mean (SEM) unless stated otherwise. *P* values below 0.05 were considered statistically significant. GraphPad Prism 5 (GraphPad Software, San Diego, CA, USA) or R (R Foundation for Statistical Computing, Vienna, Austria) was used to perform the analysis.

Results

S100A11 is up-regulated in rheumatoid arthritis synovial tissue

S100A11 protein was up-regulated in synovial tissue from patients with RA compared to synovial tissue from patients with OA, in which rather negligible S100A11 expression was observed (Fig. 1). Expression of S100A11 was markedly increased in the cells of the synovial lining layers ($p < 0.01$), interstitium ($p < 0.01$) and inflammatory infiltrates ($p < 0.01$) in samples from patients with RA compared to patients with OA. S100A11 expression in synovial tissue vessels was slightly higher in samples from patients with RA than from patients with OA ($p < 0.05$) (Table 2).

To determine which synovial cells express S100A11, we preformed double-immunofluorescence staining using fibroblast (vimentin), macrophage (CD68), B cell (CD20) and T cell (CD3) markers. We observed significant vimentin and S100A11 co-expression, indicating that the majority of S100A11-positive cells were synovial fibroblasts. We also found that S100A11 was expressed by T cells, some macrophages and only some B cells (Fig. 2a, b).

Serum and synovial fluid S100A11 levels are increased in rheumatoid arthritis

Levels of S100A11 in the synovial fluid (195.8 (20.2–974.2) vs. 26.8 (8.2–199.4) ng/ml; $p < 0.0001$) but not in the serum (14.1 (4.3–119.8) vs. 9.3 (5.0–30.2) ng/ml; $p = 0.158$) were significantly up-regulated in patients with RA compared to patients with OA when adjusted for age and sex (Fig. 3a, b). S100A11 levels in serum or synovial fluid were not affected by treatment. Synovial fluid S100A11 levels were significantly higher than systemic S100A11 levels in both RA ($p < 0.0001$) and OA ($p < 0.0001$), but there was no association between serum and synovial fluid S100A11 levels in either group.

The levels of S100A11 did not differ between double-positive (RF+/anti-CCP+) and double-negative (RF-/anti-CCP-) patients with RA in the serum or synovial fluid.

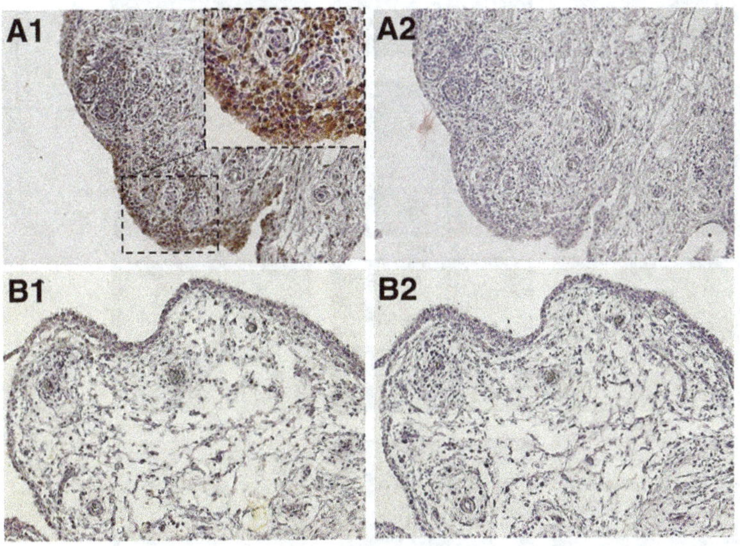

Fig. 1 S100A11 protein in rheumatoid arthritis (RA) and osteoarthritis (OA) synovial tissue assessed by immunohistochemical (IHC) analysis. Intensive staining for S100A11 was found in the synovial fibroblasts of the lining layer and within the inflammatory cell infiltrates in the RA synovial tissue (*A1*). The S100A11 expression was negligible or absent in OA synovium (*B1*). Mouse IgG was used as an isotype control (*A2*, *B2*). Representative images of IHC staining are shown at × 200 magnification. For the detailed view the × 400 magnification is shown ($n = 6$ patients with RA and $n = 6$ patients with OA)

Table 2 Expression of S100A11 related to different cellular compartments in synovial tissues from patients with rheumatoid arthritis (RA) and osteoarthritis (OA)

	RA	OA	Mann-Whitney test
Lining layer	2.58 ± 0.20	1.00 ± 0.29	$p < 0.01$
Interstitium	2.25 ± 0.11	0.25 ± 0.11	$p < 0.01$
Inflammatory infiltrate	2.42 ± 0.27	0.50 ± 0.18	$p < 0.01$
Vessels and capillaries	1.33 ± 0.17	0.33 ± 0.21	$p < 0.05$

The intensity of S100A11 expression was scored using a semiquantitative 4-point scale. A score of 0 represented no staining, 1 weak, 2 moderate and 3 strong staining intensity. Values represent mean (± SD)

Significant up-regulation of S100A11 levels in the synovial fluid but not in the serum was observed in anti-CCP-positive compared to anti-CCP-negative patients ($p = 0.007$). The levels of S100A11 did not differ between RF-positive and RF-negative patients with RA (Additional file 1).

Synovial fluid S100A11 levels are associated with inflammatory markers and with rheumatoid arthritis disease activity

In RA patients, synovial fluid S100A11 levels were significantly associated with disease activity as represented by the DAS28 ($r = 0.350$, $p = 0.027$), CRP ($r = 0.463$, $p = 0.003$) and synovial fluid leukocyte count ($r = 0.677$, $p < 0.001$) (Fig. 3c–e). Furthermore, synovial fluid S100A11 levels were correlated with serum anti-CCP levels ($r = 0.424$, $p = 0.006$) (Fig. 3f), but not IgM-RF levels ($r = 0.059$, $p = 0.719$), in patients with RA. Correlation between S100A11 and CRP ($r = 0.458$, $p = 0.004$), DAS28 ($r = 0.414$, $p = 0.011$) or synovial fluid cell count ($r = 0.703$, $p < 0.001$) was not affected by age, BMI or anti-CCP levels. As there was no association between serum and synovial fluid S100A11 levels, serum S100A11 levels were not correlated with any clinical or laboratory RA disease activity parameters.

We further analysed the selected cytokines in the synovial fluid of patients with RA and OA (Additional file 2) and their association with the levels of S100A11. Synovial fluid S100A11 was significantly correlated with the levels of IL-6 ($r = 0.578$, $p = 0.002$) and IL-8 ($r = 0.740$, $p < 0.001$) (Fig. 3g, h), but not with the levels of IL-1β, TNF-α or IL-10 in patients with RA. In patients with OA, significant association was only found between S100A11 and IL-8 in the synovial fluid ($r = 0.592$, $p = 0.005$).

Peripheral blood mononuclear cells and synovial fibroblasts from patients with rheumatoid arthritis synthesize and spontaneously release higher levels of S100A11

To identify potential S100A11 sources in patients with RA, we analysed S100A11 protein synthesis and release

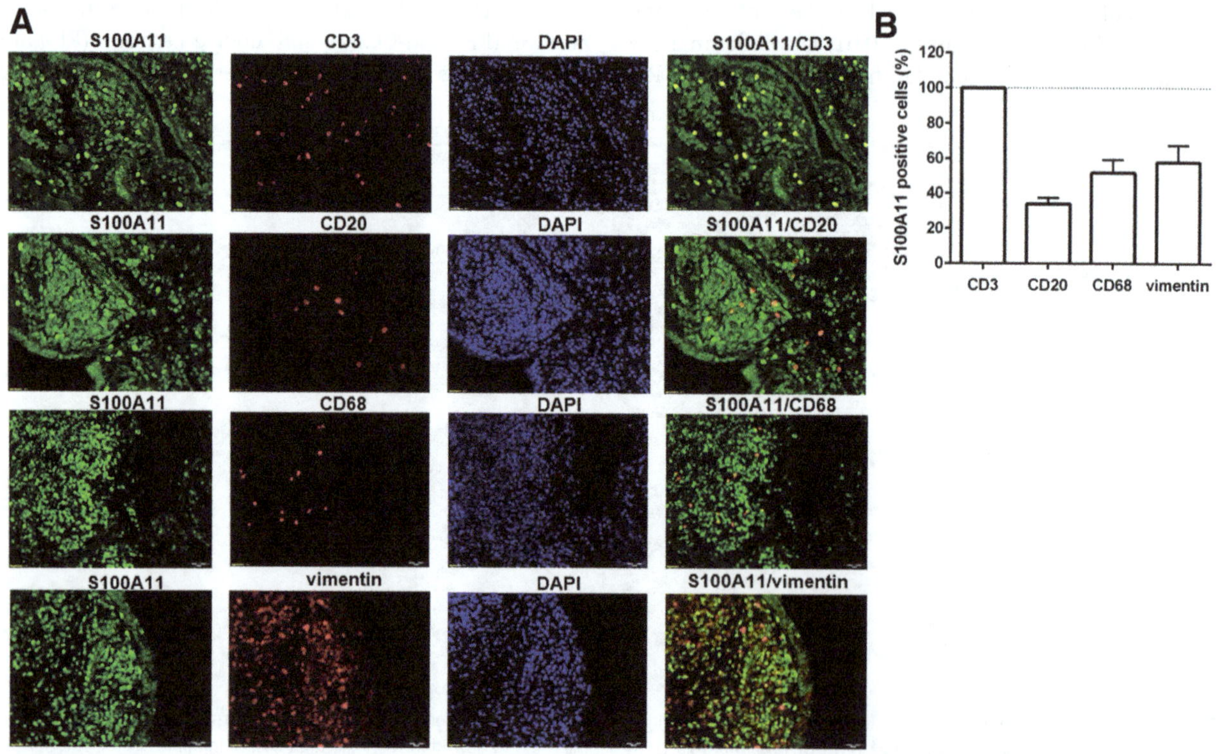

Fig. 2 Cellular distribution of the S100A11 protein in rheumatoid arthritis synovial tissue. Representative images of immunofluorescence staining (**a**) for CD68 (macrophages), CD20 (B cells), CD3 (T cells) and vimentin (cells of mesenchymal origin) are shown at × 200 magnification ($n = 4$). *DAPI* 4',6-diamidino-2-phenylindole. **b** Average percentage of S100A11-positive cells presented as mean ± SEM

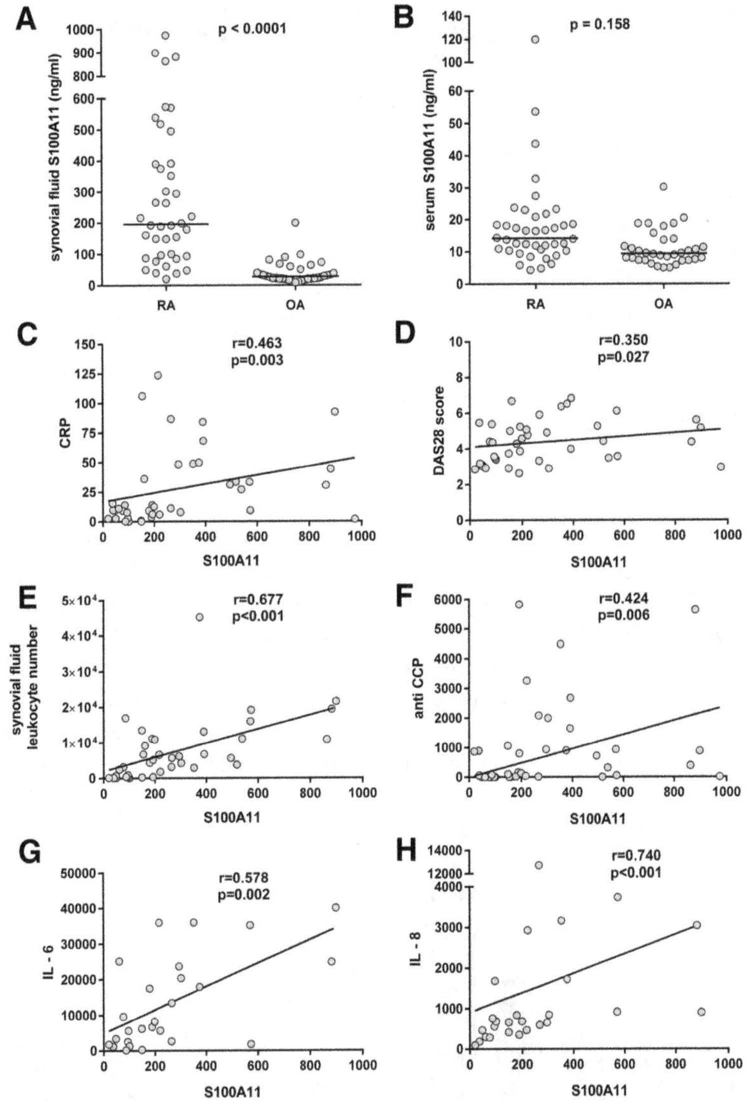

Fig. 3 S100A11 in serum and synovial fluid and its association with disease activity in rheumatoid arthritis (*RA*). Levels of S100A11 in the synovial fluid (**a**) but not in the serum (**b**) were up-regulated in patients with RA compared to patients with osteoarthritis (*OA*) when adjusted for age and sex. Levels of S100A11 in synovial fluid correlated with serum C-reactive protein (*CRP*) (**c**), disease activity score in 28 joints (*DAS28*) (**d**), synovial fluid leukocyte count (**e**), serum anti-cyclic citrullinated peptide antibodies (*anti-CCP*) (**f**), IL-6 (**g**) and IL-8 (**h**). The *horizontal line* represents the median

from selected cells. As shown by western blotting (Fig. 4a, b), S100A11 synthesis was up-regulated in PBMCs and SFs in patients with RA compared to the PBMCs and SFs in patients with OA. Consistent with these findings, we showed that PBMCs (3.12 ± 0.45 vs. 1.74 ± 0.18 ng/ml, $p = 0.011$) and SFs (1.34 ± 0.48 vs. 0.30 ± 0.06 ng/ml, $p = 0.054$) in patients with RA spontaneously released larger amounts of S100A11 into the cell culture supernatants than the cells did in patients with OA (Fig. 4c, d). Neither pro-inflammatory cytokines (IL-1β, IL-6 or TNF-α) nor LPS up-regulated the production of S100A11 by PBMCs or SFs above the spontaneous release (Additional file 3A, B). We have observed enhanced S100A11 release from SFs, but not PBMCs, upon poly I:C treatment (Additional file 3B).

S100A11 enhances pro-inflammatory cytokine release by peripheral blood mononuclear cells and synovial fibroblasts

Given the observed increases in S100A11 accumulation in patients with RA, we investigated the role of extracellular S100A11 in inflammation. PBMCs and SFs isolated from patients with RA were exposed to recombinant S100A11 for 24 h, and TNF-α, IL-1β, IL-6 and MCP-1 levels in the cell culture supernatants were analysed. S100A11 concentrations were selected based on the mean serum and synovial fluid protein levels of patients with OA or RA.

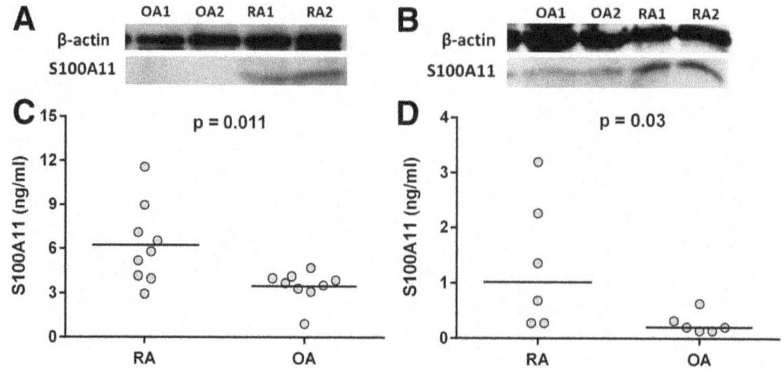

Fig. 4 Synthesis and release of S100A11 by peripheral blood mononuclear cells (PBMCs) and synovial fibroblasts (SFs). PBMCs and SFs from patients with rheumatoid arthritis (*RA*) synthesize (**a**, **b**) and spontaneously release (**c, d**) higher levels of S100A11 compared to the cells from patients with osteoarthritis (*OA*). Representative images of protein levels of S100A11 in PBMCs and SFs isolated from patients with RA ($n = 4$) and patients with OA ($n = 4$) by western blot

Exposure to recombinant S100A11 protein enhanced IL-6 release into the cell supernatant in a dose-dependent manner in PBMCs (1000 ng/ml: 33.51 (26.46–95.55), $p < 0.05$; 500 ng/ml: 25.63 (18.16–54.51), $p < 0.05$; 100 µg/ml: 16.92 (12.35–47.64), compared to unstimulated: 15.26 (9.82–39.76)) and synovial fibroblasts (1000 ng/ml: 281.6 (219.7–363.6), $p < 0.01$; 500 ng/ml: 245.3 (196.5–355.4), $p < 0.01$; 100 µg/ml: 195.2 (148.6–328.0), compared to unstimulated: 193.0 (90.08–279.0)) (Fig. 5a, b).

TNF-α production was significantly increased by exposure to higher S100A11 doses in PBMCs (1000 ng/ml: 206.5 (161.8–326.4) vs. unstimulated: 153.4 (110.7–190.0), $p < 0.01$), but not SFs (Fig. 5c, d). MCP-1 and IL-1β levels were not affected by S100A11 treatment in PBMCs or SFs (data not shown).

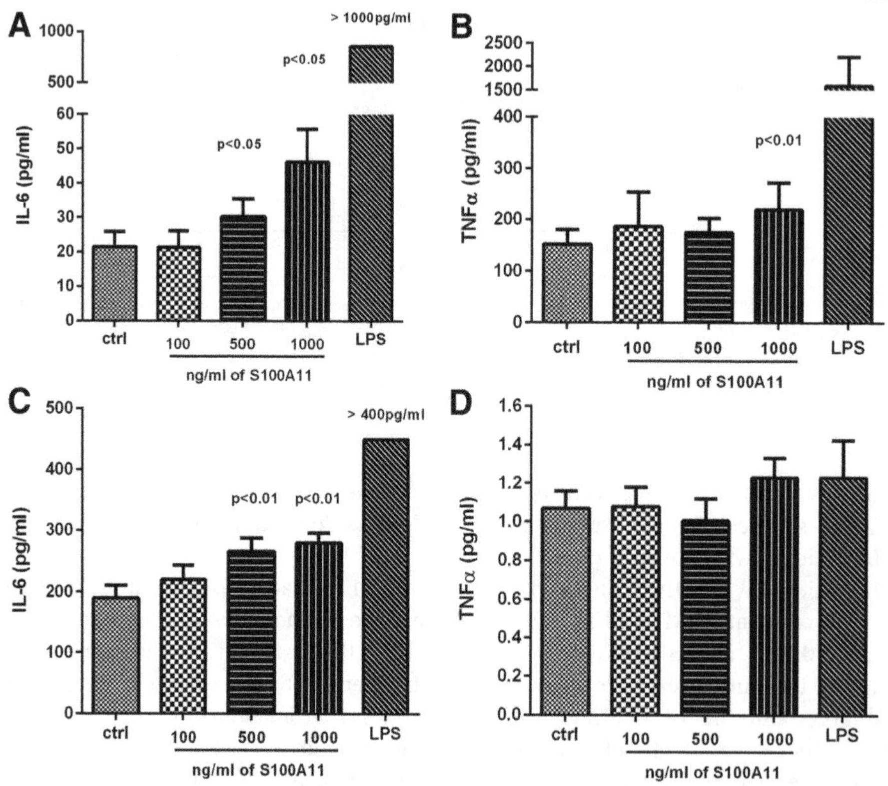

Fig. 5 Pro-inflammatory role of extracellular S100A11. S100A11 significantly enhances the release of IL-6 (**a**) and TNF-α (**b**) in peripheral blood mononuclear cells and IL-6 (**c**) in synovial fibroblasts (SFs). Levels of TNF-α were not changed in SFs treated with S100A11 protein (**d**). Protein levels in cell culture supernatants were measured after 24 h. The *horizontal line* represents the median. *Ctrl* control, *LPS* lipopolysaccharide

Discussion

In the present study, we demonstrated for the first time the up-regulation of S100A11 in patients with RA and the association between S100A11, inflammation and disease activity. Numerous studies have reported that specific members of the S100 protein family participate in immune response activation and inflammation in RA [24–27]; however, very little is known about the involvement of S100A11 in RA. The only indication of a link between S100A11 and RA was noted by Yu et al. [19], who described a rat model of adjuvant arthritis showing increased S100A11 expression during the early preclinical phase of experimental arthritis. Associations between S100A11 and low-grade inflammation and cartilage destruction have been previously described in OA [9, 18].

Here, we reported significant S100A11 accumulation in the synovial tissues of patients with RA, particularly in the synovial lining layer and inflammatory infiltrates. This finding corresponds with those of previous studies documenting the topography of other S100 proteins associated with RA [22, 24, 25]. Similar to S100A4 [22], S100A11 is strongly expressed by T cells and SFs, which therefore represent the main extracellular sources of S100A11 for the joint environment.

Consistent with the accumulation of S100A11 in RA synovial tissue was our finding of significantly elevated S100A11 expression in the synovial fluid and serum of patients with RA. The up-regulation of S100A11 in serum from patients with RA was somewhat less pronounced than the up-regulation of S100A11 in synovial fluid from patients with RA and was not significant when adjusted to age and sex. In addition, we observed no changes in serum S100A11 levels in patients with recent-onset RA compared to healthy controls (unpublished data). These findings imply that the joint microenvironment is a major source of S100A11 and that S100A11 could diffuse from the inflamed RA synovium into the circulation.

Interestingly, the serum and synovial fluid levels of S100A11 were markedly lower than the corresponding levels of other S100 family members involved in RA [22, 24, 25]. Nonetheless, synovial fluid S100A11 is significantly related to clinical disease activity in RA, reflecting a local, ongoing inflammatory process. Moreover, given the strong correlation between synovial fluid S100A11 levels and synovial fluid leukocyte count, we can speculate that the S100A11 levels may also be associated with the amount of immune cells within the inflamed synovial tissue. Accompanied by the correlation between synovial fluid S100A11 and the inflammatory status and with the synovial fluid cytokines (IL-6 and IL-8), these data further strengthen the hypothesis of S100A11 involvement in the local inflammatory process in RA. Indeed, S100A11 is significantly associated with IL-8 in synovial fluid in patients with OA. This is consistent with the up-regulation of S100A11 by human articular chondrocytes exposed to IL-8 and with its suggested role in low-grade local inflammation in OA (9). We also demonstrated association between S100A11 and anti-CCP autoantibodies and thereby with autoimmune response in RA, which is further supported by our observation of significantly higher levels of S100A11 in the synovial fluid of anti-CCP-positive compared to anti-CCP-negative patients.

Taken together, unlike other S100 proteins [24, 28–32], systemic levels of S100A11 cannot be considered a biomarker of disease activity. However the local up-regulation of S100A11 in the synovial compartment could reflect the inflammatory process and immune response in patients with RA.

In addition, we demonstrated increased S100A11 synthesis and spontaneous release by PBMCs and SFs in patients with RA. Active protein secretion has been described previously in chondrocytes [9] and keratinocytes [11]. However, in contrast to chondrocytes [9], treatment with pro-inflammatory cytokines does not up-regulate the production of S100A11 by PBMCs or SFs above the spontaneous release. This may be partly due to the lower reactivity of the chronically activated cells from patients with RA to an additional pro-inflammatory stimulus. However, in SFs exposed to the toll-like receptor 3 (TLR3) ligand poly (I:C) there were threefold increases in S100A11 production. As previously shown by Brentano et al., poly (I:C) and necrotic synovial fluid cells stimulate pro-inflammatory reactions in RA SFs via TLR3 [33].

It is likely that in RA, local destructive events in the synovial joints accompanied by the release of endogenous double stranded RNA (dsRNA) from necrotic cells can lead to the activation of tissue-resident SFs to release S100A11. On the other hand, our recent findings indicate no direct effect of S100A11 on the expression of matrix-degrading enzymes by SFs and thereby on joint destruction (data not shown). Moreover, by investigating the potential role of S100A11 as an extracellular regulatory molecule, we found that recombinant S100A11 when used in the same concentrations as in synovial fluid acts on both SFs and PBMCs to enhance IL-6 production and thus amplify inflammation. In line with that, synovial fluid levels of S100A11 correlated significantly with that of IL-6. However, it must be noted that the cytokine-like effects of S100A11 seem to be less potent than those of other S100 proteins involved in RA [26, 34]. Nevertheless, it is plausible that S100A11 in synovial fluid could enhance pro-inflammatory cytokine secretion to form a positive feedback loop in RA. The relative contributions of certain S100 proteins to the immune response in RA are different, and it is likely that S100A11 participates in several pathological processes in RA other than inflammation.

This study has some limitations. First, due to the cross-sectional study design, a longitudinal causal relationship between the modulation of S100A11 levels and changes in disease activity in time cannot be assessed. Moreover, a relatively small number of patients were enrolled in our study. Therefore, a long-term, large-scale, prospective study is warranted to further investigate the role of S100A11 in RA. Second, the relationship between histopathological scoring of levels of S100A11 in the synovium and synovial fluid could not be assessed because synovial tissue was collected from a different group of patients to those who underwent aspiration of a knee joint effusion. Similarly, the relationship between destruction in the joint at the sampling site and S100A11 levels in synovial fluid was not described because radiographic evaluation of affected knee was not available in these subjects. Third, we identified significant differences in the synthesis and release of S100A11 between RA and OA cells; however, in this study we have not focused on the determination of different conformational forms of S100A11 and their potential relationship with inflammation. Last, as other members of the S100 protein family are known to be involved in the pathogenesis of RA, further studies on their relationship and potential co-regulation with S100A11 would be extremely interesting. In spite of these limitations, this study provides novel data showing a link between S100A11 and inflammation in RA.

Conclusions

Taken together, our findings have provided us with novel insights into the involvement of S100A11 in the process of inflammation and pathogenesis of RA; however, its roles in the processes of joint inflammation and destruction seem to be complex and require further investigation.

Additional files

Additional file 1: The levels of S100A11 protein in serum and synovial fluid of seropositive and seronegative patients with RA. Values are presented as mean ± SD. *P* values were determined using the Mann-Whitney test. (JPG 59 kb)

Additional file 2: The levels of selected cytokines in the synovial fluid of patients with RA and OA. (JPG 82 kb)

Additional file 3: The release of S100A11 protein remains unchanged in PBMCs (**A**) upon the treatment with pro-inflammatory cytokines, LPS or poly I:C. Synovial fibroblasts up-regulate the release of S100A11 when stimulated with poly I:C (**B**). Protein levels in cell culture supernatants were measured after 24 h. The *horizontal line* represents the median. (TIF 85 kb)

Abbreviations

anti-CCP: Anti-cyclic citrullinated peptide antibodies; BMI: Body mass index; CRP: C-reactive protein; CXCL8: (C-X-C motif) ligand 8; DAS28: Disease activity score in 28 joints; DMARDs: disease-modifying antirheumatic drugs; DMEM: Dulbecco's modified Eagle's medium; ELISA: Enzyme immunoassay; ESR: Erythrocyte sedimentation rate; EULAR: European League Against Rheumatism; IgM-RF: IgM rheumatoid factor; IL: Interleukin; LPS: Lipopolysaccharide; MAPK: Mitogen-activated protein kinase; MCP-1: Monocyte chemotactic protein 1; MTX: Methotrexate; OA: Osteoarthritis; p21Cip1/WAF1: Cyclin-dependent kinase inhibitor 1; PBMC: Peripheral blood mononuclear cell; PBS: Phosphate-buffered saline; PCR: Polymerase chain reaction; poly I:C: Polyinosinic:polycytidylic acid; RA: Rheumatoid arthritis; RAGE: Receptor for advanced glycation end products; RIPA: Radioimmunoprecipitation assay; SD: Standard deviation; SEM: Standard error of the mean; SF: Synovial fibroblast; SJC: Swollen joints count; TLR: Toll-like receptor; TNF: Tumour necrosis factor

Acknowledgements

The authors would like to thank Růžena Paroubková and Anna Kozáková for excellent technical assistance.

Funding

This study was funded by grant 15-34065A of the Agency for Healthcare Research of the Czech Republic and by Research Project No. 023728 of the Ministry of Health of the Czech Republic.

Authors' contributions

LAC and LŠ were responsible for the study concept and design. LAC, BŠ and KP carried out the in vitro experiments and ELISAs and analysed the data. DV performed the biopsies of synovial tissues. DD performed the cytometric bead array. LAC and BŠ executed the immunohistochemistry and immunofluorescence experiments and western blotting. LAC carried out the statistical analysis. LAC, BŠ and DD were responsible for data interpretation and manuscript preparation. JV, LŠ, KP and CHN revised the manuscript and gave their final approval of the version to be published. All authors read and approved the final manuscript.

Competing interests

The authors declare that they have no competing interests.

Author details

[1]Institute of Rheumatology, Na Slupi 4, 12850 Prague, Czech Republic. [2]Department of Rheumatology, 1st Faculty of Medicine, Charles University, Prague, Czech Republic. [3]First Orthopaedic Clinic, 1st Faculty of Medicine, Charles University, Prague, Czech Republic. [4]Institute for Inflammation Research, Center for Rheumatology and Spine Diseases, Copenhagen University Hospital, Rigshospitalet, Copenhagen, Denmark.

References

1. McInnes IB, Schett G. Cytokines in the pathogenesis of rheumatoid arthritis. Nat Rev Immunol. 2007;7:42942.
2. Todoroki H, Kobayashi R, Watanabe M, Minami H, Hidaka H. Purification, characterization, and partial sequence analysis of a newly identified EF-hand type 13-kDa Ca(2+)-binding protein from smooth muscle and non-muscle tissues. J Biol Chem. 1991;266:18668–73.
3. Seemann J, Weber K, Gerke V. Annex I targets S100C to early endosomes. FEBS Lett. 1997;11(413):185–90.
4. Mailliard WS, Haigler HT, Schlaepfer DD. Calcium-dependent binding of S100C to the N-terminal domain of annexin I. J Biol Chem. 1996;12(271):719–25.
5. Seemann J, Weber K, Gerke V. Structural requirements for annexin I-S100C complex-formation. Biochem J. 1996;319:123–9.
6. Zhao XQ, Naka M, Muneyuki M, Tanaka T. Ca(2+)-dependent inhibition of actin-activated myosin ATPase activity by S100C (S100A11), a novel member of the S100 protein family. Biochem Biophys Res Commun. 2000;267:77–9.
7. Sakaguchi M, Miyazaki M, Inoue Y, Tsuji T, Kouchi H, Tanaka T, et al. Relationship between contact inhibition and intranuclear S100C of normal human fibroblasts. J Cell Biol. 2000;12(149):1193–206.
8. Makino E, Sakaguchi M, Iwatsuki K, Huh NH. Introduction of an N-terminal peptide of S100C/A11 into human cells induces apoptotic cell death. J Mol Med (Berl). 2004;82:612–20.

9. Cecil DL, Johnson K, Rediske J, Lotz M, Schmidt AM, Terkeltaub R. Inflammation-induced chondrocyte hypertrophy is driven by receptor for advanced glycation end products. J Immunol. 2005;175:8296–302.
10. Inada H, Naka M, Tanaka T, Davey GE, Heizmann CW. Human S100A11exhibits differential steady-state RNA levels in various tissues and a distinct subcellular localization. Biochem Biophys Res Commun. 1999;263:135–8.
11. Sakaguchi M, Sonegawa H, Murata H, Kitazoe M, Futami J, Kataoka K, et al. S100A11, a dual mediator for growth regulation of human keratinocytes. Mol Biol Cell. 2008;19:78–85.
12. Cross SS, Hamdy FC, Deloulme JC, Rehman I. Expression of S100 proteins normal human tissues and common cancers using tissue microarrays: S100A6, S100A8, S100A9 and S100A11 are all overexpressed in common cancers. Histopathology. 2005;46:256–69.
13. Broome AM, Eckert RL. Microtubule-dependent redistribution of a cytoplasmic cornified envelope precursor. J Invest Dermatol. 2004;122:29–38.
14. Salama I, Malone PS, Mihaimeed F, Jones JL. A review of the S100 proteins in cancer. Eur J Surg Oncol. 2008;34:357–64.
15. Sakaguchi M, Miyazaki M, Takaishi M, Sakaguchi Y, Makino E, Kataoka N, et al. S100C/A11 is a key mediator of Ca(2+)-induced growth inhibition of human epidermal keratinocytes. J Cell Biol. 2003;163:825–35.
16. Foertsch F, Teichmann N, Kob R, Hentschel J, Laubscher U, Melle C. S100A11 is involved in the regulation of the stability of cell cycle regulator p21(CIP1/WAF1) in human keratinocyte HaCaT cells. FEBS J. 2013;16:3840–53.
17. Amin AR, Islam AB. Genomic analysis and differential expression of HMG and S100A family in human arthritis: upregulated expression of chemokines, IL-8 and nitric oxide by HMGB1. DNA Cell Biol. 2014;33:550–65.
18. Cecil DL, Terkeltaub R. Transamidation by transglutaminase 2 transforms S100A11 calgranulin into a procatabolic cytokine for chondrocytes. J Immunol. 2008;180:8378–85.
19. Yu H, Lu C, Tan MT, Moudgil KD. The gene expression profile of preclinical autoimmune arthritis and its modulation by a tolerogenic disease-protective antigenic challenge. Arthritis Res Ther. 2011;13:R143.
20. Arnett FC, Edworthy SM, Bloch DA, McShane DJ, Fries JF, Cooper NS, et al. The American Rheumatism Association 1987 revised criteria for the classification of rheumatoid arthritis. Arthritis Rheum. 1988;31:315–24.
21. Damgaard D, Senolt L, Nielsen CH. Increased levels of peptidylarginine deiminase 2 in synovial fluid from anti-CCP-positive rheumatoid arthritis patients: association with disease activity and inflammatory markers. Rheumatology (Oxford). 2016;55:918–27.
22. Klingelhofer J, Senolt L, Baslund B, Nielsen GH, Skibshøj I, Pavelka K, et al. Up-regulation of metastasis-promoting S100A4 (Mts 1) in rheumatoid arthritis: putative involvement in the pathogenesis of RA. Arthritis Rheum. 2007;56:779–89.
23. Andrés Cerezo L, Kuklová M, Hulejová H, Vernerová Z, Pešáková V, Pecha O, Veigl D, Haluzík M, Pavelka K, Vencovský J, Senolt L. The level of fatty acid-binding protein 4, a novel adipokine, is increased in rheumatoid arthritis and correlates with serum cholesterol levels. Cytokine. 2013;64:441–7.
24. Foell D, Kane D, Bresnihan B, Vogl T, Nacken W, Sorg C, et al. Expression of the pro-inflammatory protein S100A12 (EN-RAGE) in rheumatoid and psoriatic arthritis. Rheumatology (Oxford). 2003;42:1383–9.
25. Sunahori K, Yamamura M, Yamana J, Takasugi K, Kawashima M, Yamamoto H, et al. The S100A8/A9 heterodimer amplifies proinflammatory cytokine production by macrophages via activation of nuclear factor kappa B and p38 mitogen-activated protein kinase in rheumatoid arthritis. Arthritis Res Ther. 2006;8:R69.
26. Cerezo LA, Remáková M, Tomčik M, Gay S, Neidhart M, Lukanidin E, et al. The metastasis-associated protein S100A4 promotes the inflammatory response of mononuclear cells via the TLR4 signalling pathway in rheumatoid arthritis. Rheumatology (Oxford). 2014;53:1520–6.
27. Oslejsková L, Grigorian M, Gay S, Neidhart M, Senolt L. The metastasis associated protein S100A4: a potential novel link to inflammation and consequent aggressive behaviour of rheumatoid arthritis synovial fibroblasts. Ann Rheum Dis. 2008;67:1499–504.
28. Oslejsková L, Grigorian M, Hulejová H, Vencovsky J, Pavelka K, Klingelhofer J, et al. Metastasis-inducing S100A4 protein is associated with the disease activity of rheumatoid arthritis. Rheumatology (Oxford). 2009;48:1590–4.
29. Andrés Cerezo L, Mann H, Pecha O, Pleštilová L, Pavelka K, Vencovsky J, et al. Decreases in serum levels of S100A8/9 (calprotectin) correlate with improvements in total swollen joint count in patients with recent-onset rheumatoid arthritis. Arthritis Res Ther. 2011;13:R122.
30. Hammer HB, Odegard S, Fagerhol MK, Landewé R, van der Heijde D, Uhlig T, et al. Calprotectin (a major leucocyte protein) is strongly and independently correlated with joint inflammation and damage in rheumatoid arthritis. Ann Rheum Dis. 2007;66:1093–7.
31. Hurnakova J, Zavada J, Hanova P, Hulejova H, Klein M, Mann H, et al. Serum calprotectin (S100A8/9): an independent predictor of ultrasound synovitis in patients with rheumatoid arthritis. Arthritis Res Ther. 2015;17:252.
32. Erlandsson MC, Forslind K, Andersson SE, Lund A, Bokarewa MI. Metastasin S100A4 is increased in proportion to radiographic damage in patients with RA. Rheumatology (Oxford). 2012;51:932–40.
33. Brentano F, Schorr O, Gay RE, Gay S, Kyburz D. RNA released from necrotic synovial fluid cells activates rheumatoid arthritis synovial fibroblasts via Toll-like receptor 3. Arthritis Rheum. 2005;52:2656–65.
34. Simard JC, Cesaro A, Chapeton-Montes J, Tardif M, Antoine F, Girard D, Tessier PA. PLoS One. S100A8 and S100A9 induce cytokine expression and regulate the NLRP3 inflammasome via ROS-dependent activation of NF-κB(1.). PLoS One. 2013;8:e72138.

8

Methotrexate upregulates circadian transcriptional factors PAR bZIP to induce apoptosis on rheumatoid arthritis synovial fibroblasts

Kohjin Suzuki[1], Kohsuke Yoshida[1], Takeshi Ueha[2], Kenta Kaneshiro[1], Ayako Nakai[1], Naonori Hashimoto[1], Koto Uchida[1], Teppei Hashimoto[3], Yoshiko Kawasaki[3], Nao Shibanuma[4], Natsuko Nakagawa[5], Yoshitada Sakai[2] and Akira Hashiramoto[1*]

Abstract

Background: Effects of methotrexate (MTX) on the proliferation of rheumatoid arthritis (RA) synovial fibroblasts are incompletely understood. We explored actions of MTX in view of circadian transcriptions of synovial fibroblasts.

Methods: Under treatment with MTX, expression of core circadian clock genes, circadian transcriptional factor proline and acidic amino acid-rich basic leucine zipper (PAR bZIP), and proapoptotic molecule Bcl-2 interacting killer (Bik) was examined by real-time polymerase chain reaction. Protein expression of circadian clock gene PERIOD2 (PER2) and CYTOCHROME C was also examined by western blotting and ELISA. Promoter activities of *Per2* and *Bik* were measured by Luciferase assay. Expression of PER2, BIK, and CYTOCHROME C and morphological changes of the nucleus were observed by fluorescent immunostaining. Synovial fibroblasts were transfected with *Per2/Bik* small interfering RNA, and successively treated with MTX to determine cell viabilities. Finally, synovial fibroblasts were treated with MTX according to the oscillation of *Per2/Bik* expression.

Results: MTX (10 nM) significantly decreased cell viabilities, but increased messenger RNA expression of *Per2, Bik*, and PAR ZIP including D site of the albumin promoter binding protein (*Dbp*), hepatic leukemia factor (*Hlf*), and thyrotroph embryonic factor (*Tef*). MTX also increased protein expression of PER2 and CYTOCHROME C, and promoter activities of *Per2* and *Bik via* D-box. Under fluorescent observations, expression of PER2, BIK, and CYTOCHROME C was increased in apoptotic cells. Cytotoxicity of MTX was attenuated by silencing of *Per2* and/or *Bik*, and revealed that MTX was significantly effective in situations where *Per2/Bik* expression was high.

Conclusions: We present here novel unique action of MTX on synovial fibroblasts that upregulates PAR bZIP to transcribe *Per2* and *Bik*, resulting in apoptosis induction. MTX is important in modulating circadian environments to understand a new aspect of pathogenesis of RA.

Keywords: Rheumatoid arthritis, Synovial fibroblasts, Methotrexate, Proline and acidic amino acid-rich basic leucine zipper, Period2, Bcl-2 interacting killer

* Correspondence: hash@med.kobe-u.ac.jp
[1]Department of Biophysics, Kobe University Graduate School of Health Sciences, Tomogaoka 7-10-2, Suma-ku, Kobe 654-0142, Japan
Full list of author information is available at the end of the article

Background

Methotrexate (MTX) is a folic acid antagonist widely used as an anchor drug in treating various cancers [1, 2], as well as rheumatoid arthritis (RA) [3]. For cancer cells, MTX competitively inhibits dihydrofolate reductase (DHFR) to block purine and pyrimidine biosynthesis, and thus it inhibits DNA replication and cell proliferation. For RA, low-dose MTX shows anti-inflammatory effects by inducing extracellular adenosine, which binds to adenosine receptors [4]. Moreover, it has been reported that MTX induced apoptosis in synovial fibroblasts in both *in-vivo* and *in-vitro* experiments [5]. Although MTX induced apoptosis in synovial fibroblast within 24–48 h [6, 7], the precise mechanism of how MTX expresses antiproliferative effects on synovial fibroblasts remains incompletely understood [8].

RA is a chronic arthritis characterized by 'tumor-like' synovial cell growth [9]. Another remarkable feature of RA is the circadian variation of disease-related symptoms, such as morning stiffness, increased production of proinflammatory cytokines at night time, and peaked secretion of immunoglobulin (Ig) A/IgM types of rheumatoid factor in the morning [10–15]. Since these rheumatic symptoms possess a daily rhythm, we have previously shown that the action of the biological clock was significantly disturbed in the mouse model of collagen antibody-induced arthritis [16] and that tumor necrosis factor (TNF)-α significantly disturbed the oscillation of biological clocks of synovial fibroblasts [17]. Fibroblasts usually demonstrate daily rhythms of circadian clock, while Haas *et al.* [18] pointed out that the expression rhythm of clock genes disappears in RA synovial fibroblasts presumably due to prolonged inflammation.

The circadian rhythm in human cells is mainly regulated by the core clock genes, including circadian locomotor output cycles kaput (*Clock*), brain and muscle Rant-like protein-1 (*Bmal1*), period (*Per*), and cryptochrome (*Cry*) [19–22]. The circadian transcriptional factor proline and acidic amino acid-rich basic leucine zipper (PAR bZIP) includes the D site of the albumin promoter binding protein (*Dbp*), hepatic leukemia factor (*Hlf*), and thyrotroph embryonic factor (*Tef*). PAR bZIP regulates gene expression by binding to a consensus sequence of D-box (5′-TTAXGTAA-3′; X = T or C) on the promoter region [23–25]. It has been reported that PAR bZIP can regulate the transcription of *Per2* gene by binding two D-box sequences existing on its promoter (D-box 1, 5′-TTATG TAA-3′, −372 to −365; and D-box 2, 5′-TTACGTAA-3′, −47 to −40) [24]. In contrast, E4-binding protein 4 (*E4bp4*) also binds to the D-box to suppress the transcription of *Per2* [26–28] (see Additional file 1).

It is noted that Bcl-2 interacting killer (Bik) possesses D-box (5′-TTAAGTCA-3′, −285 to −277) on its promoter region [28], resembling the arrangement of *Per2* genes. Bik, a member of the BH3-only subfamily, acts as an important signaling molecule upstream of the Bcl-2 and Bax subfamily [29]. The BCL-2 family has been known to be central players in regulating physiological activities of mitochondria, with Bcl-2, Bcl-xL, and Mcl-1 suppressing mitochondria-related apoptosis, whereas Bax and Bak induce it. Among these, Bik directly binds to these family proteins to induce apoptosis [29, 30].

In this study, we explored novel pharmacological effects of MTX on circadian clock genes and apoptosis induction in RA synovial fibroblasts.

Methods

Synovial fibroblast culture

Synovial tissues were obtained from RA patients (eight females and two males; aged 59.3 ± 3.4 years) during joint surgery. Eight of 10 patients took methotrexate and their average dosage was 7.4 ± 1.4 mg/week (Table 1) (see Additional file 2). This study has been approved by the ethics committee of Kobe University Graduate School of Health Sciences (#579–1) and Kobe Kaisei Hospital (#0072), in accordance with the Declaration of Helsinki. Written informed consent was obtained from each patient before study enrolment. Tissues were minced and treated with 2 mg/ml collagenase (Wako, Tokyo, Japan) in serum-free Dulbecco's modified Eagle's medium (DMEM; Nissui, Tokyo, Japan) at 37 °C for 1 h. Primary cultured synovial cell lines were established and maintained in DMEM including 10% heat-inactivated fetal bovine serum (FBS; Thermo, Waltham, MA, USA), 1% penicillin–streptomycin (100 U/ml; Life Technologies, Carlsbad, CA, USA),

Table 1 Characterization of patients

Characteristic	Value
Patients (*n*)	10
Age (years)	59.3 ± 3.4
Sex (female/male)	8/2
Disease duration (years)	22.7 ± 3.2
C-reactive protein (mg/dl)	1.2 ± 0.4
DAS28-ESR	2.6 ± 0.4
Methotrexate (mg/week)	7.4 ± 1.4
Methylprednisolone (mg)	3.7 ± 0.9
Other DMARDs	
Adalimumab	2/10
Tocilizumab	2/10
Tacrolimus	2/10 (2, 1.5 mg)
Etanercept	2/10
Infliximab	1/10
None	2/10

and 1% L-glutamine (2 mM; Life Technologies), in a humidified incubator at 37 °C in the presence of 5% CO_2. Harvested cells were continuously cultured to obtain synovial fibroblasts, and cells of passages 3–6 were used in the entire experiments.

Synchronization of synovial fibroblasts by serum shock

Synovial fibroblasts were incubated in 50% horse serum and incubated for 2 h to synchronize the expression of clock genes [17, 31].

Cell viability assay

Synovial fibroblasts (3.0×10^3 cells) were cultured in serum-free DMEM with or without MTX (1, 10, and 100 nM, 1 μM; Sigma Aldrich, St. Louis, MO, USA). After incubating for 24–72 h, cell viabilities were measured as the 450-nm absorbance of reduced WST-8 (2-(2-methoxy-4-nitrophenyl)-3-(4-nitriphenyl)–5-(2, 4-disulphonyl)-2H–tetrazolium, monosodium salt) using the Cell Counting Kit-8 (Dojindo, Kumamoto, Japan). The values were represented relative to MTX-untreated cells (control).

Real-time polymerase chain reaction

Synovial fibroblasts (8.0×10^4 cells) were cultured in serum-free DMEM with or without MTX (10, 100 nM) for 24–32 h. After incubation, total RNA was extracted using the RNeasy Mini Kit (QIAGEN, Hilden, Germany). Then, reverse transcription was performed with the ReverTra Ace® qPCR RT Kit (Toyobo, Osaka, Japan) and analyzed on the StepOnePlus™ Real-Time PCR System (Applied Biosystems, Foster City, CA, USA). The TaqMan probes used were: Hs00154147_m1 for *Bmal1*, Hs00231857_m1 for *Clock*, Hs00256143_m1 for *Per2*, Hs00172734_m1 for *Cry1*, Hs00609747_m1 for *Dbp*, Hs00171406_m1 for *Hlf*, Hs01115720_m1 for *Tef*, Hs00993282_m1 for *E4bp4*, Hs00154189_m1 for *Bik*, and Hs00427621_m1 for TATA box binding protein (*Tbp*). Expression levels were normalized to *Tbp*.

Western blotting

Synovial fibroblasts (5.0×10^5 cells) were cultured in serum-free DMEM with or without MTX (10, 100 nM) for 24–48 h, and lysed with RIPA buffer (Wako) to obtain cytoplasmic proteins. Samples were subjected to sodium dodecyl sulfate polyacrylamide gel electrophoresis (SDS-PAGE), transferred to polyvinylidene difluoride (PVDF) membrane (Millipore, Bedford, MA, USA), probed with antibodies, and developed by ImmunoStar® LD (Wako). Antibodies (Abs) used were: anti-PER2 Ab (sc-101,105; Santa Cruz, Dallas, TX, USA), anti-CYTOCHROME C Ab (ab13575; Abcam, Cambridge, UK), anti-BIK Ab (NB100–56109; Novus, Littleton, CO, USA), anti-Actin Ab (sc-1616; Santa Cruz), anti-mouse IgG Ab (NA9310; GE Healthcare, Chicago, IL, USA), and anti-rabbit IgG Ab (NA9340; GE Healthcare).

ELISA for PER2 and CYTOCHROME C

Synovial fibroblasts (3.0×10^3 cells) were cultured in serum-free DMEM with or without MTX (10, 100 nM) for 32–48 h, and protein expression of PER2 and CYTOCHROME C was measured by the In Cell ELISA test kit (3440–02; Thermo). Antibodies were as already described.

Luciferase reporter gene construction

Genomic DNA was obtained from RA synovial fibroblasts and amplified by PCR to generate the luciferase reporters. The primer pairs used for amplifying human *Bik* promoter containing D-box (−780 to +176) were 5′-TGGCCTAACTGGCCGTAAACAAGCTTTGCCGTGC-3′ (forward) and 5′-CGCCGAGGCCAGATCATGCTGGCAGCGTCTGTA-3′ (reverse). The primer pairs used for amplifying human *Bik* promoter without D-box (−260 to + 323) were 5′-TGGCCTAACTGGCCGCCTCTTGGAGCCTCGGTT-3′ (forward) and 5′-CGCCGAGGCCAGATCTTGCTGGAGCGGTAAAACC-3′ (reverse). The *KpnI* recognition sequence was added to the 5′ ends of forward primers and the *BglII* recognition sequence was added to the 5′ ends of reverse primers. The PCR products were cloned into the *KpnI* and *BglII* site of the pGL4.10 (luc2) vector (Promega, Madison, WI, USA) using In-Fusion® HD Cloning Plus (Takara, Shiga, Japan). The luciferase reporters containing *Per2* promoters were generated with reference to Yoshida *et al.* [17]. D-box motifs of *Per2* promoter were mutated from 5′-TTATGTAA-3′ to 5'-CGCCAGGC-3′ (−372 to −365) and from 5′-TTACGTAA-3′ to 5′-CAGCGTAA-3′ (−47 to −40) (see Additional file 3).

Transient transfection and luciferase reporter assay

Synovial fibroblasts (4×10^4 cells) were transfected with 500 ng of the pGL4.10 (luc2) vector containing various *Per2* and *Bik* promoters using Lipofectamine 3000 Transfection Reagent (Thermo). As an internal control, 35 ng of pRL-TK (Promega) containing the herpes simplex virus thymidine kinase promoter driving Renilla luciferase was cotransfected. After 24 h of incubation for transfection, cells were treated with 10 and 100 nM MTX for 24 h, and analyzed for luciferase activity using the Dual-Luciferase Reporter Assay (Promega). Activities of both firefly and Renilla luciferases were measured, and the activity of firefly luciferase was normalized by Renilla luciferase. The values were shown as relative variations to MTX-untreated cells.

Fluorescent immunostaining

Synovial fibroblasts (6.0×10^3 cells) were cultured in serum-free DMEM with or without MTX (10 nM) for 24 h. Then, cells were fixed with 4% formaldehyde, stained with anti-PER2 Ab, anti-BIK Ab, anti-CYTOCHROME C Ab, anti-mouse IgG (H + L), $F(ab')_2$ Fragment (Alexa Fluor® 594

Conjugate) (#8890; Cell Signaling Technology, Danvers, MA, USA), anti-rabbit IgG (H + L), F(ab′)$_2$ Fragment (Alexa Fluor® 488 Conjugate) (#4412; Cell Signaling Technology), and DAPI (0.5 μg/ml; Sigma, St. Louis, MO, USA). Protein expression and morphological changes of the nucleus were examined under fluorescence microscopy.

RNA interference

Per2 small interfering (si) RNA (s16931; Life Technologies) and *Bik* siRNA (s1990; Life Technologies) were transfected into synovial fibroblasts (3.0 × 10^3 cells) using Lipofectamine™ RNAiMAX (Life Technologies) for 48 h. Noncoding siRNA (4,390,843; Life Technologies) was also used as controls. After that, cells were cultured in serum-free DMEM with 10 nM of MTX for 24 h to measure cell viabilities using the Cell Counting Kit-8. The viabilities were represented relative to those of noncoding siRNA without MTX treatment.

Statistical analyses

In dynamite-plunger plots, values were expressed as the mean ± standard error of the mean (SEM). In boxplots, values were expressed with 10th, 25th, 50th (median), 75th, and 90th percentiles, and the single values were superimposed on the boxplots using black symbols.

For statistical analyses, a one-sample Kolmogorov–Smirnov test was used to test the normality, A one-sample *t* test was used to compare one single control value and others, a paired *t* test was used to compare differences between two experimental groups, the Tukey test was used to compare differences between more than three experimental groups, and Dunnett's test was used to compare differences between the control and others. All statistical tests were two-sided and $p < 0.05$ was considered statistically significant.

The statistical analyses were performed by EZR, based on R and R commander [32].

Results

MTX inhibited viabilities of synovial fibroblasts

We first examined the effect of MTX on viabilities of synovial fibroblasts. A lower concentration of MTX (1, 10 nM) significantly decreased cell viabilities, while cell viability was relatively weak with a higher concentration of MTX (100 nM, 1 μM) (Fig. 1). Since 10 or 100 nM was the optimum MTX concentration in human sera [33], experiments were subsequently conducted with MTX 10 nM treatment as an appropriate effective concentration and a concentration of 100 nM as a less-effective control.

MTX accelerated the expression of circadian clock gene *Per2*

We next determined the effect of MTX on expressions of circadian clock genes. Under treatment with MTX (10 nM for 24 h), the expression of *Per2* messenger RNA (mRNA) was significantly increased, while expression of *Bmal1, Clock,* and *Cry1* mRNA was not. In contrast, under treatment with MTX (100 nM for 24 h), the expression of *Per2* did not show any significant differences, while the expression of *Clock* and *Cry1* significantly decreased (Fig. 2a). In accordance with this, the expression of PER2 protein was significantly increased by 10 nM of MTX for 32 h, but not by 100 nM (Fig. 2b, c).

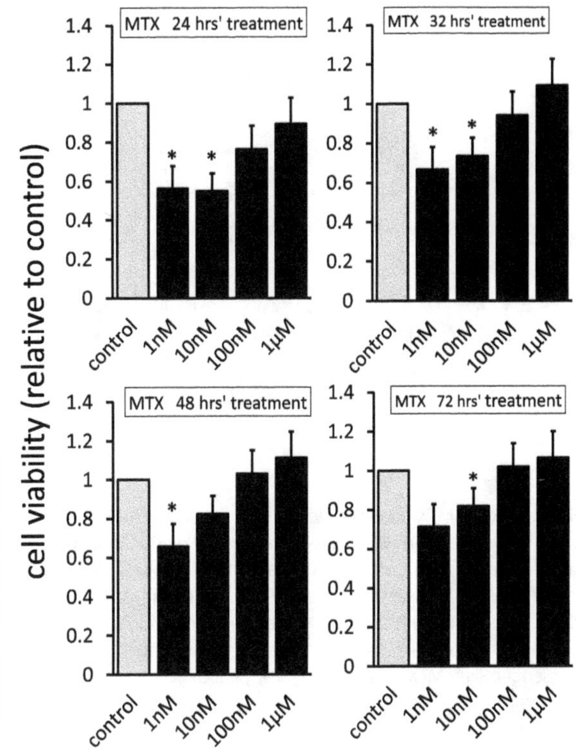

Fig. 1 Cell viabilities of MTX-treated synovial fibroblasts. Cells treated with MTX (1, 10, and 100 nM, and 1 μM) or control media for 24–72 h. Cell viabilities of MTX-untreated cells defined as 1.0, and each value shown relative to control. Values are mean ± SEM. *$p < 0.05$ *vs* control, $n = 5$. MTX methotrexate

MTX increased the expression of PAR bZIP and *Bik*

The circadian transcriptional factor PAR bZIP (*Dbp, Tef,* and *Hlf*) and *E4bp4* genes regulate *Per2* gene expression by binding to D-box on the promoter region [23–28]. We therefore examined the effect of MTX on the mRNA expression of *Dbp, Tef, Hlf,* and *E4bp4*. Expression of *Dbp, Tef,* and *Tef* mRNA was significantly increased by 10 nM MTX treatment for 24 h, while *E4bp4* mRNA expression was not. However, expression of *Dbp* and *E4bp4* significantly decreased with 100 nM of MTX treatment (Fig. 3a).

Next, we examined the mRNA expression of the proapoptotic factor *Bik,* since the PAR bZIP-binding site also exists on the promoter region of *Bik* [29]. As shown in

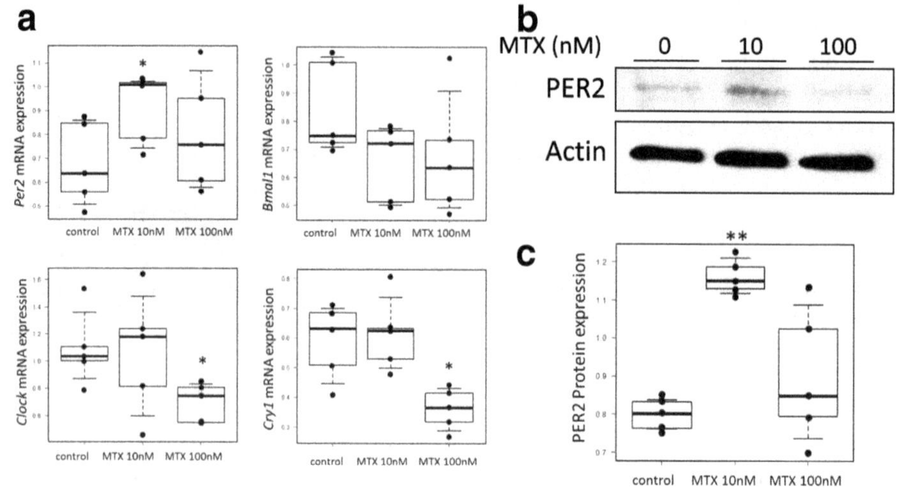

Fig. 2 Effect of MTX on expression of core circadian clock genes in synovial fibroblasts. **a** Cells treated with MTX (10, 100 nM) or control media for 24 h to measure mRNA expression of *Per2, Bmal1, Clock,* and *Cry1*. Values given with 10th, 25th, 50th (median), 75th, and 90th percentiles and single values superimposed on the boxplots using black symbols. $^*p < 0.05$ *vs* control, $n = 5$. **b** Cells treated with MTX (10, 100 nM) or control media for 32 h to observe PER2 expression. **c** Cells treated with MTX (10, 100 nM) or control media for 32 h to measure PER2 expression by ELISA. Values given with 10th, 25th, 50th (median), 75th, and 90th percentile and single values superimposed on the boxplots using black symbols. $^{**}p < 0.01$ vs control, $n = 5$. Bmal1 brain and muscle Arnt-like protein-1, Clock circadian locomotor output cycles kaput, Cry cryptochrome, mRNA messenger RNA, MTX methotrexate, Per period

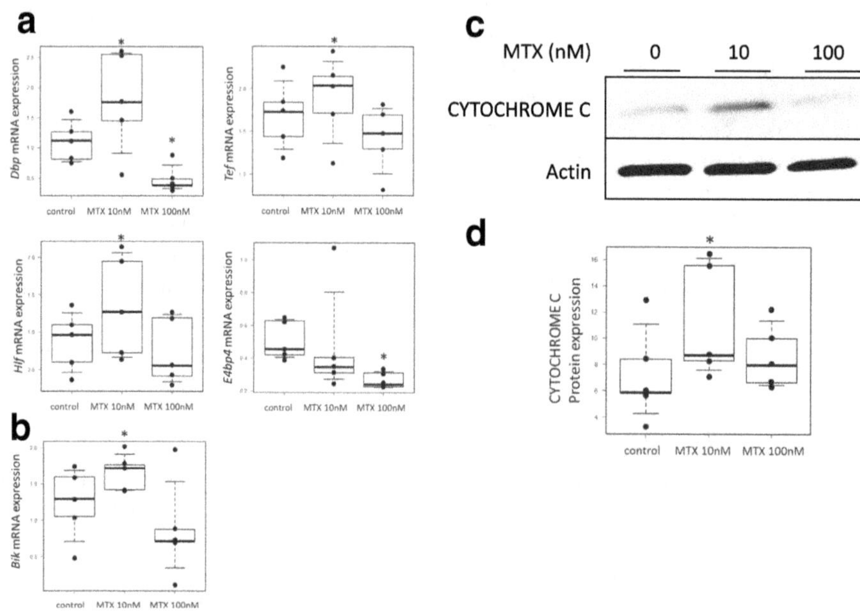

Fig. 3 Effect of MTX on expression of circadian transcriptional factors PAR bZIP and *Bik* in synovial fibroblasts. **a** Cells treated with MTX (10, 100 nM) or control media for 24 h to measure expression of PAR bZIP gene mRNA (*Dbp, Tef,* and *Hlf*) and *E4bp4*. Values given with 10th, 25th, 50th (median), 75th, and 90th percentiles and single values superimposed on boxplots using black symbols. $^*p < 0.05$ *vs* control, $n = 5$. **b** Cells treated with MTX (10, 100 nM) or control media for 24 h to measure expression of *Bik* gene mRNA. Values given with 10th, 25th, 50th (median), 75th, and 90th percentiles and single values superimposed on boxplots using black symbols. $^*p < 0.05$ *vs* control, $n = 5$. **c** Cells treated with MTX (10, 100 nM) or control media for 48 h to observe CYTOCHROME C expression. **d** Cells treated with MTX (10, 100 nM) or control media for 48 h to measure CYTOCHROME C expression by ELISA. Values given with 10th, 25th, 50th (median), 75th, and 90th percentiles and single values superimposed on boxplots using black symbols. $^*p < 0.05$ vs control, $n = 5$. Bik Bcl-2 interacting killer, Dbp D site of the albumin promoter binding protein, E4bp4 E4-binding protein 4, Hlf hepatic leukemia factor, mRNA messenger RNA, MTX methotrexate, Tef thyrotroph embryonic factor

Fig. 3b, the expression of *Bik* mRNA was significantly increased by 10 nM of MTX treatment for 32 h.

Finally, we observed cytosolic release of CYTOCHROME C since Bik interacted with BCL-2 family proteins to induce mitochondria-related apoptosis. As a result, expression of CYTOCHROME C was increased by 10 nM of MTX treatment for 48 h, but not by 100 nM (Fig. 3c, d).

Transcription of *Per2* and *Bik* was enhanced *via* D-box

To examine the roles of PAR bZIP in the transcription of *Per2* and *Bik*, we transfected luciferase reporters, constructed with or without D-box, to synovial fibroblasts. With 10 nM of MTX treatment for 24 h, D-box(+) *Per2* promoter activity was significantly increased as compared to those of the control and D-box(−) *Per2* promoter. By 100 nM of MTX treatment, D-box(−) *Per2* promoter activity was significantly decreased as compared to that of the control. *Bik* promoter activity was significantly increased after 10 nM of MTX treatment, and was higher than that of D-box(−) *Bik* promoter (Fig. 4).

PER2, BIK, and CYTOCHROME C were highly expressed in apoptotic cells

To certify the specific expression of *Per2* and *Bik* on MTX-induced apoptotic synovial fibroblasts, we used fluorescent immunostaining to examine expressions of PER2, BIK, and CYTOCHROME C and, simultaneously, morphological changes of nucleus. As a result, nuclear blebbing, shrinkage, or fragmentation were observed indicating that MTX (10 nM for 24 h) could induce cell death. PER2 was overexpressed on apoptotic cells, but not on cells with normal appearance (Fig. 5a). BIK and CYTOCHROME C were also overexpressed specifically on the apoptotic cells (Fig. 5b).

Per2 and *Bik* are critical genes for MTX-induced apoptosis

To confirm whether PER2 and BIK were responsible for MTX-induced cell death, *Per2* and *Bik* siRNA were transfected into synovial fibroblasts to examine cell viabilities. As shown in Fig. 6a, cytotoxicity of MTX was attenuated by silencing of *Per2* and *Bik*, independently and synergistically.

When we examined the long-term expression of *Per2* and *Bik* mRNA (Fig. 6b), they gradually increased from 8 h until 24 or 32 h after synchronized circadian oscillations by serum shock, consistent with our previous report that the expression of *Per2* on synovial fibroblasts was increased after synchronization and peaked at 24 h [17]. Since these genes were responsible for MTX-induced cell death, synovial fibroblasts were separately treated by 10 nM of MTX at 0–8 h (the lower *Per2/Bik* expression period) and at 24–32 h (the higher *Per2/Bik* expression period), and viabilities of synovial fibroblasts were again measured. As shown in Fig. 6c, the reduction rate of cell viabilities was

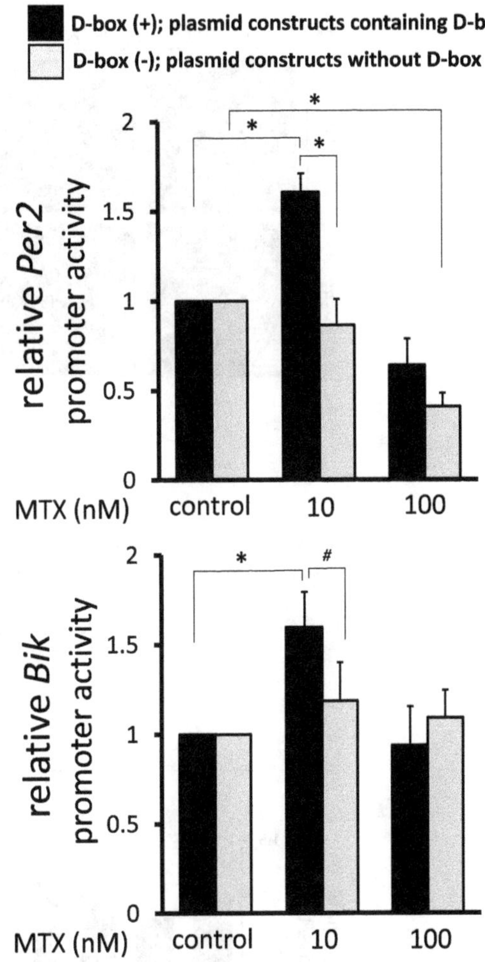

Fig. 4 Promoter activities of *Per2* and *Bik* under MTX treatment. Synovial fibroblasts transfected with vectors containing various *Per2* or *Bik* promoters for 24 h. After treatment with MTX (10, 100 nM) or control media for 24 h, luciferase reporter assay was performed. Promoter activities of MTX-untreated cells defined as 1.0, and each value shown relative to control. Values are mean ± SEM. **p* < 0.05, #*p* < 0.1, *n* = 5 (*Per2*), *n* = 6 (*Bik*). Bik Bcl-2 interacting killer, MTX methotrexate, Per period

significantly increased by 24–32 h of MTX treatment compared with 0–8 h of treatment, depending on the expression levels of *Per2* and *Bik*.

Discussion

We present here a novel pharmacological action of MTX in the viewpoint of circadian clock genes, circadian transcriptional factor PAR bZIP, and proapoptotic molecule Bik. In addition, a crucial mechanism of MTX-induced apoptosis on rheumatoid synovial fibroblasts was further traced.

In this study, the effect of MTX on cell viabilities did not show a concentration-dependent manner, with a wide range of MTX concentrations from 1 nM to 1 μM. In addition to our result, we found that MTX concentrations lower than 1 nM did not decrease cell viability (see Additional file 4). MTX is transferred almost equally to synovial fluid and sera,

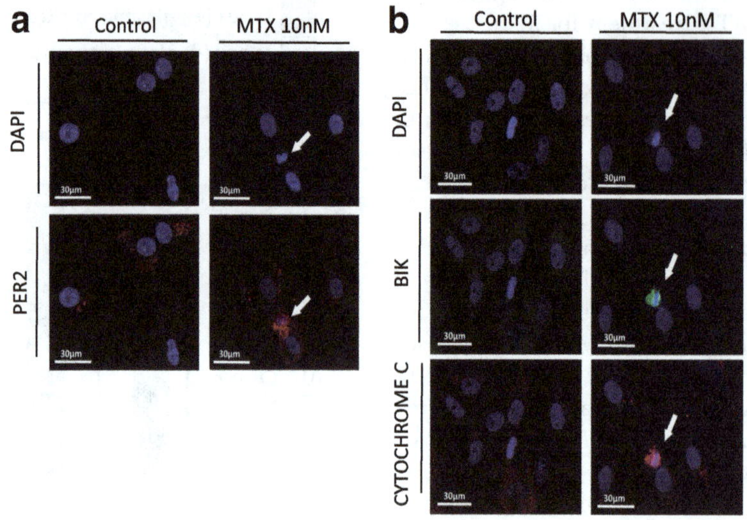

Fig. 5 PER2, BIK, and CYTOCHROME C expression and morphological changes of the nucleus. **a** Cells stained with DAPI and anti-PER2 Ab after treatment with MTX (10, 100 nM) or control media for 24 h. Arrowheads indicate apoptotic cells. **b** Cells stained with DAPI, anti-BIK Ab, and anti-CYTOCHROME C Ab after treatment with MTX (10, 100 nM) or control media for 24 h. Arrowheads indicate apoptotic cells. Bik Bcl-2 interacting killer, DAPI 4′,6-diamidino-2-phenylindole, MTX methotrexate, Per period

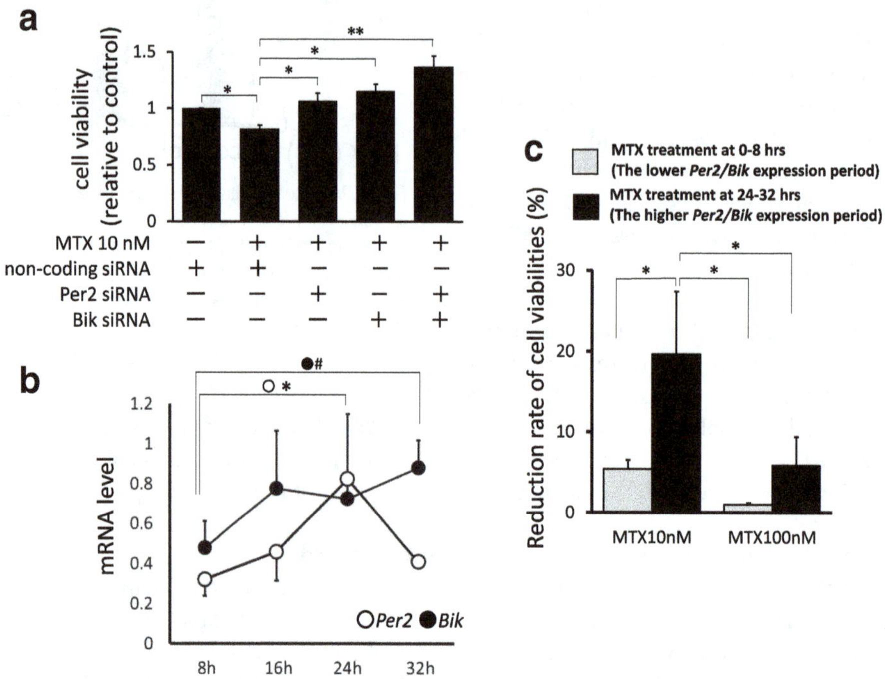

Fig. 6 Cell viabilities after RNA interfering of *Per2* and *Bik*, and long-term expression of *Per2* and *Bik* mRNA under MTX treatment. **a** After transfection with *Per2* or *Bik* siRNA, cells treated with MTX (10, 100 nM) or control media for 24 h to measure cell viabilities. Cell viabilities of control (MTX-untreated cells) defined as 1.0, and each value shown relative to control. Values are mean ± SEM. $*p < 0.05$, $**p < 0.01$, $n = 5$. **b** Long-term expression of *Per2* and *Bik*. After 8, 16, 24, and 32 h of culture in serum-free media, mRNA was extracted from synovial fibroblasts to measure expressions of *Per2* and *Bik*. Values are mean ± SEM. $*p < 0.05$, $\#p < 0.1$, $n = 5$. **c** Reduction rate of cell viabilities under time-dependent MTX treatments. Viabilities of synovial fibroblasts after treatment with 10 nM of MTX at 0–8 h (lower *Per2/Bik* expression period) or 24–32 h (higher *Per2/Bik* expression period) measured, respectively. Cell viabilities of MTX-untreated cells defined as 100%, and values are mean ± SEM. $*p < 0.05$, $n = 5$. Bik Bcl-2 interacting killer, mRNA messenger RNA, MTX methotrexate, Per period

and the concentration of MTX in human sera can reach 200 nM at the peak and immediately decreases to less than 10 nM [33], although pharmacological effects on cytotoxicity or cellular viability may not necessarily increase in a concentration-dependent manner. As reported previously, viabilities of human lymphoblastic leukemia cells and epithelial cells of rat decreased in a concentration-dependent manner at low MTX concentrations, but did not show a significant decrease at high MTX concentrations [34, 35]. Moreover, MTX did not affect viability in a concentration-dependent manner on T cells and RA synovial fibroblasts, in contrast to those of dose dependency observed in osteoarthritis synovial fibroblasts [6, 36]. Thus, further studies are required for the action of MTX correlated with drug dosage or cell types.

Since MTX concentrations below 100 nM were conceivable in sera of RA patients, we next focused on the effect of MTX on circadian clock genes and circadian transcriptional factor PAR bZIP genes and their relations to mitochondria-related apoptosis of synovial fibroblasts.

Since circadian clock genes were reported to be closely related to the pathogenesis of arthritis [16, 37] and excessive expression of *Per2* could induce apoptosis [38], we examined the effect of MTX on expression of *Per2*, *Bmal1*, *Clock*, and *Cry1* that were regarded as "core" clock genes [20–22]. We examined mRNA expression of circadian clock genes over time, and found that the controls and 10/100 nM of MTX showed almost the same expression rhythms, and MTX influenced their expression levels (see Additional file 5).

As described, both *Per2* and *Bik* genes have D-box in their promoter regions, and PAR bZIP proteins regulate the expression of these genes by binding to D-box [24, 39]. Indeed, promoter activities of *Per2* and *Bik* were upregulated by 10 nM of MTX when the D-box sequence exists and were cancelled without D-box. Moreover, both PER2 and BIK were highly expressed in MTX-induced apoptotic cells, while inhibitions of *Per2* and *Bik* synergistically attenuated the effect of MTX on cellular viabilities. As it has been reported that PAR bZIP and Bik mediate oxidative stress-induced apoptosis in fibroblasts [39], we consider *Per2* and *Bik* as essential factors for MTX-dependent synovial cell death and propose here that two independent pathways can mediate these death signals: the PAR bZIP–*Per2* transcriptional pathway and the PAR bZIP–*Bik* transcriptional pathway (see Additional file 6). However, as shown in Fig. 2a, downregulation of *Clock* and *Cry1* appeared to be less effective on cell viabilities after treatment with 100 nM of MTX. Further *in-vivo* study should be required for clinical application by investigating the cross-talk of clock genes.

Last, because of the similarity of their promoter region containing D-box, we supposed *Bik* might show oscillation as has been reported for *Per2* [17, 31]. For the further understanding of circadian manifestation in rheumatoid arthritis, we showed that the expression of *Bik*, as well as *Per2*, was gradually increased from 8 h until 24 or 32 h, and MTX was significantly effective in situations when *Per2* and *Bik* were highly expressed. It has been reported that administration of MTX at bedtime, as an optimal dosing time associated with the oscillation of TNF-α production, could reduce the disease activities of patients with RA [40, 41]. Thus, we considered that expression levels of *Per2* and *Bik* could also be a critical biomarker for chronotherapy of MTX not only for RA, but also for other diseases such as acute lymphocytic leukemia, non-Hodgkin's lymphoma, osteosarcoma, and breast cancer, in accordance with a previous report that circadian clock genes could be a biomarker for chronotherapy [42].

Conclusions

We propose here that MTX induces apoptosis in synovial fibroblasts through the binding of PAR bZIP to D-box of two different genes, *Per2 and Bik*, and these dual pathways work independently but synergistically. In consequence, MTX acts as a modulator of circadian environments of synovial fibroblasts in relation to biological clock genes and circadian transcriptional factors.

Additional files

Additional file 1: The interactions of circadian clock genes and its relative factors. BMAL/CLOCK and PER/CRY create the circadian rhythm via E-box, and DBP, TEF, HLF, E4BP4 via D-box. BMAL and CLOCK heterodimerize and bind to E-box elements on promoter regions of Per and Cry genes to induce their transcription. Thereafter, PER and CRY proteins heterodimerize to inhibit activities of their own and other E-box regulated promoters. (PDF 214 kb)

Additional file 2: Detailed information of patients with RA enrolled in this study. Joint samples obtained from 10 different patients to establish primary cultured synovial fibroblast cell lines. Age, sex, disease duration, CRP, DAS28-ESR, and treatment with MTX, PSL, and other DMARDs shown in the table. (PDF 252 kb)

Additional file 3: Plasmid constructs of *Per2/Bik* promoter. D-box(+), plasmid constructs containing D-box. D-box(−), plasmid constructs without D-box. D-box motifs of Per2 promoter were mutated from 5′-TTATGTAA-3′ to 5′-CGCCAGGC-3′ (−372 to −365), and 5′-TTACGTAA-3′ to 5′-CAGCGTAA-3′ (−47 to −40). Human Bik promoter containing D-box (−780 to +176) and human Bik promoter without D-box (−260 to +323) constructed. (PDF 215 kb)

Additional file 4: Cell viability of MTX-treated fibroblasts. Cell viability of RA synovial fibroblasts measured by WST-8 assay after 24 h of stimulation of MTX (1 pM to 1 μM). MTX (1 and 10 nM) significantly decreased cell viability as shown in Fig. 1, while 1–100 pM of MTX did not. (PDF 274 kb)

Additional file 5: The mRNA expression of circadian clock genes over time. mRNA expression of circadian clock genes measured at −4 h (before synchronization), 0 h (just before MTX stimulation), 24 h, 32 h, and 48 h. Controls and 10/100 nM of MTX showed almost the same expression rhythms, and MTX influenced their expression levels. (PDF 264 kb)

Additional file 6: Two different transcriptional pathways by which MTX induces apoptosis to synovial fibroblasts: PAR bZIP–*Per2* transcriptional pathway and PAR bZIP–*Bik* transcriptional pathway. We propose MTX induces apoptosis in synovial cells through activated binding of PAR bZIP to D-box in two different genes, *Per2* and *Bik*, and these dual pathways work independently but synergistically. (PDF 206 kb)

Abbreviations

Ab: Antibody; Bik: Bcl-2 interacting killer; Bmal1: Brain and muscle Arnt-like protein-1; Clock: Circadian locomotor output cycles kaput;
Cry: Cryptochrome; Dbp: D site of the albumin promoter binding protein; DMEM: Dulbecco's modified Eagle's medium; E4bp4: E4-binding protein 4; FBS: Fetal bovine serum; Hlf: Hepatic leukemia factor; Ig: Immunoglobulin; mRNA: Messenger RNA; MTX: Methotrexate; PAR bZIP: Proline and acidic amino acid-rich basic leucine zipper; PCR: Polymerase chain reaction;
Per: Period; PVDF: Polyvinylidene difluoride; RA: Rheumatoid arthritis; SDS-PAGE: Sodium dodecyl sulfate polyacrylamide gel electrophoresis;
SEM: Standard error of the mean; siRNA: Small interfering RNA; Tbp: TATA box binding protein; Tef: Thyrotroph embryonic factor; TNF: Tumor necrosis factor; WST-8: 2-(2-Methoxy-4-nitrophenyl)-3-(4-nitrophenyl)-5-(2,4-disulfophenyl)-2H–tetrazolium

Acknowledgements

Not applicable.

Funding

The authors declare that they have no funding.

Authors' contributions

KS performed and analyzed most of the experiments, and wrote the manuscript. KY, TU, and KK provided technical support for the experiments. AN, NH, and KU maintained synovial fibroblasts and exchanged useful arguments on this manuscript. TH, YK, NS, and NN collected synovial samples. YS supervised the project. AH conceived the idea for the project, supervised the experiments, and wrote the manuscript. All authors read and approved the final manuscript.

Competing interests

The authors declare that they have no competing interests.

Author details

[1]Department of Biophysics, Kobe University Graduate School of Health Sciences, Tomogaoka 7-10-2, Suma-ku, Kobe 654-0142, Japan. [2]Division of Rehabilitation Medicine, Kobe University Graduate School of Medicine, Kobe 650-0017, Japan. [3]Department of Rheumatology, Kobe Kaisei Hospital, Kobe 657-0068, Japan. [4]Department of Orthopedic Surgery, Kobe Kaisei Hospital, Kobe 657-0068, Japan. [5]Department of Rheumatology, Hyogo Prefectural Kakogawa Medical Center, Kakogawa 675-0003, Japan.

References

1. Jolivet J, Cowan KH, Curt GA, Clendeninn NJ, Chabner BA. The pharmacology and clinical use of methotrexate. N Engl J Med. 1983;309:1094–104.
2. Bleyer WA. The clinical pharmacology of methotrexate: new applications of an old drug. Cancer. 1978;41:36–51.
3. Cronstein BN. Low-dose methotrexate: a mainstay in the treatment of rheumatoid arthritis. Pharmacol Rev. 2005;57:163–72.
4. Cutolo M, Sulli A, Pizzorni C, Seriolo B, Straub RH. Anti-inflammatory mechanisms of methotrexate in rheumatoid arthritis. Ann Rheum Dis. 2001;60:729–35.
5. Nakazawa F, Matsuno H, Yudoh K, Katayama R, Sawai T, Uzuki M, et al. Methotrexate inhibits rheumatoid synovitis by inducing apoptosis. J Rheumatol. 2001;28:1800–8.
6. Xu K, Cai YS, Lu SM, Li XL, Liu L, Li Z, et al. Autophagy induction contributes to the resistance to methotrexate treatment in rheumatoid arthritis fibroblast-like synovial cells through high mobility group box chromosomal protein 1. Arthritis Res Ther. 2015;17:374.
7. Lee SY, Park SH, Lee SW, Lee SH, Son MK, Choi YH, et al. Synoviocyte apoptosis may differentiate responder and non-responder patients to methotrexate treatment in rheumatoid arthritis. Arch Pharm Res. 2014;37:1286–94.
8. Spurlock CF 3rd, Gass HM 4th, Bryant CJ, Wells BC, Olsen NJ, Aune TM. Methotrexate-mediated inhibition of nuclear factor κB activation by distinct pathways in T cells and fibroblast-like synoviocytes. Rheumatology. 2014;54:178–87.
9. Olsen NJ, Stein CM. New drugs for rheumatoid arthritis. N Engl J Med. 2004; 350:2167–79.
10. Arnett FC, Edworthy SM, Bloch DA, McShane DJ, Fries JF, Cooper NS, et al. The American Rheumatism Association 1987 revised criteria for the classification of rheumatoid arthritis. Arthritis Rheum. 1988;31:315–24.
11. Cutolo M, Straub RH, Buttgereit F. Circadian rhythms of nocturnal hormones in rheumatoid arthritis: translation from bench to bedside. Ann Rheum Dis. 2008;67:905–8.
12. Danis VA, Franic GM, Rathjen DA, Laurent RM, Brooks PM. Circulating cytokine levels in patients with rheumatoid arthritis: results of a double blind trial with sulphasalazine. Ann Rheum Dis. 1992;51:946–50.
13. Dasgupta B, Corkill M, Kirkham B, Gibson T, Panayi G. Serial estimation of interleukin 6 as a measure of systemic disease in rheumatoid arthritis. J Rheumatol. 1992;19:22–5.
14. Choy EH, Panayi GS. Cytokine pathways and joint inflammation in rheumatoid arthritis. N Engl J Med. 2001;344:907–16.
15. Straub RH, Cutolo M. Circadian rhythms in rheumatoid arthritis: implications for pathophysiology and therapeutic management. Arthritis Rheum. 2007; 56:399–408.
16. Hashiramoto A, Yamane T, Tsumiyama K, Yoshida K, Komai K, Yamada H, et al. Mammalian clock gene Cryptochrome regulates arthritis via proinflammatory cytokine TNF-α. J Immunol. 2010;184:1560–5.
17. Yoshida K, Hashiramoto A, Okano T, Yamane T, Shibanuma N, Shiozawa S. TNF-α modulates expression of the circadian clock gene Per2 in rheumatoid synovial cells. Scand J Rheumatol. 2013;42:276–80.
18. Haas S, Straub RH. Disruption of rhythms of molecular clocks in primary synovial fibroblasts of patients with osteoarthritis and rheumatoid arthritis, role of IL-1β/TNF. Arthritis Res Ther. 2012;14:R122.
19. Cutolo M, Villaggio B, Otsa K, Aakre O, Sulli A, Seriolo B. Altered circadian rhythms in rheumatoid arthritis patients play a role in the disease's symptoms. Autoimmun Rev. 2005;4:497–502.
20. Gibbs JE, Ray DW. The role of the circadian clock in rheumatoid arthritis. Arthritis Res Ther. 2013;15:205.
21. Cuninkova L, Brown SA. Peripheral circadian oscillators: interesting mechanisms and powerful tools. Ann N Y Acad Sci. 2008;1129:358–70.
22. Sato TK, Yamada RG, Ukai H, Baggs JE, Miraglia LJ, Kobayashi TJ, et al. Feedback repression is required for mammalian circadian clock function. Nat Genet. 2006;38:312–9.
23. Falvey E, Marcacci L, Schibler U. DNA-binding specificity of PAR and C/EBP leucine zipper proteins: a single amino acid substitution in the C/EBP DNA-binding domain confers PAR-like specificity to C/EBP. Biol Chem. 1996;377:797–809.
24. Li S, Hunger SP. The DBP transcriptional activation domain is highly homologous to that of HLF and TEF and is not responsible for the tissue type-specific transcriptional activity of DBP. Gene. 2001;263:239–45.
25. Cowell IG, Skinner A, Hurst HC. Transcriptional repression by a novel member of the bZIP family of transcription factors. Mol Cell Biol. 1992;12:3070–7.
26. Mitsui S, Yamaguchi S, Matsuo T, Ishida Y, Okamura H. Antagonistic role of E4BP4 and PAR proteins in the circadian oscillatory mechanism. Genes Dev. 2001;15:995–1006.
27. Yamajuku D, Shibata Y, Kitazawa M, Katakura T, Urata H, Kojima T, et al. Cellular DBP and E4BP4 proteins are critical for determining the period length of the circadian oscillator. FEBS Lett. 2011;585:2217–22.
28. Ohno T, Onishi Y, Ishida N. A novel E4BP4 element drives circadian expression of mPeriod2. Nucleic Acids Res. 2007;35:648–55.
29. Rashmi R, Pillai SG, Vijayalingam S, Ryerse J, Chinnadurai G. BH3-only protein BIK induces caspase-independent cell death with autophagic features in Bcl-2 null cells. Oncogene. 2008;27:1366–75.
30. Boyd JM, Gallo GJ, Elangovan B, Houghton AB, Malstrom S, Avery BJ, et al. Bik, a novel death-inducing protein shares a distinct sequence motif with Bcl-2 family proteins and interacts with viral and cellular survival-promoting proteins. Oncogene. 1995;11:1921–8.
31. Balsalobre A, Damiola F, Schibler U. A serum shock induces circadian gene expression in mammalian tissue culture cells. Cell. 1998;93:929–37.
32. Kanda Y. Investigation of the freely available easy-to-use software 'EZR' for medical statistics. Bone Marrow Transplant. 2013;48(3):452–8.
33. Shiozawa K, Tanaka Y, Yoshihara R, Imura S, Murata M, Yamane T, et al. Serum levels and pharmacodynamics of methotrexate and its metabolite 7-

hydroxy methotrexate in Japanese patients with rheumatoid arthritis treated with 2-mg capsule of methotrexate three times per week. Mod Rheumatol. 2005;15:405–9.

34. Haber M, Madafiglio J, Norris MD. Methotrexate cytotoxicity determination using the MTT assay following enzymatic depletion of thymidine and hypoxanthine. J Cancer Res Clin Oncol. 1993;119(6):315–7.
35. Horie T, Li T, Ito K, Sumi S, Fuwa T. Aged garlic extract protects against methotrexate-induced apoptotic cell injury of IEC-6 cells. J Nutr. 2006;136(3 Suppl):861S–3S.
36. Genestier L, Paillot R, Fournel S, Ferraro C, Miossec P, Revillard JP. Immunosuppressive properties of methotrexate: apoptosis and clonal deletion of activated peripheral T cells. J Clin Invest. 1998;102(2):322–8.
37. Hand LE, Hopwood TW, Dickson SH, Walker AL, Loudon AS, Ray DW, et al. The circadian clock regulates inflammatory arthritis. FASEB J. 2016;30(11): 3759–70.
38. Hua H, Wang Y, Wan C, Liu Y, Zhu B, Yang C, et al. Circadian gene mPer2 overexpression induces cancer cell apoptosis. Cancer Sci. 2006;97:589–96.
39. Ritchie A, Gutierrez O, Fernandez-Luna JL. PAR bZIP-bik is a novel transcriptional pathway that mediates oxidative stress-induced apoptosis in fibroblasts. Cell Death Differ. 2009;16:838–46.
40. To H, Irie S, Tomonari M, Watanabe Y, Kitahara T, Sasaki H. Therapeutic index of methotrexate depends on circadian cycling of tumour necrosis factor-alpha in collagen-induced arthritic rats and mice. J Pharm Pharmacol. 2009;61:1333–8.
41. To H, Yoshimatsu H, Tomonari M, Ida H, Tsurumoto T, Tsuji Y, et al. Methotrexate chronotherapy is effective against rheumatoid arthritis. Chronobiol Int. 2011;28:267–74.
42. Tang Q, Cheng B, Xie M, Chen Y, Zhao J, Zhou X, et al. Circadian clock gene Bmal1 inhibits tumorigenesis and increases paclitaxel sensitivity in tongue squamous cell carcinoma. Cancer Res. 2017;77:532–44.

9

Methotrexate inhibits effects of platelet-derived growth factor and interleukin-1β on rheumatoid arthritis fibroblast-like synoviocytes

Beatrice Bergström[1,2], Hans Carlsten[1,2] and Anna-Karin Hultgård Ekwall[1,2*]

Abstract

Background: A key feature of joints in rheumatoid arthritis (RA) is the formation of hyperplastic destructive pannus tissue, which is orchestrated by activated fibroblast-like synoviocytes (FLS). We have demonstrated that the RA risk gene and tumor suppressor Limb bud and heart development (LBH) regulates cell cycle progression in FLS. Methotrexate (MTX) is the first-line treatment for RA, but its mechanisms of action remain incompletely understood. Here, we studied the effects of MTX on mitogen-induced FLS proliferation and expression of cell cycle regulators in vitro.

Methods: Primary FLS from patients with RA or osteoarthritis were stimulated with the mitogen platelet-derived growth factor (PDGF) and the cytokine interleukin-1β (IL-1β) in the presence or absence of MTX. Cells were then subjected to qPCR for gene expression and cell cycle analysis by flow cytometry.

Results: Stimulation with PDGF and IL-1β increased the percentage of FLS in the G2/M phase and shifted the cell morphology to a dendritic shape. These effects were inhibited by MTX. Furthermore, PDGF + IL-1β reduced *LBH* mRNA expression. However, MTX treatment yielded significantly higher transcript levels of *LBH*, and of *CDKN1A* (p21) and *TP53* (p53), compared to untreated samples upon mitogen stimulation. The expression of DNA methyltransferase-1 (*DNMT1*) was also higher in the presence of MTX and there was strong correlation between *DNMT1* and *LBH* expression.

Conclusions: Therapeutic concentrations of MTX abolish the effects of PDGF and IL-1β on tumor suppressor expression and inhibit mitogen-promoted FLS proliferation. These data demonstrate novel and important effects of MTX on pathogenic effector cells in the joint, which might involve epigenetic mechanisms.

Keywords: Rheumatoid arthritis, Fibroblast-like synoviocytes, Cell cycle, Platelet-derived growth factor, Interleukin-1beta, Methotrexate

Background

The rheumatoid arthritis (RA) joint pathology is characterized by persistent inflammation and synovial hyperplasia, leading to destruction of cartilage and bone and ultimately functional disability [1]. Key players in these processes are fibroblast-like synoviocytes (FLS), which develop an aggressive, tumor-like phenotype [2] with increased invasiveness and disturbed control of cell proliferation [3]. The local FLS expansion in the synovial lining layer correlates with clinical disease activity parameters in RA [4]. Also, treatment with cell cycle inhibitors targeting FLS ameliorates arthritis in mouse models [5, 6]. Thus, studies of pathways regulating the proliferation of FLS are of considerable interest.

FLS in RA are activated to an aggressive phenotype by repeated exposure to numerous pro-inflammatory cytokines and growth factors acting on top of predisposing genetic and epigenetic factors [7, 8]. Stimulating FLS in vitro with tumor necrosis factor (TNF) and interleukin-1β (IL-1β) induces a variable expression of many of the genes characterizing the aggressive RA FLS phenotype. Platelet-

* Correspondence: ak.ekwall@rheuma.gu.se
[1]Department of Rheumatology and Inflammation Research, Institute of Medicine, The Sahlgrenska Academy, University of Gothenburg, Box 480, 405 30 Gothenburg, Sweden
[2]Centre for Bone and Arthritis Research, University of Gothenburg, Gothenburg, Sweden

derived growth factor (PDGF) is a known fibroblast mitogen and both PDGF and IL-1β have been reported to increase FLS proliferation [9, 10]. Interestingly, the cytokine (TNF or IL-1β) potentiates the effects of growth factors (PDGF and transforming growth factor (TGF)-β) on cytokine and matrix metalloproteinase production in FLS [11].

Moreover, RA FLS display intrinsic dysregulation of proliferation and apoptosis pathways, such as abnormalities of the tumor suppressor p53 [12] and its downstream mediator p21 [13] which in the normal synoviocyte induces cell cycle arrest. The number of p21-positive FLS inversely correlates with the thickness synovial lining layer in RA [13]. Recently, the transcription regulator, Limb bud and heart development (LBH), was identified as a new candidate gene for the pathogenic FLS phenotype in RA [14]. Reduced expression of this tumor suppressor in FLS has been suggested to increase the risk of RA development. LBH is regulated by growth factors and epigenetic mechanisms [15] and modulates proliferation in primary FLS by regulating cell cycle progression at the G1 to S phase transition checkpoint [16, 17]. In particular, a regulatory DNA element in the *LBH* gene region is hypomethylated in RA. This DNA element is believed to negatively regulate *LBH* transcription.

Methotrexate (MTX) is still the first-line treatment for RA, but its exact mechanisms of action and target cells remain incompletely understood. The anti-inflammatory effect of low-dose MTX used in rheumatic diseases has in part been attributed to release of adenosine [18]. Studies have also demonstrated that MTX treatment restores global DNA methylation of peripheral blood mononuclear cells [19] and increases expression of cell cycle checkpoint genes in the T cells in patients with RA [20]. However, the effects of MTX on FLS in RA are largely unknown.

In order to further understand the pharmacodynamics of MTX in RA and to identify novel drug targets and markers to predict drug response, this study aimed to investigate the effects of MTX on mitogen-induced FLS proliferation in vitro, and in particular on the expression of cell cycle regulators.

Methods

Synovial samples

Human synovial tissue specimens were obtained from patients with RA (n = 6) or osteoarthritis (OA) (n = 7) during joint replacement surgery at Sahlgrenska University Hospital in Sweden. All Patients with RA fulfilled the American College of Rheumatology 1987 revised criteria for the disease [21] and all had established seropositive and erosive disease. MTX was stopped ≥ 2 weeks before surgery. The procedures were approved by the Ethics Committee of Gothenburg, and all patients gave written informed consent.

Cell culture

Primary FLS were isolated as previously described [2] and cultured in Dulbecco's modified Eagle's medium (DMEM) GlutaMAX (Gibco, Carlsbad, CA, USA) supplemented with antibiotics (penicillin/streptomycin, gentamicin) and 10% heat-inactivated fetal bovine serum (FBS), in a humidified 5% CO_2 atmosphere. Cells at passages three to nine were seeded into 6-well or 24-well plates for experiments. Stimulation with the human recombinant proteins PDGF-BB (Invitrogen, Carlsbad, CA, USA) and IL-1β (R&D Systems, Minneapolis, MN, USA) was performed in 1% FBS medium after overnight serum starvation.

MTX dose and treatment protocol

Therapeutic doses of MTX range from 10 to 25 mg weekly among patients with RA, resulting in peak serum concentrations at 1 μM [22, 23]. Concentrations are higher in synovial tissue than in blood [24]. In previous in vitro studies of FLS, concentrations of MTX up to 100 μM have been used [25]. Treatment of FLS cultures for 48 h with 0.01–10 μM MTX had no effect on viability or apoptosis of FLS in RA [26].

Here, FLS were pretreated for 24 h with MTX (Apoteket, Sweden) or control medium, then stimulated with PDGF + IL-1β in 1% FBS medium in the presence or absence of MTX. The cells were harvested 24–48 h after mitogen stimulation for gene expression or cell cycle analysis. Only FLS lines responding to mitogen stimulation (defined by a fold change in *LBH* mRNA below 0.3 compared to the unstimulated control) under the present experimental time frame were included.

Cell cycle analysis

FLS were detached by trypsin-EDTA and resuspended in PBS, fixed in 70% ethanol and stained with the DNA label 7-amino-actinomycin D (7-AAD) (BD Pharmingen, San Diego, CA, USA). DNA content was measured using a FACSVerse flow cytometer and FACSuite software (BD Biosciences) on at least 10,000 cells/sample. Data were analyzed using FlowJo software (Tree Star, Ashland, OR, USA) and the percentages of cells in G1 and G2/M phase, respectively, were calculated from histograms of DNA content after exclusion of debris and doublets. The gating strategy is presented in Fig. 1a.

RNA extraction and gene expression analysis

Total RNA was isolated from cells using RNeasy Mini Kit (Qiagen) and quantified with a NanoDrop 100 spectrophotometer (Thermo Scientific). Complementary DNA was synthesized using TaqMan reverse transcription agents (Applied Biosystems, Carlsbad, CA, USA) with 250 ng RNA per reaction. Quantitative polymerase chain reaction (qPCR) was performed on a ViiA Real-Time PCR System using

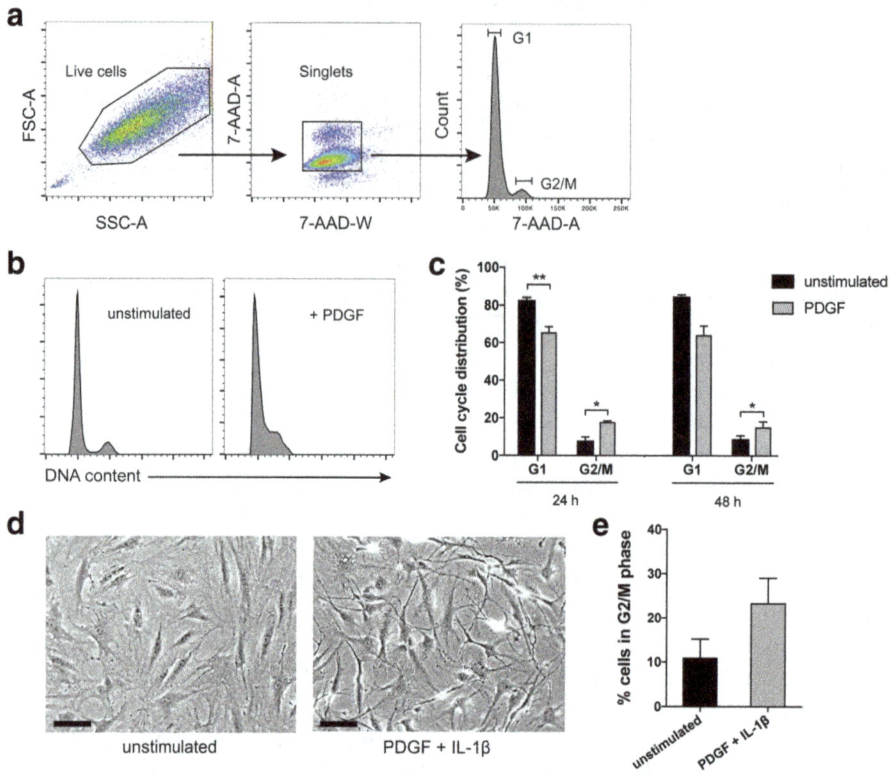

Fig. 1 Effects of mitogens on the cell cycle and cell morphology of fibroblast-like synoviocytes (FLS). Primary rheumatoid arthritis (RA) FLS were serum-starved and stimulated with platelet-derived growth factor (PDGF) or a combination of PDGF and IL-1β. The cells were then harvested and DNA-stained followed by flow cytometry. **a** Gating strategy identifying live cells and singlets and histogram gating of cell cycle analysis by DNA content. **b** Representative histograms of FLS in an unstimulated state and upon PDGF stimulation. **c** Percentage of cells in the G1 and G2/M phase, respectively, in unstimulated FLS and upon stimulation with PDGF (20 ng/mL) for 24 and 48 h, respectively. **d** Morphology of FLS in 2D culture, before stimulation and after incubation for 48 h with PDGF (20 ng/mL) + IL-1β (2 ng/mL), as visualized by light microscopy. Scale bar 20 μM. **e** Percentage of cells in the G2/M phase upon PDGF + IL-1β stimulation compared to percentage of cells without stimulation. Values are the mean ± SEM of three different FLS lines. $^*p < 0.05$, $^{**}p < 0.01$. FSC-A, forward scatter-area; SSC-A, side scatter-area

TaqMan Gene Expression Assays (Applied Biosystems) for *GAPDH* (Hs99999905_m1), *LBH* (Hs00368853_m1), *CDKN1A* (Hs00355782_m1), *CDKN2A* (Hs00923894_m1), *TP53* (Hs01034249_m1), *CCND1* (Hs00765553_m1), *CCNE1* (Hs01026536_m1), *CDC25A* (Hs00947994_m1), *DNMT1* (Hs00154749_m1), and *DNMT3A* (Hs01027 166_m1). Cycle threshold (Ct) values were normalized to *GAPDH*. Results were presented as fold changes calculated by the $2^{-\Delta\Delta Ct}$ method.

Statistical analysis

Results are presented as the mean ± SEM. Differences were evaluated by paired Student's *t* test for comparison of two groups, or one-way analysis of variance (ANOVA) followed by Tukey's post hoc test for comparison of multiple groups. Shapiro-Wilk's normality test was used to assess sample distribution. Statistical analysis of differences in gene expression was performed on ΔCt values. Correlation between fold changes in gene expression was tested with Spearman's rank correlation coefficient. The analyses were performed using GraphPad Prism software (version 7.0b; GraphPad Inc., La Jolla, CA, USA): *p* values less than 0.05 were considered significant.

Results

PDGF and IL-1β induce FLS proliferation

It has previously been reported that IL-1β enhances FLS proliferation in vitro as measured by ^{3}H-thymidine incorporation [10], and that PDGF induces colony growth of primary FLS [9]. In this study, we used cell cycle analysis by flow cytometry to assay the effects of the mitogen on cultured RA FLS. Stimulation with PDGF 20 ng/mL alone promoted cell cycle progression as expected (Fig. 1b and c), increasing the percentage of cells in the G2/M phase (18 ± 1% versus 8 ± 2% in unstimulated controls, $p = 0.03$) while reducing the percentage of cells in the G1 phase (66 ± 3% versus 83 ± 1% in unstimulated controls, $p = 0.009$), after 24 h. Similar results were observed after 48 h (Fig. 1c). Upon stimulation with a combination of PDGF 20 ng/mL and IL-1β 2 ng/mL, a pronounced shift in FLS morphology to a more dendritic cell shape was seen, with cells extending long pseudopodia

(Fig. 1d). The mean percentage of cells in the G2/M phase was also higher with this combination compared to unstimulated cells (Fig. 1e), although not statistically significant (23 ± 6% of cells in the G2/M phase versus 11 ± 4% in unstimulated controls, $p = 0.14$).

MTX inhibits the effects of mitogens on FLS proliferation

To investigate the effects of MTX on the proliferation and gene expression of RA FLS in an inflammatory setting, we developed an experimental set-up as overviewed in Fig. 2a. In cell cycle analysis by flow cytometry, MTX treatment alone did not affect the DNA content distribution seen in unstimulated cultures (Fig. 2b). Stimulation with PDGF + IL-1β could induce cell cycle progression, but this effect was abolished by the presence of MTX. Treatment with MTX resulted in only 5 ± 2% of the cell population in the G2/M phase upon mitogen stimulation, compared to 25 ± 4% on mitogen stimulation alone ($p = 0.02$) (Fig. 2c). Instead, cells were halted in the G1 phase when MTX was present upon mitogen stimulation (87 ± 3% versus 71 ± 6% in the absence of MTX, $p = 0.04$) (Fig. 2c).

PDGF and IL-1β reduce *LBH* expression

It has recently been demonstrated that LBH is a modulator of FLS proliferation and that it is regulated by growth factors implicated in RA. PDGF has been shown to reduce *LBH* expression in a dose-dependent manner and with a peak effect at 12 h [16]. We found that stimulation with IL-1β also reduced *LBH* mRNA expression in FLS and to the same extent as with PDGF (Fig. 3a). Significant effects of IL-1β were obtained at 2 ng/mL and 20 ng/mL (Fig. 3b). The combination of PDGF + IL-1β yielded the strongest effect on *LBH* expression (Fig. 3a) and was therefore employed in subsequent experiments.

MTX inhibits the effects of mitogens on *LBH* expression

Next, we examined if MTX inhibited the effects of PDGF + IL-1β on *LBH* expression in FLS. In the presence of MTX, there was a dose-dependent increase in *LBH* mRNA levels after mitogen stimulation compared to cultures without MTX. The optimal concentration was found to be 1 μM MTX (Fig. 3c), which corresponds to concentrations found in patients treated with therapeutic doses of the drug (see "Methods"). *LBH* expression was increased 3.2 ±

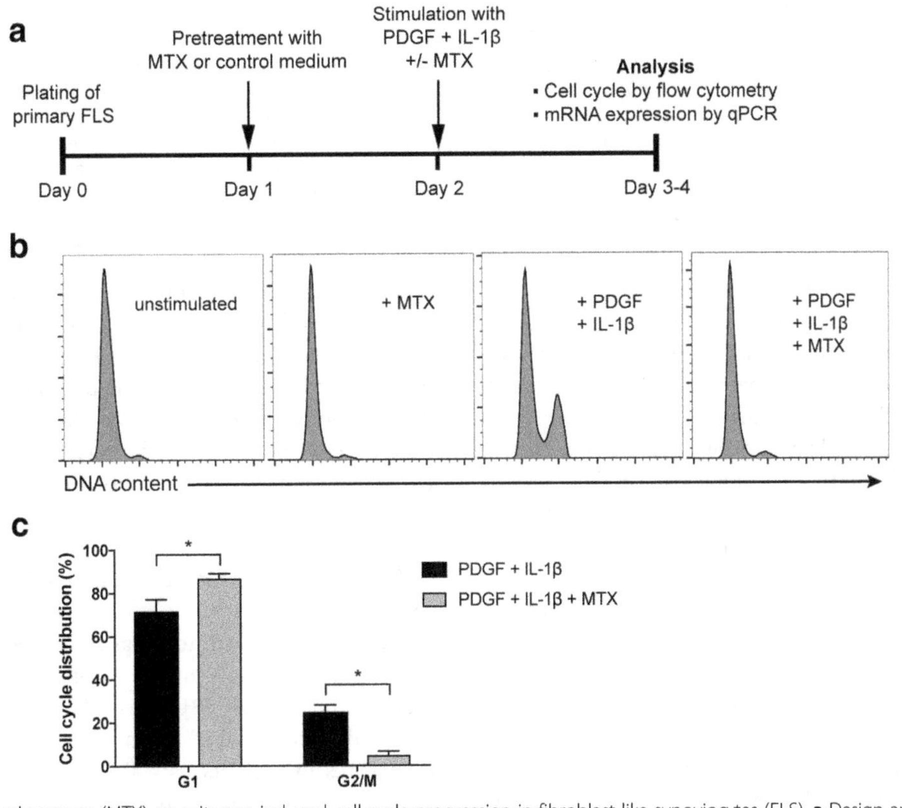

Fig. 2 Effects of methotrexate (MTX) on mitogen-induced cell cycle progression in fibroblast-like synoviocytes (FLS). **a** Design and timeline of the current MTX experiments. **b** Rheumatoid arthritis (RA) FLS were stimulated with platelet-derived growth factor (PDGF, 20 ng/mL) + IL-1β (2 ng/mL) for 24 h in the presence or absence of 1 μM MTX, or treated with MTX only. The cells were then DNA-stained followed by cell cycle analysis by flow cytometry. Representative histograms of DNA content with indicated treatments are shown. **c** Percentage of cells in the G1 and G2/M phase, respectively, in three different FLS lines. The experiments were repeated more than three times. Values are mean ± SEM. *$p < 0.05$. OA, osteoarthritis

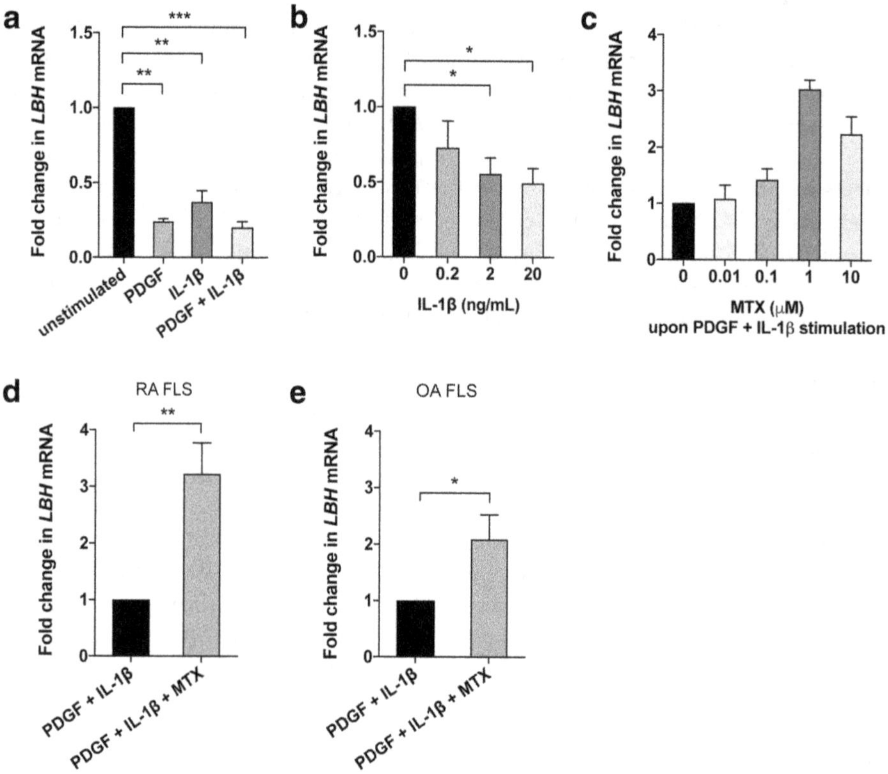

Fig. 3 *LBH* expression in fibroblast-like synoviocytes (FLS) in response to platelet-derived growth factor (PDGF) and IL-1β, with or without methotrexate (MTX). **a, b** Fold change in mRNA levels of *LBH* compared to unstimulated was assessed by qPCR in serum-starved FLS after stimulation for 12 h with PDGF (10 ng/mL) and/or IL-1β (2 ng/mL) (**a**), or IL-1β at different concentrations (0.2–20 ng/mL) (**b**). **c** Fold change in *LBH* mRNA levels was measured after 48 h of mitogen stimulation (PDGF 20 ng/mL + IL-1β 2 ng/mL) in the presence or absence of MTX at various doses (0.01–10 μM; $n = 2$). **d, e** Treatment with 1 μM MTX upon PDGF 20 ng/mL + IL-1β 2 ng/mL stimulation was evaluated in rheumatoid arthritis (RA) FLS (**d**) and in osteoarthritis (OA) FLS (**e**). Values are the mean fold change ± SEM of three to six different FLS lines. *$p < 0.05$, **$p < 0.01$, ***$p < 0.0001$

0.5 fold ($p = 0.002$) after MTX treatment in RA FLS (Fig. 3d). Since osteoarthritis (OA) FLS also can be "activated" to some extent under certain conditions in vitro [27], we repeated the experiment with OA samples. We found that stimulation with PDGF + IL-1β reduced *LBH* expression and MTX treatment increased the expression 2.2 ± 0.5 fold ($p = 0.02$) in OA FLS (Fig. 3e). The difference between RA and OA FLS was not statistically significant under the present conditions.

MTX abolishes the effects of mitogens on *CDKN1A* and *TP53* expression

We continued to study the effects of MTX on other cell cycle regulator genes in RA FLS, as presented in Fig. 4a. *CDKN1A* encodes the protein p21 (CIP1/WAF1), which regulates cell cycle progression primarily by acting as a cyclin-dependent kinase inhibitor (CDKI) at the G1 to S phase transition. Strikingly, the *CDKN1A* mRNA expression was 14.3 ± 4.4 fold higher ($p = 0.006$) in the presence of MTX upon mitogen stimulation compared to without MTX. Another CDKI, p16 encoded by the *CDKN2A* gene, was also significantly increased (2.0 ± 0.1 fold, $p = 0.002$). One of the regulators of p21 is the transcription factor p53 (encoded by *TP53*), known to inhibit cell cycle activity and inflammation. The mRNA levels of *TP53* were 1.8 ± 0.2 fold higher ($p = 0.03$) in the presence of MTX. Within the experimental time frame, we did not detect any significant effects on the transcription of *CCND1* (cyclin D1), *CCNE1* (cyclin E1) or *CDC25A* (M-phase inducer phosphatase 1).

DNMT1 expression is increased after MTX treatment and correlates with *LBH*

It has been demonstrated that IL-1β reduces the expression of DNA methylating enzymes and global DNA methylation in FLS [28]. Since MTX has previously been reported to alter DNA methylation in lymphocytes and monocytes in patients with RA, we also assessed the expression of DNA methyltransferases (DNMTs) in FLS in our experimental setting. Stimulation with PDGF + IL-1β reduced *DNMT1* mRNA expression, confirming earlier reports. However, in the presence of MTX the *DNMT1* transcript levels were significantly higher compared to mitogen-stimulated FLS without MTX treatment, both in

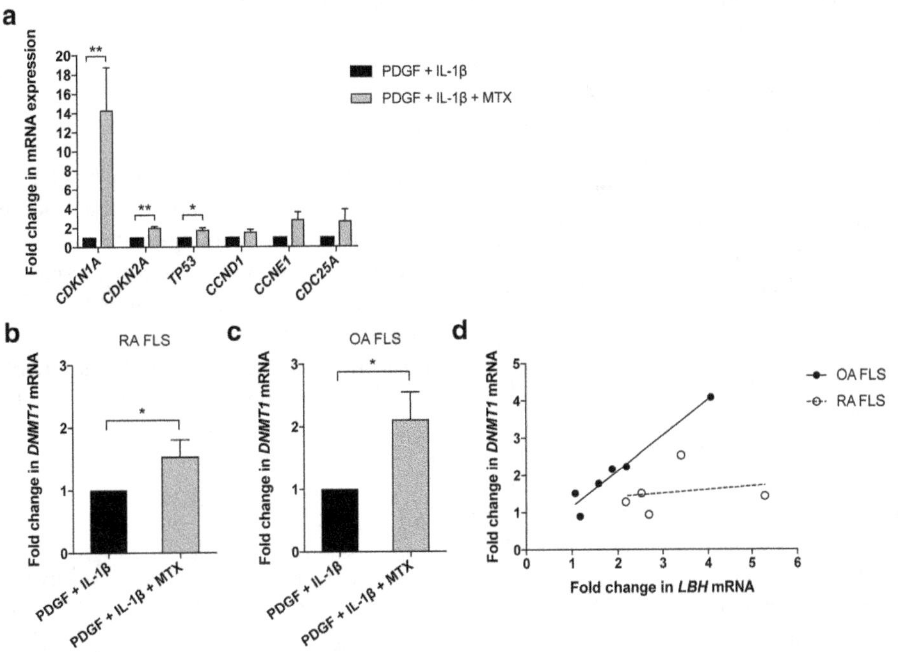

Fig. 4 Expression of cell cycle regulator genes and *DNMT1* in response to mitogens +/− methotrexate (MTX). Treatment of fibroblast-like synoviocytes (FLS) was performed according to the protocol in Fig. 2a (platelet-derived growth factor (PDGF) 20 ng/mL + IL-1β 2 ng/mL +/− MTX 1 μM). mRNA expression was analyzed by qPCR after 48 h of mitogen stimulation. **a** Fold change in mRNA levels of the indicated cell cycle regulator genes. **b**, **c** Fold change in *DNMT1* expression in rheumatoid arthritis (RA) FLS (**b**) and in osteoarthritis (OA) FLS (**c**). Values are the mean fold change ± SEM in three to six different FLS lines. *$p < 0.05$, **$p < 0.01$. **d** Correlation between *DNMT1* and *LBH* expression in OA FLS (solid circles; $n = 6$) and RA FLS (open circles; $n = 5$). Each dot represents an individual FLS line. Values are fold change in mRNA expression on PDGF + IL-1β + MTX treatment compared to PDGF + IL-1β alone. Lines show fitting of data to a linear regression

RA FLS (1.5 ± 0.3 fold, $p = 0.04$) (Fig. 4b) and OA FLS (2.1 ± 0.4 fold, $p = 0.03$) (Fig. 4c). There were no significant differences in *DNMT3A* expression (data not shown). Recent data suggest that the expression of *LBH* is in part regulated by DNA methylation in FLS [15]. We found strong correlation between fold change in *DNMT1* and *LBH* mRNA expression in the OA samples (Spearman's correlation coefficient, $r_s = 0.94$, $p = 0.017$) but not in RA FLS ($r_s = 0.30$, $p = 0.68$). Interestingly, the RA and OA samples clustered in distinct groups (Fig. 4d).

Discussion

A hallmark of the pathogenesis of RA is the formation of destructive pannus tissue in which activated FLS play a key role. This hyperplastic invasive tissue is overpopulated by FLS mediating persistent inflammation and joint destruction by production of pro-inflammatory cytokines, chemokines, growth factors and matrix degrading enzymes. Both increased resistance to apoptosis and increased proliferation is believed to cause the increased FLS number [8] and the predominant mechanism most probably varies by disease duration and between individuals. Targeting cytokines and immune cells in the treatment of RA has proven insufficient in a substantial number of patients and there is a need for more efficient treatment. Studies of the mechanisms regulating FLS proliferation are therefore of utter importance, as there is currently no therapy specifically targeting these pivotal effector cells in the joint in RA.

Low-dose MTX is the standard of care in the treatment of RA. About one third of the patients will reach low disease activity with MTX mono-therapy and another third will reach good clinical response in combination with a biologic agent [29]. The prevailing theory of the pharmacodynamic effects of MTX is that it targets the activity of immune cells. However, a recent study demonstrates the inhibitory effect of MTX on TNF-induced NF-κB activation in FLS *in vitro* [30].

We performed *in vitro* studies where the proliferative FLS phenotype was induced by PDGF + IL-1β. This is to our knowledge the only study investigating effects on cell cycle progression of FLS with this combination. IL-1β has been shown to reduce expression of DNA methylating enzymes (DNMTs) in FLS [28] and might thus act on a different regulatory level (epigenetic) than other cytokines and growth factors and could therefore potentiate or modulate their effects on gene expression. Interestingly, we found that MTX treatment inhibited cell cycle progression in PDGF + IL-1β-stimulated FLS, which suggests a new mechanism of action of this drug.

Furthermore, we studied the effects of MTX on the recently identified RA risk gene, *LBH*, which encodes a highly conserved transcription regulator and the expression of LBH in FLS is believed to be protective in RA [31]. LBH has been shown to regulate FLS growth by acting as a tumor suppressor [16]. A recent study demonstrating that LBH deficiency exacerbates arthritis in an *in vivo* model supports these findings [17]. In our experiments, the mitogens PDGF and IL-1β were found to reduce *LBH* mRNA expression in RA FLS, and MTX treatment abrogated these effects. A pronounced effect of MTX was also seen on the cell cycle checkpoint gene *CDKN1A*, encoding p21, and to some extent on *CDKN2A* (p16) and *TP53* (p53). This is consistent with earlier studies of T cells in RA, where MTX treatment induces the expression of p21 and p53 [20].

In this and earlier studies, PDGF also reduced *LBH* expression in OA FLS [16] and we demonstrated that MTX can increase expression of *LBH* and other tumor suppressor genes after mitogen stimulation not only in RA FLS but also to some extent in OA FLS. The gene expression profiles of primary FLS from patients with OA converge with those of RA FLS under high serum conditions *in vitro* [27]. This finding suggests some common intrinsic response patterns of FLS, and synovitis is common in OA [32]. However, sustained exposure to growth factors and cytokines, as in the joints in RA, has been demonstrated to prime FLS to enhanced pathogenic responses [33]. This together with genetic and epigenetic factors of RA FLS [8] might explain the differences in the degree of synovial activation and inflammation in the two diseases. Interestingly, treatment with anti-TNF agents has failed to provide symptomatic benefits in OA trials [34] but a recent study also suggests analgesic efficacy of MTX in OA [35]. It is important to point out that the RA synovial samples in this study were obtained from patients with end-stage disease and it is possible that the differences in results between RA and OA FLS would have been larger in FLS from early RA.

We have earlier demonstrated that *LBH* expression in FLS is regulated by DNA methylation [15]. Since a suggested mechanism of action of MTX in lymphocytes is interference with DNA methylation, we also studied the effects of MTX on DNA methylating enzymes in FLS. Indeed, we found that the mRNA expression of *DNMT1* was higher after MTX treatment compared to untreated PDGF + IL1β-stimulated FLS. Moreover, there was strong correlation between *DNMT1* and *LBH* expression in MTX-treated OA FLS, suggesting that MTX might mediate the effects on cell cycle regulator gene expression in FLS by restoring epigenetic patterns. In RA FLS, the samples clustered with high fold change in *LBH* expression, but the correlation with *DNMT1* expression was not present, indicating that other factors also influence gene expression. This is in agreement with our previous findings that *LBH* expression in RA FLS is regulated by growth factors as well as by DNA methylation and genetic polymorphism of a regulatory element [15].

Conclusion

We demonstrate that therapeutic concentrations of MTX abolish mitogen-promoted proliferation of RA FLS and inhibit the effects of mitogens on cell cycle regulators. This could be one hitherto unknown mode of action contributing to the efficacy of MTX in RA. Understanding the molecular mechanisms of the effects of MTX on FLS is of great importance for the development of novel, more FLS-specific drugs and for identifying biomarkers to predict response to MTX.

Abbreviations

7-AAD: 7-Amino-actinomycin D; ANOVA: Analysis of variance; CDKI: Cyclin-dependent kinase inhibitor; DNMT: DNA methyltransferase; FBS: Fetal bovine serum; FLS: Fibroblast-like synoviocytes; IL: Interleukin; LBH: Limb bud and heart development; MTX: Methotrexate; OA: Osteoarthritis; PBS: Phosphate-buffered saline; PDGF: Platelet-derived growth factor; qPCR: Quantitative polymerase chain reaction; RA: Rheumatoid arthritis; TGF: Transforming growth factor; TNF: Tumor necrosis factor

Acknowledgements

We gratefully acknowledge Dr Thomas Eisler and Dr Christian Anderberg for participating in the recruitment of patients and establishment of the synovial tissue biobank.

Funding

This work was supported by grants from the Swedish Society of Medicine, the King Gustaf V:s 80-year Foundation, the Professor Nanna Svartz Foundation, the Rune and Ulla Amlöv Foundation, the Gothenburg Region Foundation for Rheumatology Research, and the Swedish Rheumatism Foundation.

Authors' contributions

AKE directed the research. AKE and BB collected the patient samples and established the biobank. AKE and BB designed the experiments. BB and AKE conducted the experiments and acquired the data. AKE, BB and HC analyzed the data. BB drafted the manuscript. All authors read and approved the final manuscript.

Competing interests

The authors declare that they have no competing interests.

References

1. Firestein GS, McInnes IB. Immunopathogenesis of rheumatoid arthritis. Immunity. 2017;46:183–96.
2. Ekwall A-KH, Eisler T, Anderberg C, Jin C, Karlsson N, Brisslert M, et al. The tumour-associated glycoprotein podoplanin is expressed in fibroblast-like synoviocytes of the hyperplastic synovial lining layer in rheumatoid arthritis. Arthritis Res Ther. 2011;13:R40.
3. Bartok B, Firestein GS. Fibroblast-like synoviocytes: key effector cells in rheumatoid arthritis. Immunol Rev. 2010;233:233–55.

4. Izquierdo E, Cañete JD, Celis R, Del Rey MJ, Usategui A, Marsal S, et al. Synovial fibroblast hyperplasia in rheumatoid arthritis: clinicopathologic correlations and partial reversal by anti-tumor necrosis factor therapy. Arthritis Rheum. 2011;63:2575–83.
5. Sekine C, Sugihara T, Miyake S, Hirai H, Yoshida M, Miyasaka N, et al. Successful treatment of animal models of rheumatoid arthritis with small-molecule cyclin-dependent kinase inhibitors. J Immunol. 2008;180:1954–61.
6. Hosoya T, Iwai H, Yamaguchi Y, Kawahata K, Miyasaka N, Kohsaka H. Cell cycle regulation therapy combined with cytokine blockade enhances antiarthritic effects without increasing immune suppression. Ann Rheum Dis. 2016;75:253–9.
7. Croft AP, Naylor A, Zimmermann B, Desanti G, Hardie D, Muller-Ladner U, et al. Synovial fibroblasts differentiate into distinct functional subsets in the presence of cytokines and cartilage. Arthritis Res Ther. 2016;18:270.
8. Bottini N, Firestein GS. Duality of fibroblast-like synoviocytes in RA: passive responders and imprinted aggressors. Nat Rev Rheumatol. 2013;9:24–33.
9. Lafyatis R, Remmers EF, Roberts AB, Yocum DE, Sporn MB, Wilder RL. Anchorage-independent growth of synoviocytes from arthritic and normal joints. Stimulation by exogenous platelet-derived growth factor and inhibition by transforming growth factor-beta and retinoids. J Clin Invest. 1989;83:1267–76.
10. Lacey D, Sampey A, Mitchell R, Bucala R, Santos L, Leech M, et al. Control of fibroblast-like synoviocyte proliferation by macrophage migration inhibitory factor. Arthritis Rheum. 2003;48:103–9.
11. Rosengren S, Corr M, Boyle DL. Platelet-derived growth factor and transforming growth factor beta synergistically potentiate inflammatory mediator synthesis by fibroblast-like synoviocytes. Arthritis Res Ther. 2010;12:R65.
12. Han Z, Boyle DL, Shi Y, Green DR, Firestein GS. Dominant-negative p53 mutations in rheumatoid arthritis. Arthritis Rheum. 1999;42:1088–92.
13. Perlman H, Bradley K, Liu H, Cole S, Shamiyeh E, Smith RC, et al. IL-6 and matrix metalloproteinase-1 are regulated by the cyclin-dependent kinase inhibitor p21 in synovial fibroblasts. J Immunol. 2003;170:838–45.
14. Whitaker JW, Boyle DL, Bartok B, Ball ST, Gay S, Wang W, et al. Integrative omics analysis of rheumatoid arthritis identifies non-obvious therapeutic targets. PLoS One. 2015;10:e0124254.
15. Hammaker D, Whitaker JW, Maeshima K, Boyle DL, Ekwall A-KH, Wang W, et al. LBH Gene transcription regulation by the interplay of an enhancer risk allele and DNA methylation in rheumatoid arthritis. Arthritis Rheumatol. 2016;68:2637–45.
16. Ekwall AKH, Whitaker JW, Hammaker D, Bugbee WD, Wang W, Firestein GS. The rheumatoid arthritis risk gene LBH regulates growth in fibroblast-like synoviocytes. Arthritis Rheumatol. 2015;67:1193–202.
17. Matsuda S, Hammaker D, Topolewski K, Briegel KJ, Boyle DL, Dowdy S, et al. Regulation of the cell cycle and inflammatory arthritis by the transcription cofactor LBH gene. J Immunol. 2017;199:2316–22.
18. Cronstein BN, Naime D, Ostad E. The antiinflammatory mechanism of methotrexate. Increased adenosine release at inflamed sites diminishes leukocyte accumulation in an in vivo model of inflammation. J Clin Invest. 1993;92:2675–82.
19. de Andres MC, Perez-Pampin E, Calaza M, Santaclara FJ, Ortea I, Gomez-Reino JJ, et al. Assessment of global DNA methylation in peripheral blood cell subpopulations of early rheumatoid arthritis before and after methotrexate. Arthritis Res Ther. 2015;17:233.
20. Spurlock CF, Tossberg JT, Fuchs HA, Olsen NJ, Aune TM, Aune TM. Methotrexate increases expression of cell cycle checkpoint genes via JNK activation. Arthritis Rheum. 2012;64:1780–9.
21. Arnett FC, Edworthy SM, Bloch DA, McShane DJ, Fries JF, Cooper NS, et al. The American Rheumatism Association 1987 revised criteria for the classification of rheumatoid arthritis. Arthritis Rheum. 1988;31:315–24.
22. Edelman J, Biggs DF, Jamali F, Russell AS. Low-dose methotrexate kinetics in arthritis. Clin Pharmacol Ther. 1984;35:382–6.
23. Combe B, Edno L, Lafforgue P, Bologna C, Bernard JC, Acquaviva P, et al. Total and free methotrexate pharmacokinetics, with and without piroxicam, in rheumatoid arthritis patients. Br J Rheumatol. 1995;34:421–8.
24. Bologna C, Edno L, Anaya J-M, Canovas F, Vanden BM, Jorgensen C, et al. Methotrexate concentrations in synovial membrane and trabecular and cortical bone in rheumatoid arthritis patients. Arthritis Rheum. 1994;37:1770–3.
25. Revu S, Neregård P, af Klint E, Korotkova M, Catrina AI. Synovial membrane immunohistology in early-untreated rheumatoid arthritis reveals high expression of catabolic bone markers that is modulated by methotrexate. Arthritis Res Ther. 2013;15:R205.
26. Xu K, Cai Y, Lu S-M, Li X-L, Liu L, Li Z, et al. Autophagy induction contributes to the resistance to methotrexate treatment in rheumatoid arthritis fibroblast-like synovial cells through high mobility group box chromosomal protein 1. Arthritis Res Ther. 2015;17:374.
27. Filer A, Antczak P, Parsonage GN, Legault HM, O'Toole M, Pearson MJ, et al. Stromal transcriptional profiles reveal hierarchies of anatomical site, serum response and disease and identify disease specific pathways. PLoS One. 2015;10:e0120917.
28. Nakano K, Boyle DL, Firestein GS. Regulation of DNA methylation in rheumatoid arthritis synoviocytes. J Immunol. 2013;190:1297–303.
29. Smolen JS, Aletaha D. Rheumatoid arthritis therapy reappraisal: strategies, opportunities and challenges. Nat Rev Rheumatol. 2015;11:276–89.
30. Spurlock CF, Gass HM, Bryant CJ, Wells BC, Olsen NJ, Aune TM. Methotrexate-mediated inhibition of nuclear factor κB activation by distinct pathways in T cells and fibroblast-like synoviocytes. Rheumatology (Oxford). 2015;54:178–87.
31. Kim K, Bang S-Y, Lee H-S, Cho S-K, Choi C-B, Sung Y-K, et al. High-density genotyping of immune loci in Koreans and Europeans identifies eight new rheumatoid arthritis risk loci. Ann Rheum Dis. 2015;74:e13.
32. Mathiessen A, Conaghan PG. Synovitis in osteoarthritis: current understanding with therapeutic implications. Arthritis Res Ther. 2017;19:18.
33. Crowley T, O'Neil JD, Adams H, Thomas AM, Filer A, Buckley CD, et al. Priming in response to pro-inflammatory cytokines is a feature of adult synovial but not dermal fibroblasts. Arthritis Res Ther. 2017;19:35.
34. Dimitroulas T, Lambe T, Klocke R, Kitas GD, Duarte RV. Biologic drugs as analgesics for the management of osteoarthritis. Semin Arthritis Rheum. 2017;46:687–91.
35. Wenham CYJ, Grainger AJ, Hensor EMA, Caperon AR, Ash ZR, Conaghan PG. Methotrexate for pain relief in knee osteoarthritis: an open-label study. Rheumatology. 2013;52:888–92.

10

Is synovial hypertrophy without Doppler activity sensitive to change? Post-hoc analysis from a rheumatoid arthritis ultrasound study

Lene Terslev[1*], Mikkel Østergaard[1,2], Joe Sexton[3] and Hilde Berner Hammer[3]

Abstract

Background: To explore to what extent synovial hypertrophy in joints *without* Doppler activity is a sign of active disease, we investigated the sensitivity to change of synovial hypertrophy *without* Doppler activity during biological disease-modifying antirheumatic drug (bDMARD) treatment in rheumatoid arthritis (RA) patients.

Method: RA patients initiating or switching bDMARD treatment had ultrasound (US) performed on 36 joints at baseline, and at 3 and 6 months. Synovial hypertrophy by grayscale US and Doppler activity were graded separately from 0 to 3 at the joint level for all time points. Changes in synovial hypertrophy in joints without Doppler activity during treatment were assessed and compared with changes in synovial hypertrophy in joints with Doppler activity.

Results: We included 151 patients (82.8% women, 80.1% seropositive for anticyclic citrullinated peptide) with a mean ± standard deviation age of 51.4 ± 13.2 years, a disease duration of 9.9 ± 7.9 years, and baseline Disease Activity Score 28-joint count C-reactive peptide (DAS28-CRP) of 4.14 ± 1.32. At baseline, 44.8% of all joints examined ($n = 5225$) had synovial hypertrophy ≥ 1 and 50.7% of these had synovial hypertrophy *without* Doppler activity. The improvement in synovial hypertrophy was similar in joints with and without Doppler activity but, when adjusting for the baseline score of synovial hypertrophy, joints with synovial hypertrophy *without* Doppler had a higher tendency towards a decrease than joints with synovial hypertrophy *with* Doppler activity independent of grade (3 months: $p < 0.0001$; 6 months: $p = 0.0003$).

Conclusion: Joints *with* synovial hypertrophy *without* Doppler activity improve during treatment, independent of the grade. Thus, SH *without* Doppler activity is not a sign of inactive disease. These findings indicate that joints *with* synovial hypertrophy *without* Doppler activity should also be taken in to account when assessing disease activity by US.

Keywords: Ultrasound, Synovitis, Rheumatoid arthritis, Doppler, Sensitivity-to-change

Background

The treatment strategy and treatment options for rheumatoid arthritis (RA) have improved considerably over the past years. The strategy is to "treat-to-target" (with a target of remission or low disease activity (LDA)) and includes early and aggressive treatment with mono- or combination therapy using disease-modifying antirheumatic drugs (DMARDs). Furthermore, rapid treatment escalation is recommended when there is insufficient clinical response, including the addition of biological DMARDs (bDMARDs). The aim of this strategy is to gain rapid disease control and avoid inflammation, thereby preventing pain and joint destruction and improving physical function [1, 2].

In addition to conventional clinical monitoring of treatment in RA patients, ultrasound (US) has been increasingly applied over the last decade to assess disease activity and the response to therapy. As US has been proven to be

* Correspondence: terslev@dadlnet.dk
[1]Copenhagen Center for Arthritis Research and Center for Rheumatology and Spine Diseases, Centre of Head and Orthopaedics, Rigshospitalet, Copenhagen, Denmark
Full list of author information is available at the end of the article

more sensitive than clinical joint evaluation [3, 4], the addition of US to clinical joint evaluation has allowed for a more elaborate joint involvement, helping in correctly classifying and diagnosing RA patients [5]. When assessing synovitis by US, two components are evaluated: synovial hypertrophy by grayscale (GS) US and hyperemia by Doppler US. Scoring systems have been developed for the two components, with each scored individually [6–10]. Most emphasis in the clinical studies/trials has been on changes in Doppler activity as this is considered to reflect the inflammatory activity, i.e., disease activity [10–12], and hence the primary aim has been the elimination of signs of Doppler activity [13–17].

Joints with synovial hypertrophy *without* Doppler activity are generally believed to be inactive changes [12] and without the ability to change when optimizing treatment [18], thereby being of minimal clinical importance. However, very little is known about how GS synovial hypertrophy *without* Doppler activity behaves in joints during treatment, i.e., if these joints have the potential to improve. The fact that GS synovial hypertrophy per se (though weaker than Doppler activity) is a predictor of erosive progression in patients in remission [19, 20] suggests that GS synovial hypertrophy is important and possibly should be part of imaging remission, and that elimination of Doppler per se is potentially not the only treatment goal in RA patients when considering treatment escalation.

It is therefore of great importance to explore the reversibility of synovial hypertrophy in joints *without* Doppler activity as this—if sensitive to change—may impact decisions to optimize or change treatment in both clinically active RA patients and in patients in remission/LDA.

The aim of the present paper is to explore if synovial hypertrophy in joints *without* Doppler activity is sensitive to change, as compared with synovial hypertrophy in joints *with* Doppler activity, when initiating or switching treatment with bDMARDs in patients with RA. Furthermore, the relationship between the presence of synovial hypertrophy *with and without* Doppler activity and clinical evaluation of disease activity is investigated.

Methods

The study cohort comprised of patients with RA fulfilling the American College of Rheumatology (ACR) 1987 criteria [21] initiating or switching bDMARD treatment in the period from January 2010 to June 2013 (Anzctr.org.au identifier, ACTRN12610000284066). Clinical evaluation (number of tender and swollen joints (= 28), patient and assessor global visual analogue scale (VAS), C-reactive protein (CRP), and US examinations of 36 joints) were performed at baseline, and at 3 and 6 months. Two trained study nurses with longstanding experience in evaluating tender and swollen joints performed the clinical evaluations blinded to the US findings. Disease Activity Score 28-joint count (DAS28)-CRP was calculated for each visit.

US examinations (blinded for the results of the clinical assessments) were performed by the same experienced sonographer (HBH) throughout the study using a Siemens Antares, Excellence version (Siemens Medical Solutions, CA, USA) equipped with a 5–13 MHz linear probe. Power Doppler settings were optimized for inflammatory flow with pulse repetition frequency 391 Hz, Doppler frequency 7.3 MHz, and gain just below the level of noise according to guidelines [22]. The same ultrasound machine with the same settings was used throughout the study and no software upgrade was done.

At each visit, US examination for signs of synovitis was performed for the following 18 joints bilaterally: metacarpophalangeal joints 1–5, proximal interphalangeal joints 2–3, wrist (scoring radiocarpal, intercarpal, and radioulnar joints separately), elbow, knee, talocrural, and metatarsophalangeal joints 1–5. Each joint at each visit was scored semiquantitatively from 0–3 for GS and power Doppler (PD) according to the US atlas of Hammer et al. [8]. Joints with recent surgery, prosthesis, or overlying skin infections were not examined at time of inclusion or during follow-up. The performing sonographer has previously demonstrated a high intra-observer reliability (weighted kappa 0.83 [8]) for the included joints using this atlas [8] for scoring.

The study was approved by the Regional Committee for Medical and Health Research Ethics, South-East Norway, and all patients gave written consent according to the Declaration of Helsinki.

A post-hoc analysis was carried out on those patients from the original cohort [23] fulfilling all follow-up visits. Only joints with follow-up at all time points were included in the analysis.

The primary endpoint of the study was to assess the relative frequency of a synovial hypertrophy score change ≥ 1 in joints *without* Doppler activity versus joints *with* Doppler activity in all joints having a baseline synovial hypertrophy of grade 1 or above. The changes were assessed from baseline to 3-month follow-up and baseline to 6-month follow-up. The secondary endpoint was the correlation between the change in mean synovial hypertrophy score in joints *without* Doppler activity and the change in mean synovial hypertrophy score in joints *with* Doppler activity in joints with baseline synovial hypertrophy of grade 1 or above. This was assessed from baseline to 3-month follow-up and baseline to 6-month follow-up. The tertiary outcome was the association between the mean grade of synovial hypertrophy in joints and the presence/absence of clinical joint tenderness and presence/absence of clinical joint swelling in joints as follows: 1) at 3 months in joints with baseline

Doppler activity; 2) at 6 months in joints *with* baseline Doppler activity; 3) at 3 months in joints *without* baseline Doppler activity; and 4) at 6 months in joints *without* baseline Doppler activity. Finally, we assessed the correlation between changes in mean synovial hypertrophy in Doppler-negative joints, Doppler-positive joints, and changes in DAS28-CRP from baseline to 3-month follow-up and baseline to 6-month follow-up.

Statistics

R statistical software version 3.3.2 was used for analyses. To assess differences in the tendency of synovial hypertrophy to decrease between Doppler-positive versus Doppler-negative joints, the corresponding odds ratio between these two groups was estimated. This was performed using a logistic mixed-effects model, where the dependent variable was decrease in synovial hypertrophy from baseline ≥ 1 point, coded as a binary variable equal to 1 if a decrease was observed (for a given joint at a given time point) and 0 otherwise. The independent variable was Doppler status of the joint at baseline (0 if Doppler = 0, 1 if Doppler > 0), further adjusting for both baseline synovial hypertrophy level of each joint as well as the observation time (treated as a categorical variable). To account for dependencies between observations from the same patient, as well as from the same joint, random intercepts for both terms were included in the model. Only joints with synovial hypertrophy at baseline were included in the analysis, and the model was fit using data at both 3 and 6 months. The difference in mean grade synovial hypertrophy between tender and non-tender joints was evaluated using a bootstrap test. The same was performed for joint swelling. Correlation between change in mean synovial hypertrophy across joints and change in DAS28-CRP was calculated using Spearman's correlation.

Results

Of the original cohort of 212 patients [23], 151 completed both baseline and 3- and 6-month follow-up. Baseline demographics for the included patients are listed in Table 1.

In total, 5225 joints were evaluated at baseline and, of these, 1191 joints had synovial hypertrophy *without* Doppler activity but only 1172 had follow-up at both 3 and 6 months. At baseline, 1154 had synovial hypertrophy *with* Doppler activity, but only 1122 had follow-up at 3 and 6 months. The reasons that joints were unavailable for US examination at 3 and/or 6 months included recent surgery, including prosthesis surgery, joint trauma, or overlying skin infections.

Joints with synovial hypertrophy *without* Doppler activity had overall lower grades of synovial hypertrophy (1.3 ± 0.3 (mean ± standard deviation (SD)) than joints with synovial hypertrophy *with* Doppler activity (2.1 ± 0.5) at baseline. In general, joints with lower levels of synovial hypertrophy had lower tendency towards change (Table 2).

Table 1 Demographic data for the 151 patients

Patients	82.8% women
Age (years)	51.4 ± 13.2
Anti-CCP	80.1% positive
Rheumatoid factor	75.2% positive
Disease duration (years)	9.9 ± 7.9
Number of swollen joints	6.49 ± 5.5
Number of tender joints	5.98 ± 6.4
bDMARDs initiated in the study cohort	Infliximab (*n* = 19), etanercept (*n* = 59), adalimumab (n = 8), certolizumab (*n* = 12), golimumab (*n* = 8), rituximab (*n* = 30), tocilizumab (n = 8), and abatacept (*n* = 5); 8% of the patients were biologic naive
Prednisolone treated	50.7%
Prednisolone dose	7.8 ± 4.68 mg
DAS28-CRP score	4.14 ± 1.32)
Total number of joints examined, *n*	5225
Joints with SH and no Doppler at baseline, *n* (%)	1191 (23%)
Joints with SH and Doppler at baseline, *n* (%)	1151 (22%)

Values are shown as mean ± standard deviation unless otherwise indicated
bDMARD biological disease-modifying antirheumatic drug, *CCP* cyclic citrullinated peptide, *DAS28-CRP* Disease Activity Score 28-joint count C-reactive peptide, *SH* synovial hypertrophy

Improvement in synovial hypertrophy during treatment

The overall frequency of change in synovial hypertrophy in joints *without* Doppler activity and joints *with* Doppler activity was similar at both 3 months (0.54 and 0.53, respectively) and 6 months (0.56 and 0.60, respectively) (Table 2). However, when adjusting for the baseline grade of synovial hypertrophy, the change was significantly different between joints *with and without* Doppler activity. The adjusted odds ratios were 0.35 at 3 months and 0.39 at 6 months, showing that joints with synovial hypertrophy *with* Doppler activity were significantly less likely to change than joints with synovial hypertrophy *without* Doppler activity for all grades (3 months: $p < 0.0001$; 6 months $p = 0.0003$).

The mean ± SD synovial hypertrophy in joints *without* Doppler activity at both 3 and 6 months was 1.3 ± 0.3 with a change from baseline of −0.5 ± 0.4 and −0.6 ± 0.4, respectively. In joints with synovial hypertrophy *with* Doppler activity, the synovial hypertrophy score at both 3 and 6 months was 2.1 ± 0.5 with a change at 3 months of −0.7 ± 0.6 and at 6 months of −0.8 ± 0.6. The change in mean synovial hypertrophy score in joints *with and without* Doppler activity correlated significantly at both

Table 2 Improvement in synovial hypertrophy (SH) in joints with and without Doppler activity

Time	Grades	Joints with SH without Doppler activity			Joints with SH with Doppler activity			Adjusted odds ratio	p value
		Number of joints		Frequency of improvement	Number of joints		Frequency of improvement		
		Baseline	With improvement		Baseline	With improvement			
3 months	All grades	1172	637	0.54	1122	594	0.53	0.35	< 0.0001
	Grade 1	863	441	0.51	169	58	0.35		
	Grade 2	269	164	0.61	494	271	0.55		
	Grade 3	40	32	0.80	459	265	0.58		
6 months	All grades	1172	657	0.56	1122	669	0.60	0.39	0.0003
	Grade 1	863	457	0.53	169	58	0.34		
	Grade 2	269	167	0.62	494	312	0.63		
	Grade 3	40	33	0.82	459	299	0.65		

The table shows the frequency of improvement in joints at 3 and 6 months for all grades overall and separately for each grade
The relative frequency of a SH score decrease ≥ 1 were analyzed using a generalized linear mixed model adjusting for baseline SH score using a separate coefficient per time point

3 and 6 months ($r = 0.37$, $p < 0.0001$, and $r = 0.34$, $p < 0.0001$, respectively).

Of the joints with synovial hypertrophy *without* Doppler activity included in the analysis, 43% had achieved a synovial hypertrophy score of 0 at 3 months and 45% at 6 months while, for the joints with synovial hypertrophy *with* Doppler activity, this was found in 20% and 24% at 3 and 6 months, respectively. The frequency of different synovial hypertrophy grades at different time points are shown in Table 3.

The mean synovial hypertrophy grade in different joint groups were comparable (mean 1.23, range 1.15–1.53, at baseline in joints with synovial hypertrophy *without* Doppler activity). All joint groups showed an improvement in synovial hypertrophy at both 3 and 6 months compared with baseline (data not shown).

Association between mean grade of synovial hypertrophy and clinical evaluation

Joint swelling

When evaluating the joints with synovial hypertrophy *without* Doppler activity there was a significantly higher grade of synovial hypertrophy in joints with clinical joint swelling compared with joints without clinical joint swelling at all time points ($p < 0.0001$). At baseline, the mean grade of synovial hypertrophy was 0.81 in clinical swollen joints as opposed to 0.22 in non-swollen joints; at 3 months it was 0.92 versus 0.19, and at 6 months 1.07 versus 0.20. Similar findings were seen in the joints with synovial hypertrophy *with* Doppler activity but with higher mean synovial hypertrophy score at all time points (2.56 in swollen versus 2.12 in non-swollen joints at baseline, 2.49 versus 1.95 at 3 months, and 2.53 versus 1.86 at 6 months).

Table 3 The frequency of different synovial hypertrophy (SH) grades at different time points

Time	SH grade 0	SH grade 1	SH grade 2	SH grade 3
Baseline	53.9%	19.1%	14.2%	9.3%
3 months	61.1%	19%	11%	5%
6 months	61.6%	19.1%	10%	4.3%

Joint tenderness

When evaluating the joints with synovial hypertrophy *without* Doppler activity, there was a significant difference in mean synovial hypertrophy score in clinically tender joints compared with non-tender joints at all time points ($p < 0.0001$). At baseline the mean synovial hypertrophy score was 0.50 in clinically tender joints as opposed to 0.24 in non-tender joints; at 3 months the results were 0.44 versus 0.22, and at 6 months 0.48 versus 0.23, respectively. However, in joints with synovial hypertrophy *with* Doppler activity there was no statistically significant difference in mean synovial hypertrophy score between clinically tender and non-tender joints at any time point (2.45 in tender versus 2.45 in non-tender joints at baseline, 2.29 versus 2.31 at 3 months, and 2.38 versus 1.33 at 6 months).

Correlation between synovial hypertrophy and DAS28-CRP remission

There was a weak but statistically significant correlation between change in the mean synovial hypertrophy score across all joints and the change in DAS28-CRP for joints with synovial hypertrophy with as well as *without* Doppler activity. The correlation coefficient for joints with synovial hypertrophy *without* Doppler activity was 0.28 ($p = 0.001$) at 3 months and 0.17 ($p = 0.03$) at 6 months. For joints with synovial hypertrophy *with* Doppler activity, the correlation coefficient was 0.23 ($p = 0.007$) at 3 months and 0.34 ($p = 0.001$) at 6 months.

Discussion

The present study reveals that joints with synovial hypertrophy *without* Doppler activity are sensitive to change during bDMARD treatment and, when taking into account the baseline score of the synovial hypertrophy, joints with synovial hypertrophy *without* Doppler activity have a higher tendency towards change than joints with synovial hypertrophy *with* Doppler activity, independent of the grade.

Even though the treatment effect is evaluated by both GS and Doppler, the main focus is often on the changes in Doppler activity since the Doppler activity is believed to reflect the inflammatory component of the disease [11, 12, 14, 16, 18]. Although the two components in synovitis (i.e., synovial hypertrophy and hyperemia) are likely to change in parallel when treatment is initiated [10, 24, 25], there has been a lack of evidence of the ability for joints with initial synovial hypertrophy without signs of hyperemia to change per se during treatment. In 2013, Witt et al. [18] showed that synovial hypertrophy grade 1 in cohorts of both early and late RA patients was less likely to respond to treatment and, furthermore, grade 1 was also found in healthy controls. These grade 1 findings were not associated with swelling or tenderness in either RA patients or healthy controls. Padovano et al. reported similar frequent findings of grade 1 synovial hypertrophy among healthy controls [26]. In the current study, we have demonstrated that, in RA patients, synovial hypertrophy both *with and without* Doppler activity has the ability to improve when initiating effective treatment, even grade 1 synovial hypertrophy. Similar results have been seen for tenosynovitis, where grade 1 tenosynovitis without Doppler improves during treatment [27]. The US changes were also compared with changes in DAS28-CRP (i.e., to clinical assessment of treatment response). A weak but significant correlation was found between changes in DAS28-CRP and changes in mean synovial hypertrophy score for both joints *with and without* Doppler activity, indicating that the improvements in the joints are in line with the overall disease improvement during treatment. Furthermore, in the current study, the mean grade of synovial hypertrophy was higher in joints *with* than *without* Doppler activity, both in tender and swollen joints, supporting that both measures reflect aspects of disease activity.

The present study shows that synovial hypertrophy is susceptible to change during treatment but does not indicate which of the two components is the most important. In a recent publication from the Outcome Measures in Rheumatology (OMERACT) US group [9, 28], a consensus-based scoring system for synovitis in RA patients has been developed taking both components of the synovitis complex into account in a combined score. The relevance of including the GS synovial hypertrophy in this scoring is further substantiated by the findings in the present study.

The impact of Doppler sensitivity on scoring has previously been investigated and it has been shown that suboptimal settings and suboptimal equipment may result in lack of Doppler activity in inflamed joints [29]. In the present study, high-end US equipment was used to make sure that the detected joints with synovial hypertrophy but no Doppler activity truly reflected a lack of hyperemia in the joints.

Conclusion

Our study shows that joints with synovial hypertrophy *without* Doppler activity improve during bDMARD treatment, demonstrating that synovial hypertrophy *without* Doppler activity is a sign of active disease. These findings indicate that joints with synovial hypertrophy *without* Doppler activity should be taken into account when assessing disease activity by ultrasound.

Abbreviations

ACR: American College of Rheumatology; bDMARD: Biological disease-modifying antirheumatic drug; CRP: C-reactive protein; DAS28: Disease Activity Score 28-joint count; DMARD: Disease-modifying antirheumatic drug; GS: Grayscale; LDA: Low disease activity; OMERACT: Outcome Measures in Rheumatology; RA: Rheumatoid arthritis; SD: Standard deviation; US: Ultrasound; VAS: Visual analogue scale

Funding

The ULRABBIT trial was supported by AbbVie, Pfizer and Roche in form of study grants to the Department of Rheumatology, DiakonHjmmet Hospital, Oslo, Norway.

Authors' contributions

LT and MO performed the post-hoc study design, HBH carried out data acquisition, and JS performed the statistical analyses. LT, MO, and HBH carried out data interpretation and manuscript preparation. All authors read and approved the final manuscript.

Competing interests

LT declares speakers fees from Roche, MSD, BMS, Pfizer, AbbVie, Novartis, and Janssen. MO declares research support and/or consultancy/speaker fees from Abbvie, BMS, Boehringer-Ingelheim, Celgene, Eli-Lilly, Centocor, GSK, Hospira, Janssen, Merck, Mundipharma, Novartis, Novo, Orion, Pfizer, Regeneron, Roche, Takeda, UCB, and Wyeth. HBH declares study grants from AbbVie/Pfizer and Roche. JS declares that he has no competing interests.

Author details

[1]Copenhagen Center for Arthritis Research and Center for Rheumatology and Spine Diseases, Centre of Head and Orthopaedics, Rigshospitalet, Copenhagen, Denmark. [2]Department of Clinical Medicine, University of Copenhagen, Copenhagen, Denmark. [3]Department of Rheumatology, Diakonhjemmet Hospital, Oslo, Norway.

References

1. Smolen JS, Aletaha D, Bijlsma JW, Breedveld FC, Boumpas D, Burmester G, et al. Treating rheumatoid arthritis to target: recommendations of an international task force. Ann Rheum Dis. 2010;69(4):631–7.
2. Smolen JS, Landewé R, Breedveld FC, Dougados M, Emery P, Gaujoux-Viala C, et al. EULAR recommendations for the management of rheumatoid

arthritis with synthetic and biological disease-modifying antirheumatic drugs. Ann Rheum Dis. 2010;69(6):964–75.

3. Wakefield RJ, Green MJ, Marzo-Ortega H, Conaghan PG, Gibbon WW, McGonagle D, et al. Should oligoarthritis be reclassified? Ultrasound reveals a high prevalence of subclinical disease. Ann Rheum Dis. 2004;63:382–5.
4. Salaffi F, Filippucci E, Carotti M, Naredo E, Meenagh G, Ciapetti A, et al. Inter-observer agreement of standard joint counts in early rheumatoid arthritis: a comparison with grey scale ultrasonography—a preliminary study. Rheumatology (Oxford). 2008;47:54–8.
5. Aletaha D, Neogi T, Silman AJ, Funovits J, Felson DT, Bingham CO 3rd, et al. 2010 rheumatoid arthritis classification criteria: an American College of Rheumatology /European league against rheumatism collaborative initiative. Arthritis Rheum. 2010;62(9):2569–81.
6. Qvistgaard E, Rogind H, Torp-Pedersen S, Terslev L, Danneskiold-Samsøe B, Bliddal H. Quantitative ultrasonography in rheumatoid arthritis: evaluation of inflammation by Doppler technique. Ann Rheum Dis. 2001;60:690–3.
7. Szkudlarek M, Court-Payen M, Jacobsen S, Klarlund M, Thomsen HS, Østergaard M. Interobserver agreement in ultrasonography of the finger and toe joints in rheumatoid arthritis. Arthritis Rheum. 2003;48:955–62.
8. Hammer HB, Bolton-King P, Bakkeheim V, Berg TH, Sundt E, Kongtorp AK, et al. Examination of intra and interrater reliability with a new ultrasonographic reference atlas for scoring of synovitis in patients with rheumatoid arthritis. Ann Rheum Dis. 2011;70(11):1995–8.
9. D'Agostino MA, Terslev L, Aegerter P, Backhaus M, Balint P, Bruyn GA, et al. Scoring ultrasound synovitis in rheumatoid arthritis: a EULAR-OMERACT ultrasound taskforce-part 1: definition and development of a standardised, consensus-based scoring system. RMD Open. 2017;3(1):e000428.
10. Larché MJ, Seymour M, Lim A, Eckersley RJ, Pétavy F, et al. Quantitative power Doppler ultrasonography is a sensitive measure of metacarpophalangeal joint synovial vascularity in rheumatoid arthritis and declines significantly following a 2-week course of oral low-dose corticosteroids. J Rheumatol. 2010;37(12):2493–501.
11. Taylor PC, Steuer A, Gruber J, Cosgrove DO, Blomley MJ, Marsters PA, et al. Comparison of ultrasonographic assessment of synovitis and joint vascularity with radiographic evaluation in a randomized, placebo-controlled study of infliximab therapy in early rheumatoid arthritis. Arthritis Rheum. 2004;50(4):1107–16.
12. Brown AK, Quinn MA, Karim Z, Conaghan PG, Peterfy CG, Hensor E, et al. Presence of significant synovitis in rheumatoid arthritis patients with disease-modifying antirheumatic drug-induced clinical remission: evidence from an imaging study may explain structural progression. Arthritis Rheum. 2006;54(12):3761–73.
13. Dale J, Stirling A, Zhang R, Purves D, Foley J, Sambrook M, et al. Targeting ultrasound remission in early rheumatoid arthritis: the results of the TaSER study, a randomised clinical trial. Ann Rheum Dis. 2016;75(6):1043–50.
14. Haavardsholm EA, Aga AB, Olsen IC, Lillegraven S, Hammer HB, Uhlig T, et al. Ultrasound in management of rheumatoid arthritis: ARCTIC randomised controlled strategy trial. BMJ. 2016;354:i4205.
15. Wakefield RJ, Freeston JE, Hensor EM, Bryer D, Quinn MA, Emery P. Delay in imaging versus clinical response: a rationale for prolonged treatment with anti-tumor necrosis factor medication in early rheumatoid arthritis. Arthritis Rheum. 2007;57(8):1564–7.
16. Filippucci E, Iagnocco A, Salaffi F, Cerioni A, Valesini G, Grassi W. Power Doppler sonography monitoring of synovial perfusion at the wrist joints in patients with rheumatoid arthritis treated with adalimumab. Ann Rheum Dis. 2006;65(11):1433–7.
17. Terslev L, Torp-Pedersen S, Qvistgaard E, Kristoffersen H, Røgind H, Danneskiold-Samsøe B, et al. Effects of treatment with etanercept (Enbrel, TNRF:fc) on rheumatoid arthritis evaluated by Doppler ultrasonography. Ann Rheum Dis. 2003;62(2):178–81.
18. Witt M, Mueller F, Nigg A, Reindl C, Leipe J, Proft F, et al. Relevance of grade 1 gray-scale ultrasound findings in wrists and small joints to the assessment of subclinical synovitis in rheumatoid arthritis. Arthritis Rheum. 2013;65(7):1694–701.
19. Brown AK, Conaghan PG, Karim Z, Quinn MA, Ikeda K, Peterfy CG, et al. An explanation for the apparent dissociation between clinical remission and continued structural deterioration in rheumatoid arthritis. Arthritis Rheum. 2008;58(10):2958–67.
20. Saleem B, Brown AK, Keen H, Nizam S, Freeston J, Karim Z, et al. Disease remission state in patients treated with the combination of tumor necrosis factor blockade and methotrexate or with disease-modifying antirheumatic drugs: a clinical and imaging comparative study. Arthritis Rheum. 2009;60(7):1915–22.
21. Arnett FC, Edworthy SM, Bloch DA, McShane DJ, Fries JF, Cooper NS, et al. The American Rheumatism Association 1987 revised criteria for the classification of rheumatoid arthritis. Arthritis Rheum. 1988;31:315–24.
22. Torp-Pedersen ST, Terslev L. Settings and artefacts relevant in colour/power Doppler ultrasound in rheumatology. Ann Rheum Dis. 2008;67(2):143–9.
23. Hammer HB, Uhlig T, Kvien TK, Lampa J. Pain catastrophizing is strongly associated with subjective outcomes, but not with inflammatory assessments in rheumatoid arthritis patients. Arthritis Care Res (Hoboken). 2018;70(5):703–12.
24. Døhn UM, Ejbjerg B, Boonen A, Hetland ML, Hansen MS, Knudsen LS, et al. No overall progression and occasional repair of erosions despite persistent inflammation in adalimumab-treated rheumatoid arthritis patients: results from a longitudinal comparative MRI, ultrasonography, CT and radiography study. Ann Rheum Dis. 2011;70(2):252–8.
25. D'Agostino MA, Wakefield RJ, Berner-Hammer H, Vittecoq O, Filippou G, Balint P, Iagnocco A, Naredo E, Østergaard M, Boers M, Gaillez C, van Holder K, Le Bars M, OMERACT-EULAR Ultrasound task force. Value of ultrasonography as a marker of early response to abatacept in patients with rheumatoid arthritis and an inadequate response to methotrexate: results from the APPRAISE study. Ann Rheum Dis. 2016;75(10):1763–9.
26. Padovano I, Costantino F, Breban M, D'Agostino MA. Prevalence of ultrasound synovial inflammatory findings in healthy subjects. Ann Rheum Dis. 2016;75(10):1819–23.
27. Ammitzbøll-Danielsen M, Østergaard M, Naredo E, Terslev L. Validity and sensitivity to change of the semi-quantitative OMERACT ultrasound scoring system for tenosynovitis in patients with rheumatoid arthritis. Rheumatology (Oxford). 2016;55(12):2156–66.
28. Terslev L, Naredo E, Aegerter P, Wakefield RJ, Backhaus M, Balint P, et al. Scoring ultrasound synovitis in rheumatoid arthritis: a EULAR-OMERACT ultrasound taskforce-part 2: reliability and application to multiple joints of a standardised consensus-based scoring system. RMD Open. 2017;3(1):e000427.
29. Torp-Pedersen S, Christensen R, Szkudlarek M, Ellegaard K, D'Agostino MA, Iagnocco A, et al. Power and color Doppler ultrasound settings for inflammatory flow: impact on scoring of disease activity in patients with rheumatoid arthritis. Arthritis Rheumatol. 2015;67(2):386–95.

11

Sequence of joint tissue inflammation during rheumatoid arthritis development

R. M. ten Brinck[1*], H. W. van Steenbergen[1] and A. H. M. van der Helm–van Mil[1,2]

Abstract

Objective: Subclinical joint inflammation in patients with arthralgia is predictive for progression to rheumatoid arthritis (RA). However, the time course of progression for bone marrow edema (osteitis), synovitis, and/or tenosynovitis is unsettled. This longitudinal study assessed the course of magnetic resonance imaging (MRI)-detected subclinical joint inflammation during progression to RA.

Methods: Patients that progressed from clinically suspect arthralgia (CSA) to RA underwent 1.5-T MRI of the metacarpophalangeal (MCP), wrist, and metatarsophalangeal (MTP) joints at presentation with arthralgia and at first identification of synovitis assessed through physical examination ($n = 31$). MRIs were evaluated for osteitis, synovitis, tenosynovitis, and erosions by two readers, blinded for clinical data and order in time. To estimate changes in MRI scores between the asymptomatic state and CSA onset, scores of MRI features at CSA baseline were compared with scores from age-matched symptom-free persons.

Results: At presentation with CSA, synovitis and tenosynovitis scores were higher than scores from age-matched symptom-free persons ($p = 0.004$ and $p = 0.001$, respectively). Anti-citrullinated protein antibody (ACPA)-positive arthralgia patients also had increased osteitis scores ($p = 0.04$). Median duration between presentation with arthralgia and RA development was 17 weeks. During progression to RA, synovitis and osteitis increased significantly ($p = 0.001$ and $p = 0.036$, respectively) in contrast to tenosynovitis and erosion scores. This pattern was similar in both ACPA subsets, although statistical significance was reached for synovitis and osteitis in ACPA-negative but not ACPA-positive RA.

Conclusion: Increased tenosynovitis and synovitis scores at CSA onset and the increase in synovitis and osteitis during progression to RA suggest an 'outside-in' temporal relationship of arthritis development, in particular for ACPA-negative RA. For ACPA-positive RA, further studies are needed.

Keywords: Rheumatoid arthritis, Inflammation, Imaging

Background

Rheumatoid arthritis (RA) can be diagnosed at the time patients present with clinically detectable inflammatory arthritis (swollen joints). It is known that immunological alterations are present long before that [1]. For instance, magnetic resonance imaging (MRI)-detected subclinical inflammation is present weeks to months before arthritis becomes clinically apparent in patients presenting with clinically suspect arthralgia (CSA) and has been shown to be predictive for RA development [2]. Nonetheless, a long-standing question is where inflammation starts in the joint, or in what order the different tissues of the joints (synovium, tenosynovium, and bone) become inflamed during the development of RA.

Several hypotheses on the chronology of arthritis development prevail. Firstly, it has been postulated that synovitis is an initial process that is succeeded by bone involvement. This is the traditional 'outside-in hypothesis,' presuming that inflammation of the synovium precedes bone marrow edema (or osteitis) [3–7]. Alternatively, it has been suggested that RA is a primary bone marrow disease which subsequently encroaches upon the synovial membrane; this is the 'inside-out hypothesis,' with osteitis preceding synovitis, a hypothesis that has become popular after imaging and histological studies revealed the presence of osteitis at

* Correspondence: r.m.ten_brinck@lumc.nl
[1]Department of Rheumatology C1-R, Leiden University Medical Centre, PO Box 9600, Leiden 2300RC, the Netherlands
Full list of author information is available at the end of the article

locations with MRI-detected osteitis in patients with RA [4, 7, 8]. It has also been hypothesized that these processes could emerge and progress simultaneously with microscopic bone canals allowing transduction of inflammation from the outside (synovium) to the inside (bone marrow) and vice versa [4, 7, 9]. Finally, mouse models of arthritis development have shown that tenosynovitis was the initial preclinical change [10]. Extrapolation to humans would suggest that tenosynovitis rather than synovitis or osteitis is the primary feature of joint inflammation [10]. For the development of bone erosions (instead of the development of clinically apparent inflammatory arthritis) similar hypotheses have been postulated, with the primary inflammation located inside [11, 12] or outside the bone [13], respectively. Altogether, temporal relationships are yet unknown and can be discovered by longitudinal imaging studies that start in pre-arthritis phases of the disease.

To address the question about the chronological order in which the different tissues of the joints become inflamed, this longitudinal MRI study investigated the course of MRI-detected subclinical joint inflammation (synovitis, tenosynovitis, osteitis) and erosions in patients that presented with arthralgia and progressed to RA. MRIs were performed longitudinally at presentation with arthralgia and at development of RA. Although no MRIs were made in the asymptomatic phase of these patients, the MRI data obtained at presentation with arthralgia were compared with data obtained in age-matched symptom-free persons to estimate the course of inflammation before presentation with arthralgia. Finally, as anti-citrullinated protein antibody (ACPA)-positive and ACPA-negative RA are considered as different disease subsets with differences in the underlying pathophysiology, analyses were stratified for ACPA-positive and ACPA-negative RA to explore if there are differences in the chronological order in which different articular tissues become inflamed.

Patients and methods

Patients

We longitudinally followed patients that presented with CSA between April 2012 and September 2016. The Leiden CSA cohort consecutively included patients that presented at the rheumatology outpatient clinic of the Leiden University Medical Centre without clinically evident arthritis, but with recent-onset (< 1 year) arthralgia of small joints that was considered at risk for RA by their rheumatologists based on the clinical presentation [14]. A detailed description of the inclusion and exclusion criteria of the Leiden CSA cohort and the study protocol are described in [15]. Absence of clinical arthritis at baseline was ascertained through physical examination by an experienced rheumatologist.

Regular follow-up visits in the cohort were planned at 4, 12, and 24 months. If necessary (for instance, when the patient experienced more symptoms or noticed a swollen joint), patients were seen in between scheduled visits by their rheumatologist. Hence, logistics were arranged such that patients in this cohort had very easy access to rheumatology care, and clinically evident inflammatory arthritis was identified at the first opportunity. The outcome was clinically apparent arthritis, identified at joint examination by an experienced rheumatologist. Previous studies revealed that ~ 20% of patients that presented with CSA progressed to clinically apparent inflammatory arthritis [2].

For this study we selected the patients included in the CSA cohort that developed clinically apparent RA. A flowchart is provided in Fig. 1. From a total of 416 patients included in the CSA cohort during the studied period, 76 were diagnosed with RA. Serial MRI was performed at baseline and at arthritis development (but before disease-modifying antirheumatic drugs (DMARDs) were started). Of the 76 RA patients, serial MRIs were available in 35 patients. In 41 patients serial imaging was not available because four patients had contraindications for gadolinium contrast, three patients progressed to RA in a very short period of time, and 34 patients were lacking serial MRI due to logistical reasons.

Thirty-five patients were diagnosed with RA and had serial MRI available. Four out of these 35 patients did not receive a prescription for a DMARD at the visit when clinical arthritis was identified (three patients subsequently had resolution of arthritis, one patient received a prescription at the next visit). Thus, in total 31 patients with a clinical diagnosis of RA and immediate prescription of DMARDs were studied. Notably, fulfilment of the 2010 classification criteria was not required to define RA since ACPA-negative patients require > 10 involved joints to fulfil these criteria [16] and this can be hampered by DMARD initiation. Nonetheless, despite this theoretical threshold, 21 patients (68%) fulfilled the 2010 criteria for RA at arthritis development. It is important to note that DMARDs (including corticosteroids) were not prescribed in the phase of arthralgia.

Symptom-free persons

Serial MRIs were not made in the period preceding presentation with CSA. To infer the course of MRI-detected subclinical inflammation over time before the phase of CSA, the MRI data from the 31 CSA patients were compared with data from symptom-free persons [17]. Symptom-free persons were matched based on age in a 1:2 ratio. These 62 symptom-free persons had no history of inflammatory rheumatic diseases, no joint symptoms during the previous month, and no evidence of synovitis at physical examination. The persons were retrieved from

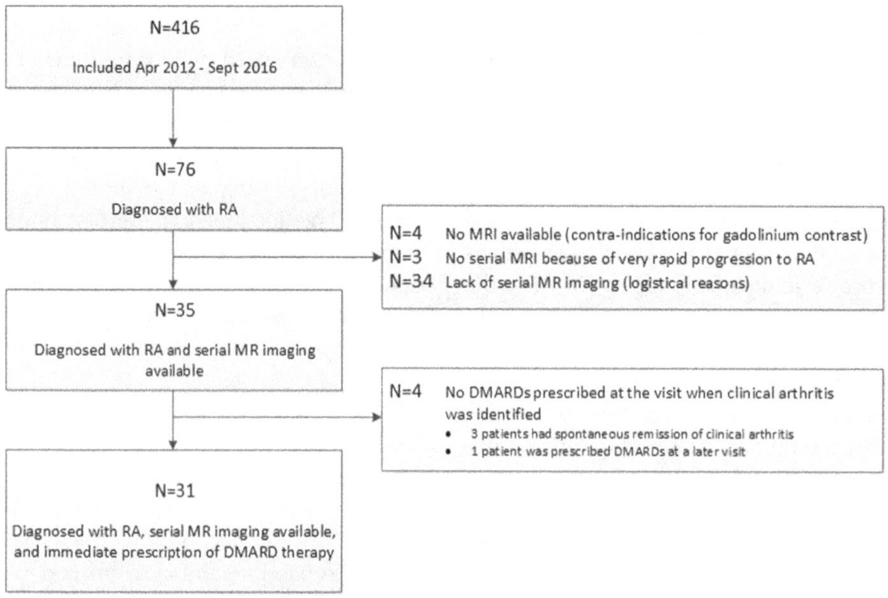

Fig. 1 Flowchart of selection of rheumatoid arthritis (RA) patients studied from the total CSA cohort. Patient characteristics of the different groups are provided in Additional file 1 (Table S2). DMARD disease-modifying antirheumatic drug, MR magnetic resonance, MRI magnetic resonance imaging

the general population; the recruitment procedure is described elsewhere [17]. Since gender ($p = 0.10$), increased body mass index (BMI) ($p = 0.59$) [18], and smoking ($p = 0.21$) had no effect on MRI-detected inflammation, matching was not performed on these factors.

MRI

Unilateral MRIs of the wrist, metacarpophalangeal (MCP) joints 2–5, and metatarsophalangeal (MTP) joints 1–5 were performed at presentation with CSA (on the most painful side) and at first presentation with clinical synovitis (the same side as scanned at baseline). A total of 18 tenosynovitis locations were scored in each patient: 10 at the wrist, including 6 extensor compartments and 4 regions on the volar side (the flexor digitorum profundus and flexor digitorum superficialis, the flexor pollicis longus, the flexor carpi ulnaris, and the flexor carpi radialis), and 8 locations at MCP joints 2–5 (paired flexor tendons and extensor tendons of the fingers). An ONI MSK Extreme 1.5-T MRI scanner (GE Healthcare, Wisconsin, USA) was used as described previously [2] and in Additional file 1 (Supplementary methods). All patients were instructed not to use nonsteroidal anti-inflammatory drugs (NSAIDs) 24 h prior to MRI, with only seven patients (23%) reporting the daily use of NSAIDs at baseline. The serial MRIs were scored blinded for clinical data and order in time by two readers for osteitis, erosions, and synovitis as described in [19] and tenosynovitis as described in [20]. The mean scores of two readers were studied. Additional information on the scoring is provided in Additional file 1 (Supplementary methods). Three readers contributed to the scoring of the MRIs. Within-reader intraclass correlation coefficients (ICCs) and between-reader ICCs were all > 0.90 and are also presented in Additional file 1 (Table S1). Results of MRI were not shared with the treating rheumatologists.

Analyses

Paired t tests were used. Longitudinal modeling was performed using generalized estimating equations (GEE); the scores of the different inflammatory features and erosions were studied over time. The GEE models, utilizing an unstructured correlation matrix, corrected for the influence of age, gender, and time to progression to RA and baseline score per feature. Residuals of GEE modeling were checked for normal distribution. Statistical analyses were performed using the Statistical Package for the Social Sciences (SPSS, version 23.0). P values < 0.05 were considered significant.

Results

Patients

Characteristics of the 31 RA patients studied were similar to the total group of 76 patients diagnosed with RA, except for a lower frequency of ACPA positivity in the studied group (Additional file 1: Table S2). Baseline characteristics of the 31 patients studied are presented in Table 1. The mean age was 44 years, 71% were female, the median tender joint count (68-TJC) was 5 (interquartile range (IQR) 4–10), 42% were rheumatoid factor-positive, and 29% were

Table 1 Characteristics of the RA patients at presentation with clinically suspect arthralgia and at first identification of clinical arthritis and age-matched symptom-free volunteers

	At presentation with arthralgia ($n = 31$)	At presentation with RA ($n = 31$)	Age-matched symptom-free volunteers ($n = 62$)
Age (years), mean (SD)	44 (14)	–	44 (13)
Female sex, *n* (%)	22 (71)	–	38 (61)
Symptom duration (weeks), median (IQR)	17 (9–32)	–	n/a
Presence of morning stiffness ≥ 60 min, *n* (%)	11 (35)	24 (77)	0 (0)
68-TJC, median (IQR)	5 (4–10)	7 (5–12)	0 (0–0)
66-SJC, median (IQR)	0 (0–0)	2 (1–5)	0 (0–0)
Increased CRP (≥ 5 mg/L), *n* (%)	6 (19)	7 (29)	n/a
Autoantibody status			
IgM-RF-positive (≥ 3.5 IU/mL), *n* (%)	13 (42)	13 (42)	n/a
ACPA-positive (≥ 7 U/mL), *n* (%)	9 (29)	9 (29)	n/a
Any antibody-positive (either RF or ACPA)	16 (52)	16 (52)	n/a

ACPA anti-citrullinated peptide antibody, *CRP* C-reactive protein, *IgM-RF* immunoglobulin M rheumatoid factor, *IQR* interquartile range, *n/a* not applicable or not assessed, *RA* rheumatoid arthritis, *RF* rheumatoid factor, *SD* standard deviation, *SJC* swollen joint count, *TJC* tender joint count

ACPA-positive. These characteristics are in line with previous research in CSA patients [15]. The median interval between presentation with arthralgia and progression to RA was 17 weeks. The characteristics of the 31 patients at the time of identification of RA are also presented in Table 1. The DMARDs that were initiated after RA development are presented in Additional file 1 (Table S3).

MRI data at presentation with arthralgia compared with that of age-matched symptom-free controls

Compared with age-matched symptom-free persons from the general population, CSA patients had increased tenosynovitis (mean 1.7 versus 0.27; $p < 0.001$) and synovitis scores (2.2 versus 0.93; $p < 0.001$; Fig. 2). Osteitis scores (1.9 versus 1.4; $p = 0.35$) and erosion scores (1.7 versus 1.8; $p = 0.53$) were not significantly elevated (Fig. 2) at presentation with arthralgia.

Inflammation increased during progression from arthralgia to rheumatoid arthritis

During progression from arthralgia to RA, the mean osteitis score increased from 1.9 to 2.7 ($p = 0.036$), and the mean synovitis score from 2.2 to 3.4 ($p = 0.001$; Fig. 2). Tenosynovitis and erosion scores did not increase significantly (mean 1.7 to 2.0, $p = 0.35$, and 1.7 to 1.9, $p = 0.092$, respectively; Fig. 2). Next, GEE models were constructed, allowing longitudinal data comparisons of MRI inflammatory scores. These models corrected for gender, age at inclusion, time interval to RA, and the score of each feature (e.g., osteitis) at presentation with CSA. GEE modeling demonstrated that only synovitis scores ($\beta = 1.0$; $p = 0.004$) were significantly higher at the time of RA development than at presentation with arthralgia.

Stratification for ACPA status

Finally, we explored if results were different in ACPA-positive and ACPA-negative RA patients, although absolute numbers were small ($n = 9$ and $n = 22$, respectively). ACPA-positive patients had higher osteitis scores ($p = 0.04$), synovitis scores ($p < 0.001$), and tenosynovitis scores ($p < 0.001$) at presentation with arthralgia compared with age-matched symptom-free persons. ACPA-negative patients had higher synovitis scores ($p = 0.02$) and tenosynovitis scores ($p = 0.001$), but the osteitis score was not different ($p = 0.24$). Erosion scores were not different from age-matched symptom-free persons in both ACPA-positive and ACPA-negative patients at presentation with arthralgia.

Over time, during progression from arthralgia to RA, ACPA status did not change for any of the patients. In ACPA-negative patients, osteitis and synovitis score increased significantly (1.1 to 1.7, $p = 0.03$, and 1.8 to 2.9, $p = 0.003$, respectively) during progression from arthralgia to RA, whereas tenosynovitis and erosion scores remained stable (Fig. 3). In ACPA-positive patients, no statistical significance was obtained but osteitis scores increased from 3.6 to 5.2 ($p = 0.22$) and synovitis from 3.1 to 4.5 ($p = 0.13$). Tenosynovitis scores were 1.7 and 2.3 ($p = 0.32$) and erosion scores were 2.4 and 2.6 at presentation with arthralgia and RA, respectively ($p = 0.62$; Fig. 3).

Finally, analyses were repeated for autoantibody-positive (positive for either rheumatoid factor and/or ACPA; $n = 16$) and autoantibody-negative patients ($n = 15$). Similar results were obtained as for ACPA-positive and ACPA-negative RA patients as described above (data not shown).

Discussion

To increase our understanding of the chronological order of joint inflammation during the development of RA, serial MRIs were made in RA patients at the time of

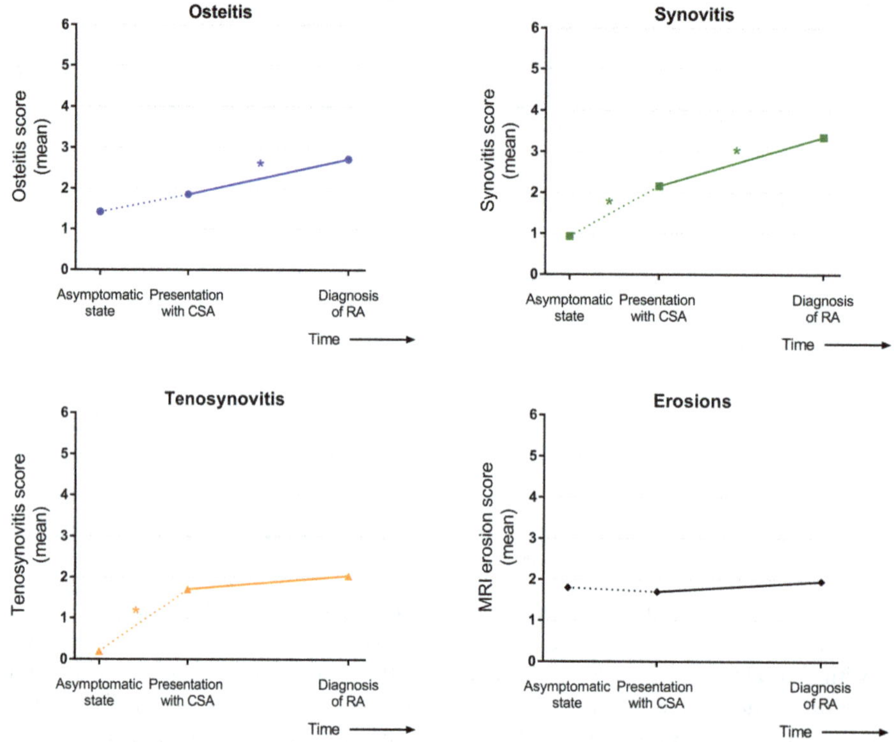

Fig. 2 Magnetic resonance imaging (MRI) features of joint inflammation and erosions in patients that developed rheumatoid arthritis (RA). MRI was performed at presentation with arthralgia and at diagnosis of RA. MRIs were not made in the asymptomatic phase but the course of local inflammation before presentation with arthralgia was estimated by comparisons with age-matched symptom-free persons (1:2 ratio to patients). Since these data were not measured longitudinally, data are presented in dashed lines. *$p < 0.05$. CSA clinically suspect arthralgia

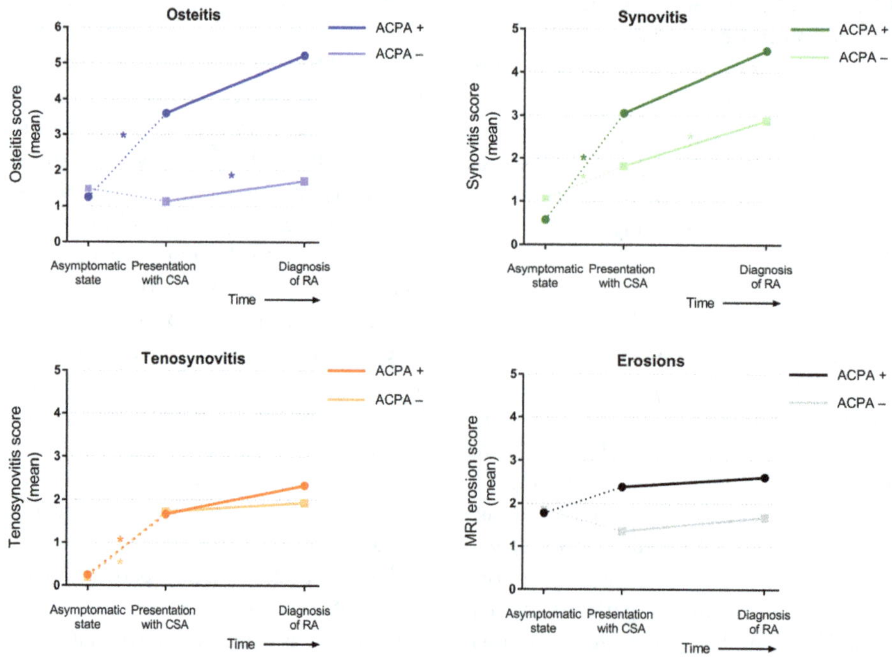

Fig. 3 Magnetic resonance imaging (MRI) features of joint inflammation and erosions in patients that developed rheumatoid arthritis (RA) stratified for anti-citrullinated protein antibody (ACPA) status. MRI was performed at presentation with arthralgia and at diagnosis of RA. MRIs were not made in the asymptomatic phase but the course of local inflammation before presentation with arthralgia was estimated by comparisons with age-matched symptom-free persons (1:2 ratio to patients). Since these data were not measured longitudinally, data are presented in dashed lines. *$p < 0.05$ by paired t test. CSA clinically suspect arthralgia

presentation with arthralgia and at first identification of RA. This revealed that synovitis and osteitis increased during the symptomatic pre-arthritis phase. In addition, data on MRI-detected subclinical inflammation obtained at presentation with arthralgia were compared with data from age-matched symptom-free persons. This showed that synovitis and tenosynovitis scores were higher in patients with arthralgia, suggesting that these features had already increased at presentation with arthralgia. The erosion scores did not increase, neither in the asymptomatic nor during the symptomatic phase preceding the identification of RA. Together, these results suggest that tenosynovitis and synovitis are the earliest inflammatory features. Subsequently, synovitis and osteitis increased over time in the symptomatic pre-arthritis phase, whereas erosions did not increase before RA had become apparent. This implies that inflammation mainly starts outside the bone (fitting the outside-in hypothesis), after which osteitis develops, which puts the joint at risk for structural damage development in the phase of clinically evident RA (if left insufficiently treated).

Stratification for ACPA status showed that synovitis and osteitis progressed similarly during the symptomatic pre-arthritis phase in both ACPA subsets, but that ACPA-positive arthralgia patients already had higher osteitis scores at presentation with arthralgia. This could be explained by a longer symptom duration of ACPA-positive patients at presentation with arthralgia: median symptom duration at baseline was 22 weeks in ACPA-positive CSA patients and 15 weeks in ACPA-negative CSA patients (Additional file 1: Table S3). As established previously, ACPA-positive RA has a more gradual onset of symptoms [21]. ACPA-positive patients may therefore have presented in a slightly later phase of the disease. Alternatively, this finding could also imply a different chronology of joint inflammation in ACPA-negative and ACPA-positive RA, with osteitis being one of the first inflammatory features in ACPA-positive RA. This could be in line with the associations of autoantibody status and osteitis scores observed in the phase of classifiable RA [22].

There are several limitations to this study. One limitation is that the analyses were performed on the sum of synovitis, osteitis, and tenosynovitis scores observed in 310 joints, 1023 bones, and 868 tendons. Whilst it would be interesting to perform similar analyses at the individual joint/bone/tendon level, this was not done because of low numbers of joints/bones/tendons with subclinical inflammation. Larger studies are needed to this end.

Another limitation is the sample size. Although all patients that developed RA from a total cohort of consecutive CSA patients (with serial MRI available) were studied, the absolute number ($n = 31$) is rather small. Future longitudinal imaging studies are therefore required to validate the results. Nonetheless, the present study is the largest longitudinal MRI study in a population of patients that converted from arthralgia to RA that is available to date.

Analyses were stratified for ACPA to explore differences between these subgroups, although the ACPA-positive subgroup especially was rather small. This may be explained by more intramuscular corticosteroid injections in ACPA-positive patients, preventing the performance of an MRI before DMARD initiation. Larger future studies, especially in ACPA-positive convertors, are needed.

Another limitation is that MRIs were made at first presentation with CSA and at development of RA, but no scans were made in between. Furthermore, patients were included at first presentation with clinically suspect arthralgia and were not scanned in an asymptomatic phase. Although some information on the chronology of joint inflammation in this disease phase was obtained by comparison of data obtained in age-matched symptom-free persons, this analysis was cross-sectional in nature and therefore less reliable than longitudinally collected data. Hence, future longitudinal imaging studies would be still highly relevant to further increase our understanding of RA development.

In our study, T1-weighted fat-suppressed sequences were obtained. These were previously demonstrated to have a strong correlation with T2-weighted fat-suppressed sequences in three studies [23–25]. Furthermore, persistent osteitis was strongly associated with erosive progression using these sequences [11]. Taken together, these findings demonstrate that osteitis is an established risk factor for the development of articular bone erosions regardless of the acquired sequence. The lack of a significant increase in osteitis scores between asymptomatic persons and arthralgia patients is more likely to be caused by the (early) disease stage in which the patients were assessed rather than a difference due to the scanning protocol. Nevertheless, replication of our results using T2-weighted fat-suppressed sequences is warranted.

Future serial imaging studies performed in the asymptomatic phase until development of RA would be useful to further elucidate the chronology in which the different articular tissues become inflamed. However, this cannot be easily accomplished as the 5-year positive predictive value of ACPA in the general population is approximately 5% [26, 27]. Consequently, 20 symptom-free ACPA-positive persons would need to be followed for several years with serial MRIs to acquire longitudinal data of one RA patient. Studying 30 ACPA-positive RA patients already in the asymptomatic phase would require serial imaging in ~ 600 ACPA-positive symptom-free persons during several years of follow-up. Hence, although challenging, studying temporal relationships of inflammatory features during progression from the asymptomatic to the symptomatic pre-arthritis phase is a subject for follow-up research.

Animal studies have demonstrated that tenosynovitis is the earliest inflammatory joint feature in murine models [10]. Studies in CSA patients have also revealed that, of all three inflammatory features, tenosynovitis is the strongest predictor for RA development [2]. The current data, showing that tenosynovitis is a very early phenomenon, denote the importance of inflammation of synovial tendon sheaths in very early phases of RA development.

The erosion score did not increase in the pre-arthritis phase, in contrast with the osteitis score. Previous research has revealed that osteitis that persisted in the early clinical phase of RA was strongly associated with erosion development (odds ratio ~ 60) at the same location [11]. CSA patients in this study had very early access to rheumatologic care in case of symptom deterioration or if they suspected joint swelling. Therefore, we expect that patients were seen very shortly after clinical synovitis had developed. In addition, the median duration to development of RA was relatively short (17 weeks). Both factors may explain why articular bone erosions were not (yet) increased during the studied period. Based on MRI data collected in early arthritis patients [11], we anticipate that the bones with osteitis at RA presentation were at risk for development of erosions, but the time period was too brief for actual erosive progression. This is in line with previous studies showing that MRI-detected erosions predominantly developed in joints with persistent osteitis [11].

Imaging using ultrasound (US) can be used to assess the presence of synovitis and tenosynovitis. Our data, obtained in the earliest disease phases, could suggest that US could suffice for assessment of these features. However, US cannot depict osteitis which may also provide valuable information. Studies in larger patient groups are needed before the present findings can be translated to clinical practice, although the present data contribute to our understanding of clinical arthritis and RA development.

Conclusions

In summary, the data provided on RA patients suggest an increase of tenosynovitis and synovitis scores before the onset of arthralgia. Our study demonstrated that synovitis and osteitis scores increased during progression from arthralgia to clinical arthritis, suggesting an 'outside-in' temporal relationship of arthritis development, particularly in ACPA-negative RA. For ACPA-positive RA further studies are needed.

Additional file

Additional file 1: Table S1. Matrix of ICC scores of three readers who contributed to the data; each MRI was evaluated by two readers. **Table S2.** Comparison of patient characteristics between all patients converting to clinically apparent arthritis, those with serial MRIs, and the final selection of RA patients studied. **Table S3.** Patient characteristics of ACPA-positive and ACPA-negative patients studied at presentation with CSA. **Table S4.** Disease-modifying antirheumatic drugs prescribed when clinical arthritis was identified. **Supplementary methods.** MRI scanning protocol and scoring.

Abbreviations

ACPA: Anti-citrullinated protein antibody; BMI: Body mass index; CSA: Clinically suspect arthralgia; DMARD: Disease-modifying antirheumatic drug; GEE: Generalized estimating equations; ICC: Interclass correlation coefficient; IQR: Interquartile range; MCP: Metacarpophalangeal; MRI: Magnetic resonance imaging; MTP: Metatarsophalangeal; NSAID: Nonsteroidal anti-inflammatory drug; RA: Rheumatoid arthritis; SPSS: Statistical Package for the Social Sciences; TJC: Tender joint count; US: Ultrasound

Acknowledgments

The authors would like to thank L. Mangnus and D. Boeters for their scoring of the magnetic resonance images.

Funding

This work was supported by a Vidi grant by the Netherlands Organisation of Health Research and Development and a Starting Grant of the European Research Council. The funding sources had no role in design or conduction of the study, nor the decision to submit the manuscript for publication.

Authors' contributions

RMtB and AHMvdHvM contributed to the conception and study design. RMtB analyzed the data. RMtB, HWvS, and AHMvdHvM contributed to the interpretation of the data. RMtB and AHMvdHvM wrote the first version of the manuscript and RMtB, HWvS, and AHMvdHvM revised it critically. RMtB, HWvS, and AHMvdHvM read and approved the final manuscript.

Authors' information

Not applicable.

Competing interests

The authors declare that they have no competing interests.

Author details

[1]Department of Rheumatology C1-R, Leiden University Medical Centre, PO Box 9600, Leiden 2300RC, the Netherlands. [2]Department of Rheumatology, Erasmus Medical Centre, Rotterdam, The Netherlands.

References

1. Choy E. Understanding the dynamics: pathways involved in the pathogenesis of rheumatoid arthritis. Rheumatology (Oxford). 2012;51(Suppl 5):v3–11. https://doi.org/10.1093/rheumatology/kes113.
2. Van Steenbergen HW, Mangnus L, Reijnierse M, et al. Clinical factors, anticitrullinated peptide antibodies and MRI-detected subclinical

inflammation in relation to progression from clinically suspect arthralgia to arthritis. Ann Rheum Dis. 2016;75(10):1824–30. https://doi.org/10.1136/annrheumdis-2015-208138.
3. Jimenez-Boj E, Nöbauer-Huhmann I, Hanslik-Schnabel B, et al. Bone erosions and bone marrow edema as defined by magnetic resonance imaging reflect true bone marrow inflammation in rheumatoid arthritis. Arthritis Rheum. 2007;56(4):1118–24.
4. Schett G, Firestein GS. Mr Outside and Mr Inside: classic and alternative views on the pathogenesis of rheumatoid arthritis. Ann Rheum Dis. 2010; 69(5):787–9. https://doi.org/10.1136/ard.2009.121657.
5. Kishimoto Y, Fukumoto S, Nishihara S, et al. Gene expression relevant to osteoclastogenesis in the synovium and bone marrow of mature rats with collagen-induced arthritis. Rheumatology (Oxford). 2004;43(12):1496–503.
6. Jimenez-Boj E, Redlich K, Türk B, et al. Interaction between synovial inflammatory tissue and bone marrow in rheumatoid arthritis. J Immunol. 2005;175(4):2579–88.
7. Bugatti S, Manzo A, Caporali R, Montecucco C. Inflammatory lesions in the bone marrow of rheumatoid arthritis patients: a morphological perspective. Arthritis Res Ther. 2012;14(6):229. https://doi.org/10.1186/ar4115.
8. Haavardsholm EA, Bøyesen P, Østergaard M, et al. Magnetic resonance imaging findings in 84 patients with early rheumatoid arthritis: bone marrow oedema predicts erosive progression. Ann Rheum Dis. 2008;67(6): 794–800.
9. Marinova-Mutafchieva L, Williams RO, Funa K, et al. Inflammation is preceded by tumor necrosis factor-dependent infiltration of mesenchymal cells in experimental arthritis. Arthritis Rheum. 2002;46(2):507–13.
10. Hayer S, Redlich K, Korb A, et al. Tenosynovitis and osteoclast formation as the initial preclinical changes in a murine model of inflammatory arthritis. Arthritis Rheum. 2007;56(1):79–88.
11. Nieuwenhuis WP, van Steenbergen HW, Stomp W, et al. The course of bone marrow edema in early undifferentiated and rheumatoid arthritis; a longitudinal MRI study on bone level. Arthritis Rheum. 2016;68(5):1080–8. https://doi.org/10.1002/art.39550.
12. Hetland ML, Ejbjerg B, Hørslev-Petersen K, et al. MRI bone oedema is the strongest predictor of subsequent radiographic progression in early rheumatoid arthritis. Results from a 2-year randomised controlled trial (CIMESTRA). Ann Rheum Dis. 2009;68(3):384–90. https://doi.org/10.1136/ard.2008.088245.
13. Tan AL, Tanner SF, Conaghan PG, et al. Role of metacarpophalangeal joint anatomic factors in the distribution of synovitis and bone erosion in early rheumatoid arthritis. Arthritis Rheum. 2003;48(5):1214–22.
14. Ten Brinck RM, van Steenbergen HW, Mangnus L, et al. Functional limitations in the phase of clinically suspect arthralgia are as serious as in early clinical arthritis; a longitudinal study. RMD Open. 2017;3(1):e000419. https://doi.org/10.1136/rmdopen-2016-000419.
15. Van Steenbergen HW, Van Nies JAB, Huizinga TWJ, et al. Characterising arthralgia in the preclinical phase of rheumatoid arthritis using MRI. Ann Rheum Dis. 2015;74(6):1225–32. https://doi.org/10.1136/annrheumdis-2014-205522.
16. Van Der Helm-van Mil AHM, Zink A. What is rheumatoid arthritis? Considering consequences of changed classification criteria. Ann Rheum Dis. 2017;76(2):315–7. https://doi.org/10.1136/annrheumdis-2016-209629.
17. Mangnus L, Van Steenbergen HW, Reijnierse M, Van der Helm-van Mil AHM. Magnetic resonance imaging-detected features of inflammation and erosions in symptom-free persons from the general population. Arthritis Rheumatol. 2016;68(11):2593–602. https://doi.org/10.1002/art.39749.
18. Mangnus L, Nieuwenhuis WP, van Steenbergen HW, et al. Body mass index and extent of MRI-detected inflammation: opposite effects in rheumatoid arthritis versus other arthritides and asymptomatic persons. Arthritis Res Ther. 2016;18(1):245.
19. Østergaard M, Edmonds J, McQueen F, et al. An introduction to the EULAR–OMERACT rheumatoid arthritis MRI reference image atlas. Ann Rheum Dis. 2005;64(Suppl 1):i3–7.
20. Haavardsholm EA, Østergaard M, Ejbjerg BJ, et al. Introduction of a novel magnetic resonance imaging tenosynovitis score for rheumatoid arthritis: reliability in a multireader longitudinal study. Ann Rheum Dis. 2007;66(9): 1216–20 Epub 2007 Mar 28.
21. Burgers LE, van Steenbergen HW, Ten Brinck RM, et al. Differences in the symptomatic phase preceding ACPA-positive and ACPA-negative RA: a longitudinal study in arthralgia during progression to clinical arthritis. Ann Rheum Dis. 2017;76(10):1751–4. https://doi.org/10.1136/annrheumdis-2017-211325.
22. Boeters DM, Nieuwenhuis WP, Verheul MK, et al. MRI-detected osteitis is not associated with the presence or level of ACPA alone, but with the combined presence of ACPA and RF. Arthritis Res Ther. 2016;18(1). https://doi.org/10.1186/s13075-016-1076-0.
23. Stomp W, Krabben A, van der Heijde D, et al. Aiming for a shorter rheumatoid arthritis MRI protocol: can contrast-enhanced MRI replace T2 for the detection of bone marrow oedema? Eur Radiol. 2014;24:2614–22. https://doi.org/10.1007/s00330-014-3272-0.
24. Schmid MR, Hodler J, Vienne P, et al. Bone marrow abnormalities of foot and ankle: STIR versus T1-weighted contrast-enhanced fat-suppressed spin-echo MR imaging. Radiology. 2002;224:463–9. https://doi.org/10.1148/radiol.2242011252.
25. Mayerhoefer ME, Breitenseher MJ, Kramer J, et al. STIR vs. T1-weighted fat-suppressed gadolinium-enhanced MRI of bone marrow edema of the knee: computer-assisted quantitative comparison and influence of injected contrast media volume and acquisition parameters. J Magn Reson Imaging. 2005;22:788–93. https://doi.org/10.1002/jmri.20439.
26. Hensvold AH, Frisell T, Magnusson PK, et al. How well do ACPA discriminate and predict RA in the general population: a study based on 12,590 population-representative Swedish twins. Ann Rheum Dis. 2017;76(1):119–25. https://doi.org/10.1136/annrheumdis-2015-208980.
27. Nielen MM, van Schaardenburg D, Reesink HW, et al. Specific autoantibodies precede the symptoms of rheumatoid arthritis: a study of serial measurements in blood donors. Arthritis Rheum. 2004;50(2):380–6.

TNFα expressed on the surface of microparticles modulates endothelial cell fate in rheumatoid arthritis

Cristiana Barbati[1*], Marta Vomero[1], Tania Colasanti[1], Marco Diociaiuti[2], Fulvia Ceccarelli[1], Sara Ferrigno[1], Annacarla Finucci[1], Francesca Miranda[1], Lucia Novelli[1], Carlo Perricone[1], Francesca Romana Spinelli[1], Simona Truglia[1], Fabrizio Conti[1], Guido Valesini[1] and Cristiano Alessandri[1]

Abstract

Background: Rheumatoid arthritis (RA) is associated with a high prevalence of atherosclerosis. Recently increased levels of microparticles (MPs) have been reported in patients with RA. MPs could represent a link between autoimmunity and endothelial dysfunction by expressing tumor necrosis factor alpha (TNFα), a key cytokine involved in the pathogenesis of RA, altering endothelial apoptosis and autophagy. The aim of this study was to investigate TNFα expression on MPs and its relationship with endothelial cell fate.

Methods: MPs were purified from peripheral blood from 20 healthy controls (HC) and from 20 patients with RA, before (time (T)0) and after (T4) 4-month treatment with etanercept (ETA). Surface expression of TNFα was performed by flow cytometry analysis. EA.hy926 cells, an immortalized endothelial cell line, were treated with RA-MPs purified at T0 and at T4 and also, with RA-MPs in vitro treated with ETA. Apoptosis and autophagy were then evaluated.

Results: RA-MPs purified at T0 expressed TNFα on their surface and this expression significantly decreased at T4. Moreover, at T0 RA-MPs, significantly increased both apoptosis and autophagy levels on endothelial cells, in a dose-dependent manner. RA-MPs did not significantly change these parameters after 4 months of in vivo treatment with ETA.

Conclusions: Our data demonstrate that MPs isolated from patients with RA exert a pathological effect on endothelial cells by TNFα expressed on their surface. In vivo and in vitro treatment with ETA modulates this effect, suggesting anti-TNF therapy protects against endothelial damage in patients with RA.

Keywords: Rheumatoid arthritis, Microparticles, Autophagy, Endothelial cells

Background

Microparticles (MPs) are small membrane vesicles (0.1–1.0 μm) released by many cell types under physiological and pathological conditions. In the past these particles were considered as inert cell debris, but recently many studies have demonstrated they could be involved in intercellular communication. Generation and scattering of MPs occurs during different biological processes, including apoptosis and cellular activation [1–3]. Due to their formation, MPs have an array of surface markers derived from their parental cell that can be used to assess their origin. Thus, MPs can transfer biological messages from parental to target cells by direct interaction with the ligands expressed on the surface of target cells and activate cascade signaling; or they can transfer proteins, messenger RNA (mRNA), micro RNA (miRNA), and bioactive lipids by fusion or internalization with target cells [4].Thus, MPs are able to modulate various biological phenomena such as cell proliferation, angiogenesis, immune response, and coagulation [5, 6].

Increased levels of MPs have been reported in various pathological conditions including infections, malignancies,

* Correspondence: cristiana.barbati1@gmail.com
[1]Arthritis Center, Department of Internal Medicine and Medical Specialties, Sapienza University of Rome, Rome, Italy
Full list of author information is available at the end of the article

and autoimmune diseases, such as rheumatoid arthritis (RA) [7]. RA is an autoimmune systemic inflammatory disease characterized by chronic synovial inflammation, resulting in cartilage and bone damage with accelerated atherosclerosis and increased mortality [8]. Tumor necrosis factor alpha (TNFα) is the main cytokine involved in the pathogenesis of RA and many studies agree on the pro-atherogenic effect of TNFα in patients with RA. TNF-inhibitors are effective treatments for joint inflammation in RA; however, very little is known about their effect on atherosclerosis and endothelial dysfunction, which occur in this disease. Previous studies have shown that TNF-inhibitors can improve endothelial function and decrease cardiovascular events in responder patients, highlighting the pro-atherogenic effect of TNFα in RA [9, 10].

According to the literature, MPs could also have a role in endothelial dysfunction, contributing to atherosclerosis in patients with RA [11]. Moreover, an imbalance between apoptosis and autophagy mechanisms seems to be involved in endothelial dysfunction. Apoptosis is programmed cell death and many studies suggest the involvement of endothelial apoptosis in the atherosclerosis process [12]. Autophagy is a reparative process by which cytoplasmic components are sequestered in double-membrane vesicles and degraded on fusion with lysosomal compartments. It has been shown that basal autophagy is essential to proper vascular function [13].

Taking into account these considerations, the aim of this study was to analyze MP subsets in patients with RA and their contribution to endothelial dysfunction, with special focus on apoptosis and autophagy pathways, and to investigate if biological therapy could modulate these effects.

Materials and methods

Patients and controls

We enrolled 20 patients with RA fulfilling the 2010 American College of Rheumatology RA criteria [14], recruited from the Rheumatology Unit of Sapienza University of Rome at time zero (T0) and after 4 months (T4) of therapy with the TNF-inhibitor etanercept (ETA). The main clinical and laboratory variables assessed were the erythrocyte sedimentation rate (ESR), C-reactive protein (CRP), rheumatoid factor (RF) and anti-cyclic citrullinated peptide (anti-CCP) titer, tender and swollen joint count, patient's assessment of pain, patient's assessment of disease activity, physician's global assessment of disease activity, and the health assessment questionnaire (HAQ). The European League Against Rheumatism (EULAR) response to therapy was also recorded before and after treatment. All patients had a history of failed treatment with at least one disease-modifying antirheumatic drug (DMARD). Patients were allowed to continue DMARDs, steroids, and non-steroidal anti-inflammatory drugs at a stable dose for at least 4 weeks before and during ETA treatment. Patients received ETA at a dose of 50 mg given by subcutaneous injection (sc) weekly. Methotrexate (MTX) was given at a dose of 10–20 mg weekly. In addition to MTX, hydroxychloroquine (200–400 mg daily) and steroids (maximum daily dose 10 mg of oral prednisone or equivalent) were also permitted.

Simultaneously, 20 healthy controls (HC) within a similar age range and gender as the patients were recruited. Also 10 patients with RA who had only been treated with traditional DMARDs were enrolled.

The protocol of study was approved by the Ethics Committee of Sapienza University of Rome (Protocol number 109/18), and informed written consent was obtained from all patients prior to enrollment.

Isolation of MPs

A fasting blood sample was obtained from patients with RA, at T0 and T4, and from HC by venipuncture in 5-ml tubes containing citrate, which were centrifuged two times at 2500 g for 15 min at room temperature, to obtain platelet-poor plasma (PPP), rich in MPs. The resulting plasma was divided into five aliquots and stored at − 80 °C until analysis [15, 16].

Energy-filtered transmission electron microscopy (EF-TEM)

For electron microscopy analysis MPs were centrifuged at 14000 rpm for 1 h at 4 °C and pellets were fixed. The samples were observed using a Zeiss EM902 transmission electron microscope, operating at 80 kV and equipped with an "in column" electron energy filter. The filter was set to collect only elastic electrons (ΔE 1/4 0), with the result of enhancing image contrast and resolution, thanks to the elimination of inelastic electrons in the image formation (reduction of the chromatic aberration). The sample was stained with 2% (*w*/*v*) phosphotungstic acid (PTA) in buffered aqueous solution at pH 7.3 (NaOH), previously filtered by polycarbonate 0.2-µm filters to eliminate impurities. Images were acquired with a digital charge-coupled device camera, model PROSCAN HSC2 (1 K × 1 K pixels), thermostated by a Peltier unit. The analysis was performed using a digital analyzer SIS 3.0. The overall resolution is in the range of 2 nm [16].

Assessment of MP subsets and surface expression of TNFα by flow cytometry

MPs were analyzed using a FACS Calibur cytometer (Becton Dikinson, BD). Forward scatter (FSC) and side scatter (SSC) were adjusted to logarithmic gain. MP gating was accomplished using 1-µm beads (SIGMA) for setting upper limits in both FSC and SSC signals, and a lower limit was placed to exclude buffer noise.

Antibodies anti-CD41a–(Percp), anti-CD45–(APC) anti-CD31–(PE) were added to MP samples to identify specific MP subsets: platelet MPs (PMP ($CD41a^+$ $CD31^+$)), leukocyte MPs (LMP ($CD45^+$)) and endothelial MPs (EMP ($CD41a^-$ $CD31^+$)) [17]. To evaluate the surface expression of TNFα, MPs were incubated with antibodies anti-TNFα–(fluorescein isothiocyanate (FITC)). MPs were also labeled using FITC-conjugated Annexin-V (AV). Fluorescent-conjugated isotype mAbs were used as controls. Incubation was performed at room temperature for 30 min in AV buffer and then MP suspensions were transferred into count tubes that were immediately processed by flow cytometry. MP number was calculated as described [18, 19]. All antibodies were purchased from BD Biosciences, San Josè, CA, USA.

RA-MP incubation with ETA

In vitro treatment of MPs was performed with ETA. Briefly, $2*10^6$ MPs/ml RA-MPs purified at T0 were cultured in Dulbecco's modified Eagle's medium (DMEM) containing 10% fetal bovine serum (FBS), and treated with ETA at different concentrations (1, 3, 5, and 10 μg/ml) for 30 min, 2 h and 4 h. Surface expression of TNFα was evaluated at the end of each time period.

In vitro culture of EA.hy926 cells

The in vitro effects of plasma-isolated MPs on the endothelium were evaluated using human umbilical vein cell line EA.hy926. Cells were cultured in DMEM containing 10% FBS, 50 IU/ml penicillin, 50 μg/ml streptomycin and 2 mM l-glutamine at 37 °C under an atmosphere of 5% CO2. To this end, MP suspensions purified from patients with RA at T0 and T4 and from HC were prepared. Briefly, MPs were centrifuged at 14000 rpm for 1 h at room temperature and resuspended in DMEM 10% FBS to obtain the desired concentration. Cells were cultured with MP suspensions at different concentrations (0.5, 2 and $8*10^6$ MPs/ml) for 6 h, 16 h, 24 h, 48 h, and 72 h. Cells were also treated with RA-MPs pre-incubated with ETA. Where indicated, cells were treated in the presence of lysosomal inhibitors E64d and pepstatin A (PepA) (both at 10 μg/ml; Sigma-Aldrich) for 2 h before the end of the culture. For inhibition of autophagy, cells were treated with 10 mM 3-methyladenine (3MA), which pharmacologically blocks this catabolic process (Sigma-Aldrich). Apoptosis and autophagy were evaluated at the end of experiments.

Evaluation of EA.hy926 cell apoptosis

After in vitro treatment with MPs, EA.hy926 cell apoptosis was analyzed by flow cytometry using a FITC-conjugated Annexin V and propidium iodide apoptosis detection kit [20] according to the manufacturer's instructions (MBL).

Analysis of autophagy and TNF pathway by western blot

For analysis of autophagy EA.hy926 lysates (30 μg) were loaded on SDS-PAGE and expression levels of the autophagic markers LC3-II and P62 were analyzed by western blot [21]. Rabbit anti-human p65 antibody was used for NF-kB-p65 protein detection,. All antibodies were purchased from Cell Signaling Technology, Beverly, MA, USA.

Statistical analysis

Normal distribution of variables was assessed using the Kolmogorov-Smirnov test. Statistical analysis was performed using the program GraphPad Prism Version 6 (GraphPad Software, San Diego, CA, USA). The Mann–Whitney unpaired test or Student's t test was used to compare quantitative variables in different groups. Statistical correlation was examined using Spearman's rank correlation coefficient. Values of $p < 0.05$ were considered statistically significant.

Results

Patients and controls

The demographic, serological and clinical characteristics of patients with RA and of HC are summarized in Table 1.

Electron microscopy

Transmission electron microscopy of PPP confirms the purity of the samples used to conduct all our in vitro experiments. The images show vesicles that are heterogeneous in terms of shape and density, with the majority in the range of between 0.2 μm and 1 μm. Those sizes represent the typical size of MPs that differ from exosomes and apoptotic bodies in size, composition and mechanism of formation (Fig. 1).

Evaluation of MP subsets and surface expression of TNFα

The number of MPs in serum from patients with RA and HC was quantified by flow cytometry analysis. The strategy used to identify MP morphology, MP subsets and TNFα expression is shown in Fig. 2a, b, and c.

Our study showed that at baseline the total number of MPs was significantly increased in patients with RA compared to HC ($p < 0.0001$) (Fig. 3a). Only the EMP subset was significantly increased in patients with RA compared to HC ($p = 0.0049$) (Fig. 3a). Interestingly, after 4 months of in vivo treatment with ETA, the total number of MPs and of the EMPs were both significantly decreased compared to baseline ($p < 0.0001$ and $p = 0.03$, respectively) (Fig. 3b). Moreover, after in vivo treatment with ETA, the percentage of EMPs that were AV-positive decreased, demonstrating downregulation of apoptosis of endothelial cells in vivo ($p = 0.03$) (Fig. 3c). There were no differences between seropositive and seronegative patients with RA with regard to the levels of MPs (data not shown). As shown in Fig. 3d the percentage of TNFα expressed on the surface of MPs (sTNFα) was significantly increased in

Table 1 Clinical, demographic, serological, and therapeutic characteristics of patients with RA and HC

	Patients with RA (n = 20)	HC (n = 20)
Demographic parameters		
Female/male	19/1	20/0
Age, years (median (IQR))	58.5 (50–67)	58 (50–65)
Disease duration, years (mean ± SD),	5.3 ± 5.6	
Disease activity		
DAS28 (mean ± SD)	4.1 ± 1.7	
TJ, n (mean ± SD)	6.16 ± 5.9	
SJ, n (mean ± SD)	2.79 ± 2.7	
CDAI (mean ± SD)	18.8 ± 10.7	
HAQ (mean ± SD)	1.15 ± 0.8	
Laboratory parameters	N (%)	
RF+	15 (75)	
ACPA+	15(75)	
ESR, mm/h (mean ± SD)	16.5 ± 10.3	
CRP, mg/dl (mean ± SD)	0.7 ± 0.73	
Therapy		
Concurrent csDMARDs (n (%))	20 (100)	
ETA (n (%))	20 (100)	

RA rheumatoid arthritis, *HC* healthy controls, *SD* standard deviation, *DAS28* Disease Activity Score in 28 joints, *TJ* tender joints, *SJ* swollen joints, *CDAI* Clinical Disease Activity Index, *HAQ* Health Assessment Questionnaire, *RF* rheumatoid factor, *ACPA* anti-citrullinated peptide antibodies, *ESR* erythrocyte sedimentation rate, *CRP* C-reactive protein, *csDMARDs* conventional synthetic disease-modifying antirheumatic drugs

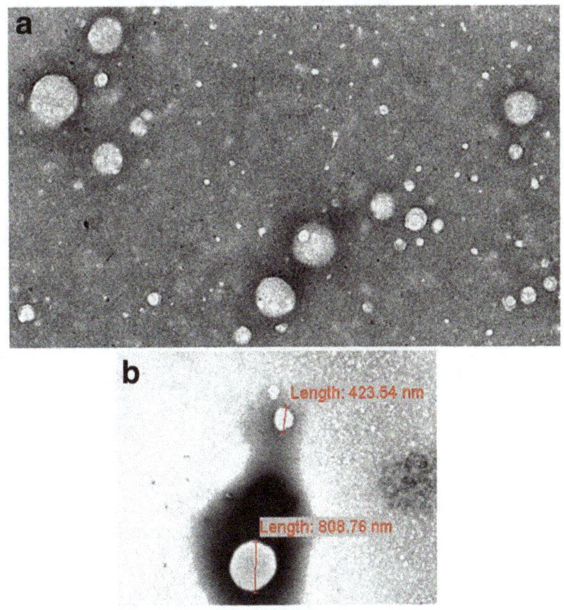

Fig. 1 Transmission electron microscopy (TEM) of microparticles (MPs). Micrographs show the negative staining of a typical sample observed by the TEM. **a** White particles of different sizes ranging from a few nanometers to 1 mm were present. As expected, all particles appeared as white structures in the dark background, due to phosphotungstic acid (PTA) negative staining. They were round-shaped and sometimes superimposed. This observation suggests that the smallest nanoparticles and MPs coexist in our sample, because it is well-known that MP size ranges from 100 to 1000 nm. **b** Two MPs of about 500 nm in diameter are shown, together with their measured diameters. (Images from Miranda F. PhD Thesis)

patients with RA compared to HC (p = 0.0009). After 4 months of in vivo treatment with ETA the percentage of sTNFα was significantly decreased with respect to baseline (p = 0.0002) (Fig. 3e). Instead, there was no significant change in the percentage of sTNFα-MPs after therapy in patients treated only with traditional DMARDs (data not shown).This result corroborated our hypothesis on the capacity of ETA to bind TNFα carried on the surface of the MPs, as explained in the next paragraph. Moreover, as shown in Additional file 1, in relation to the expression of sTNF on MP subsets, we observed that EMPs expressed a greater percentage of TNFα than PMPs. LMPs expressed a high percentage of TNFα but this was not significantly different to the percentage in the other subsets.

Finally, to compare the percentage of TNFα expressed on the surface of the MPs and the serum TNFα, we also performed ELISA of serum TNF on the same patients in whom we evaluated the surface expression of TNFα on MPs, as shown in Additional file 1.

Surface expression of TNFα on MPs after incubation with ETA

We demonstrated for the first time the expression of TNF on the surface of human MPs. On the basis of this result we decided to incubate MPs with ETA at different concentrations in order to demonstrate that the drug was able to bind and inhibit surface MP-TNFα expression. ETA, a fully soluble, human dimeric fusion protein, functions as a TNF inhibitor by competitively binding to TNF and preventing its activation of the inflammatory cascade. ETA is a soluble form of the p75 receptor that inhibits TNFα, by blocking its interaction with cell-surface TNF receptors and is different from adalimumab and infliximab, which are monoclonal antibodies to TNF. Moreover, its peculiarity with respect to the other TNFα inhibitors, is that besides recognizing soluble TNFα, it also recognizes the membrane-related portion.

For this reason, we hypothesized that ETA, in addition to the soluble portion, recognizes and binds the portion transported on the membrane of the MPs, preventing the link with its receptor and then the inflammatory cascade. Results obtained confirmed our hypothesis, in fact, in vitro experiments showed that the percentage of sTNFα expressed on RA-MPs significantly decreased, in a dose-dependent manner, after incubation with ETA at each timepoint of the experiment. In particular, the major effect was at 10 μg/ml of ETA at (Fig. 4).

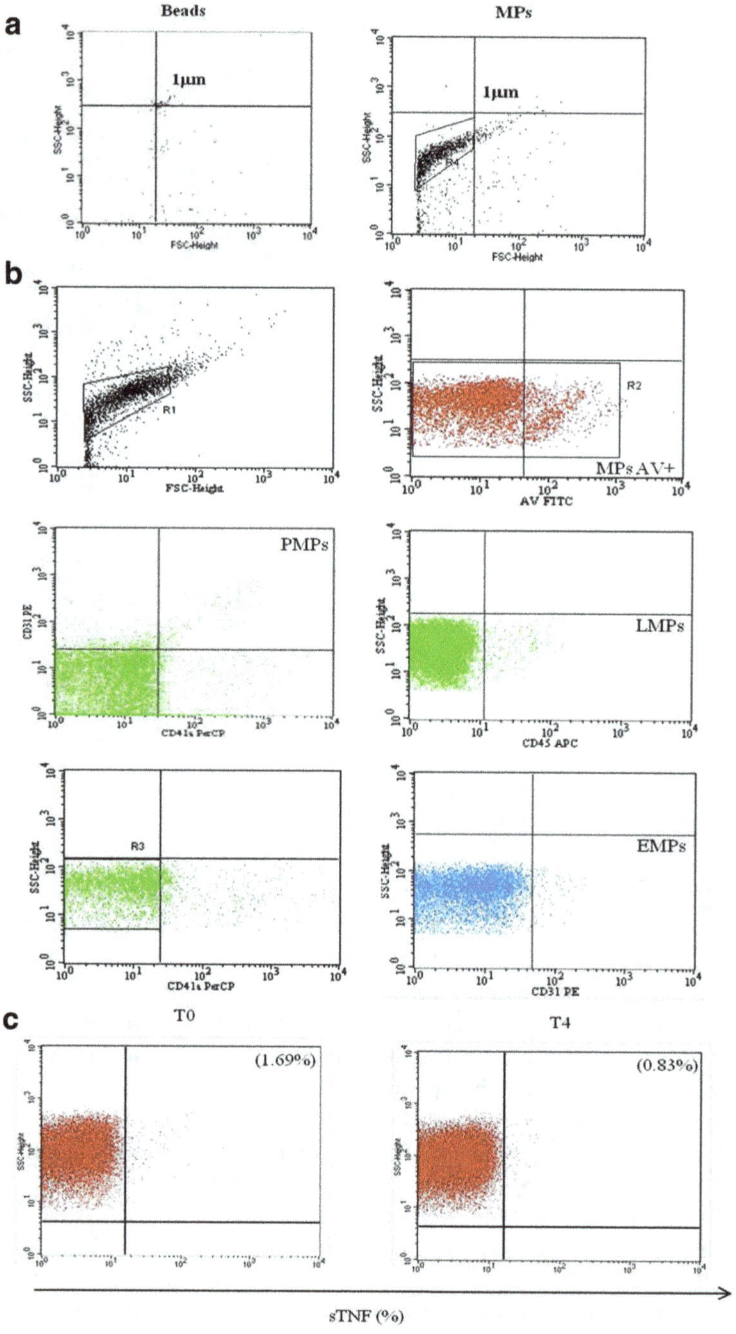

Fig. 2 Gating strategy for flow cytometric analysis. **a** All microparticles (MPs) were gated as described in "Materials and methods". **b** Flow cytometry analysis of specific binding of antibodies to MPs derived from platelets, leukocytes and endothelial cells and annexin-V (AV). **c** MPs were also labeled for the surface expression of TNFα. SSC, side scatter; FSC, forward scatter; FITC, fluorescein isothiocyanate; PMP, platelet MPs; LMP, leukocyte MPs; EMP, endothelial MPs; APC, allophycocyanin; PE, phycoerythrin; PerCP, peridin chlorophyll protein; T0, time zero (baseline); T4, 4 months after treatment

The percentage of sTNFα correlates with clinical parameters of patients with RA

The purpose of our study was to test for correlation between MPs and endothelial damage. However, observing a decrease in the surface expression of MP-TNFα and a concomitant improvement in the parameters of disease activity in patients after therapy with ETA, we decided to test correlation between them. When we compared the sTNFα of RA-MPs and clinical parameters, such as the Disease Activity Score in 28 joints (DAS28), tender joints (TJ), swollen joints (SW), CDAI and HAQ, identified significant correlation between these parameters as shown in Fig. 5. These results lead us to suppose there is a link between sTNFα on MPs and the status of patients' disease.

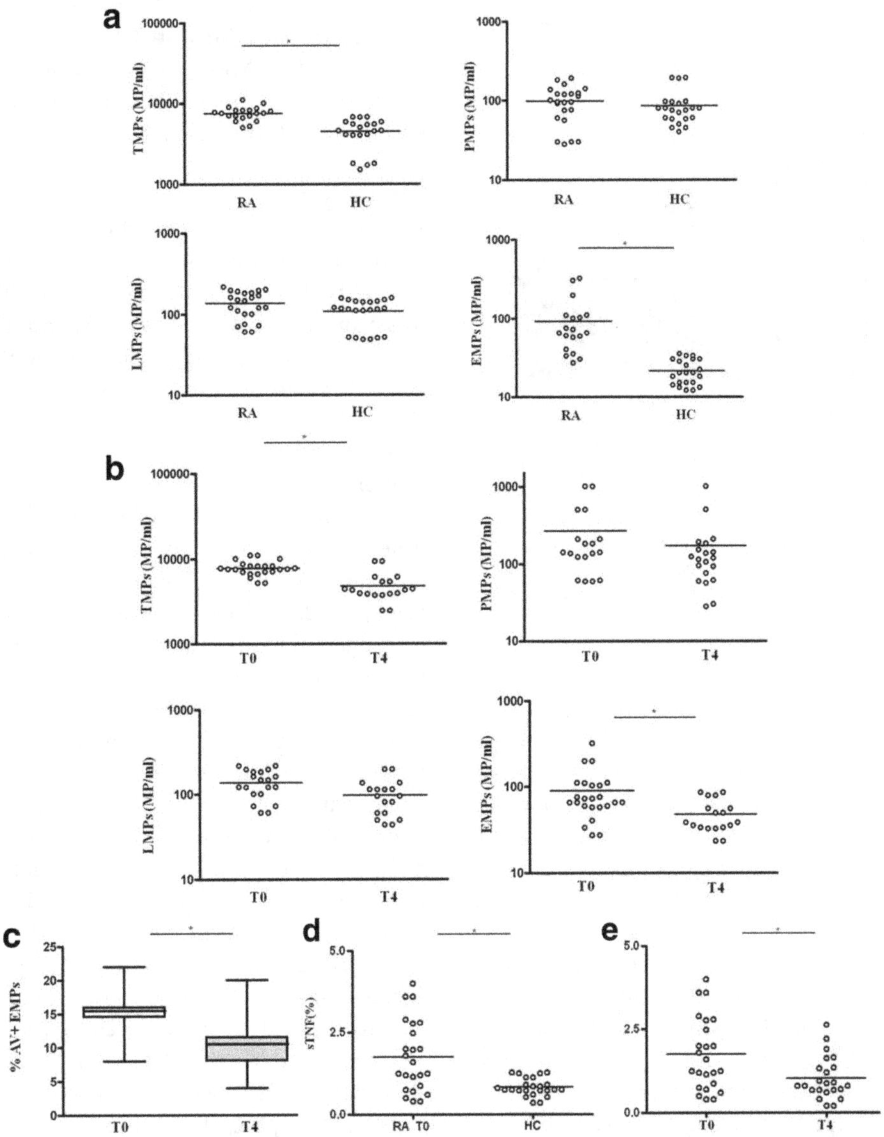

Fig. 3 Plasma levels of microparticles (MPs) in patients with rheumatoid arthritis (RA) at time zero (baseline (T0)) and after 4 months of treatment (T4) and in healthy controls (HC) and surface expression of TNFα. **a** Relative distribution of total MPs (TMPs), platelet MPs (PMPs), leukocyte MPs (LMPs) and endothelial MPs (EMPs) in 20 patients with rheumatoid arthritis (RA) and 20 healthy controls (HC). **b, c** Relative distribution of TMPs, PMPs, LMPs, EMPs (**a**) and EMPs annexin-V (AV)+ (**c**) in patients with RA at time zero (baseline (T0) and 4 months after treatment (T4). **d** Relative distribution of the percentage of the expression of TNFα on the surface of MPs from patients with RA and HC. **e** Relative distribution of TNFα expression on MPs from patients with RA at T0 and T4. Each data point represents a single subject; horizontal lines show the median. Groups were compared using Student's *t* test; $*p < 0.05$

sTNFα of RA-MPs mediates in vitro induction of apoptosis and autophagy in EA.hy926 cells

TNFα is the main cytokine involved in RA pathogenesis and has a pathogenic effect, with a direct effect on endothelial cells. Earlier studies have shown that TNFα inhibitors are able to improve endothelial function and decrease cardiovascular events in those patients who respond clinically [9, 10]. After demonstrating the expression of TNFα on the surface of MPs we decided to investigate whether MPs induce apoptosis and autophagy on endothelial cells and whether TNFα carried on their surface was responsible for this effect. Our in vitro results on EA.hy926 cells showed that at baseline (T0), serum RA-MPs significantly increased both apoptosis and autophagy levels compared to untreated cells, in a dose-dependent manner ($p = 0.005$ and $p = 0.02$, respectively) (Fig. 6a–d).

After 4 months of in vivo treatment with ETA, RA-MPs did not significantly change these parameters ($p > 0.05$ versus untreated cells for both parameters) (Fig. 6e, f). These effects were comparable to those

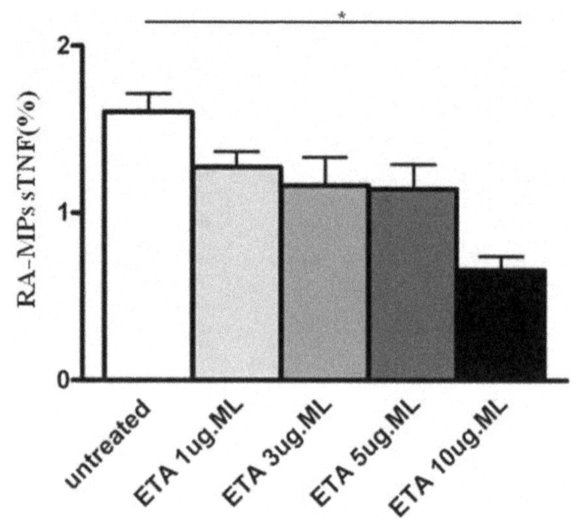

Fig. 4 Surface expression of TNFα after incubation of rheumatoid arthritis (RA)-microparticles (MPs) with etanercept (ETA). Percentage of surface (s)TNFa expression on RA-MPs is shown after in vitro incubation with ETA at different concentrations for 2 h. Values are expressed as means ± SD; *$p < 0.05$

obtained with the same number of MPs from HC (Fig. 6e, f). Interestingly, in the same experiment described above, treatment with the 3MA restored a situation comparable to that at T0, with an increase in endothelial apoptosis after autophagy block in EA.hy926 cells treated with MPs at T4, asserting the protective role of autophagy (Fig. 6e, f). The experiments reported above showed the results at 16 h, but a cellular response, comparable to that obtained at 16 h, had begun by 6 h when the cells were incubated with RA-MPs, (data not shown). However, at 24 h, 48 h, and 72 h the cellular response in terms of apoptosis and autophagy gave rise to confused and uninterpretable results, probably because, after some hours, other surface molecules started a cellular response, or the MPs fused themselves with the cells or were internalized, and so the molecular content of MPs may have altered the initial response (data not shown).

Moreover, in vitro studies showed that RA-MPs treated with ETA were no longer able to significantly modulate apoptosis and autophagy in EA.hy926 cells. In particular, when MPs were treated with ETA at 10 µg/ml, both endothelial apoptosis and autophagy reached levels comparable to those of untreated cells ($p = 0.01$ and $p = 0.02$, respectively versus cells treated with RA-MPs at T0), to confirm possible involvement of TNFα carried on MPs in the induction of apoptosis and autophagy (Fig. 6g, h).

Finally, the result of western blot for NF-kB showed a significant decrease in p65 protein when endothelial cells were incubated with RA-MPs purified at T0 and treated with ETA at 10 µg/ml ($p = 0.02$ versus cells treated with RA-MPs at T0). This result confirms the hypothesis that MPs carry TNFα on their surface, which activates TNF-signaling pathways by interaction with its surface receptors (Fig. 7).

Discussion

In our study, for the first time we demonstrated TNFα expression on the surface of MPs from patients with RA [22]. Higher circulating levels of TNFα are present in serum from patients with RA, and TNFα itself is able to directly damage endothelial function triggering NF-κB activation and accumulation of reactive oxygen species (ROS) [23].

Some evidence indicates a beneficial effect of TNF inhibitors on vascular wall physiology, increasing the possibility that TNF blockade may improve endothelial function, with consequent improvement of arterial stiffness and reduced progression of subclinical atherosclerosis [24, 25]. However, clinical studies conducted to investigate the effect of anti-TNF therapy on endothelial function in patients with RA have had contradictory results, generating controversy on this subject.

Based on our results and these considerations, we hypothesized that TNFα carried on the surface of RA-MPs could participate in the atherosclerotic process in patients with RA. Impaired endothelial cell function is a hallmark of atherosclerosis. The endothelial dysfunction is directly associated with the development of atherosclerosis, and it is present during all stages of the disease. Moreover, alterations in endothelial function precede morphological atherosclerotic changes [26]. Injury to the endothelium is believed to be a preliminary event in most vascular diseases [27]. Furthermore, those alterations could include an imbalance between apoptosis and autophagy pathways.

Endothelial apoptosis has been associated with multiple cardiovascular events that cause vascular wall damage and atherosclerotic plaque, and consequently it promotes vascular injury [28]. MPs have been shown to initiate cell death when applied to cultured primary rat brain microvascular endothelial cells (RBMVECs) and a variety of different mechanisms have been identified [29].

Previous studies showed that MPs derived from human umbilical vein endothelial cells [30] and platelets [31] contain caspase 3, and Schneider et al. [32] have suggested that circulating MPs induce apoptosis by the transfer of caspases into target cells. In relation to this, Abid Hussein et al. [30] suggest that MPs could be phagocytosed by cells, causing the release of caspase 3 within the cell itself and initiating apoptosis. In this study, treatment of MPs with a caspase 3 inhibitor significantly improved cell survival, indicating that the MPs impart pro-apoptotic caspase 3 signals.

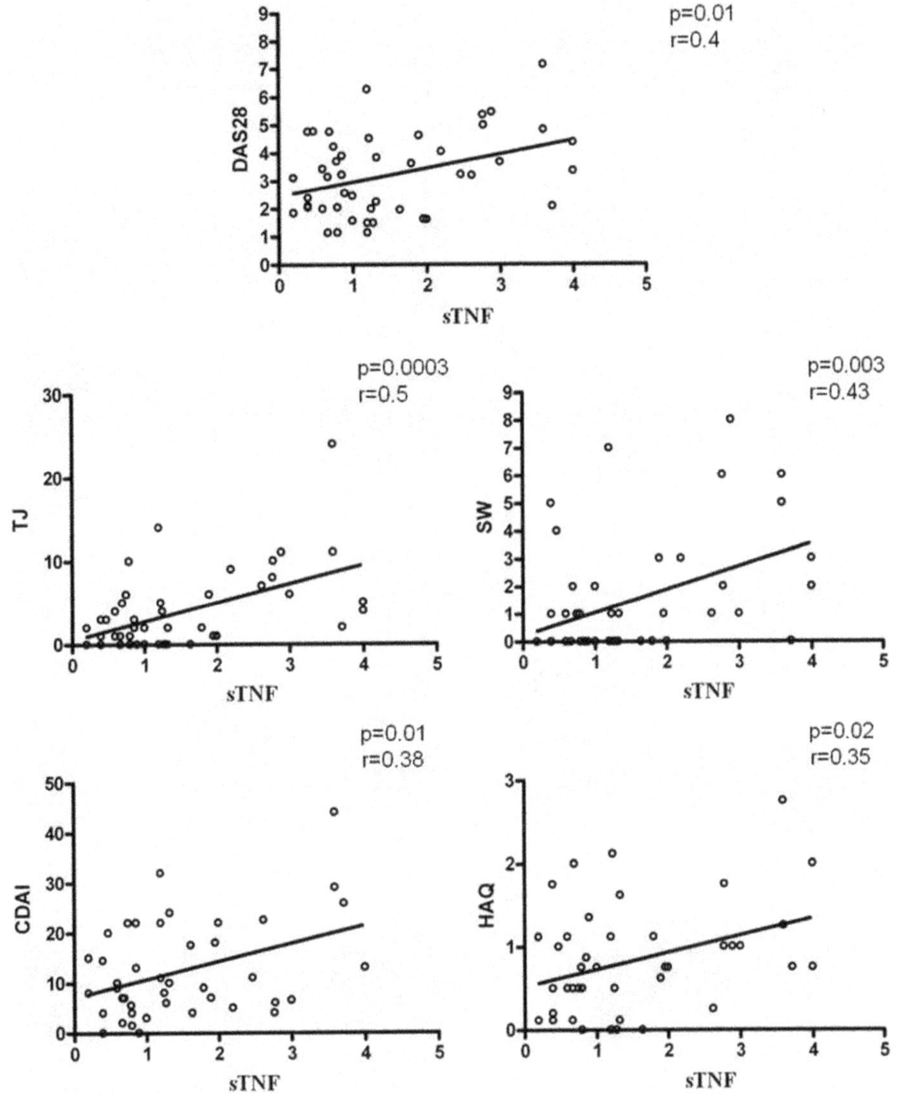

Fig. 5 Correlation between the percentage of surface (s)TNFα expression on rheumatoid arthritis (RA)-microparticles (MPs) and clinical parameters of patients with RA. Correlation and linear regression analysis of sTNFα expression on MPs from patients with RA and Disease Activity Score in 28 joints (DAS 28), tender joints (TJ), swollen joints (SW), Clinical Disease Activity Index (CDAI) and Health Assessment Questionnaire (HAQ) (*r* and *p* values are shown on each diagram)

Moreover, many studies showed that basal levels of autophagy are protective for the endothelium, continuously stimulated by mechanical and physical stress [33]. During injury, endothelial cell autophagy may occur to protect the cells from damage, while the failure of autophagy results in endothelial cell apoptosis, leading to the breakdown of the integrity of endothelium to induce the local lipid deposition into atheroma, plaque instability, and even acute coronary occlusion and death [34–37]. Nevertheless, the mechanisms that control the autophagy of endothelial cells are still limited. Moreover, autophagy has been shown to play an important role in endothelial cells to prevent development of atherosclerosis.

From the discovery of MPs up to now there has been no scientific evidence of the involvement of MPs in the regulation of autophagy pathway. Thus, in light of the numerous reported data, we can assume that MPs could be involved in alteration of apoptosis and autophagy, which together could contribute to the formation and progression of atherosclerotic plaque [38]. On the basis of this observation, after investigating surface expression of TNFα on MPs purified from patients with RA, we evaluated if MPs were able to modulate endothelial apoptosis and autophagy in vitro, and if TNFα carried on the surface of MPs could be involved in these cellular processes. In this regard Schock and coworkers identified three independent pro-apoptotic

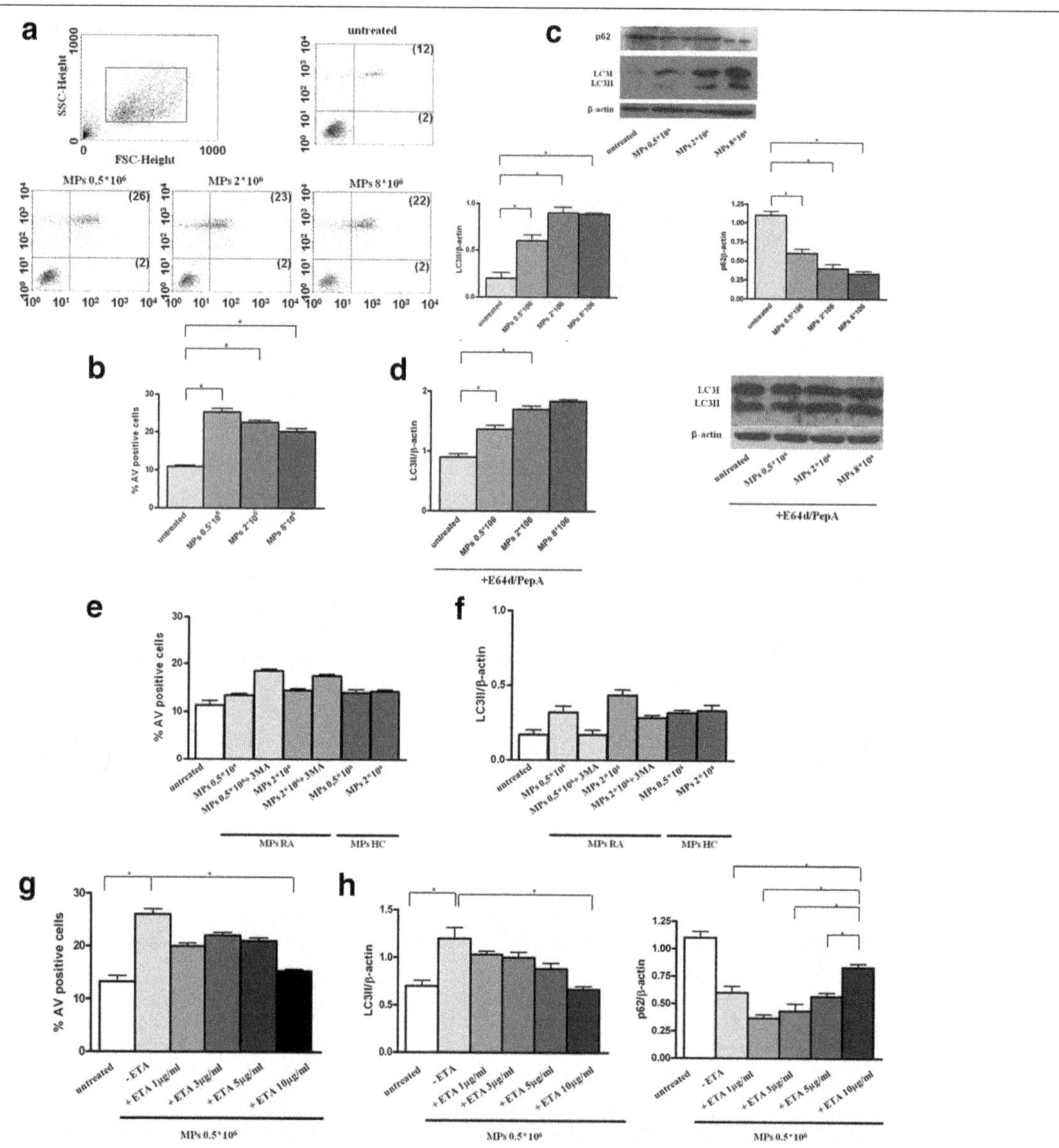

Fig. 6 Induction of apoptosis and autophagy in EA.hy926 cells by microparticles (MPs) isolated from patients with rheumatoid arthritis (RA) after in vivo and in vitro treatment with etanercept (ETA) and by MPs isolated from healthy controls (HC). **a** Flow cytometry analysis of apoptosis in untreated MPs and MPs treated with EA.hy926 cells. Results obtained in a representative experiment are shown. Numbers in the upper and bottom right quadrants of each plot refer to annexin-V (AV)/propidium iodide (PI) double-positive cells and to AV single-positive cells, respectively. **b** Mean ± SD of the percentages of AV-positive cells obtained in three independent experiments; **p* < 0.05. **c**, **d** Western blot analysis of LC3-II (left panel) and p62 (right panel) levels in EA.hy926 cells cultured with MPs purified from patients with RA at time zero (baseline (T0)), in the absence (**c**) or in the presence (**d**) of lysosomal inhibitors E64d and pepstatin A (PepA). Blot shown is representative of three independent experiments. **e**, **f** Flow cytometry analysis of apoptosis (**e**) and western blot analysis (**f**) of LC3-II in EA.hy926 cells cultured with (i) MPs purified from patients with RA after 4 months of treatment with ETA, (ii) MPs purified from HC, and (iii) in the presence or absence of the autophagy inhibitor 3MA. **g**, **h** Flow cytometry analysis of apoptosis (**g**) and western blot analysis (**h**) of LC3-II (left panel) and p62 (right panel) levels in EA.hy926 cells cultured with MPs purified from patients with RA at T0 and with MPs from patients with RA at T0 in vitro-treated with ETA. **e**-**h** Mean ± SD of the percentages of AV-positive cells obtained in three independent experiments is reported and densitometry analysis of LC3-II and p62 levels relative to β-actin is shown. Values are expressed as means ± SD; **p* < 0.05. FSC, forward scatter; SSC, side scatter

signals induced by MPs on RBMVECs cells: caspase 3 and activation of TNF-related apoptosis-inducing ligand (TRAIL) and TNF receptors. To support our last point on the induction of apoptosis by sTNF-MPs on EC, this study showed that treatment with a neutralizing antibody to TRAIL and TNF receptor blocker did improve cell survival. Genetic analysis confirmed that Tumor necrosis factor receptor 1 and 2 (TNFR1, TNFR2) and TRAIL receptor 4 are present in the cells. TRAIL may activate the extrinsic apoptotic pathway, but in some circumstances may activate

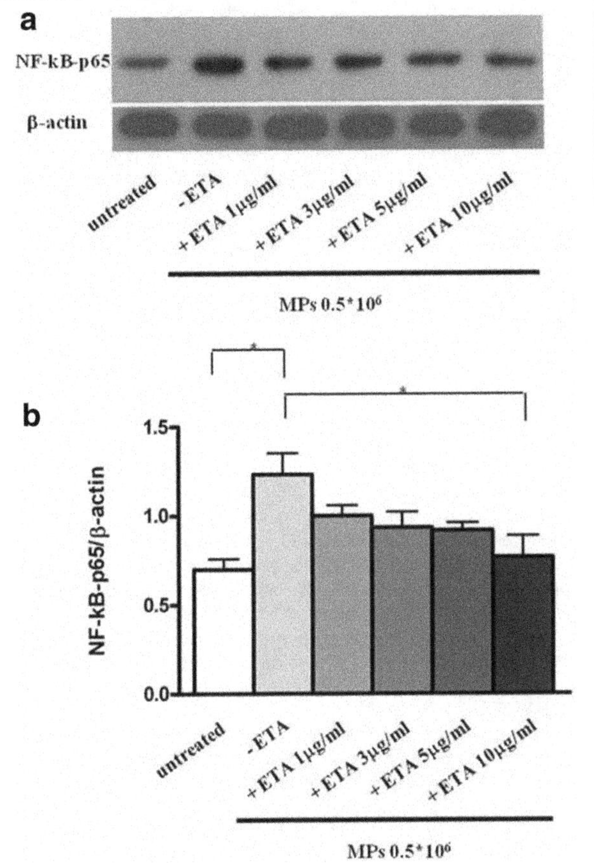

Fig. 7 Activation of the TNFα pathway by microparticles (MPs). **a** Western blot analysis of NF-kB levels in EA.hy926 cells cultured with MPs purified from patients with rheumatoid arthritis (RA) at time zero (baseline (T0) and with MPs from patients with RA at T0 in vitro-treated with etanercept (ETA). Blot shown is representative of three independent experiments. **b** Densitometry analysis of NF-kB relative to β-actin. Values are expressed as means ± SD; $^{*}p < 0.05$

pro-survival or proliferative pathways [29]. TNF is synthesized as a type-2 transmembrane protein and cleaved by the tumor necrosis factor-alpha-converting enzyme (TACE) ADAM17 to release soluble TNF, which may then activate TNF receptors. The authors showed that treating MPs with the TACE inhibitor (TAPI-0) prior to applying MPs to cultured cells provides a significant improvement in cell survival. This result indicates that TACE is present and active in MP membranes. Given the small size of MPs it is uncertain whether they are able to shed soluble TNF for an extended period of time.

According to these reported data, our results confirm that MPs from RA at T0 significantly increased apoptosis in endothelial cells. Interestingly, MPs purified from RA at T4, after in vivo treatment with ETA, and RA-MPs after in vitro treatment with ETA, were no longer able to significantly modify this parameter.

We obtained the same results for autophagy; indeed MPs obtained from RA at T0 significantly increased autophagy in endothelial cells and MPs purified from RA after in vivo treatment with ETA, and RA-MPs after in vitro treatment with ETA, were no longer able to significantly modify the autophagy pathway. The experiments with the 3MA, which is able to block autophagy and increase apoptosis of endothelial cells treated with RA-MPs, led us to suppose that MPs, if they induce cell death on one side, on the other side they induce cells to upregulate autophagy as a protective mechanism, at least at an early stage.

Furthermore, we demonstrated that RA-MPs induced an increase in NF-kB expression in endothelial cells, and that RA-MPs in vitro treated with ETA did not. These conclusive results support the concept, already proposed in other studies [39, 40], that the TNF transported on the surface of MPs interacts with TNF receptors on endothelial cells and activates the TNF-signaling cascade, including apoptosis and autophagy pathways.

Moreover, we observed significant correlation between DAS28 and TNFα expression on the surface of RA-MPs. This result supports other clinical observations that demonstrated the efficacy and safety of ETA in patients with active RA.

Finally, the interpretation of the ELISA results, i.e. that serum TNF does not change or increase after therapy, as demonstrated in other studies [41, 42], induced us to hypothesize the possibility of using surface expression of TNF on MPs as a possible therapy response marker. Obviously, to confirm this statement we need a far greater cohort of patients.

Conclusions

Our results suggest that MPs isolated from patients with RA could exert their pathological effect on endothelial cells by TNFα expressed on their surface. In vivo treatment with ETA attenuates this effect, probably binding and blocking the TNF carried on the surface of MPs, as confirmed by our in vitro studies. To conclude, these results show a new pathway of endothelial damage mediated by MPs and confirm the protective effect of anti-TNF therapy against endothelial damage in patients with RA.

Certainly, we cannot assume that sTNF on MPs is the only architect of a cellular response; we hypothesize that it acts in synergy with multiple factors, some of which are already widely discussed in the literature, like serum TNF.

Abbreviations

3MA: 3-Methyladenine; AV: Annexin-V; anti-CCP: Anti-cyclic citrullinated peptide; APC: Allophycocyanin; CDAI: Clinical Disease Activity Index; CRP: C-reactive protein; DAS28: Disease Activity Score in 28 joints; DMARD: Disease-modifying antirheumatic drug; DMEM: Dulbecco's modified Eagle's medium; EA.hy926: Human umbilical vein cell line; EF-TEM: Energy-filtered transmission electron microscopy; ELISA: Enzyme-linked immunosorbent assay; EMPs: Endothelial-derived microparticles; ESR: Erythrocyte sedimentation rate; ETA: Etanercept; FBS: Fetal bovine serum; FITC: Fluorescein isothiocyanate; FSC: Forward scatter; HAQ: Health Assessment Questionnaire; HC: Healthy controls; LMPs: Leukocyte-derived microparticles; mAbs: Monoclonal antibodies; MPs: Microparticles; PE: Phycoerythrin; PepA: Pepstatin A; PerCP: Peridin chlorophyll protein; PMPs: Platelet-derived microparticles; PTA: Phosphotungstic acid; RA: Rheumatoid arthritis; SJ: Swollen joints; SSC: Side scatter; STNFα: TNFα expressed on the surface of microparticles; T0: Time zero (before treatment); T4: Four months after treatment; TJ: Tender joints; TNFα: Tumor necrosis factor alpha

Acknowledgements
None.

Funding
None.

Disclosures
None

Authors' contributions
CB and CA collected the clinical data, examined and interpreted the data, performed statistical analyses, and wrote and revised the manuscript. FCe, AF, FM, FRS, and ST recruited patients. CB, TC, and MV carried out the laboratory experiments. CP and LN revised the manuscript. AF and SF collected the clinical data. MD performed EF-TEM experiments. CA, FCo, and GV designed, coordinated and supervised the study, and wrote and revised the manuscript. All authors read and approved the final manuscript.

Authors' information
Cristiana Barbati, Marta Vomero, Tania Colasanti, Marco Diociaiuti: PhD. Fulvia Ceccarelli, Francesca Miranda, Carlo Perricone, Francesca Romana Spinelli, Simona Truglia: MD, PhD. Annacarla Finucci, Lucia Novelli: MD. Fabrizio Conti, Guido Valesini and Cristiano Alessandri: MD, PhD, professor. Sara Ferrigno: medical student

Competing interests
The authors declare that they have no competing interests.

Author details
[1]Arthritis Center, Department of Internal Medicine and Medical Specialties, Sapienza University of Rome, Rome, Italy. [2]Technology and health Department, Istituto Superiore di Sanità, Rome, Italy.

References
1. Raposo G, Stoorvogel W. Extracellular vesicles: exosomes, microvesicles, and friends. J Cell Biol. 2013;200:373–83.
2. Piccin A, Murphy WG, Smith OP. Circulating microparticles: pathophysiology and clinical implications. Blood Rev. 2007;21:157–71.
3. Morel O, Toti F, Hugel B, Freyssinet J-M. Cellular microparticles: a disseminated storage pool of bioactive vascular effectors. Curr Opin Hematol. 2004;11:156–64.
4. Loyer X, Vion AC, Tedgui A, Boulanger CM. Microvesicles as cell-cell messengers in cardiovascular diseases. Circ Res. 2014;114:345–53.
5. Connor DE, Exner T, Ma DD, Joseph JE. Detection of the procoagulant activity of microparticle-associated phosphatidylserine using XACT. Blood Coagul Fibrinolysis. 2009;20:558–64.
6. Morel O, Toti F, Freyssinet JM. Markers of thrombotic disease: procoagulant microparticles. Ann Pharm Fr. 2007;65:75–84.
7. Boilard E, Nigrovic PA, Larabee K, Watts GF, Coblyn JS, Weinblatt ME. Platelets amplify inflammation in arthritis via collagen-dependent microparticle production. Science. 2010;327:580–3.
8. Aviña-Zubieta JA, Choi HK, Sadatsafavi M, Etminan M, Esdaile JM, Lacaille D. Risk of cardiovascular mortality in patients with rheumatoid arthritis: a meta-analysis of observational studies. Arthritis Rheum. 2008;59:1690–7.
9. Hürlimann D, Forster A, Noll G, Enseleit F, Chenevard R, Distler O, et al. Anti-tumor necrosis factor-a treatment improves endothelial function in patients with rheumatoid arthritis. Circulation. 2002;106:2184–7.
10. Irace C, Mancuso G, Fiaschi E, Madia A, Sesti G, Gnasso A. Effect of antiTNF-a therapy on arterial diameter and wall shear stress and HDL cholesterol. Atherosclerosis. 2004;177:113–8.
11. Pamuk GE, Vural O, Turgut B, Demir M, Pamuk ON, Cakir N. Increased platelet activation markers in rheumatoid arthritis: are they related with subclinical atherosclerosis? Platelets. 2008;19:146–54.
12. Fukuo K, Nakahashi T, Nomura S, Hata S, Suhara T, Shimizu M, et al. Possible participation of Fas-mediated apoptosis in the mechanism of atherosclerosis. Gerontology. 1997;1:35–42.
13. Salabei JK, Hill BG. Implications of autophagy for vascular smooth muscle cell function and plasticity. Free Radic Biol Med. 2013;65:693–703.
14. Shanthini K, Barbara LG, Susan M, Elizabeth WK, Karen HC. Comparison of the 1987 American College of Rheumatology and the 2010 American College of Rheumatology/European League against Rheumatism Criteria for Classification of Rheumatoid Arthritis in the Nurses' Health Study Cohorts. Rheumatol Int. 2014;34:407–11.
15. Biró É, Nieuwland R, Sturk A. Measuring circulating cell-derived microparticles. J Thromb Haemost. 2004;2:1843–54.
16. Jy W, Horstman LL, Jimenez JJ, Ahn YS. Measuring circulating cell-derived microparticles. J Thromb Haemost. 2004;2:1842–51.
17. Diociaiuti M. Electron energy loss spectroscopy microanalysis and imaging in the transmission electron microscope: example of biological applications. J Electron Spectrosc Relat Phenom. 2005;143:189–203.
18. Ayers L, Kohler M, Harrison P, Sargent I, Dragovic R, Schaap M, et al. Measurement of circulating cell-derived microparticles by flow cytometry: sources of variability within the assay. Thromb Res. 2011;127:370–7.
19. Niccolai E, Squatrito D, Emmi G, Silvestri E, Emmi L, Ciucciarelli L, et al. A new cytofluorimetric approach to evaluate the circulating microparticles in subjects with antiphospholipid antibodies. Thromb Res. 2015;136:1252–8.
20. Alessandri C, Barbati C, Vacirca D, Piscopo P, Confaloni A, Sanchez M, et al. T lymphocytes from patients with systemic lupus erythematosus are resistant to induction of autophagy. FASEB J. 2012;26:4722–32.
21. Barbati C, Alessandri C, Vomero M, Vona R, Colasanti T, Vacirca D, et al. Autoantibodies specific to D4GDI modulate Rho GTPase mediated cytoskeleton remodeling and induce autophagy in T lymphocytes. J Autoimmun. 2015;58:78–89.
22. Beyer C, Pisetsky DS. The role of microparticles in the pathogenesis of rheumatic diseases. Nat Rev Rheumatol. 2010;6:21–9.
23. Gao X, Belmadani S, Picchi A, Xu X, Potter BJ, Tewari-Singh N, et al. Tumor necrosis factor-α induces endothelial dysfunction in Lepr(db) mice. Circulation. 2007;115:245–54.
24. Libby P. Inflammation in atherosclerosis. Nature. 2002;420:868–74.
25. Brezinski EA, Follansbee MR, Armstrong EJ, Armstrong AW. Endothelial dysfunction and the effects of TNF inhibitors on the endothelium in psoriasis and psoriatic arthritis: a systematic review. Curr Pharm Des. 2014; 20:513–28 Review.
26. Tam LS, Kitas GD, Gonzalez-Gay MA. Can suppression of inflammation by anti-TNF prevent progression of subclinical atherosclerosis in inflammatory arthritis? Rheumatology. 2014;53:1108–19.
27. Bonetti PO, Lerman LO, Lerman A. Endothelial dysfunction: a marker of atherosclerotic risk. Arterioscler Thromb Vasc Biol. 2003;23:168–75.
28. Vita JA. Endothelial function. Circulation. 2011;124:e906–12.
29. Deanfield JE, Halcox JP, Rabelink TJ. Endothelial function and dysfunction: testing and clinical relevance. Circulation. 2007;115:1285–95.
30. Schock SC, Edrissi H, Burger D, Cadonic R, Hakim A, Thompson C. Microparticles generated during chronic cerebral ischemia deliver proapoptotic signals to cultured endothelial cells. Biochem Biophys Res Commun. 2014;450:912–7.
31. Abid Hussein MN, Nieuwland R, Hau CM, Evers LM, Meesters EW, Sturk A. Cell-derived microparticles contain caspase 3 in vitro and in vivo. J Thromb Haemost. 2005;3:888–96.
32. Böing AN, Hau CM, Sturk A, Nieuwland R. Platelet microparticles contain active caspase 3. Platelets. 2008;19:96–103.
33. Schneider J, Chromik AM, Uhl W, Mügge A, Bulut D. Apoptosis in esophagus and pancreas carcinoma cells induced by circulating microparticles is related to phosphatidyl serine and microparticle-associated caspases. Med Oncol. 2012;29:962–9.

34. Torisu K, Singh KK, Torisu T, Lovren F, Liu J, Pan Y. Intact endothelial autophagy is required to maintain vascular lipid homeostasis. Aging Cell. 2016;15:187–91.
35. Ding Z, Liu S, Wang X, Dai Y, Khaidakov M, Romeo F, et al. Lox-1, oxidant stress, mtDNA damage, autophagy, and immune response in atherosclerosis. Can J Physiol Pharmacol. 2014;92:524–30.
36. Martinet W, De Meyer GR. Autophagy in atherosclerosis. Curr Atheroscler Rep. 2008;10:216–23.
37. Wang L, Li H, Zhang J, Lu W, Zhao J, Su L, et al. Phosphatidylethanolamine binding protein 1 in vacular endothelial cell autophagy and atherosclerosis. J Physiol. 2013;591:5005–15.
38. Ding Z, Liu S, Wang X, Khaidakov M, Dai Y, Mehta JL. Oxidant stress in mitochondrial DNA damage, autophagy and inflammation in atherosclerosis. Sci Rep. 2013;3:1077.
39. Mesri M, Altieri DC. Endothelial cell activation by leukocyte microparticles. J Immunol. 1998;161:4382–7.
40. Distler JH, Huber LC, Gay S, Distler O, Pisetsky DS. Microparticles as mediators of cellular cross-talk in inflammatory disease. Autoimmunity. 2006;39:683–90.
41. Kotyla P, Jankiewicz-Ziobro K, Owczarek A, Kucharz EJ. Etanercept increases tumor necrosis factor-alpha level but not sFas level in patients with rheumatoid arthritis. Isr Med Assoc J. 2015;17:14–8.
42. Berthold E, Månsson B, Gullstrand B, Geborek P, Saxne T, Bengtsson AA, Kahn R. Tumour necrosis factor-α/etanercept complexes in serum predict long-term efficacy of etanercept treatment in seronegative rheumatoid arthritis. Scand J Rheumatol. 2018;47:22–6.

13

Models solely using claims-based administrative data are poor predictors of rheumatoid arthritis disease activity

Brian C. Sauer[1,4*], Chia-Chen Teng[1], Neil A. Accortt[2], Zachary Burningham[1], David Collier[2], Mona Trivedi[2] and Grant W. Cannon[3]

Abstract

Background: This study developed and validated a claims-based statistical model to predict rheumatoid arthritis (RA) disease activity, measured by the 28-joint count Disease Activity Score (DAS28).

Method: Veterans enrolled in the Veterans Affairs Rheumatoid Arthritis (VARA) registry with one year of data available for review before being assessed by the DAS28, were studied. Three models were developed based on initial selection of variables for analyses. The first model was based on clinically defined variables, the second leveraged grouping systems for high dimensional data and the third approach prescreened all possible predictors based on a significant bivariate association with the DAS28. The least absolute shrinkage and selection operator (LASSO) with fivefold cross-validation was used for variable selection and model development. Models were also compared for patients with <5 years to those ≥5 years of RA disease. Classification accuracy was examined for remission (DAS28 < 2.6) and for low (2.6–3.1), moderate (3.2–5.1) and high (>5.1) activity.

Results: There were 1582 Veterans who fulfilled inclusion criteria. The adjusted *r*-square for the three models tested ranged from 0.221 to 0.223. The models performed slightly better for patients with <5 years of RA disease than for patients with ≥5 years of RA disease. Correct classification of DAS28 categories ranged from 39.9% to 40.5% for the three models.

Conclusion: The multiple models tested showed weak overall predictive accuracy in measuring DAS28. The models performed poorly at predicting patients with remission and high disease activity. Future research should investigate components of disease activity measures directly from medical records and incorporate additional laboratory and other clinical data.

Keywords: Disease activity, Statistical methods, Rheumatoid arthritis

Background

The estimated prevalence of rheumatoid arthritis (RA) among US adults is approximately 0.6% (1.5 million people age ≥18 years) [1, 2]. Administrative claims databases continue to serve as one of the largest sources of data to study RA treatment and patient outcomes. Nevertheless, the utility of these studies is limited as disease activity is not directly captured in claims databases and there is no method to directly measure disease activity in relation to treatment modification and patient outcomes that are captured in claims data. Researchers have attempted to overcome this limitation by developing claims-based indexes of disease severity. Studies have typically used a Delphi approach to identify variables thought to be associated with disease activity and tested correlation between their approach and clinical information obtained from the electronic health record [3] or existing measures of RA disease activity [4]. A recent study by Desai et al. (2015) [5] attempted to validate the Claims-based Index for Rheumatoid

* Correspondence: brian.sauer@utah.edu
[1]Salt Lake City Veterans Affairs Medical Center, Health Services Research and Development (IDEAS) Center and University of Utah Division of Epidemiology, Salt Lake City, UT, USA
[4]Salt Lake IDEAS Center, VA; Salt Lake City Health Care System, 500 Foothill Drive Bldg. 182, Salt Lake City, UT 84148-0001, USA
Full list of author information is available at the end of the article

Arthritis Severity (CIRAS) developed by Ting et al. [3], who used the Delphi approach, against the C-reactive-protein-based 28-joint Disease Activity Score (DAS28-CRP) in a relatively small population (n = 315) of patients enrolled in the Brigham Women's Hospital Rheumatoid Arthritis Sequential Study (BRASS) and Medicare [5]. Unfortunately, they found the correlation between CIRAS and DAS28-CRP was poor and attempts to improve the performance by adding additional claims-derived variables also performed poorly ($R^2 = 0.23$).

These findings highlight the need to develop an algorithm to measure disease activity/severity in observational studies, as claims data are regularly used to evaluate disease progression and response to RA therapies. The ability to measure disease activity is also important in understanding how clinicians make therapeutic decisions, determining whether patients who may benefit from more aggressive treatment are escalating treatment, and providing real-world evidence of adoption of treatment guidelines.

The goal of this study was to develop and validate claims-based statistical models to predict disease activity measured by DAS28 in a larger population of Veteran patients enrolled in the Veterans Affairs Rheumatoid Arthritis (VARA) registry.

Methods

Design and data

A cohort study design was used on historical data available in the VARA registry and the Veterans Administration (VA) Informatics and Computing Infrastructure (VINCI), which houses the VA Corporate Data Warehouse (CDW) data available for research. This study used VARA and VINCI data from 1 January 2006 until 31 December 2014 to predict disease activity using data typically available in administrative claims databases. The gold standard clinical DAS28 was measured in Veteran patients enrolled in the VARA registry as part of routine care.

The VARA registry is a prospective, multicenter, observational registry involving 11 VA medical centers (Birmingham, AL; Brooklyn, NY; Dallas, TX; Denver, CO; Jackson, MS; Iowa City, IA; Little Rock, AR; Omaha, NE; Portland, OR; Salt Lake City, UT; and Washington, DC). Clinical disease activity measures (i.e., DAS28 and duration of disease) were obtained from the VARA registry, which has been described elsewhere [6, 7].

All administrative claims data were obtained from VINCI [8], which contains both CDW and Managerial Cost Accounting (MCA) system data. VINCI is a research and development environment jointly funded by Health Services Research & Development Service (HSR&D) and the Office of Information and Technology (OIT). VINCI contains rich clinical data in addition to administrative claims data. As the focus of this analysis was on developing a claims-based predictor of the DAS28 we limited our predictor variables to those available in patient tables, inpatient and outpatient procedure, diagnosis and pharmacy data domains.

Study population

Veteran patients had to be enrolled in the VARA registry to be included in the study, and had to be 18+ years of age, have a DAS28, and have at least 365 days of enrollment in the VA health care system prior to the DAS28 measurement. To ensure Veteran patients were actively using the system they were required to have had at least two encounters with the system during the 365-day baseline period. The first encounter with a DAS28 measurement that fulfilled other inclusion and exclusion criteria was eligible as the index date for training and testing the prediction model.

Veteran patients were excluded if they met any of the following criteria because their RA medications and treatment may be modified to treat cancer, transplant or other autoimmune disorders:

1. Diagnosed with any active cancer (Healthcare Cost and Utilization Project (HCUP) Single-level Clinical Classification System (CCS) [9] Diagnosis Category 11-45)
2. Undergone a transplant (HCUP CCS Procedure Category 64, 105, 176)
3. Diagnosed with other autoimmune disorders (HCUP CCS Diagnosis Category: 57, 210)

The index date was defined as the first encounter with a DAS28 after 1 January 2006 and before 31 December 2014 that fulfilled inclusion and exclusion criteria. The baseline period was defined as the 365-day observational period prior to the index date, which is the time we allowed comorbidities to accrue and contribute to the prediction of patient-level DAS.

Study variables

Dependent variables

The dependent variable was the continuous DAS28, which was collected at enrollment in the VARA registry and routinely thereafter. The DAS28 is a widely used disease activity assessment tool that affects treatment decisions by rheumatologists in daily clinical practice [10]. The DAS28 is a statistically derived composite index that takes into account the patient's number of swollen joints, number of tender joints, erythrocyte sedimentation rate (ESR), and general health using patient global assessment [11].

Our secondary endpoint was to determine if the predicted DAS28 could be correctly categorized to reflect typical clinical classification of disease, which includes remission (<2.6), low (2.6–3.1), moderate (3.2–5.1), and high (>5.1) disease activity.

Predictor variables

Potential predictor variables for model development were established using three distinct but complementary approaches. The first approach identified a list of potential predictors from literature review and discussion with clinical domain experts (GWC, DC, and MT). The second approach utilized hierarchical grouping software to generate drug categories, medical conditions and procedures at a feasible level for model development - described as the "all predictor" model. The third approach started with all possible predictors (i.e., *a priori* clinically defined variables and potential predictors based on hierarchical grouping systems) then used a prescreening approach that preselected variables exhibiting significant correlation with the DAS28 (p value <0.05). An automatic variables selection technique, described in the "Statistical approach" section, was then used to identify final sets of predictor variables for the three approaches used to identify the initial pool of potential predictor variables.

Table 4 in Appendix 1 lists the *a priori* clinically defined potential predictors used for model development. It is important to keep in mind that we restricted potential predictors to information available in administrative claims databases. For example, we recorded when specific laboratory measurements occurred but did not attempt to make use of the laboratory results. The potential baseline predictors involved patient demographics, whether specific laboratory tests or radiographs were performed, counts of clinic visits for primary, rheumatology, orthopedic, physical rehabilitation, occupational therapy, and emergency care. Hospital admissions and the number of unique drug classes served as proxies for healthcare utilization. Administrative codes were used to identify surgical procedures, hand surgery, orthopedic surgery and joint injections. Surgical procedures were identified using the Healthcare Cost and Utilization Project (HCUP) Surgical Flag Software [12, 13]. We measured specific comorbidities and implemented the Rheumatic Disease Comorbidity Index (RDCI) to account for comorbidities [14]. Procedure codes were also used to measure the use of assistive devices, such as a cane, crutch, or wheelchair.

Careful attempts were made to accurately measure disease modifying anti-rheumatic drug (DMARD) use during the baseline period and up to 14 days following the index date to reflect treatment changes in response to the DAS28. Three variables were produced for each generic ingredient and by therapeutic classes to represent: (1) days since start of therapy from the beginning of the baseline period, (2) days since ending a course of therapy from the index date (e.g., a value of 25 means the drug was discontinued 25 days before the index date), and (3) the proportion of days covered during the baseline year. Initiation and discontinuation of these therapies was also tracked during the 14 days post index date to account for the potential association between treatment modification and changes in disease activity.

In addition to the *a priori* defined potential predictors of disease activity, we leveraged existing grouping software to organize procedures, diagnoses and pharmacy claims into levels of aggregation that support prediction of RA disease activity. Specifically, we used counts of all single-level HCUP Clinical Classification System (CCS) condition and procedure groups [9]. We also used counts of all VA drug class codes (e.g., CV200: calcium channel blocker, CV300: antiarrhythmic, etc.) to account for pharmaceutical exposures, dispensed vitamins and dispensed prosthetics/supplies/devices during the baseline period (http://www.pbm.va.gov/nationalformulary.asp. - VA National Formulary by Class April 2016 Excel Spreadsheet). Dichotomous variables were required to have >1% prevalence in the population to be included in the statistical models.

Statistical approach

Least absolute shrinkage and selection operator (LASSO) is a widely used regularization technique used for developing high-dimensional prediction models without high variance [15]. LASSO selection arises from a form of ordinary least squares regression where the sum of the absolute value of the regression coefficients is constrained to be smaller than a specified parameter. Let $X = (x_1, x_2, x_3 \ldots x_m)$ denote the matrix of predictor variables (e.g., Table 1 with 250+ predictors) and let y denote the DAS28, (i.e., the response variable), where the x_is have been centered and scaled to have unit standard deviation and mean zero and y has a mean of zero. For a given tuning parameter t, the LASSO regression coefficients minimize: $\|y - X\beta\|^2$ ***subject to*** $\sum_{j=1}^{m} |\beta_j| \le t$

Provided that the LASSO parameter t is small enough, some of the regression coefficients will be exactly zero. Therefore, the LASSO can be viewed as having a built-in variable selection technique. By increasing the LASSO parameter in discrete steps a sequence of regression coefficients is obtained, where the non-zero coefficients at each step correspond to selected parameters. The LASSO method produces a series of models, M_0, M_1 ….M_k, with each model being the solution for a unique tuning parameter value. In this series, M_0 can be thought of as the least complex model, for which the maximum penalty is imposed on the regression coefficient, and M_k is the most complex model, for which no

Table 1 Attrition table for model development

	Inclusion/exclusion criteria	Population and encounters
1.	VARA registry patients April 1, 2015	2161 Veterans, 25,464 Encounters
2.	At least one valid DAS28	2063 Veterans, 19,064 Encounters
3.	Study period of interest (Jan 1, 2006 to Dec 31, 2014)	2002 Veterans, 17,000 Encounters
4.	Meet 365 days of enrollment criteria with ≥2 visits during baseline period	1976 Veterans with index date
5.	Remove patients with cancer	1631 Veterans
6.	Remove patients with transplant	1631 Veterans
7.	No other autoimmune disorders	1582 Veterans

VARA Veterans Affairs Rheumatoid Arthritis, *Das28* 28-joint disease activity score

penalty is imposed. The prediction error is then computed for each model and the model that yields the minimum prediction error is chosen.

Cross-validation is important in guarding against overfitting the model to the data, meaning the model is fit to random error instead of true underlying relationships among the variables. Overfitting reduces model performance when applied to an independent dataset that was not involved in the training of the model. Fivefold "external" cross-validation was applied using randomly selected folds to train and test the statistical model. Every fold was used for both training and testing, e.g., when fold 0 was the testing set then folds 1–4 were used for training and when fold 4 was the testing set then folds 0–3 were used for training. SAS GLMSELECT (SAS version 9.4 with Enterprise Guide version 6.1 (Cary, NC, USA)) was used to implement the cross-validated LASSO procedure and the model that minimizes the cross-validated external predicted sum of squares was used as the primary model selection criterion [16].

Classification analysis

As the secondary study endpoint, we attempted to use the predicted DAS28 to correctly classify patients who were categorized into typical clinical categories of remission and low, moderate, and high disease activity using the actual DAS28.

The correct classification rate (CCR) was used to determine how well the predicted values were classified into the four clinical groups based on the clinical DAS28. CCR is the percentage of correct observations (suitability with the expected value). CCR can be calculated using the following formula:

$$CCR = \frac{number\ of\ correct\ prediction}{number\ of\ observation}\ x\ 100\%$$

The higher percentage of CCR shows higher accuracy [17]. Exact binomial 95% confidence internals were computed for the CCR [18].

Sensitivity analysis

We developed three models that varied by the initial pool of variables available for model development. As described above, the first model comprised the clinically defined variables identified from our comprehensive literature review and use of clinical domain experts. The second model comprised these same clinically defined variables, plus HCUP CCS condition and procedure codes, and Veterans Health Administration (VHA) drug class codes. The third model comprised variables from the second model; however, only those variables statistically associated with the DAS28 were included (prescreening). Additional sensitivity analysis was applied on duration of RA disease. Models were compared for RA patients with <5 years of disease and ≥5 years of disease.

Results

Population

During the observation period from 1 January 2006 to 31 December 2014 there were 1582 VARA patients meeting all inclusion criteria for the model development phase. Study attrition is presented in Table 1. The average age at index for the population was 63 years (standard deviation (SD): 11) and 90% (95% CI: 88–91%) of the population were male. The DAS28 was normally distributed with an average DAS28 of 3.8 (SD: 1.54) and average Rheumatoid Disease Comorbidity Index (RDCI) of 2.2 (SD: 1.6).

Model development and testing

The clinical experts identified 253 *a priori* claims-based variables representing clinical concepts thought to be associated with the DAS28. After applying the restriction that variables must be present in >1% of the population we ended up with 175 potential predictor variables. After model development with the LASSO regularized regression, the final model contained 32 variables and the adjusted *R*-square was 0.221 (Table 2). The "all predictors" and prescreening models started with different initial potential predictor variables but produced similar cross-validated adjusted *R*-square values, 0.221 and 0.223, respectively.

Review of the scatter plots presented in Fig. 1a-c show that the predicted DAS28 did not contain the same range of values as the true DAS28. The predicted DAS28 overestimated those with low DAS28 and underestimated the predicted value for Veteran patients with high DAS28.

Model-retained predictor variables

Variables selected and their standardized estimates for each model are presented in Appendix 2: Tables 5-7. Variables are ordered by the magnitude of the standardized estimate. Healthcare utilization (total visit count,

Table 2 Model validation by initial set of predictor variables

Variable sets	All clinical predictors	All predictors	Prescreening
Potential predictors	253	1275	279
Potential predictors with ≥1% prevalence (i.e., predictors put into model)	175	567	230
Predictors in final model	32	45	46
Fivefold cross-validated *R*-square (test)	0.237	0.243	0.246
Fivefold cross-validated Adj *R*-square (test)	0.221	0.221	0.223
<5 Years of RA disease Adj *R*-square	0.218	0.190	0.196
≥5 years of RA disease Adj *R*-square	0.186	0.185	0.185

RA rheumatoid arthritis, *Adj* adjusted

primary care visits and occupational health visits) were relatively strong predictors of higher DAS28. Starting a new DMARD (biologic or non-biologic) 14 days after the DAS28 measurement was also consistently associated with higher DAS28. Higher baseline proportion of days covered (PDC) for DMARDs during the prior year was associated with lower DAS28. Measures indicating higher comorbidity, such as the RDCI and number of distinct VA drug classes were associated with higher DAS28. In the two models that used grouping software, we found analgesics, antidepressants and other agents acting on the central nervous system to be associated with higher DAS28. Please review Appendix 2 for a complete list of variables retained in each model.

Secondary analysis: correct classification of disease activity categories

The overall CCR for correctly classifying patients with the predicted DAS28 into clinical categories based on the true DAS28 ranged from 39.9% to 40.5% (Table 3). The true positive rate (TPR), which essentially represents measurement sensitivity, was fairly low in the group classified as having high disease activity by the predicted DAS28 and ranged from 9.9% to 10.8% (Table 3), while the positive predicted value (PPV) ranged from 57.9% to 63.0%. The TPR for those classified as having moderate disease ranged from 84.6% to 87.6%, while the PPV ranged from 42.5% to 43.0%. The TPR for low disease acitivity ranged from 17.9% to 20.2%, while the PPV ranged from 21.0% to 21.6%. None of the prediction models developed and tested accurately classified patients with remission. The TPR ranged from 0.0% to 0.3%, while the PPV ranged from 100% to 0%. Attempts to statistically define the cut points for the predicted DAS28 to optimize correct classification did not meaningfully improve the CCR. The optimized CCR only increased by approximately 3% (not presented).

Discussion

This study developed and internally validated statistical models to predict RA disease activity using data available in administrative claims data but was not successful in establishing a high level of predictive value. The relatively low adjusted *R*-square value and the inability to accurately classify patients into categories of disease activity using the predicted DAS28, draw into question the ability of a claims-based predictor to successfully represent patient disease activity in RA.

The sensitivity analysis focused on development of multiple models based on the initial pool of variables and applying these models to subsets of patients with <5 years of RA disease and ≥5 years of disease. This cut point was chosen because it has been used in other studies (e.g., TICORA 2004 study) [19] to represent early disease and because the data did not support comparisons with earlier cut-points.

The initial pool of predictors did not impact predictive accuracy, as the three models had similar adjusted *R*-square values. The models performed slightly better for patients with <5 year of disease. Similar results were found for patients with <2 years of disease (not presented). Duration of RA disease was recorded at VARA enrollment and would not be available in claims data, but could be approximated based on duration of enrollment and indicators of disease in claims-based data.

Variables retained in the three models were intuitive and interpretable. Variables indicating increased healthcare utilization, comorbidities, the use of agents that act on the central nervous system, and new DMARD prescriptions after the DAS28 measurement were associated with higher DAS28. Variables indicating longer exposure and a higher proportion of days covered by DMARDs in the baseline period were associated with lower DAS28. Even though many variables were associated with DAS28 the models poorly explained the variation in DAS28.

The classification accuracy of predicted DAS28 was evaluated by categorizing the true DAS28 and predicted DAS28 into remission (<2.6), low disease activity (2.6–3.1), moderate disease activity (3.2–5.1), and high disease activity (>5.1). The overall classification accuracy across the three models was modest. The models were poor predictors of remission and high levels of disease activity, which is likely due to the relatively small number of Veterans in the lower and higher end of the DAS28 scale. They performed best at classifying patients with moderate disease activity, which is the range for the majority of the population. In an additional

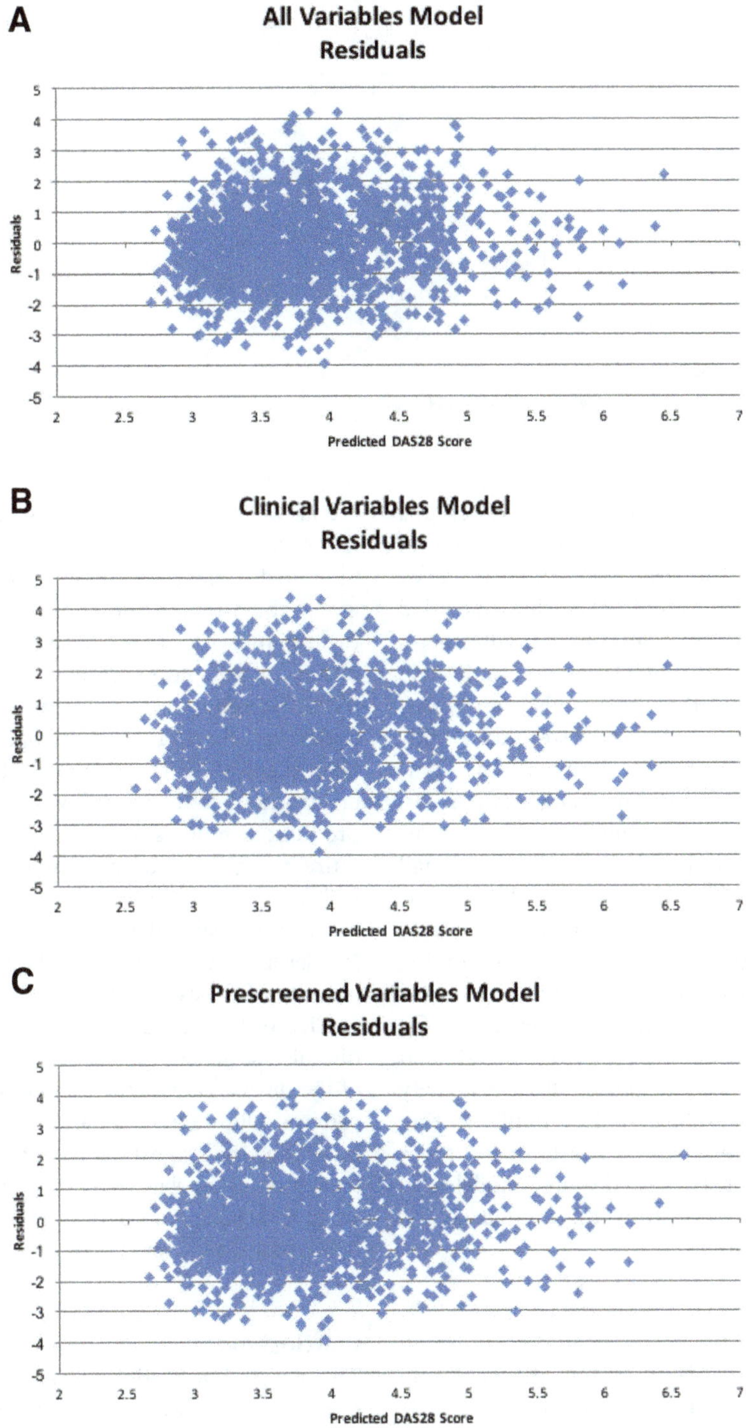

Fig. 1 Predicted 28-joint disease activity score (DAS28) vs true DAS28 for test data. **a** Clinical predictors. **b** All predictors. **c** Pre-screened variables

analysis (not presented), we identified the optimal cut points of the predicted DAS28 to correctly classify patients by true DAS28 category of disease activity but were only able to increase classification accuracy to 43% across the three models.

A recent study evaluating the accuracy of a claims-based model to predict DAS28-CRP also performed poorly and found other claims-based measures of RA disease severity were not well correlated with true DAS28-CRP. Desai et al. (2015) [5] evaluated the

Table 3 Classification accuracy by disease activity category

			All clinical predictors	All predictors	Prescreening
4 Categories	High (>5.1)	TPR	10.5%	9.9%	10.8%
		PPV	57.9%	62.0%	63.0%
	Moderate (3.2–5.1)	TPR	84.6%	87.6%	86.9%
		PPV	42.5%	43.0%	43.0%
	Low (2.6–3.1)	TPR	20.2%	17.9%	18.3%
		PPV	21.6%	21.2%	21.0%
	Remission (<2.6)	TPR	0.3%	0.0%	0.0%
		PPV	100.0%	0.0%	0.0%
	CCR (95% CI)		39.9% (37.5–42.3%)	40.5% (38.1–43.0%)	40.5% (38.1–43.0%)

CCR correct classification rate, *TPR* true positive rate, *PPV* positive predicted value

claims-based index for RA severity (CIRAS) developed by Ting et al. [3] using a Delphi panel and found poor correlation with the true DAS28-CRP. They added additional variables to CIRAS that included medical claims for rheumatoid lung involvement, hand surgery, tuberculin test ordered and anti-CCP test orders. Furthermore, they also added pharmacy claims for steroids, opioids, non-steroidal anti-inflammatory drugs (NSAIDs), number of non-biologic DMARDs, and number of biologic DMARDs, and found the model *R*-square value (0.23) was similar to ours, even though they had a relatively small sample of Medicare patients (n = 315). They concluded that CIRAS may not approximate RA disease in observational cohorts and its use for confounding adjustment should be carefully considered. They also concluded that claims-based algorithms developed for clinical disease activity should be rigorously tested in a population with actual measures of disease activity to establish their generalizability before implementing in research. Our study leveraged a substantially larger population and rigorously tested our models to reduce the likelihood of overfitting the models to the data, yet had similar results.

Strength and limitations

The primary strength of this study was the access to DAS28 in a relatively large number of patients. This is the largest study that attempted to train and validate a claims-based predictor of RA disease activity using the actual DAS28. In addition, we used statistical methods that supported high-dimensional variable selection and prevented overfitting the model to the actual data. Of note, we replicated model development and classification accuracy using the Clinical Disease Activity Index (CDAI) and found similar adjusted *R*-square values and classification accuracy (results not presented).

One weakness of this study is that the population studied may not represent average RA patients. Veterans tend to be older and more likely male than the general population. Another weakness of this study was the reliance on claims-based predictors. Even though observational comparative effectiveness and safety studies often rely on commercial and Federal claims databases there is a new paradigm for population health analytics that involves the integration of the electronic health record with claims data. Accurate prediction models of disease activity will likely require integration of clinical data, such as laboratory test results and information captured in structured electronic health data or in medical notes. The use of standardized templates would be required to extract components of disease activity scores, such as the number of swollen or tender joints, and used in models to predict future disease activity and to better understand what features of the disease activity score influence changes in treatment patterns. Our future work aims to develop natural language processing tools to extract components of the DAS28 from templated notes within the VA and use this information along with other clinical data in the development of future RA disease activity prediction models.

Conclusions

The prediction models developed and tested found a relatively low level of predictive accuracy, drawing into question their use for confounding adjustment or to evaluate treatment decisions in patients with predicted DAS28. Our findings are consistent with other recent studies that attempted to use claims-based data to predict RA disease activity. Future work to predict disease activity in patient populations should incorporate clinical data from the electronic health record in addition to key variables available in administrative claims data.

Appendix 1

Table 4 List of *a priori* Clinically Defined Predictors and their Measurement

Measurement	Value	Variable	Table
Laboratory			
Number ESR tests	85651, 85652	CPT	CDW.OutpatProcedure
Number CRP tests	86140	CPT	CDW.OutpatProcedure
aCCP – (Y/N)	86200	CPT	CDW.OutpatProcedure
RF – (Y/N)	86431	CPT	CDW.OutpatProcedure
Number. complete blood counts	85025	CPT	CDW.OutpatProcedure
Number. chemistry panels ordered or any electrolyte	80053, 82248, 82465, 82977, 83540, 83615, 84100, 84478, 84550	CPT	CDW.OutpatProcedure
Radiology			
Radiographs (Y/N)	70010-79999	CPT	CDW.OutpatProcedure
Number radiographs	Count of 70010-79999	CPT	CDW.OutpatProcedure
Hand or foot (Y/N) (toes, fingers, wrist)	73620, 73630, 73650, 73660, 73100, 73110,73120, 73130	CPT	CDW.OutpatProcedure
C-spine (Y/N)	72040, 75052	CPT	CDW.OutpatProcedure
Other bone x-ray (Y/N)	Master file	CPT	CDW.OutpatProcedure
Clinic Visits			
Any visit	Any	stopcode	CDW.outpatVisit
Rheumatology	314	stopcode	CDW.outpatVisit
Primary care	323, 342	stopcode	CDW.outpatVisit
Orthopedic	60, 509	stopcode	CDW.outpatVisit
Physical Rehabilitation	201, 250	stopcode	CDW.outpatVisit
Occupational Therapy	21, 206, 460	stopcode	CDW.outpatVisit
Number ED visits	130, 101	stopcode	CDW.outpatVisit
Utilization			
Number Inpatient stay	Row count per person	Admission date	Inpatient.inpatient
Unique Drug class codes	Row count per person	VAdrugclasscode	CDW.Rxoutpat
Procedures			
Any surgery	10021-6990	CPT	
Any surgery	Master file	ICD9	CDW.outpatProcedure, inpatProcedure, inpatientCPT
Hand surgery	26500, 26502, 26504, 26494, 26989	CPT	CDW.Outpat.Procedure, inpatientCPT
Hand surgery	Master file[a]	ICD9	CDW.inpatientProcedure
Any orthopedic (include spine) surgery	Master file	CPT	CDW.inpatientCPT, Outpat.Procedure
Joint injections	Master file	Jcode	CDW.Outpat.Procedure, inpatientCPT
Comorbidity			
RDCI RA comorbidity score	See published paper	ICD9	CDW.outpatDiagnosis
Rheumatoid lung involvement	714.81	ICD9	CDW.outpatDiagnosis
Felty's syndrome	714.1	ICD9	CDW.outpatDiagnosis
Sjogrens	710.2	ICD9	CDW.outpatDiagnosis

Table 4 List of *a priori* Clinically Defined Predictors and their Measurement *(Continued)*

Assistive Devices			
Cane (Y/N)	Master file	CPT/ICD9 procedure	CDW.outpatProcedure, inpatProcedure
Crutch (Y/N)	Master file	CPT/ICD9 procedure	CDW.outpatProcedure, inpatProcedure
Walker (Y/N)	Master file	CPT/ICD9 procedure	CDW.outpatProcedure, inpatProcedure
Wheelchair (Y/N)	Master file	CPT/ICD9 procedure	CDW.outpatProcedure, inpatProcedure
Other Assist Device (Y/N)	Master file	CPT/ICD9 procedure	CDW.outpatProcedure, inpatProcedure
Medications dispensed			
Number NSAID	MS102	VA drug Class	CDW.Rxoutpatfill
Number Non-biologic DMARD	String search - list below	drugnamewithoutdose	CDW.Rxoutpatfill
Methotrexate (Y/N)	String search	drugnamewithoutdose	CDW.Rxoutpatfill
Leflunomide (Y/N)	String search	drugnamewithoutdose	CDW.Rxoutpatfill
Sulfasalazine (Y/N)	String search	drugnamewithoutdose	CDW.Rxoutpatfill
Hydroxychloroquine (Y/N)	String search	drugnamewithoutdose	CDW.Rxoutpatfill
Azathioprine (Y/N)	String search	drugnamewithoutdose	CDW.Rxoutpatfill
TNFi (Y/N)	String search: etanercept, adalimumab, infliximab, golimumab, certolizumab	drugnamewithoutdose	CDW.MCA, Rxoutpatfill, outpatProcedure, TIU notes
Other biologics	rituximab, abatacept, anakinra, tocilizumab,	drugnamewithoutdose	CDW.MCA, Rxoutpatfill, outpatProcedure, TIU notes
Tofacitinib (Y/N)	String search	drugnamewithoutdose	CDW.Rxoutpatfill
Glucocorticosteroids (Y/N and Dose)	HS051	VA drug Class	CDW.MCA and Rxoutpatfill
Minor DMARDs (Any Y/N)	Doxycyline, minocycline, auranofin, d-penicillamine, cyclosporine	drugnamewithoutdose	CDW.Rxoutpatfill
Smoking cessation medication (Y/N)	Chantix Nicotine substitutes	Drugnamewithoutdose	CDW.Rxoutpatfill
Processed Medication Data for DMARDs			
Days since start med	All meds	drugnamewithoutdose	CDW.Rxoutpatfill
Days since end med (90-day gap to end)	All meds	drugnamewithoutdose	CDW.Rxoutpatfill
PDC from start therapy to end of observation period	All meds	drugnamewithoutdose	CDW.Rxoutpatfill
Demographics			
Age	Age	DOB	CDW.patient
Gender	M/F	Gender	CDW.patient

[a]Master File = primary excel workbook containing all measured concepts and is available by request (brian.sauer@utah.edu)
ESR erythrocyte sedimentation rate, *CRP* c-reactive protein, *PDC* proportion of days covered

Appendix 2

Table 5 Model Generated from Clinically Defined Predictors

Effect	Estimate	Standardized Est
Intercept	4.639526	0
Baseline Visit Count	0.001981	0.02366
Baseline RDCI Score	0.005026	0.00521
Baseline Labtest Days for Chem Panel	-0.001423	-0.0026
Baseline Primary Care Visit Count	0.005222	0.01475
Baseline Occupational Visit Count	0.010707	0.01553
Bupropion Rx in Baseline (Y/N)	0.106174	0.0135
Distinct VA Drug Class Rx	0.030526	0.13957
Joint Injection Count	0.019454	0.0097
Rheumatism, Unspecified And Fibrosis Dx Count (ICD:729)	0.008102	0.00519
Baseline Surgery Count	-0.058006	-0.0162
Days End of Prednisone	-0.000912	-0.09845
Days End of Sulfasalazine	-0.000063599	-0.00505
Baseline PDC for Etanercept	-0.152669	-0.02073
Days Start of Golimumab	-0.001374	-0.00927
Baseline PDC for Non-Biologic DMARDs	-0.708075	-0.16342
Start Methotrexate in 14 Days after Index Date (Y/N)	0.077462	0.01148
Start Leflunomide in 14 Days after Index Date (Y/N)	0.073709	0.00598
Start in TNFi Biologic DMARDs in 14 Days after Index Date (Count of distinct Rx)	0.542521	0.06171
Start in Non-Biologic DMARDs in 14 Days after Index Date (Count of distinct Rx)	0.380811	0.09612
Start in Steroid in 14 Days after Index Date (Count of distinct Rx)	0.45952	0.06632
Rheumatism, Unspecified And Fibrosis Dx (ICD:729) (Y/N)	0.003294	0.00075
Baseline Labtest for Chem Panel (Y/N)	-0.482788	-0.0294
Baseline Labtest for RF (Y/N)	0.022162	0.00714
Baseline Foot Surgery (Y/N)	0.037806	0.01158
Baseline Hand Surgery (Y/N)	0.105081	0.02942
Baseline Occupational Visit (Y/N)	0.116702	0.02344
Baseline Rheumatology Visit (Y/N)	-0.033104	-0.00143
Start in Non-Biologic DMARDs in 14 Days after Index Date (Y/N)	0.340854	0.07459
Start in DMARDs in 14 Days after Index Date (Y/N)	0.590044	0.08356
Baseline Use of Sulfasalazine (Y/N)	0.158241	0.03893
Baseline Use of Rituximab (Y/N)	0.112073	0.00872
Baseline Use of Infliximab (Y/N)	0.003816	0.00057

Table 6 Model Generated from All Predictors

Effect	Estimate	Standardized Est
Intercept	4.027342	0
Baseline Visit Count	0.002189	0.02615
Baseline Occupational Visit Count	0.008477	0.01229
Bupropion Rx in Baseline (Y/N)	0.020813	0.00265
Non-Opioid Analgesics Rx Count (CN103)	0.001982	0.005
Sedative/Hypnotics, Other Rx Count (CN309)	0.002925	0.00222
Tricyclic Antidepressants Rx Count (CN601)	0.001475	0.00207
Local Anesthetics, Topical Rx Count (DE700)	0.016648	0.00492
Calcium Rx Count (TN402)	-0.050907	-0.01654
Decongestants, Systemic Rx Count (RE200)	0.030669	0.00639
Platelet Aggregation Inhibitors Rx Count (BL700)	0.001719	0.00095
Distinct VA Drug Class Rx	0.017323	0.07921
Baseline Surgery Count	-0.007242	-0.00202
Days End of Prednisone	-0.000873	-0.09417
Baseline PDC for Etanercept	-0.102578	-0.01393
Days Start of Golimumab	-0.000198	-0.00133
Baseline PDC for Non-Biologic DMARDs	-0.662683	-0.15295
Start Methotrexate in 14 Days after Index Date (Y/N)	0.037588	0.00557
Start in TNFi Biologic DMARDs in 14 Days after Index Date (Count of distinct Rx)	0.446665	0.05081
Start in Non-Biologic DMARDs in 14 Days after Index Date (Count of distinct Rx)	0.352313	0.08893
Start in Steroid in 14 Days after Index Date (Count of distinct Rx)	0.173564	0.02505
Disease of Mouth Excluding Dental Dx Count in Baseline (CCS137)	0.03199	0.00289
Calculus of Urinary Tract Dx Count in Baseline (CCS160)	-0.013249	-0.00541
Other Non-Traumatic Joint Disorders Dx Count in Baseline (CCS204)	0.000382	0.00074
Other Connective Tissue Disease Dx Count in Baseline (CCS211)	0.00293	0.00464
Disease of White Blood Cells Dx Count in Baseline (CCS63)	0.044243	0.00827
Conditions Associated With Dizziness or Vertigo Dx Count in Baseline (CCS93)	0.005453	0.00187
Baseline Labtest for Chem Panel (Y/N)	-0.314001	-0.01912
Baseline Foot Surgery (Y/N)	0.006726	0.00206
Baseline Hand Surgery (Y/N)	0.106317	0.02977
Opioid Analgesics Rx (CN101) (Y/N)	0.183042	0.05861
Non-Opioid Analgesics Rx (CN103) (Y/N)	0.065908	0.02006
Tricyclic Antidepressants Rx (CN601) (Y/N)	0.080738	0.01271
Antidepressants, Other Rx (CN609) (Y/N)	0.059894	0.01824
CNS Medications, Other Rx (CN900) (Y/N)	0.047949	0.00365
Loop Diuretics Rx (CV702) (Y/N)	0.073401	0.01455
Diagnostics, Other Rx (DX900) (Y/N)	0.142061	0.03273
Insulin Rx (HS051) (Y/N)	0.002114	0.00069
Thyroid Supplements Rx (HS851) (Y/N)	0.00651	0.0013
Immune Suppressants Rx (IM600) (Y/N)	0.033029	0.0059
Calcium Rx (TN420) (Y/N)	-0.080805	-0.01165
Baseline Occupational Visit (Y/N)	0.045223	0.00908
Start in Non-Biologic DMARDs in 14 Days after Index Date (Y/N)	0.375004	0.08206
Start in DMARDs in 14 Days after Index Date (Y/N)	0.816375	0.11562
Baseline Use of Sulfasalazine (Y/N)	0.144504	0.03555
Baseline Use of Rituximab (Y/N)	0.028977	0.00226

Table 7 Model Generated from Pre-screened Predictors

Effect	Estimate	Standardized Est
Intercept	4.268844	0
Baseline Visit Count	0.001667	0.01991
Baseline Primary Care Visit Count	0.000924	0.00261
Baseline Occupational Visit Count	0.011031	0.016
Bupropion Rx in Baseline (Y/N)	0.052414	0.00666
Non-Opioid Analgesics Rx Count (CN103)	0.003163	0.00798
Anti-rheumatics, Other Rx Count (MS190)	-0.000129	-0.00032
Sedative/Hypnotics, Other Rx Count (CN309)	0.00711	0.0054
Tricyclic Antidepressants Rx Count (CN601)	0.002659	0.00374
Local Anesthetics, Topical Rx Count (DE700)	0.026352	0.00779
Soaps/Shampoos/Soap-Free Cleansers Rx Count (DE400)	0.012432	0.00283
Decongestants, Systemic Rx Count (RE200)	0.055989	0.01166
Distinct VA Drug Class Rx	0.014658	0.06702
Joint Injection Count	0.003921	0.00196
Days End of Prednisone	-0.000913	-0.09852
Baseline PDC for Etanercept	-0.131689	-0.01788
Days Start of Golimumab	-0.000651	-0.00439
Baseline PDC for Non-Biologic DMARDs	-0.672468	-0.1552
Start Methotrexate in 14 Days after Index Date (Y/N)	0.04705	0.00697
Start Leflunomide in 14 Days after Index Date (Y/N)	0.013983	0.00113
Start in TNFi Biologic DMARDs in 14 Days after Index Date (Count of distinct Rx)	0.471838	0.05367
Start in Non-Biologic DMARDs in 14 Days after Index Date (Count of distinct Rx)	0.364512	0.09201
Start in Steroid in 14 Days after Index Date (Count of distinct Rx)	0.175888	0.02539
Varicose Veins of Lower Extremity (CCS119)	0.020937	0.00268
Disease of Mouth Excluding Dental Dx Count in Baseline (CCS137)	0.064254	0.00581
Other Connective Tissue Disease Dx Count in Baseline (CCS211)	0.003949	0.00625
Disease of White Blood Cells Dx Count in Baseline (CCS63)	0.066725	0.01247
Conditions Associated With Dizziness or Vertigo Dx Count in Baseline (CCS93)	0.013165	0.0045
Baseline Lab test for Chem Panel (Y/N)	-0.378938	-0.02308
Baseline Lab test for RF (Y/N)	0.001583	0.00051
Baseline Foot Surgery (Y/N)	0.019935	0.00611
Baseline Hand Surgery (Y/N)	0.10473	0.02932
Opioid Analgesics Rx (Y/N)	0.190656	0.06105
Non-Opioid Analgesics Rx (CN103) (Y/N)	0.070215	0.02137
Tricyclic Antidepressants Rx (CN601) (Y/N)	0.098618	0.01553
Antidepressants, Other Rx (CN609) (Y/N)	0.064811	0.01974
CNS Medications, Other Rx (CN900) (Y/N)	0.095795	0.00729
Loop Diuretics Rx (CV702) (Y/N)	0.084218	0.01669
Diagnostics, Other Rx (DX900) (Y/N)	0.15962	0.03678
Insulin Rx (HS501) (Y/N)	0.013138	0.00212
Thyroid Supplements Rx (HS851) (Y/N)	0.02656	0.00532
Antigout Agents Rx (MS400) (Y/N)	0.003596	0.00046
Baseline Occupational Visit (Y/N)	0.052566	0.01056
Start in Non-Biologic DMARDs in 14 Days after Index Date (Y/N)	0.357809	0.0783
Start in DMARDs in 14 Days after Index Date (Y/N)	0.834045	0.11812
Baseline Use of Sulfasalazine (Y/N)	0.157077	0.03865
Baseline Use of Rituximab (Y/N)	0.08026	0.00625

Abbreviations

BRASS: Brigham Women's Hospital Rheumatoid Arthritis Sequential Study; CCR: Correct classification rate; CCS: Clinical Classification System; CDAI: Clinical Disease Activity Index; CDW: Corporate Data Warehouse; CIRAS: Claims-base Index for Rheumatoid Arthritis Severity; DAS28: 28-Joint Disease Activity Score; DAS28-CRP: C-reactive protein-based 28-Joint Disease Activity Score; DMARD: Disease modifying anti-rheumatic drug; ESR: Erythrocyte sedimentation rate; HCUP: Healthcare Cost and Utilization Project; HSR&D: Health Services Research & Development Service; LASSO: Least absolute shrinkage and selection operator; MCA: Managerial Cost Accounting; OIT: Office of Information and Technology; PDC: Proportion of days covered; PPV: Positive predicted value; RA: Rheumatoid arthritis; RDCI: Rheumatic Disease Comorbidity Index; SEAC: Scientific, Ethical, and Advisory Committee; TPR: True positive rate; VA: Veterans Administration; VARA: Veterans Affairs Rheumatoid Arthritis; VINCI: Veterans Administration (VA) Informatics and Computing Infrastructure

Acknowledgements

This material is based upon work supported by Amgen, the Department of Veterans Affairs, Veterans Health Administration, Office of Research and Development and Value and Epidemiology Research using Causal Inference and Data Science (VERITAS). The authors would like to thank Tina Huynh for her administrative support.

Funding

This work was funded by Amgen Inc. Supplemental funding was provided by a Veterans Affairs Health Services Research and Development Award.

Authors' contributions

All authors contributed to the design and interpretation of the study. BCS, GWC, C-CT, and ZB accessed and analyzed the data. BCS and GWC obtained funding and provided project management. BCS provided the initial draft of the manuscript. All authors read and contributed to revisions and approved the final manuscript.

Competing interests

Brian C. Sauer is employed by the University of Utah and Salt Lake City Veterans Affairs Medical Center and received research grant funding from Amgen Inc. Chia-Chen Teng is employed by the University of Utah and received research grant funding from Amgen Inc. Neil A. Accortt is employed by Amgen Inc. and holds stock in Amgen Inc. Zachary Burningham is employed by the University of Utah and Salt Lake City Veterans Affairs Medical Center and received research grant funding from Amgen Inc. David Collier and Mona Trivedi are employed by Amgen Inc. and hold stock in Amgen Inc. Grant W. Cannon is employed by the University of Utah and Salt Lake City Veterans Affairs Medical Center and received research grant funding from Amgen Inc.

Disclaimer

The views expressed in this article are those of the authors and do not necessarily reflect the position or policy of the Department of Veterans Affairs or the United States government.

Author details

[1]Salt Lake City Veterans Affairs Medical Center, Health Services Research and Development (IDEAS) Center and University of Utah Division of Epidemiology, Salt Lake City, UT, USA. [2]Amgen, Thousand Oaks, CA, USA. [3]Salt Lake City Veterans Affairs Medical Center, Health Services Research and Development (IDEAS) Center and University of Utah Division of Rheumatology, Salt Lake City, UT, USA. [4]Salt Lake IDEAS Center, VA; Salt Lake City Health Care System, 500 Foothill Drive Bldg. 182, Salt Lake City, UT 84148-0001, USA.

References

1. Scott DL, Wolfe F, Huizinga TWJ. Rheumatoid arthritis. Lancet. 2010; 376(9746):1094–108. doi:10.1016/S0140-6736(10)60826-4.
2. Helmick CG, Felson DT, Lawrence RC, et al. Estimates of the prevalence of arthritis and other rheumatic conditions in the United States. Part I. Arthritis Rheum. 2008;58(1):15–25. doi:10.1002/art.23177.
3. Ting G, Schneeweiss S, Scranton R, Katz J, Weinblatt M, Young M, et al. Development of a health care utilisation data-based index for rheumatoid arthritis severity: a preliminary study. Arthritis Res Ther. 2008;10:R95. doi:10.1186/ar2482. [PMC free article] [PubMed] [Cross Ref].
4. Baser O, Du J, Xie L, Wang H, Dysinger AH, Wang L. Derivation of severity index for rheumatoid arthritis and its association with healthcare outcomes. J Med Econ. 2012;15(5):918–24. doi:10.3111/13696998.2012.688905.
5. Desai RJ. An external validation study reporting poor correlation between the claims-based index for rheumatoid arthritis severity and the disease activity score. Arthritis Res Ther. 2015;17(1):1–5. doi:10.1186/s13075-015-0599-0.
6. Mikuls TR, Reimold A, Kerr GS, Cannon GW. Insights and implications of the VA Rheumatoid Arthritis Registry. Fed Pract. 2015;32:24–9.
7. Cannon GW, Mikuls TR, Hayden CL, et al. Merging Veterans Affairs rheumatoid arthritis registry and pharmacy data to assess methotrexate adherence and disease activity in clinical practice. Arthritis Care Res (Hoboken). 2011;63(12):1680–90. doi:10.1002/acr.20629.
8. Fihn SD, Francis J, Clancy C, et al. Insights from advanced analytics at the Veterans Health Administration. Health Aff. 2014;33(7):1203–11. doi:10.1377/hlthaff.2014.0054.
9. HCUP. HCUP CCS. Healthcare Cost and Utilization Project (HCUP). www.hcup-us.ahrq.gov/toolssoftware/ccs/ccs.jsp. Accessed 24 Apr 2017.
10. Sato M, Schneeweiss S, Scranton R, et al. The validity of a rheumatoid arthritis medical records-based index of severity compared with the DAS28. Arthritis Res Ther. 2006;8(3):R57. doi:10.1186/ar1921.
11. Prevoo ML, Hof MA v 't, Kuper HH, van Leeuwen MA, van de Putte LB, van Riel PL. Modified disease activity scores that include twenty-eight-joint counts. Development and validation in a prospective longitudinal study of patients with rheumatoid arthritis. Arthritis Rheum. 1995;38(1):44–8.
12. HCUP. Surgical Flag Software. Healthcare Cost and Utilization Project (HCUP). www.hcup-us.ahrq.gov/toolssoftware/surgflags/surgeryflags.jsp. Accessed 24 Apr 2017.
13. Weiser TG, Semel ME, Simon AE, et al. In-hospital death following inpatient surgical procedures in the United States, 1996–2006. World J Surg. 2011; 35(9):1950–6. doi:10.1007/s00268-011-1169-5.
14. England BR, Sayles H, Mikuls TR, Johnson DS, Michaud K. Validation of the Rheumatic Disease Comorbidity Index. Arthritis Care Res (Hoboken). 2015;67(6):865–72. doi:10.1002/acr.22456.
15. Tibshirani R. Regression shrinkage and selection via the lasso. J R Stat Soc Ser B. (…. 1996. https://statweb.stanford.edu/~tibs/lasso/lasso.pdf.
16. Gunes F. Penalized regression methods for linear models in SAS/STAT®. https://support.sas.com/rnd/app/stat/papers/2015/PenalizedRegression_LinearModels.pdf.
17. David W, Hosmer J, Lemeshow S, Sturdivant RX. Applied logistic regression. Hoboken: John Wiley & Sons; 2013. doi:10.1002/9781118548387
18. Agresti A. Dealing with discreteness: making 'exact' confidence intervals for proportions, differences of proportions, and odds ratios more exact. Stat Methods Med Res. 2003;12(1):3–21. doi:10.1191/0962280203sm311ra.
19. Grigor C, Capell H, Stirling A, et al. Effect of a treatment strategy of tight control for rheumatoid arthritis (the TICORA study): a single-blind randomised controlled trial. Lancet. 2004;364(9430):263–9. doi:10.1016/S0140-6736(04)16676-2.

Pregnancy-induced gene expression changes in vivo among women with rheumatoid arthritis

Dana E. Goin[1,2], Mette Kiel Smed[3], Lior Pachter[2,4], Elizabeth Purdom[2], J. Lee Nelson[5,6], Hanne Kjærgaard[3^], Jørn Olsen[7,8], Merete Lund Hetland[9,10], Vibeke Zoffmann[3,10], Bent Ottesen[3] and Damini Jawaheer[1,8,11*]

Abstract

Background: Little is known about gene expression changes induced by pregnancy in women with rheumatoid arthritis (RA) and healthy women because the few studies previously conducted did not have pre-pregnancy samples available as baseline. We have established a cohort of women with RA and healthy women followed prospectively from a pre-pregnancy baseline. In this study, we tested the hypothesis that pregnancy-induced changes in gene expression among women with RA who improve during pregnancy ($pregDAS_{improved}$) overlap substantially with changes observed among healthy women and differ from changes observed among women with RA who worsen during pregnancy ($pregDAS_{worse}$).

Methods: Global gene expression profiles were generated by RNA sequencing (RNA-seq) from 11 women with RA and 5 healthy women before pregnancy (T0) and at the third trimester (T3). Among the women with RA, eight showed an improvement in disease activity by T3, whereas three worsened. Differential expression analysis was used to identify genes demonstrating significant changes in expression *within* each of the RA and healthy groups (T3 vs T0), as well as *between* the groups at each time point. Gene set enrichment was assessed in terms of Gene Ontology processes and protein networks.

Results: A total of 1296 genes were differentially expressed between T3 and T0 among the 8 $pregDAS_{improved}$ women, with 161 genes showing at least two-fold change (FC) in expression by T3. The majority (108 of 161 genes) were also differentially expressed among healthy women ($q<0.05$, FC≥2). Additionally, a small cluster of genes demonstrated contrasting changes in expression between the $pregDAS_{improved}$ and $pregDAS_{worse}$ groups, all of which were inducible by type I interferon (IFN). These IFN-inducible genes were over-expressed at T3 compared to the T0 baseline among the $pregDAS_{improved}$ women.

Conclusions: In our pilot RNA-seq dataset, increased pregnancy-induced expression of type I IFN-inducible genes was observed among women with RA who improved during pregnancy, but not among women who worsened. These findings warrant further investigation into expression of these genes in RA pregnancy and their potential role in modulation of disease activity. These results are nevertheless preliminary and should be interpreted with caution until replicated in a larger sample.

Keywords: Rheumatoid arthritis, Pregnancy, RNA-seq, Gene expression, Type I interferon

* Correspondence: djawaheer@chori.org
^Deceased
[1]UCSF Benioff Children's Hospital Oakland, Children's Hospital Oakland Research Institute, 5700 Martin Luther King Jr. Way, Oakland, CA, USA
[8]Aarhus University, Aarhus, Denmark
Full list of author information is available at the end of the article

Background

Rheumatoid arthritis (RA) is a systemic inflammatory disease characterized by inflammation of the joints that continues to contribute significantly to the global burden of disease [1]. To date, its etiopathogenesis remains unknown, and despite major advancements in treatment, a cure remains elusive. Intriguingly, however, it is well documented that pregnancy can induce significant changes in RA disease activity. During pregnancy, 50–75% of women with RA experience a natural and often dramatic improvement in disease, whereas others may worsen or show no change [2–5]. Some pregnancy-related factors, including maternal-fetal disparity at the human leukocyte antigen locus [6] and fetal microchimerism [7, 8], have been associated with the pregnancy-induced improvement of RA symptoms. Nonetheless, the biology of human pregnancy in terms of the overall systemic changes that it induces, how those may differ between RA and healthy women, and how the pregnancy-induced changes may have an impact on RA remain unknown.

Gene expression studies, more specifically comparison of gene expression profiles (third trimester vs pre-pregnancy baseline) from women followed longitudinally from the pre-pregnancy state to the third trimester, can provide information about biological changes that are induced during pregnancy. Unfortunately, there have been no gene expression studies in which women — healthy or with RA — were studied before they became pregnant as well as during pregnancy to examine such pregnancy-induced changes. Only few studies of gene expression have been conducted in the context of RA pregnancy, using microarray technology [9–12]. In these studies, pregnancy-related changes with respect to the pre-pregnancy state were not examined, due to pre-pregnancy samples not being available [9–11], or pregnancy profiles were compared to profiles of unrelated non-pregnant women [12].

We have established a cohort of RA and healthy women enrolled before pregnancy and followed prospectively through pregnancy. Using state-of-the-art RNA sequencing (RNA-seq) technology, we examined systemic global gene expression in peripheral blood in a subset of women from this cohort as a pilot. We previously identified genes whose expression are modulated by pregnancy in both RA and healthy women, and we showed that a few genes are modulated differently in RA compared to healthy women [13]. We have now used differential expression analysis to further investigate pregnancy-induced gene expression patterns and fold-changes (FCs) in expression within our pilot dataset, taking into account whether the women with RA improved or worsened during pregnancy. We hypothesized that pregnancy-induced changes in gene expression among women with RA who improve during pregnancy may overlap substantially with those observed among healthy women and may differ from changes among women with RA who worsen during pregnancy.

Methods

Study subjects

Women with RA and healthy women of Danish descent were recruited and enrolled in a pregnancy cohort in Denmark, as previously described [13]. A subset of 20 women with RA and 5 healthy women from this cohort were included in the pilot dataset. Subjects with RA fulfilled the 1987 revised American College of Rheumatology criteria for RA [14]. The study was approved by the ethics committee for Region Hovedstaden (Denmark), the Danish Data Protection Agency, and the Children's Hospital Oakland Research Institute Institutional Review Board. All subjects provided written informed consent prior to enrollment.

Data

Data collected before pregnancy (T0) and at the third trimester (T3) were included in the present study. Therefore, women who had missing data at the T0 baseline or at T3 (eight women with RA) were excluded from further analyses. At both time points, the women with RA were examined by trained study nurses. Disease activity measures including tender and swollen joint counts based on a total of 28 joints (TJC28 and SJC28, respectively) and patient global health (GH) scores were recorded, and a serum sample was collected for measurement of C-reactive protein (CRP) levels. Data on medication use during the 3 months prior to both visits were also recorded. At each visit, blood samples from the women with RA and healthy women were collected in PAXgene RNA tubes (PreAnalytiX, Hombrechtikon, Switzerland).

Assessment of RA disease activity

RA disease activity was assessed using the Disease Activity Score based on 28 joints and 4 variables (DAS28-CRP4, abbreviated henceforth as DAS28), as follows [15]:

$$\begin{aligned}\text{DAS28} &= \left(0.56*\sqrt{TJC28}\right) + \left(0.28*\sqrt{SJC28}\right)\\ &\quad + (0.36*ln(CRP+1)) + 0.014*\text{GH} + 0.96\end{aligned}$$

Change in DAS28 from T0 to T3 was calculated as: $\Delta\text{DAS28} = \text{DAS28}_{T3} - \text{DAS28}_{T0}$.

The women with RA were categorized into two subsets: those with negative ΔDAS28 values were considered to show an improvement in DAS28 score at T3 compared to the T0 baseline (referred to as the pregDAS$_{improved}$ subset), whereas those with positive ΔDAS28 values were included in the "worsened" subset, referred to as pregDAS$_{worse}$. Any improvement in DAS28 scores (ΔDAS28 < 0) was used as a surrogate for improvement in disease activity. This was done to capture even small changes in disease activity that may correlate with biological changes observed at the gene expression level. Disease activity categories (remission, low, moderate, or high) were assessed using previously defined criteria [16].

Sample processing and bioinformatic analyses

Total RNA was isolated from frozen blood samples, and barcoded cDNA libraries were prepared as previously described [13]. Pseudo-alignment of the de-multiplexed raw sequence reads (FASTQ format) to the Ensembl reference human GRCh38 transcriptome assembly, and quantification of transcript abundances was performed using kallisto (version 0.42.4) [17]. BioMart annotations were used to combine transcript-level counts into gene-level estimates. Pseudogenes, genes with no annotations, and genes with very low read counts (<1 count per million) in at least 25% of all samples were filtered out. Any globin genes and ribosomal RNA (rRNA) transcripts still present were also filtered out. To adjust for variable sequencing depths across samples, the gene-level counts were normalized using the Trimmed Mean of M values (TMM) algorithm as implemented in the edgeR package (version 3.10.5) [18, 19]. To assess batch effects, normalized gene counts from each pair of technical replicates were plotted, and correlations were assessed.

Statistical analyses

Differential gene expression analysis was performed using edgeR (version 3.10.5) [18] to compare normalized gene-level counts between the T3 and T0 time points *within* each group of women (i.e., pregDAS$_{improved}$, pregDAS$_{worse}$ and healthy women). A model with a paired-sample design was used for these *within*-group comparisons. *Between*-group comparisons (pregDAS$_{improved}$ vs pregDAS$_{worse}$, and pregDAS$_{improved}$ vs healthy) at each time point were also performed using differential expression analyses. A negative binomial distribution was used to handle the over-dispersion in RNA-seq gene counts. Differential expression was tested using generalized linear model (GLM) likelihood ratio tests. To correct for any batch effects, batch was included as a covariate in the model. A *q* value threshold of 0.05 was used to assess significance. Because sample sizes were small, FCs in expression were also used in the interpretation of results, focusing on genes with at least a two-fold change in expression from T0 to T3.

Functional analysis

Differentially expressed genes were analyzed for over-representation of Gene Ontology (GO) categories using a hypergeometric test implemented in the Web-based Gene Set Analysis Toolkit (WebGestalt) with a threshold of at least five genes per category [20]. A significance threshold of $q<0.05$ was used to define enrichment. Functional enrichment of gene sets was examined using the STRING database of known and predicted interactions among proteins [21, 22].

Results

Study subjects

Of the 12 women with RA who had data at both T0 and T3, 8 were in the pregDAS$_{improved}$ group and 3 were in the pregDAS$_{worse}$ group. One woman was excluded because, although she had an increase in DAS28 at T3, she was in remission at both time points and hence did not fit into the pregDAS$_{worse}$ group. The DAS28 scores of the 11 women included in the analyses are shown in Fig. 1. The average disease duration among the women with RA was (mean ± SD) 5.9±4.4 years for pregDAS$_{improved}$ and 8.7 ±1.0 years for pregDAS$_{worse}$. The average age at conception was 30.3±5.7 years for pregDAS$_{improved}$, 33.2±1.9 years for pregDAS$_{worse}$, and 31.2±5.7 years for the healthy women.

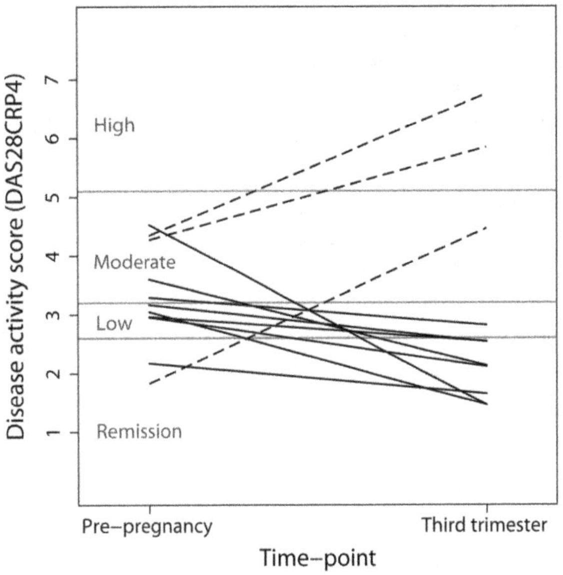

Fig. 1 Disease activity before pregnancy and at the third trimester among the women with rheumatoid arthritis. Disease Activity Scores based on 28 joints and 4 variables (DAS28-CRP4) are shown for the eight women who improved during pregnancy (solid lines) and the three women who worsened (dashed lines), at the pre-pregnancy baseline and at the third trimester. (The straight lines between time-points are included for graphical purposes only and do not imply a linear change in score.)

Among the eight pregDAS$_{improved}$ women, three did not take any medications at T0 and only one of these three women started taking medications by T3 (prednisolone + sulfasalazine). The remaining five women were taking prednisolone and/or sulfasalazine at both time points; one of them was also on anti-tumor necrosis factor (anti-TNF) therapy at T0, and another was taking methotrexate at T0. The three pregDAS$_{worse}$ women were all on anti-TNF therapy and taking prednisolone and/or sulfasalazine (except for one) at T0; at T3, one was taking prednisolone + sulfasalazine, one remained on anti-TNF therapy, and one stopped taking medications.

Genes differentially expressed between T3 and T0 in the pregDAS$_{improved}$ subset

A total of 1296 genes showed significant differential expression between T3 and T0 in the pregDAS$_{improved}$ subset, of which 161 displayed two-fold or more change in expression (*see* Additional file 1). These 161 genes were enriched in a number of immune-related pathways, as shown in Table 1. Similar results were obtained when the woman who was receiving anti-TNF therapy at T0 was excluded from the analysis.

Overlap with genes differentially expressed among healthy women

A large proportion of the 161 genes that exhibited at least two-fold change in expression between T3 and T0 among the pregDAS$_{improved}$ women were also differentially expressed among healthy women ($q<0.05$), mostly ($n=108$) with two-fold or more change in expression (*see* Additional files 1 and 2), although some ($n=33$) showed more modest FCs in expression ($1.5 \le FC < 2.0$). In addition, another 77 genes differentially expressed ($q<0.05$) in both the pregDAS$_{improved}$ and healthy groups showed lower FCs among the pregDAS$_{improved}$ women ($1.5 \le FC < 2.0$) than among the healthy women ($FC \ge 2$). The genes with $FC \ge 2$ in both the women with RA and healthy women were enriched in immune-related pathways such as immune system process ($q = 7.9\times10^{-9}$), response to other organism ($q = 2.7\times10^{-7}$), and defense response to bacterium ($q = 9.3\times10^{-6}$).

Overlap with genes differentially expressed in the pregDAS$_{worse}$ subset

Of the 161 genes differentially expressed in the pregDAS$_{improved}$ subset, some ($n=31$) were also differentially expressed ($q<0.05$, $FC \ge 2$) among pregDAS$_{worse}$ women, with most of these genes overlapping with those differentially expressed among healthy women ($n=30$) (*see* Additional file 2). The FCs in expression from T0 to T3 were correlated between the two RA subsets (Pearson correlation coefficient $r=0.86$, $p<0.00005$).

Differences in genes differentially expressed (T3 vs T0) between the pregDAS$_{improved}$ and pregDAS$_{worse}$ subsets

The remaining 130 genes that were differentially expressed (T3 vs T0: $FC \ge 2$, $q<0.05$) in our data among the pregDAS$_{improved}$ women, but not among the pregDAS$_{worse}$ women, were significantly enriched in several immune-related GO processes, such as immune system process ($q=4.7\times10^{-10}$), defense response ($q=9.6\times10^{-6}$), immune response ($q=5.0\times10^{-5}$), and innate immune response ($q=8.0\times10^{-6}$), among others (Table 2). Of these 130 genes, 78 were also differentially expressed among

Table 1 Gene Ontology (GO) biological processes enriched in genes differentially expressed among women with RA who improved during pregnancy

GO biological process	Gene count	*q* value
Immune system process	55	7.9×10^{-14}
Response to stress	54	9.1×10^{-6}
Defense response	35	1.5×10^{-8}
Immune response	34	2.2×10^{-8}
Multiorganism process	34	6.7×10^{-6}
Response to other organism	27	1.4×10^{-9}
Response to biotic stimulus	27	2.9×10^{-9}
Innate immune response	22	5.6×10^{-7}
Response to bacterium	16	9.0×10^{-6}
Erythrocyte differentiation	10	6.5×10^{-7}

Of the 161 genes differentially expressed (with $FC \ge 2$) between T0 and T3 among pregDAS$_{improved}$ women, several were enriched in GO biological processes relating to immune functions. (*Note*: These 161 genes included some that were also differentially expressed among healthy women and pregDAS$_{worse}$ women.)

Table 2 Gene Ontology biological processes enriched in genes differentially expressed among women with RA who improved during pregnancy, but not among those who worsened

GO biological process	Gene count	*q* value
Immune system process	43	4.7×10^{-10}
Defense response	26	9.6×10^{-6}
Immune response	24	5.0×10^{-5}
Innate immune response	18	8.0×10^{-6}
Response to other organism	17	6.7×10^{-5}
Response to biotic stimulus	17	1.0×10^{-4}
Hemopoiesis	15	2.0×10^{-4}
Homeostasis of number of cells	11	6.9×10^{-6}
Myeloid cell differentiation	11	7.1×10^{-5}
Erythrocyte differentiation	10	2.5×10^{-7}

The 130 genes that were differentially expressed (with $FC \ge 2$) between T0 and T3 among pregDAS$_{improved}$, but not among pregDAS$_{worse}$ women, included several that were enriched in GO biological processes relating to immune functions

healthy women (*see* Additional files 1 and 2). A comparison of the FCs in expression from T0 to T3 within each of the RA subsets revealed a small cluster of genes that were significantly over-expressed at T3 among pregDAS$_{improved}$ women and under-expressed (FC≥2, not significant) among pregDAS$_{worse}$ women (Fig. 2). By T3, mean normalized expression levels of these genes were higher among the pregDAS$_{improved}$ women than among the pregDAS$_{worse}$ women. Interestingly, all of the genes in this cluster were type I interferon (IFN)-inducible (*IFI44, IFI44L, IFIT1, HERC5, CMPK2, RSAD2*, and *SIGLEC1*). Among these, only the *RSAD2* gene was differentially expressed (under-expressed) at T3 compared to T0 among healthy women (q<0.05, FC≥2). A number of other type I IFN-inducible genes (*STAT1, IFI16, IFIT2, IFIT5, IFIH1*, and *MX1*) also exhibited similar patterns of expression, being over-expressed at T3 (q<0.05) among pregDAS$_{improved}$ women, though FCs were more modest (1.5- to 1.9-fold), and under-expressed among pregDAS$_{worse}$ women. The *PLSCR1* gene, which can enhance the type I IFN response, also showed a significant increase in expression (FC≥2) in the pregDAS$_{improved}$ women by T3, but no change was observed in the pregDAS$_{worse}$ women. Of interest, a comparison of normalized expression levels of these genes at T0 between pregDAS$_{improved}$ and healthy women revealed that some of the IFN signature genes (*IFI44, IFI44L, HERC5, CMPK2, SIGLEC1*, and *MX1*) were significantly under-expressed in the pregDAS$_{improved}$ subset compared to healthy women at T0 (q<0.05, FC≥2). However, by T3, there were no significant differences in expression of these genes between the two groups of women. The IFN-inducible genes that were over-expressed at T3 among pregDAS$_{improved}$ women, but not among in the pregDAS$_{worse}$ women, belong to a common functional network, as shown by known and predicted protein interactions from the STRING database (Fig. 3). Other than *RSAD2*, none of the genes shown in this network were differentially expressed (T3 vs T0) among healthy women.

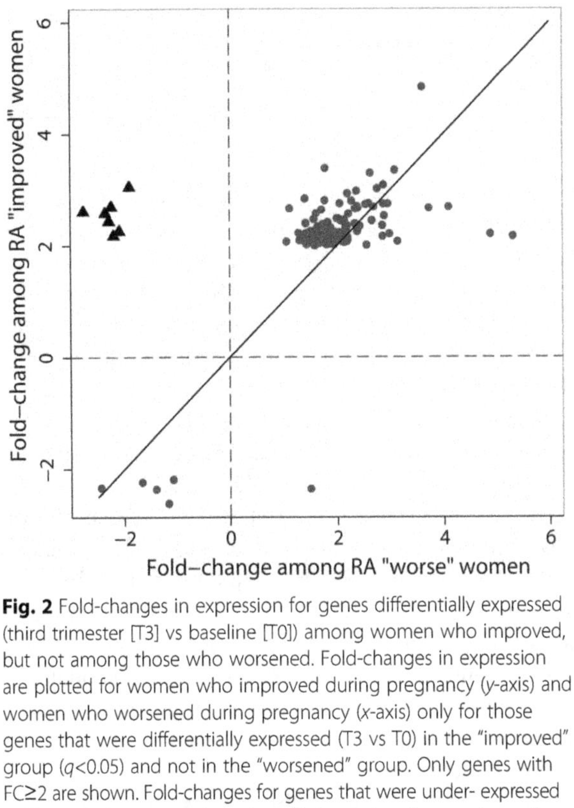

Fig. 2 Fold-changes in expression for genes differentially expressed (third trimester [T3] vs baseline [T0]) among women who improved, but not among those who worsened. Fold-changes in expression are plotted for women who improved during pregnancy (*y*-axis) and women who worsened during pregnancy (*x*-axis) only for those genes that were differentially expressed (T3 vs T0) in the "improved" group (q<0.05) and not in the "worsened" group. Only genes with FC≥2 are shown. Fold-changes for genes that were under- expressed at T3 are shown as negative values. The majority of genes showed similar expression changes in both groups of women with RA, as shown by the *gray dots* around the $y = x$ line (*solid line*). A small cluster of genes (*black triangles*), however, was over-expressed among women who improved and under-expressed among women who worsened. Genes in this cluster were *IFI44, IFI44L, IFIT1, HERC5, CMPK2, RSAD2*, and *SIGLEC1*

Discussion

There have been no previous reports of pregnancy-induced changes in gene expression in RA or healthy women from pre-pregnancy to the third trimester, other than our own published findings from our pilot RNA-seq dataset [13]. Gene expression changes that accompany improvement or worsening of RA disease activity during pregnancy, relative to a pre-pregnancy baseline, have also not been investigated. Thus, our findings are novel.

In our data, genes showing similar differential expression from T0 to T3 in both the pregDAS$_{improved}$ and pregDAS$_{worse}$ women were also similarly differentially expressed among healthy women, suggesting that these were normal pregnancy-related changes. The observation that a cluster of type I IFN-inducible genes demonstrated contrasting changes in expression from T0 to T3 between the pregDAS$_{improved}$ and pregDAS$_{worse}$ women was particularly interesting. These genes were over-expressed at T3 among the pregDAS$_{improved}$ women, compared to the T0 baseline, even though at T3 five of the eight pregDAS$_{improved}$ women were on corticosteroid therapy, which has been shown to inhibit type I IFN signaling [23, 24]. Over-expression of IFN-inducible genes has also been observed in RNA-seq profiles of neutrophils among patients with juvenile idiopathic arthritis (JIA) who were in drug-induced remission compared to those with active disease [25]. Neutrophils appear to be activated during pregnancy, as reported by us [13] and others [26–28]. However, neutrophil-related genes were over-expressed in both the pregDAS$_{improved}$ and pregDAS$_{worse}$ groups; yet, levels of the IFN-inducible genes (except *IFI27*) decreased from T0 to T3 in the pregDAS$_{worse}$ subset (not significantly). Thus, over-expression of IFN-inducible genes during pregnancy among pregDAS$_{improved}$ women may not be due to

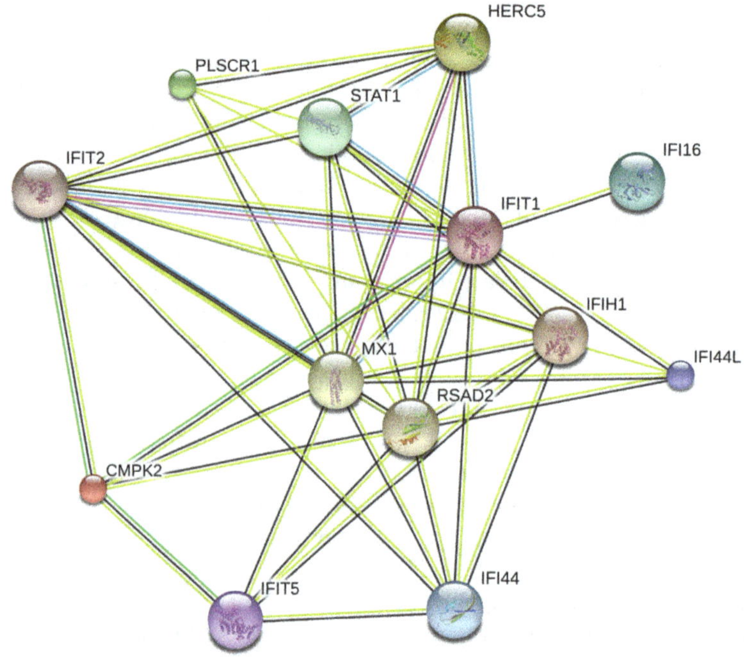

Fig. 3 Network graph showing associations between proteins encoded by genes with contrasting changes in expression from the pre-pregnancy baseline to the third trimester between RA women who improved and those who worsened. The nodes in the network represent proteins encoded by genes. The edges represent known as well as predicted interactions between the proteins, suggesting that they are part of a common functional network. Proteins that were not joined in the network are not shown. Variations at the levels of transcripts or post-translational modification are also not shown. Nodes with unknown 3D structure are shown by smaller size

neutrophil activation. Of interest, the three women who worsened during pregnancy were all on anti-TNF therapy at baseline, and non-responders to anti-TNF therapy have been reported to produce lower levels of IFNγ than good responders [29, 30]. Although we might also expect type I IFN genes to be differentially expressed in concert with type I IFN-inducible genes, we found no such evidence in our data.

The significance of the type I IFN signature in the $pregDAS_{improved}$ subset is not entirely clear. Type I IFNs appear to have conflicting roles in autoimmune diseases. Whereas a type I IFN signature in lupus is associated with active disease [31], it correlates with an alleviation of symptoms in multiple sclerosis (MS) [32], and IFNβ therapy has been used successfully to treat patients with MS [33]. In vitro studies as well as studies of animal models of arthritis suggest that type I IFN most likely has a protective role in RA [32, 34], although translation of the findings from the animal models to treat human RA using IFNβ therapy has thus far not been successful [34]. The majority of the IFN-inducible genes identified in our data were under-expressed in the $pregDAS_{improved}$ subset compared to healthy women at T0, which may suggest that expression patterns of these genes in RA could be deregulated as a consequence of the disease. Type I IFNs appear to promote down-regulation of pro-inflammatory cytokines and up-regulation of anti-inflammatory cytokines in organ-targeted autoimmune diseases [32, 35]. It is thus possible that the lower levels of IFN-inducible genes in the $pregDAS_{improved}$ women before pregnancy may reflect lower systemic IFNβ levels, which favor a pro-inflammatory state. Furthermore, while expression levels of the IFN-inducible genes did not change significantly from T0 to T3 among healthy women, they changed significantly in the $pregDAS_{improved}$ women, and by T3, they were no longer differentially expressed between the two groups (data not shown). These observations support the notion that increased levels of the IFN-inducible genes identified in our pilot data may help shift the immunomodulatory balance to an anti-inflammatory state during pregnancy. We speculate that specific levels of these gene products may be crucial to maintaining a healthy pregnancy, explaining why expression levels at T3 among $pregDAS_{improved}$ women became comparable to those of healthy women.

Some of the IFN-inducible genes that were over-expressed at T3 in our data (*IFI44*, *IFI44L*, and *SIGLEC1*) have been reported to show increased expression in pregnant RA women compared to unrelated non-pregnant RA women [12]. That study found no association between expression levels of these genes and disease activity. However, pre-pregnancy data on both disease activity and expression levels were not available for comparison with pregnancy data. Although in the present study we did not test for associations between expression of IFN-inducible genes and disease activity, we cannot exclude the possibility that they may be involved.

The strengths of our study include the availability of paired time-dependent data from the same women at both time points. This allowed global gene expression changes induced by pregnancy to be compared to a pre-pregnancy baseline, while at the same time controlling for unmeasured confounders. The use of RNA-seq technology to assess gene expression was also an advantage over microarray data. Our study does have some limitations. First, the sample sizes were small, especially for the women who worsened during pregnancy. However, the availability of data from the same women before and during pregnancy, as well as the ethnic homogeneity of the study population, enabled us to overcome some of the limitations of having a small sample size. Nevertheless, observations relating to the $\text{pregDAS}_{\text{worse}}$ subset should be interpreted with caution until they can be replicated in a larger sample. Because samples were processed in two batches, we used sample replicates in both batches to assess and mitigate batch effects. We did not examine changes in proportions of different cell types in blood samples across time points, because our goal was to identify overall systemic gene expression changes resulting either from altered expression of specific genes or from differences in cell proportions. Although there is a possibility that anti-TNF and/or other medications may have influenced the results, the lack of variation in medication use within each subset of women with RA precluded us from determining if this was the case. Nevertheless, in the $\text{pregDAS}_{\text{improved}}$ group, exclusion of the woman on anti-TNF therapy did not significantly change the results, suggesting that the findings were not influenced by anti-TNF. We did not adjust for dosage and/or specific medications.

Conclusions

The results from our pilot study suggest that genes demonstrating significant changes in expression in the $\text{pregDAS}_{\text{improved}}$ women, but not the $\text{pregDAS}_{\text{worse}}$ women, during pregnancy — that is, those showing similar patterns of expression as in healthy pregnancy or those among the IFN signature — could be involved in the natural amelioration of RA. These findings warrant further investigations into expression of these genes in RA pregnancy, but are nevertheless preliminary, and should be interpreted with caution until replicated in a larger sample.

Additional files

Additional file 1: Table S1. Within-group differential expression results (T3 vs T0) for the 161 genes that showed significant differential expression (q<0.05, FC≥2) among the $\text{pregDAS}_{\text{improved}}$ women. Fold changes (FCs) in expression, p values (unadjusted), and q values are shown for each of the three groups of women (i.e., $\text{pregDAS}_{\text{improved}}$, $\text{pregDAS}_{\text{worse}}$, and healthy women). Given the small sample sizes, we recommend that the q values be interpreted with caution, especially among the three $\text{pregDAS}_{\text{worse}}$ women. (PDF 153 kb)

Additional file 2: Figure S1. Numbers of genes differentially expressed (q<0.05, FC≥2) in the three groups of women. (*Note*: These numbers are provided only to give context, given the small sample sizes). (PDF 5 kb)

Abbreviations

CRP: C-reactive protein; DAS28-CRP4: Disease Activity Score based on 28 joint counts and 4 variables, including C-reactive protein ; FC: Fold-change; GH: Patient global health; GLM: Generalized linear model; GO: Gene Ontology; IFN: Interferon; JIA: Juvenile idiopathic arthritis; MS: Multiple sclerosis; $\text{pregDAS}_{\text{improved}}$: Women with rheumatoid arthritis whose disease activity improved during pregnancy; $\text{pregDAS}_{\text{worse}}$: Women with rheumatoid arthritis whose disease activity worsened during pregnancy; RA: Rheumatoid arthritis; RNA-seq: RNA sequencing; rRNA: Ribosomal RNA; SJC28: Swollen joint count based on 28 joints; T0: Pre-pregnancy; T3: Third trimester; TJC28: Tender joint count based on 28 joints; TMM: Trimmed Mean of M values; TNF: Tumor necrosis factor

Acknowledgements

We are immensely grateful to the study subjects for their participation in the study. We thank Mr. Kurt Stig Jensen at the Juliane Marie Center for his support. The Rheumatology departments at the following hospitals in Denmark facilitated collection of data and samples: Rigshospitalet (Glostrup), Odense Universitetshospital, Kong Christian X's Gigthospital (Gråsten), Aarhus University Hospital NBG, and Regionshospitalet Viborg. We thank all members of our project team for making this work possible: Anne-Grethe Rasmussen, Charlotte Schön Frengler, Dorte Heide, Randi Petersen, Tove Thorup Rasmussen, Lone Thomasen, Britta Hvidberg Nielsen, Teresa Rozenfeldt, Kirsten Junker, Lis Kastberg Schubert, Lis Lund, Jette Barlach, Helle Bendtsen, Helle Andersen, and Marjo Westerdahl for their contribution to data and sample collection; and Rikke Godtkjær Andersen, Mie Rams Rasmussen, Pia Pedersen, Stine Birkelund, Louise Mielke, and Andreas Smed for management of data and samples. We also greatly appreciate the valuable assistance provided by Majbritt Norman Nielsen and DANBIO personnel.

Funding

This work was supported in part by funds from the National Institute of Arthritis, Musculoskeletal and Skin Diseases (NIAMS), USA (grant R21 AR057931); Gigtforeningen, Denmark (grant R87-A1477-B512); and the Juliane Marie Center, Rigshospitalet (Denmark). These funders did not have any role in conducting this study or in the interpretation and reporting of results.

Authors' contributions

DEG analyzed the data, interpreted the results, and contributed to manuscript writing. MKS was responsible for acquisition of the data. LP and EP contributed to the analysis and interpretation of the data. JLN, HK, and JO contributed to the conception and design of the study. HK was also responsible for data acquisition. MLH, VZ, and BO contributed to the data acquisition. DJ was involved in the conception and design of the experiments, in the analysis and interpretation of the data, and in writing the manuscript. All authors contributed to critically revising the manuscript for important intellectual content. All authors read and approved the final manuscript. HK passed away before the submission of the final version of the manuscript; DJ accepts responsibility for the integrity and validity of the data collected and analyzed.

Competing interests

The authors declare that they have no competing interests.

Author details

[1]UCSF Benioff Children's Hospital Oakland, Children's Hospital Oakland Research Institute, 5700 Martin Luther King Jr. Way, Oakland, CA, USA. [2]University of California, Berkeley, Berkeley, CA, USA. [3]Juliane Marie Center, Copenhagen University Hospital, Rigshospitalet, Copenhagen, Denmark. [4]California Institute of Technology, Pasadena, CA, USA. [5]Fred Hutchinson Cancer Research Center, Seattle, WA, USA. [6]University of Washington, Seattle, WA, USA. [7]University of California, Los Angeles, Los Angeles, CA, USA. [8]Aarhus University, Aarhus, Denmark. [9]DANBIO Registry and Copenhagen Centre for Arthritis Research, Centre for Rheumatology and Spine Diseases (VRR), Rigshospitalet, Glostrup, Denmark. [10]Faculty of Health and Medical Sciences, University of Copenhagen, Copenhagen, Denmark. [11]University of California, San Francisco, San Francisco, CA, USA.

References

1. Cross M, Smith E, Hoy D, Carmona L, Wolfe F, Vos T, et al. The global burden of rheumatoid arthritis: estimates from the global burden of disease 2010 study. Ann Rheum Dis. 2014;73(7):1316–22.
2. Hench PS. The ameliorating effect of pregnancy on chronic atrophic (infectious rheumatoid) arthritis, fibrositis, and intermittent hydrarthrosis. Mayo Clin Proc. 1938;13:161–7.
3. Nelson JL, Ostensen M. Pregnancy and rheumatoid arthritis. Rheum Dis Clin North Am. 1997;23(1):195–212.
4. de Man YA, Dolhain RJ, van de Geijn FE, Willemsen SP, Hazes JM. Disease activity of rheumatoid arthritis during pregnancy: results from a nationwide prospective study. Arthritis Rheum. 2008;59(9):1241–8.
5. Barrett JH, Brennan P, Fiddler M, Silman AJ. Does rheumatoid arthritis remit during pregnancy and relapse postpartum? Results from a nationwide study in the United Kingdom performed prospectively from late pregnancy. Arthritis Rheum. 1999;42(6):1219–27.
6. Nelson JL, Hughes KA, Smith AG, Nisperos BB, Branchaud AM, Hansen JA. Maternal-fetal disparity in HLA class II alloantigens and the pregnancy-induced amelioration of rheumatoid arthritis. N Engl J Med. 1993;329(7):466–71.
7. Yan Z, Lambert NC, Ostensen M, Adams KM, Guthrie KA, Nelson JL. Prospective study of fetal DNA in serum and disease activity during pregnancy in women with inflammatory arthritis. Arthritis Rheum. 2006; 54(7):2069–73.
8. Adams Waldorf KM, Nelson JL. Autoimmune disease during pregnancy and the microchimerism legacy of pregnancy. Immunol Invest. 2008;37(5):631–44.
9. Haupl T, Ostensen M, Grutzkau A, Burmester GR, Villiger PM. Interaction between rheumatoid arthritis and pregnancy: correlation of molecular data with clinical disease activity measures. Rheumatology (Oxford). 2008;47 Suppl 3:iii19–22.
10. Haupl T, Ostensen M, Grutzkau A, Radbruch A, Burmester GR, Villiger PM. Reactivation of rheumatoid arthritis after pregnancy: increased phagocyte and recurring lymphocyte gene activity. Arthritis Rheum. 2008;58(10):2981–92.
11. Weix J, Forger F, Haupl T, Surbek D, Ostensen M, Villiger PM. Influence of pregnancy on the adipocytokine and peroxisome proliferator-activated receptor pathways in peripheral blood mononuclear cells from healthy donors and rheumatoid arthritis patients. Arthritis Rheum. 2012;64(7):2095–103.
12. Weix J, Haupl T, Raio L, Villiger PM, Forger F. The physiologic increase in expression of some type I IFN-inducible genes during pregnancy is not associated with improved disease activity in pregnant patients with rheumatoid arthritis. Transl Res. 2013;161(6):505–12.
13. Mittal A, Pachter L, Nelson JL, Kjaergaard H, Smed MK, Gildengorin VL, et al. Pregnancy-induced changes in systemic gene expression among healthy women and women with rheumatoid arthritis. PLoS One. 2015;10(12):e0145204.
14. Arnett FC, Edworthy SM, Bloch DA, McShane DJ, Fries JF, Cooper NS, et al. The American Rheumatism Association 1987 revised criteria for the classification of rheumatoid arthritis. Arthritis Rheum. 1988;31(3):315–24.
15. Home of the Disease activity score and DAS28. http://www.das-score.nl/.
16. van Gestel AM, Anderson JJ, van Riel PL, Boers M, Haagsma CJ, Rich B, et al. ACR and EULAR improvement criteria have comparable validity in rheumatoid arthritis trials. J Rheumatol. 1999;26(3):705–11.
17. Bray NL, Pimentel H, Melsted P, Pachter L. Near-optimal probabilistic RNA-seq quantification. Nat Biotechnol. 2016;34(5):525–7.
18. Robinson MD, McCarthy DJ, Smyth GK. edgeR: a Bioconductor package for differential expression analysis of digital gene expression data. Bioinformatics. 2010;26(1):139–40.
19. Robinson MD, Oshlack A. A scaling normalization method for differential expression analysis of RNA-seq data. Genome Biol. 2010;11(3):R25.
20. Zhang B, Kirov S, Snoddy J. WebGestalt: an integrated system for exploring gene sets in various biological contexts. Nucleic Acids Res. 2005;33 Suppl 2:W741–8.
21. von Mering C, Jensen LJ, Snel B, Hooper SD, Krupp M, Foglierini M, et al. STRING: known and predicted protein-protein associations, integrated and transferred across organisms. Nucleic Acids Res. 2005;33(Database issue):D433–7.
22. Jensen LJ, Kuhn M, Stark M, Chaffron S, Creevey C, Muller J, et al. STRING 8—a global view on proteins and their functional interactions in 630 organisms. Nucleic Acids Res. 2009;37(Database issue):D412–6.
23. Flammer JR, Dobrovolna J, Kennedy MA, Chinenov Y, Glass CK, Ivashkiv LB, et al. The type I interferon signaling pathway is a target for glucocorticoid inhibition. Mol Cell Biol. 2010;30(19):4564–74.
24. de Jong TD, Vosslamber S, Blits M, Wolbink G, Nurmohamed MT, van der Laken CJ, et al. Effect of prednisone on type I interferon signature in rheumatoid arthritis: consequences for response prediction to rituximab. Arthritis Res Ther. 2015;17:78.
25. Jiang K, Sun X, Chen Y, Shen Y, Jarvis JN. RNA sequencing from human neutrophils reveals distinct transcriptional differences associated with chronic inflammatory states. BMC Med Genomics. 2015;8:55.
26. Sacks GP, Studena K, Sargent K, Redman CW. Normal pregnancy and preeclampsia both produce inflammatory changes in peripheral blood leukocytes akin to those of sepsis. Am J Obstet Gynecol. 1998;179(1):80–6.
27. Wang Y, Gu Y, Philibert L, Lucas MJ. Neutrophil activation induced by placental factors in normal and pre-eclamptic pregnancies in vitro. Placenta. 2001;22(6):560–5.
28. Luppi P, Haluszczak C, Trucco M, Deloia JA. Normal pregnancy is associated with peripheral leukocyte activation. Am J Reprod Immunol. 2002;47(2):72–81.
29. Cacciapaglia F, Buzzulini F, Arcarese L, Ferraro E, Afeltra A. The use of an interferon-gamma release assay as a biomarker of response to anti-TNF-alpha treatment. Drug Dev Res. 2014;75 Suppl 1:S50–3.
30. Wright HL, Thomas HB, Moots RJ, Edwards SW. Interferon gene expression signature in rheumatoid arthritis neutrophils correlates with a good response to TNFi therapy. Rheumatology (Oxford). 2015;54(1):188–93.
31. Bennett L, Palucka AK, Arce E, Cantrell V, Borvak J, Banchereau J, et al. Interferon and granulopoiesis signatures in systemic lupus erythematosus blood. J Exp Med. 2003;197(6):711–23.
32. Kalliolias GD, Ivashkiv LB. Overview of the biology of type I interferons. Arthritis Res Ther. 2010;12 Suppl 1:S1.
33. Buttmann M, Rieckmann P. Interferon-beta1b in multiple sclerosis. Expert Rev Neurother. 2007;7(3):227–39.
34. Aalbers CJ, Bevaart L, Loiler S, de Cortie K, Wright JF, Mingozzi F, et al. Preclinical potency and biodistribution studies of an AAV5 vector expressing human interferon-β (ART-I02) for local treatment of patients with rheumatoid arthritis. PLoS One. 2015;10(6):e0130612.
35. Crow MK. Type I interferon in organ-targeted autoimmune and inflammatory diseases. Arthritis Res Ther. 2010;12 Suppl 1:S5.

15

Drug safety analyses in a rheumatoid arthritis registry: application of different approaches regarding timing of exposure and confounder measurement

Daniel H. Solomon[1,2*], Nancy A. Shadick[1], Michael E. Weinblatt[1], Agnes Zak[1], Michelle Frits[1] and Jessica M. Franklin[2]

Abstract

Background: Patient registry data serves an increasing role in drug safety and comparative effectiveness research, but registry databases often do not contain confounder information measured at the same time that treatments begin. This study evaluated a set of approaches for estimating confounder values at treatment initiation using actual data from a rheumatoid arthritis (RA) registry to examine the risk of infection associated with different biologic DMARDs (bDMARDs).

Methods: We examined the risk of infection associated with starting a TNF inhibitor (TNFi) versus any of the other non-TNFi bDMARDs. Different confounder assessment approaches were tested. All approaches were tested in Cox proportional hazard regression models that used a propensity score (PS). The confounder of interest was the disease activity score (DAS28-CRP). The confounder assessment approaches utilized different temporal relationships between the DAS28-CRP measurement and the start of the treatments of interest.

Results: We included 219 subjects with RA with 269 initiations of either a TNFi or a different bDMARD or both. Among this group, 305 infections were reported and confirmed through chart review. The hazard ratio (HR) for the risk of infection associated with use of a non-TNFi bDMARD ranged from 1.17 to 3.03 using 13 different approaches; only the approach with the highest HR produced results significantly different than one, but this approach included the fewest subjects and infections.

Conclusions: The relative risk of infection for TNFi and other non-TNFi bDMARDs was similar using various approaches regarding which DAS28-CRP score should be used as the baseline measure in adjusted analyses.

Keywords: Rheumatoid arthritis, Comparative effectiveness research, Disease-modifying antirheumatic drugs, TNF antagonist, Infection

Background

Clinical registries have grown in popularity over the last decade [1]. Their growth can be attributed to several factors. First, clinical registries allow for systematic collection of real-world practice data. Second, registry data provide evidence for comparative effectiveness and comparative safety evaluations. Third, registries facilitate patient-reported outcome data. The systematic collection of disease activity and patient-reported outcomes facilitates control for confounders in epidemiologic analyses. However, the confounders are not always measured at the ideal time.

For example, if one is interested in the relationship between a medication and an adverse outcome, it is ideal to have potential confounders measured at the time the medication was started. However, medications may be started between the time of registry visits and

* Correspondence: dsolomon@partners.org
[1]Division of Rheumatology, Brigham and Women's Hospital, 75 Francis Street, Boston, MA 02115, USA
[2]Division of Pharmacoepidemiology, Brigham and Women's Hospital, Boston, MA 02120, USA

confounder collection. This raises the question of how to use confounder information collected at visits prior to or after the start of a given intervention.

We considered this methodologic question using a simulation study [2]. In the simulation, we examined 13 different approaches, including using confounder data from prior to the start of treatment, after the start of treatment, an average value, a weighted average value, and restricted cohorts based on proximity of the confounder measurement to the start of the intervention. In these simulations, we confirmed theoretical work showing that using the value of an important confounder measured after exposure start introduces bias for estimating the total effect of exposure on outcome if the confounder mediates part of the effect [3]. However, adjusting for the value measured from a visit prior to the start of exposure can also introduce bias, especially when measured long before exposure initiation. When selecting a time point for the confounder, analysts should carefully consider the timing of confounder measurements relative to exposure initiation and the rate of change in the confounder to choose the most relevant measure.

In the current set of analyses, we applied the simulation results using actual registry data to answer a relevant clinical question in the care of patients with rheumatoid arthritis (RA); namely, is use of non-tumor necrosis factor inhibitor (TNFi) biologic disease-modifying antirheumatic drugs (bDMARDs) associated with a higher risk of infection than use of a TNFi? Since patients with RA have a higher than expected risk of infection, [4] selecting treatments that minimize risk is a priority for patients and providers. The two strategies – use of a TNFi versus a non-TNFi bDMARD – are commonly considered strategies among patients with RA who have failed first-line disease-modifying antirheumatic drugs (DMARDs) [5]. While there are some data comparing these strategies in randomized controlled trials, those trials were relatively small and focused on efficacy not adverse events [6]. Since RA disease activity appears to be associated with infection risk, such analyses should include disease activity as a potential confounder. Thus, we have pursued study of this question in a registry of patients with RA.

Methods

Study design and cohort

The analyses conducted follow a simulation study examining different approaches to the measurement of confounders that change over time and may change in response to treatment. We tested a variety of scenarios and assumptions in a previous simulation study [2], and now apply the simulation results using actual data from the BRASS registry. BRASS is a single-center registry of patients with RA followed over the last 12 years [7]. Patients seen during routine clinical care who meet criteria for RA have been recruited and follow-up is conducted every 6 months. Follow-up includes standardized patient-reported outcome instruments, such as global arthritis activity, fatigue, functional status, and comorbid conditions [7–10].

Subjects selected for this analysis began either a TNFi (adalimumab, certolizumab pegol, etanercept, golimumab, infliximab) or non-TNFi bDMARD (e.g., abatacept, rituximab, tocilizumab) during BRASS follow-up. Four patients started tofacitinib, a newer synthetic DMARD, but not typically used first-line; these starts were not included. We required at least one BRASS visit prior to the start of the drug of interest as well as after.

Data collection: outcomes and confounders

Since infections are an important potential adverse event in BRASS, we specifically ask about any infections since the last registry visit in the patient and physician questionnaires. Details such as type of infection, hospitalization, and treatments are collected. The dataset includes information on all patient- and physician-reported infections, from minor to severe. As part of this project, we performed a chart review on all such reported infections to assess which could be confirmed using the medical records from our health care system. This method would not necessarily ascertain information about infections that occur outside of our health care system. In the total cohort, we found medical record evidence to confirm (i.e., a provider note mentioning infection, microbiologic or radiographic information, or antibiotic prescriptions) an infection for 768 of the 1254 (61%) reported events. The primary outcome for this study was the confirmed infections and all reported infections were considered a secondary outcome.

The confounder of interest that we examined in these analyses using multiple assessment approaches is RA disease activity, as measured by the disease activity score based on 28 joints - C-reactive protein (DAS28-CRP) [11, 12]. This measure has been widely used in RA clinical research and includes four components: tender joint count, swollen joint count, patient global arthritis activity, and the C-reactive protein (CRP) level. When all components of the DAS28-CRP were not available, chart reviews were performed to extract missing data from the medical record. In 21 subjects, we were able to fill this information in from chart review. In one subject, last observation carried forward was used. For this confounder, we used 13 different approaches (see "Statistical analyses" below) for selecting the value to be used for adjustment.

For all other confounders, we used confounder information from the visit at the time the treatments of interest were started. However, in most instances, the treatments were started between registry visits. Thus, the covariates were assessed at the most proximal visit prior to the start of the treatment of interest.

Statistical analyses

We examined the relationship between non-TNFi bDMARD use and infection, setting TNFi use as the reference exposure in a series of Cox proportional hazard regressions. To better balance baseline covariates, a propensity score was estimated using logistic regression [13]. The propensity score is the probability of one treatment or another, ranging from 0 to 1, based on a logistic regression that includes all of the potential confounders. We excluded subjects from the analysis with propensity scores that fell outside the distribution of the other exposure.

Separate Cox proportional hazard regression models were estimated for the various assessment approaches for the DAS28-CRP (see Table 1). The regression model included the exposure indicator, the propensity score as quintiles, as well as the DAS28-CRP. The adjusted hazard ratios were plotted for the primary outcome using an as-treated approach, in which patients are followed until the first censoring event. These included: first infection outcome; 30 days after the last dosage of a TNFi or a non-TNFi bDMARD; or loss to follow-up. A secondary analysis followed patients for a maximum of 6 months or one of the censoring events, whichever occurred first.

Cox proportional hazard assumptions were tested by including time-dependent covariates in the Cox model. Interaction terms of each predictor and a function of survival time were added to the original Cox model and a proportionality test was performed. All time-dependent covariates were non-significant, as was the p value for the proportionality test, indicating that there is no evidence of violation of model assumptions. All analyses were conducted using SAS version 9.4 (SAS Institute Inc., Cary, NC, USA).

Results

From the 1395 participants in BRASS, we identified 294 (21%) who were eligible for this study. Because of some baseline imbalance in covariates (see Additional file 1 for full cohort prior to trimming), a propensity score was calculated and the cohorts trimmed. Characteristics at the visit prior to the start of the medication of interest for the trimmed cohorts used in analyses are shown in Table 2. The two groups are well matched with respect to age, gender, serologic status, DAS28-CRP, concomitant non-biologic DMARDs, cigarette use, and diabetes. However, they differ in several baseline variables, including disease duration (other bDMARD 19 years vs TNFi 12 years), modified health assessment questionnaire (HAQ) (other bDMARD 0.6 vs TNFi 0.4), current glucocorticoid use (other bDMARD 57% vs TNFi 41%), and prior TNFi use (other bDMARD 92% vs TNFi 59%).

The types of infections reported in BRASS by providers and patients are displayed in Table 3. Most of the infections were not severe and would not have required hospitalization. We found medical record evidence to confirm (i.e., a provider note mentioning infection, microbiologic or radiographic information, or antibiotic prescriptions) an infection for 305 of the 472 (65%) reported events in the trimmed cohort. The confirmed infections serve as the primary outcomes and the reported infections as the secondary outcomes for the regression analyses described below. For the primary outcome, the incidence rates per 100 person-years for infection for the

Table 1 Thirteen different approaches tested based on prior simulation results [2]

Approaches for DAS28-CRP adjustment	Description
1. No adjustment	No inclusion of any DAS28-CRP values.
2. Most recent prior measurement	Adjust for most recent DAS28-CRP value prior to start of treatment.
3. Most recent after measurement	Adjust for most recent DAS28-CRP value after start of treatment.
4. Arithmetic mean	Adjust for the arithmetic mean of the two nearest DAS28-CRP measurements.
5. Nearest measurement	Adjust for nearest DAS28-CRP measurement.
6. Weighted mean	Adjust for the weighted mean of the two nearest DAS28-CRP measurements, accounting for proximity.
7. Restricted to within 4 months	Only include subjects with DAS28-CRP within 4 months of start of treatment, prior or post.
8. Restricted to within 2 months	Only include subjects with DAS28-CRP within 2 months of start of treatment, prior or post.
9. Restricted to within 10 months prior	Only include subjects with DAS28-CRP within 10 months prior to start of treatment.
10. Restricted to within 8 months prior	Only include subjects with DAS28-CRP within 8 months prior to start of treatment.
11. Restricted to within 6 months prior	Only include subjects with DAS28-CRP within 6 months prior to start of treatment.
12. Restricted to within 4 months prior	Only include subjects with DAS28-CRP within 4 months prior to start of treatment.
13. Restricted to within 2 months prior	Only include subjects with DAS28-CRP within 2 months prior to start of treatment.

DAS28-CRP disease activity score based on 28 joints - C-reactive protein

Table 2 Baseline characteristics in trimmed cohort

	Anti-TNF (n = 175)	Other bDMARD (n = 94)
	Mean (± SD) or median (IQR) or %	
Age, years	58 (±12)	60 (±11)
Female	86%	88%
Disease duration, years	12 (5, 26)	19 (10, 30)
Seropositive, RF or CCP	79%	85%
DAS28-CRP at T0	4.0 (2.9, 5.3)	4.4 (3.0, 5.4)
DAS28-CRP at T1	3.4 (2.4, 4.7)	3.9 (2.5, 5.2)
Modified HAQ score at T0	0.4 (0.1, 0.6)	0.6 (0.1, 1.0)
Modified HAQ score at T1	0.3 (0, 0.8)	0.5 (0.1, 0.8)
Corticosteroid use		
Current	41%	57%
In past 6 months	58%	79%
Ever	90%	96%
Cumulative glucocorticoid, mg	2464 (336, 12156)	6592 (1230, 17,546)
Prior TNF use	59%	92%
Concomitant non-biologic DMARD	69%	60%
Cigarette use, pack-years	0 (0, 13)	2.3 (0, 14)
Smoking status		
Never smoker	51%	47%
Past smoker	41%	51%
Current smoker	8%	2%
Diabetes	7%	9%

The only missing data were for cigarette use where nine subjects had missing values. T0 = visit immediately before start of treatment of interest; T1 = visit immediately after start of treatment of interest
TNF tumor necrosis factor, *bDMARD* biologic disease-modifying antirheumatic drug, *RF* rheumatoid factor, *CCP* cyclic citrullinated peptide, *DAS28-CRP* disease activity score based on 28 joints - C-reactive protein, HAQ health assessment questionnaire

Table 3 Infections reported in BRASS and confirmed through chart review

Infection type	Reported in BRASS[a]	Confirmed by chart review In total cohort	Confirmed by chart review In trimmed cohort[b]
	N (column %)		
Upper respiratory infection	274 (36%)	188 (25%)	84 (28%)
Sinus infection	207 (27%)	100 (13%)	48 (16%)
Genitourinary tract	163 (21%)	90 (12%)	34 (11%)
Bronchitis/pneumonia	154 (20%)	96 (12%)	46 (16%)
Skin, soft tissue	123 (16%)	173 (23%)	64 (21%)
Otitis media	33 (4%)	12 (2%)	4 (1%)
Bone or joint	27 (4%)	23 (3%)	4 (1%)
Blood stream	9 (1%)	10 (1%)	4 (1%)
Gastrointestinal	—	26 (3%)	4 (1%)
Oral/dental	—	15 (2%)	4 (1%)
Ophthamalogic	—	9 (1%)	2 (1%)
Lyme disease	—	7 (1%)	4 (1%)
Unknown source	264 (34%)	19(3%)	3 (1%)
Total	1254	768	305

[a]The infections reported in BRASS, by patients or rheumatology providers, were used in the sensitivity analysis reported in Fig. 2a. Columns may not add up to 100% because of rounding
[b]This column only includes infections occurring after the start of a new DMARD; these infections were used in the main analysis

TNFi group was 36.0 (95% CI 31.3 to 41.4) and 40.3 (95% CI 33.4 to 48.7) for non-TNFi bDMARDs.

We examined the distribution of DAS28-CRP measures recorded before and after the start of the medications of interest. The time between the visit immediately before the start of the medication of interest was similar in the two groups, 20–22 weeks ($p = 0.37$). Similarly, the time after the start of medication until the next study visit was similar in the two groups, 24–32 weeks ($p = 0.39$). In addition, we show the distribution of the actual DAS28-CRP scores before and after the start of the medications of interest (see Table 4 and Additional file 2). These show that DAS28-CRP did not change over time during the 12 months before the initiation of the treatment of interest, but there was a small decrease on average during the year after initiation. Therefore, measuring disease activity up to 12 months prior to treatment start may provide adequate confounding adjustment, while measurements after treatment start may deserve more scrutiny, as the observed decrease may be due to treatment.

Using Cox proportional hazards regression, we estimated the hazard ratios across the 13 approaches for infection comparing TNFi (reference) to non-TNFi bDMARDs. Unadjusted risk was 1.17 (95% CI 0.75–1.82) (see Fig. 1). The approaches that included all subjects (scenarios 2–6) found very similar HRs. However, the HRs varied in approaches 7–13 when the analyses were restricted to smaller subsets of subjects with DAS28-CRP measured within a given proximity to the start of treatment. The most restrictive approach that only included patients with a DAS measurement 2 months prior to treatment start had just 70 observations and 36 infections, resulting in a strongly protective estimated effect of TNFi, but with poor precision.

The HRs and patterns observed in the primary analyses remained stable in sensitivity analyses that included the secondary outcome of reported infection (see Fig. 2a) and the extended follow-up period (see Fig. 2b).

Discussion

Registries are playing an increasing role in determining the post-marketing comparative safety of drugs. They have contributed important information to understanding the

Table 4 Distribution of DAS28-CRP scores used in analyses

Months BEFORE start of DMARD of interest	N	Mean DAS28-CRP (± SD)
0	46	4.1 ± 1.6
1	19	4.8 ± 1.5
2	18	4.7 ± 1.3
3	21	4.0 ± 1.6
4	28	3.6 ± 1.6
5	13	3.8 ± 1.8
6	11	3.8 ± 1.5
7	21	4.0 ± 1.9
8	21	4.1 ± 1.2
9	22	4.3 ± 1.3
10	15	4.2 ± 1.4
11	16	4.1 ± 1.4
12+	18	4.3 ± 1.9
Months AFTER start of DMARD of interest	N	Mean DAS28-CRP (± SD)
0	3	5.6 ± 0.8
1	21	4.2 ± 1.5
2	29	4.2 ± 1.5
3	25	3.8 ± 1.5
4	20	4.3 ± 1.3
5	16	3.6 ± 1.6
6	12	2.7 ± 1.0
7	14	3.4 ± 1.6
8	26	3.7 ± 1.3
9	25	3.8 ± 1.6
10	20	3.0 ± 1.2
11	19	4.0 ± 1.6
12+	39	3.1 ± 1.4

DAS28-CRP disease activity score based on 28 joints - C-reactive protein, *DMARD* disease-modifying antirheumatic drug

safety of various treatments for rheumatoid arthritis (RA). However, many methodologic questions regarding optimal analytic strategies have not been adequately answered for registries. Registries often include data on potential confounders measured at time points separate from when drugs are started. To assess the effect of different assumptions regarding how to estimate confounders in such circumstances, we focused on the comparative risk of infections among patients with RA starting different bDMARDs – any TNFi versus non-TNFi bDMARDs – using data from a single-center RA registry. We found that all approaches that estimated treatment effect using adjusted models in the full sample (approaches 2–6), regardless of the confounder assessment approach, gave very similar estimates. However, using restricted populations with disease activity measured in close temporal relationship before the start of drug (approaches 9–13) gave less precise estimates because of smaller sample sizes that indicated a stronger protective effect than other estimates. Similar results were also seen in the prior simulation study [2] and suggest that the risk of adverse effects of drugs differs across study populations in important ways, but based on subtle differences in the subpopulations of patients. While it may not be "incorrect" to estimate risks in subpopulations, the risks may differ substantially from the risk observed in the broader population.

The findings of this study have several methodologic implications. First, it is likely the case that the findings in this example apply to other registries and other clinical scenarios. We anticipate that whenever there is the possibility of a strong confounder, timing of its measurement with relation to the start of interventions is important and may influence estimates of association. Second, if one restricts analyses to subpopulations, even based on seemingly uninformative issues like when a confounder is measured, findings may not generalize to all subjects exposed to a given drug. This also may be due to the fact that the propensity score, estimated in the full sample, does not balance the confounder distributions as well in the subgroups identified in methods 7–13 (see Additional file 3: Table S2). Finally, as shown in the companion simulation study [2], it may be preferred to use confounder values from visits after the start of interventions if they are closer than any visit pre-intervention, especially if confounder values are changing rapidly prior to treatment initiation. This may seem to violate basic epidemiologic teaching that suggests that confounder measurement should always come before the start of an exposure [14].

Limitations of the current study include incomplete medical record data on all infections. However, analyses using the broader outcome of all reported infections gave us very similar results. As well, there were some missing data in the registry regarding disease activity. This was minimal. Patients may have differentially reported infections based on the time between starting a medication and the follow-up visit. Six months was the standard follow-up and this may have limited our ability to detect later effects of drug. It is also possible that disease activity was not a strong confounder in the clinical scenario under question. Prior data suggest disease activity impacts infection risk but the effect on treatment choice may not be as dramatic when choosing between different DMARDs. Strengths include the ability to test a prior set of simulation analyses in real data, the clinical relevance of the study question, the consistency of results across primary and secondary analyses, as well as the ability to confirm infections using medical records.

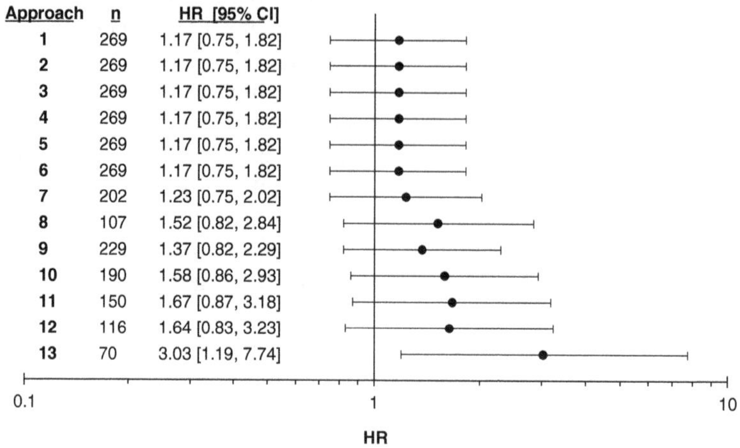

Fig. 1 This graph displays the hazard ratios (*black circles*) and 95% confidence intervals (*lines through circles*) for each approach, using our primary outcome and analysis strategy

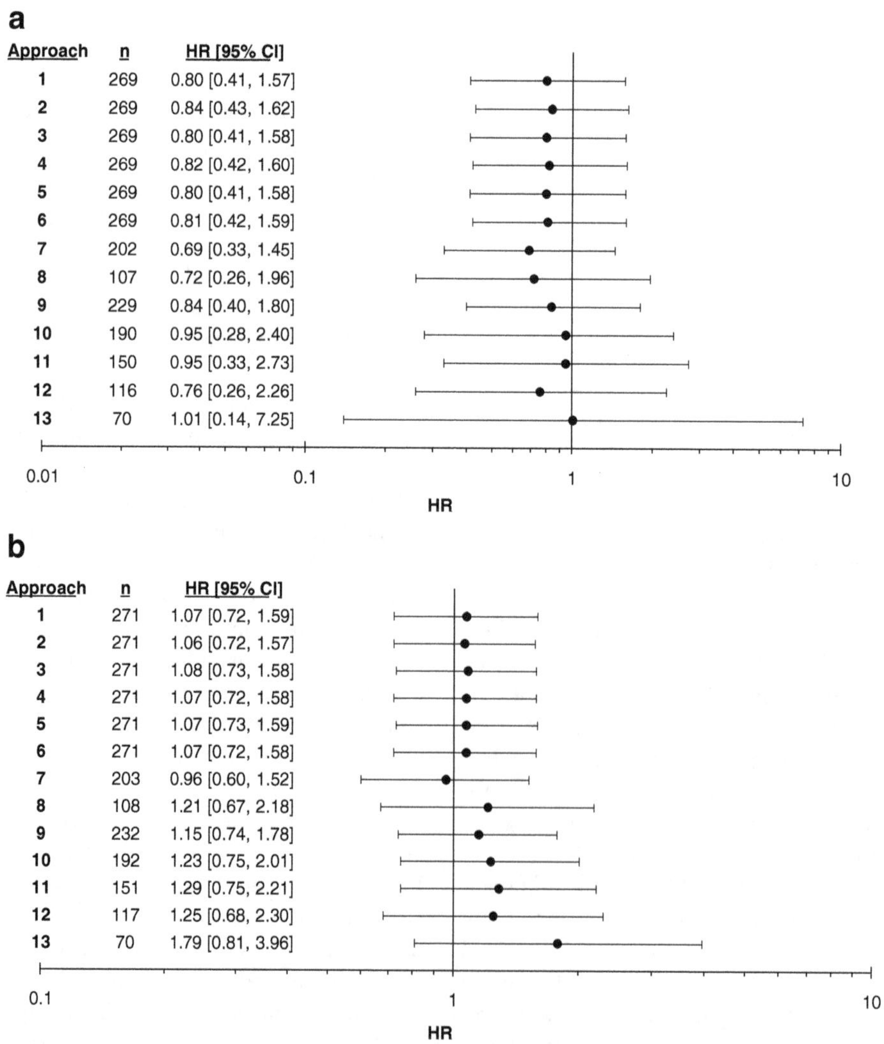

Fig. 2 This graph displays the hazard ratios (*black circles*) and 95% confidence intervals (*lines through circles*) for each approach, using our secondary outcome (panel **a**) and secondary analysis strategy (panel **b**)

In addition to the methodologic implications of our findings, we must consider the potential clinical ramifications. The infection risk in this well-characterized cohort of RA patients starting new treatments did not differ between patients starting a TNFi and those starting other bDMARDs. These results are similar to a recently published large claims-based Medicare analysis that examined infection risk for each bDMARD separately [15]. This larger analysis found that infliximab and rituximab users had higher infection risk than abatacept, while other agents were similar in risk. The current study cohort included few infliximab and rituximab users. Our findings' agreement with prior work is useful as a replication study using different methodology.

Conclusions

In conclusion, we examined the risk of infection among patients with RA starting a TNFi versus a non-TNFi bDMARD. The analyses were conducted in the setting of a large single-center registry where the measurement of disease activity, a key potential confounder, often occurred at a different visit than the start of RA treatments. We tested various methods of estimating disease activity at treatment start and found that the risk of infection was similar for the two groups in nearly all approaches. This is in general agreement with prior estimates of risk [16]. Using all patients with the most proximal disease activity measurements, whether prior to or after the start of bDMARD, were most consistent, while analyses that restricted to subgroups with confounder data measured in very close proximity to the start of treatment appeared to give biased estimates with the least precision. The methods pursued in this study provide a template for how to evaluate the measurement of an important time-varying confounder in other registry analyses.

Abbreviations

bDMARD: Biologic disease-modifying antirheumatic drug; CRP: C-reactive protein; DAS28: Disease activity score based on 28 joints; DMARD: Disease-modifying antirheumatic drug; RA: Rheumatoid arthritis; TNF: Tumor necrosis factor

Acknowledgements

None.

Funding

Support: PCORI ME-1303-5602.

Authors' contributions

DHS contributed to design, analysis, writing, revising, and approval of the final manuscript. NAS contributed to design, analysis, revising, and approval of the final manuscript. MEW contributed to design, revising, and approval of the final manuscript. AZ contributed to analysis, revising, and approval of the final manuscript. MF contributed to design, analysis, revising, and approval of the final manuscript. JMF contributed to design, analysis, revising, and approval of the final manuscript.

Competing interests

The authors declare that they have no competing interests.

References

1. Travers K, Sallum RH, Burns MD, Barr CE, Beattie MS, Pashos CL, et al. Characteristics and temporal trends in patient registries: focus on the life sciences industry, 1981-2012. Pharmacoepidemiol Drug Saf. 2015; 24(4):389–98.
2. Franklin J, Schneeweiss S, Solomon DH. Assessment of patient-reported confounders in comparative effectiveness studies from registry data. Am J Epidemiol. 2017;185(6):474–8.
3. Rothman KJ, Greenland S, Lash LT. Modern epidemiology. 3rd ed. Philadelphia: Lippincott Williams & Wilkins; 2008.
4. Doran MF, Crowson CS, Pond GR, O'Fallon WM, Gabriel SE. Frequency of infection in patients with rheumatoid arthritis compared with controls: a population-based study. Arthritis Rheum. 2002;46(9):2287–93.
5. Singh JA, Saag KG, Bridges Jr SL, Akl EA, Bannuru RR, Sullivan MC, et al. 2015 American College of Rheumatology guideline for the treatment of rheumatoid arthritis. Arthritis Rheumatol. 2016;68(1):1–26.
6. Schiff M, Weinblatt ME, Valente R, van der Heijde D, Citera G, Elegbe A, et al. Head-to-head comparison of subcutaneous abatacept versus adalimumab for rheumatoid arthritis: two-year efficacy and safety findings from AMPLE trial. Ann Rheum Dis. 2014;73(1):86–94.
7. Iannaccone CK, Lee YC, Cui J, Frits ML, Glass RJ, Plenge RM, et al. Using genetic and clinical data to understand response to disease-modifying anti-rheumatic drug therapy: data from the Brigham and Women's Hospital Rheumatoid Arthritis Sequential Study. Rheumatology (Oxford). 2011;50(1):40–6.
8. Pincus T, Swearingen C, Wolfe F. Toward a multidimensional Health Assessment Questionnaire (MDHAQ): assessment of advanced activities of daily living and psychological status in the patient-friendly health assessment questionnaire format. Arthritis Rheum. 1999;42(10):2220–30.
9. Lorig K, Chastain RL, Ung E, Shoor S, Holman HR. Development and evaluation of a scale to measure perceived self-efficacy in people with arthritis. Arthritis Rheum. 1989;32(1):37–44.
10. Fransen J, Langenegger T, Michel BA, Stucki G. Feasibility and validity of the RADAI, a self-administered rheumatoid arthritis disease activity index. Rheumatology (Oxford). 2000;39(3):321–7.
11. Prevoo ML, Hof MA v 't, Kuper HH, van Leeuwen MA, van de Putte LB, van Riel PL. Modified disease activity scores that include twenty-eight-joint counts. Development and validation in a prospective longitudinal study of patients with rheumatoid arthritis. Arthritis Rheum. 1995;38(1):44–8.
12. Paulus HE, Ramos B, Wong WK, Ahmed A, Bulpitt K, Park G, et al. Equivalence of the acute phase reactants C-reactive protein, plasma viscosity, and Westergren erythrocyte sedimentation rate when used to calculate American College of Rheumatology 20% improvement criteria or the Disease Activity Score in patients with early rheumatoid arthritis. Western Consortium of Practicing Rheumatologists. J Rheumatol. 1999; 26(11):2324–31.
13. Rosenbaum PR, Rubin DB. The central role of the propensity score in observational studies for causal effects. Biometrika. 1983;70(1):41–55.
14. Rothman KJ, Greenland S, Lash TL. Modern Epidemiology. 3rd ed. Philadelphia: Lippincott Williams & Wilkins; 2008.
15. Yun H, Xie F, Delzell E, Levitan EB, Chen L, Lewis JD, et al. Comparative risk of hospitalized infection associated with biologic agents in rheumatoid arthritis patients enrolled in Medicare. Arthritis Rheumatol. 2016;68(1):56–66.
16. Curtis JR, Xie F, Chen L, Baddley JW, Beukelman T, Saag KG, et al. The comparative risk of serious infections among rheumatoid arthritis patients starting or switching biological agents. Ann Rheum Dis. 2011;70(8):1401–6.

16

Genetic deficiency of Wnt5a diminishes disease severity in a murine model of rheumatoid arthritis

Susan MacLauchlan[1], Maria A. Zuriaga[1], José J. Fuster[1], Carla M. Cuda[2], Jennifer Jonason[3], Fernanda Behzadi[1], Jennifer Parker Duffen[1], G. Kenneth Haines III[5], Tamar Aprahamian[4], Harris Perlman[2] and Kenneth Walsh[1*]

Abstract

Background: Rheumatoid arthritis (RA) is a common autoimmune disease characterized by chronic inflammation of the joints, leading to bone erosion and joint dysfunction. Despite the recent successes of disease-modifying anti-rheumatic drugs (DMARDs), there is still clinical need for understanding the development and molecular etiology of RA. Wnts are developmental morphogens whose roles in adult pathology are poorly characterized. Wnt5a is a member of the non-canonical family of Wnts that modulates a wide range of cell processes, including differentiation, migration, and inflammation. Wnt5a has been implicated as a possible contributor to arthritis and it is upregulated in synovial fibroblasts from RA patients.

Methods: We investigated the role of endogenous Wnt5a in RA. Tamoxifen-inducible, Wnt5a knockout (Wnt5a cKO) mice and littermate controls were monitored for arthritis development and joint pathology using the K/BxN serum transfer-induced arthritis (STIA) model. To explore a role of Wnt5a in osteoclast fusion, bone marrow-derived monocytes (BMDMs) were differentiated in vitro.

Results: Wnt5a cKO mice were resistant to arthritis development compared to control littermates as assessed by ankle thickness and histologic measurements. Some parameters of inflammation were reduced in the Wnt5a cKO mice, including the extent of polymononuclear cell infiltration and extra-articular inflammation. Wnt5a cKO mice also exhibited less cartilage destruction and a reduction in osteoclast activity with concomitant reduction in *tartrate-resistant acid phosphatase* (*TRAP*), *cathepsin K* (*CTSK*), *macrophage colony-stimulating factor* (*MCSF*), *matrix metalloproteinase* (*MMP*)*2* and *MMP9* in the arthritic joints. Treatment of BMDMs with Wnt5a enhanced osteoclast fusion and increased the expression of *dendrocyte-expressed seven transmembrane protein* (*DCSTAMP*) and *MMP9*, that are necessary for osteoclast formation and activity.

Conclusions: These data suggest that Wnt5a modulates the development of arthritis by promoting inflammation and osteoclast fusion, and provide the first mouse genetic evidence of a role for endogenous Wnt5a in autoimmune disease.

Keywords: Rheumatoid arthritis, Wnt5a, Inflammation, Osteoclast fusion

* Correspondence: kxwalsh@bu.edu; kwalsh@theworld.com
[1]Molecular Cardiology, Whitaker Cardiovascular Institute, Boston University School of Medicine, 700 Albany Street, W-611, Boston, MA 02118, USA
Full list of author information is available at the end of the article

Background

Rheumatoid arthritis (RA) is a common chronic autoimmune disease that leads to significant morbidity and mortality. The prevalence of this disease is between 0.5 and 1% in the USA, with greater risk of incidence among women [1]. The molecular cues that trigger RA are complex and likely require a combination of genetic and environmental factors. Ultimately, the loss of self-tolerance to self-proteins, typically citrullinated-proteins, results in disease progression through inflammation, synovial hyperplasia, and osteoclast activation [2]. These processes lead to the recognizable hallmarks of the disease, including joint swelling, pain, and dysfunction. Although joint involvement is the major clinical manifestation of the autoimmune process, RA patients suffer from a number of co-morbidities including increased risk of cardiovascular disease even when accounting for the increased inflammatory state [3, 4]. Significant strides have been made in the treatment of RA. Standard therapy for RA includes methotrexate and one of several disease-modifying anti-rheumatic drugs (DMARDs) that target the key inflammatory molecules that promote RA, including TNFα (infliximab, etanercept) and IL6 (tocilizumab). These treatments allow many patients to achieve disease-free status, but their use is associated with significant side effects and these biologic agents do not confer sustained remission after drug cessation [1, 5]. Thus, there remains a clinical need for improved understanding of novel targets for drugs in the process of RA development.

The Wnt family proteins are developmental regulators that are becoming appreciated for their diverse roles in adult physiology. Wnt5a is the archetypal non-canonical Wnt, the subset of Wnts whose functions are independent of beta-catenin [6]. In post-natal tissue, the functions of Wnt5a are diverse and include modulation of cell fate decisions and inflammation. Previous work has established Wnt5a as a pro-inflammatory molecule in a number of settings including vascular dysfunction [7, 8], peripheral arterial disease [9], and cardiometabolic disease [10–12]. Wnt5a has also been demonstrated to promote expression of various cytokines that may contribute to RA progression [13–16]. However, studies on the role of Wnt5a in immune regulation can be confounded by the likely presence of TLR4 agonists in commercial Wnt5a protein preparations [17]. Thus, analyses of Wnt5a function using mouse genetic models are warranted as they are not subject to this potential confounder.

Wnt5a is increased in the synovium in patients with RA and osteoarthritis (OA) [18], and inhibition of Wnt5a is reported to block the activation of cultured synovial fibroblasts from RA patients [19]. In addition, the delivery of a soluble form of receptor-tyrosine orphan receptor 2 (ROR2), a candidate decoy receptor for Wnt5a, leads to reduced radiographic severity in mice undergoing collagen-induced arthritis (CIA) [20]. These data underscore the potential clinical value of Wnt5a in the pathogenesis of RA. However, there is as yet no direct genetic evidence to support that endogenous Wnt5a plays a contributory role in the development of RA.

In the present study, we used inducible Wnt5a knockout (Wnt5a cKO) and littermate control mice in the K/BxN serum transfer-induced arthritis (STIA) model. Wnt5a cKO mice were protected from development of RA, both in terms of ankle thickness and other markers of disease severity. Histologic examination demonstrated reduced inflammation in the Wnt5a cKO, including reduced PMN infiltrate into the inflamed joints. Less osteoclast activity was also observed in the arthritic Wnt5a cKO joints compared to the controls. Mechanistically, this may result from decreases in osteoclast fusion as Wnt5a promoted osteoclast fusion in an in vitro culture of bone marrow-derived macrophage (BMDM) differentiation. Wnt5a increased the expression of critical molecules for osteoclast differentiation and fusion, specifically *dendrocyte-expressed seven transmembrane protein* (*DCSTAMP*) and *matrix metalloproteinase 9* (*MMP9*). These data suggest Wnt5a signaling as a modulator of inflammation and osteoclast fusion could represent a component of disease activity in RA patients.

Methods

Animals

All animal protocols were approved by the Institutional Animal Care and Use Committee (IACUC), Boston University School of Medicine (BUSM). Wnt5a whole body inducible cKO mice (Wnt5a cKO) were generated as previously described [10] by selective breeding of the *Wnt5a* floxed mice [21] with the *UBC* cre promoter mice (Jackson Labs, Bar Harbor, ME, USA, stock number 007001). Female littermate *Wnt5a* floxed cre-negative mice (control) and cre-positive mice (Wnt5a cKO) were used for this study. *Wnt5a* recombination was induced in the mice at 6 weeks of age by five daily intraperitoneal injections of tamoxifen delivered in corn oil (80ug tamoxifen per g body weight each day). Both control and Wnt5a cKO mice were treated with tamoxifen. Baseline mice (at least four per genotype) were euthanized following 2 weeks of tamoxifen wash out. Tissue was collected and processed as described in the following section. Mice were used in the arthritis model following 2 weeks of tamoxifen wash out ($n = 13$ per genotype for RA studies). Female C57BL6J (Jackson Laboratories) mice 10 – 12 weeks of age were used for the in vitro fusion assays ($n = 3$).

K/BxN serum transfer-induced arthritis (STIA) model

Rheumatoid arthritis development was induced in control and Wnt5a cKO mice using the K/BxN serum transfer model of arthritis as previously described [22]. Briefly, serum from K/BxN mice (the offspring of mice expressing the KRN T cell receptor transgene and the major histocompatibility complex (MHC) class II molecule A(g7), which develop spontaneous arthritis) was isolated at 8 weeks of age. Passive transfer of arthritis was induced in control and Wnt5a cKO mice by intraperitoneal injection of 150 µl of K/BxN serum at day 0 (d0) and d2. Severity of arthritis was monitored by two measures prior to serum injection and every other day for 28 days. The clinical score of each joint was determined using a well-established scoring metric [22–24]. The reported clinical score is the summation of the scores for all four appendages. Ankle thickness was measured at the thickest point of the ankle using digital Vernier calipers (Fine Science Tools). Significance for the clinical score and ankle thickness measurements was determined using the statistical package in Prism GraphPad using two-way analysis of variance (ANOVA). Significance was determined using the Sidak post-hoc test. Tissues were collected at d7 ($n = 6$ per genotype) or d28 ($n = 7$ per genotype) following induction of arthritis. Serum was collected by cardiac puncture after euthanasia by carbon dioxide inhalation. Paw joints were snap frozen for mRNA isolation and ankle joints were fixed in 10% formalin and decalcified in 0.375 M EDTA.

Paw joints were pooled for each individual animal prior to mRNA extraction. The joints were cleaned of skin, homogenized with Qialyzer (Qiagen) and mRNA was isolated with the Qiagen RNeasy Fibrous tissue kit according to the manufacturer's directions. cDNA was transcribed from 1 µg of RNA using High Capacity cDNA Kit (Applied Biosystems) and quantitative PCR (qPCR) was performed using SYBR-based detection (primer sequences are shown in Table 1). Fold changes were calculated after normalization of the average *hypoxanthine guanine phosphoribosyl transferase* (*HPRT*) and beta-actin relative to baseline mice. *P* values ≤0.05 from

Table 1 Sequences for SYBR qPCR

Gene ID	Forward primer	Reverse primer
CAR2	TCC CAC CAC TGG GGA TAC AG	CTC TTG GAC GCA GCT TTA TCA TA
CD68	TGT CTG ATC TTG CTA GGA CCG	GAG AGT AAC GGC CTT TTT GTG A
CLCN7	CGC CAG TGT CAT TCT GCA CT	GCT TCT CGT TGT GTG GAA TCT
CTSK	GAA GAA GAC TGA CCA GAA GCA G	TCC AGG TTA TGG GCA GAG ATT
DCSTAMP	GGG GAC TTA TGT GTT TCC ACG	ACA AGG CAA CAG ACT CCC AAA T
F4/80	CTT TGG CTA TGG GCT TCC AGT C	GCA AGG AGG ACA GAG TTT ATC GTG
GAPDH	TGA CCA CCA TGG AGA AGG C	GCT AAG CAG TTG GTG GTG CA
HPRT	TCA GTC AAC GGG GGA CAT AAA	GGG GCT GTA CTG CTT AAC CAG
IL1β	TGA CAG TGA TGA GAA TGA CCT GTT C	TTG GAA GCA GCC CTT CAT CT
IL6	GCT ACC AAA CTG GAT ATA ATC AGG A	CCA GGT AGC TAT GGT ACT CCA GAA
MCP1	GCC TAC TCA TTG GGA TCA TCT TG	CAG CCA GAT GCA GTT AAC GC
MCSF	GGC TTG GCT TGG GAT GAT TCT	GAG GGT CTG GCA GGT ACT C
MMP2	CAG GGT GGT GGT CAT AGC TAC TT	GAG ACT TTG GTT CTC CAG CTT CA
MMP9	CAA GTG GGA CCA TCA TAA CAT CA	CTC GCG GCA AGT CTT CAG A
MMP14	AGT GAC AGG CAA GGC TGA TTT	AGG GGT GTA ATT CTG AAT GCA G
NFATc1	CAG GGC GAG TTC GAC TTC G	TGA CAC TAG GGG ACA CAT AAC TG
OPG	ACC CAG AAA CTG GTC ATC AGC	CTG CAA TAC ACA CAC TCA TCA CT
OSCAR	CCT AGC CTC ATA CCC CCA G	CGT TGA TCC CAG GAG TCA CAA
RANKL	CAG CAT CGC TCT GTT CCT GTA	CTG CGT TTT CAT GGA GTC TCA
RANK	GGA CGG TGT TGC AGC AGA T	GCA GTC TGA GTT CCA GTG GTA
RCAN2	CCA CTC TGG TCG CCT GTG T	CGG AAC AGT CCC TCG AAT TTT TCC TTA
TBP	CTT CCT GCC ACA ATG TCA CAG	CCT TTC TCA TGC TTG CTT CTC TG
TNFα	CGG AGT CCG GGC AGG	GCT GGG TAG AGA ATG GAT GAA
TRAP	CAC TCC CAC CCT GAG ATT TGT	CAT CGT CTG CAC GGT TCT G
Wnt5a Ex2	CAA ATA GGC AGC CGA GAG AC	CTC TAG CGT CCA CGA ACT CC
18S	AAT CAA GAA CGA AAG TCG GAG G	GCG GGT CAT GGG AAT AAC G
36B4	GCT CCA AGC AGA TGC AGC A	CCG GAT GTG AGG CAG CAG

the t test calculated using GraphPad Prism were considered significant.

Histopathologic assessment

Paraffin-embedded tissue sections were stained with hematoxylin and eosin (H&E). Disease severity was analyzed by a pathologist (KGH) blinded to the genotypes as previously described [25] (n = 6 per genotype). Clinical score, cartilage destruction, bone erosion, inflammation, polymononuclear (PMN) infiltration, extra-articular inflammation, lymphocyte infiltration, pannus formation and synovial lining average were evaluated as previously described [23, 25–28]. Tartrate acid resistant phosphatase (TRAP) staining was performed as specified by the manufacturer (Sigma Kit) ($n = 6$ per genotype at d7 and at least 4 per genotype for baseline analysis). Stained sections were visualized on a Keyence BZ-X700 and analyzed with the on-board image processing software to identify total TRAP + area in at least four fields per mouse in both ankle joints.

L cell conditioned media

L control cells (ATCC, CRL-2648) and L Wnt5a cells (ATCC, CRL-2814) were used to generate controls and Wnt5a conditioned media as previously described [29]. L cells were maintained in DMEM with 10% FBS and pen/strep/Lglut. Conditioned medium for the fusion assays were generated in complete alpha-MEM with 10% FBS and pen/strep/Lglut. This conditioned medium was diluted 1:4 with fresh complete alpha-MEM medium for the fusion assays.

In vitro analysis of fusion

BMDM were isolated from female C57BL6J mice (Jackson Laboratories) and cultured in alpha-MEM with 10% FBS and pen/strep/Lglut. Following differential plating to purify monocyte cells in the presence of macrophage colony-stimulating factor (MCSF) (100 ng/mL), 10^5 cells per well were plated in 24 well plates in the presence of diluted L cell control or diluted Lcell Wnt5a-treated medium. BMDM were induced to fuse with the stimulation cocktail (MCSF (50 ng/mL) and RANKL (50 ng/mL)), which was replenished at d2 and d4. RNA was isolated at d2 and d5 using the miRNeasy Micro Kit (Qiagen) and 1 μg of RNA was transcribed using the Quantitect kit (Qiagen). SYBR chemistry was used to detect transcripts and these were analyzed on a ViiA7 using the primers listed in Table 1. Significance was determined in GraphPad Prism using two-way ANOVA with the Tukey post-hoc test, considering p values ≤0.05 as significant. To enumerate osteoclasts, d5 cultures were stained for TRAP (Sigma) and co-stained with 4',6-diamidino-2-phenylindole (DAPI) (Thermo Fisher Scientific). Cultures were visualized using a Keyence microscope. Osteoclasts were identified as TRAP+ multinucleated cells (3 nuclei or more). Total nuclei, total TRAP+ cells, total osteoclasts and total nuclei in osteoclasts were enumerated in at least six random high powered fields per condition per experiment. The osteoclast frequency per 1000 cells was calculated as the ratio of total osteoclasts per high-powered field (HPF) divided by total nuclei in the same HPF. The percentage of cells in osteoclasts is the total nuclei in osteoclasts per HPF divided by the total nuclei in the same image. Statistical significance for enumeration tests was performed using Prism Software and the unpaired t test and considering significance at $p \leq 0.05$. All in vitro studies were performed three times. Enumeration studies were performed in duplicate three times.

Results

Wnt5a-deficiency attenuates the development of RA-like disease

Due to the association of Wnt5a with clinical arthritis, we sought to determine its role in the murine STIA model of RA. In apparent contrast to clinical arthritis [18], *Wnt5a* transcript levels were reduced at d7 after RA induction (Additional file 1: Figure S1). However, active RA induced the levels of the Wnt5a co-receptor *ROR2* mRNA at this time point (Additional file 1: Figure S1). To further evaluate the role of Wnt5a in the development of RA, a murine model of Wnt5a deficiency was subjected to the STIA model. Using primers that hybridize within the floxed Exon 2 of *Wnt5a* (Additional file 1: Figure S2A), the Wnt5a cKO mice exhibited >90% decrease in *Wnt5a* in the paws of Wnt5a cKO mice after 2 weeks of tamoxifen-induced ablation (Additional file 1: Figure S2A) compared with littermate controls. Baseline measures in healthy Wnt5a cKO mice did not demonstrate alterations in inflammatory markers (Additional file 1: Figure S2B), in ankle morphology (Additional file 1: Figure S3), or in osteoclast activation (Additional file 1: Figure S4). Following STIA induction of RA, there was attenuated development of arthritis in the Wnt5a cKO mice in terms of ankle thickness, which plateaued below the thickness developed in the littermate controls and resolved in a similar timeframe (Fig. 1a). In a separate cohort of animals, the arthritic process was examined in control and Wnt5a cKO mice at the earliest peak of inflammation (d7). Measurement of the disease severity was performed by a pathologist blinded to genotype using previously established histopathologic scoring metrics [23, 24], using H&E stained sections from control and Wnt5a cKO mice at d7 (Fig. 2a). The Wnt5a cKO mice displayed statistically significant reduction in overall disease severity (overall H&E score) and this cohort exhibited a significant reduction in clinical score (Fig. 2b). Histologic analysis of the arthritic joints also revealed that Wnt5a cKO mice exhibit significant

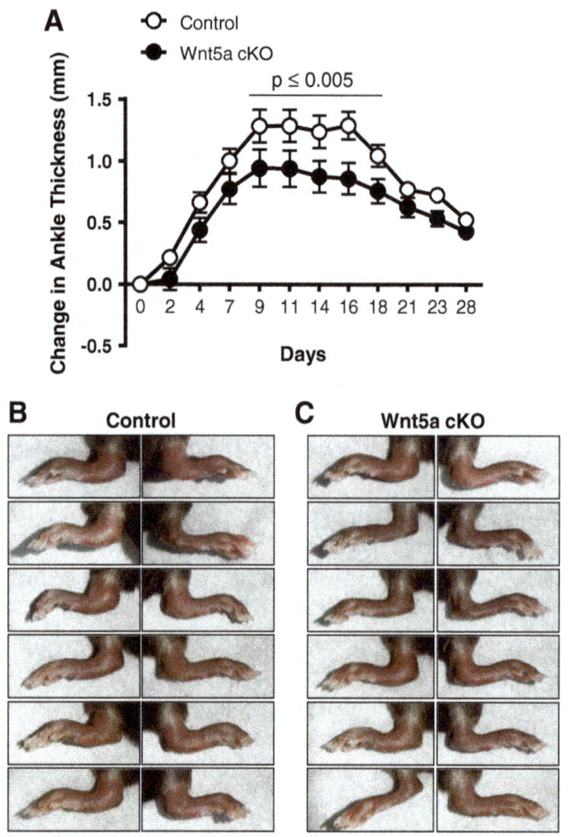

Fig. 1 Whole body inducible Wnt5a knockout (*Wnt5a cKO*) mice display attenuated rheumatoid arthritis development in the serum transfer model. **a** The change in ankle thickness was monitored in Wnt5a cKO and littermate control mice following a period of 28 days after induction of arthritis by serum transfer. Images of the ankles at day 7 indicate that there is more inflammation and arthritis in the limbs of control mice (**b**) compared to the Wnt5a cKO mice (**c**)

reductions in some parameters of inflammation, including measures of reduced extra-articular inflammation and PMN infiltration (Fig. 2b). Although not statistically different, trends of reduced pannus formation, synovial lining average and bone erosion were also observed in the Wnt5a cKO mice compared to control mice (Fig. 2b and Additional file 1: Figure S5). Numerous studies have reported that Wnt5a promotes cytokine expression [13–16]. However, only trends of decreased *TNFα*, *IL6*, and *IL1β* were observed in Wnt5a cKO at day 7 following RA induction (Additional file 1: Figure S6A), which were not statistically significant.

Decreased osteoclast activity in arthritic Wnt5a cKO mice

We next evaluated the osteoclast activity in the arthritic ankles from control and Wnt5a cKO mice. TRAP staining (Fig. 3a) demonstrated robust activity in the control mice, with obvious staining at multiple destruction pits, whereas Wnt5a cKO mice displayed a markedly reduced TRAP-positive area as quantified in Fig. 3b. Consistent with these findings, decreased levels of TRAP and *cathepsin K* (*CTSK*) mRNA were detected in the arthritic paws of Wnt5a cKO mice (Fig. 3c), but there were no changes in the *calcitonin receptor* (*CAL*) or *carbonic anhydrase 2* (*CAR2*) mRNA in Wnt5a cKO mice (Additional file 1: Figure S6B). There was a trend toward lower expression of the osteoclast differentiation signal *RANKL* and reduction in the expression of *MCSF* observed in the arthritic paws of Wnt5a cKO mice (Fig. 3c). Consistent with their roles both in inflammation and in osteoclast activity, levels of *MMP2* and *MMP9* mRNA were significantly decreased in the arthritic paws of Wnt5a cKO mice (Fig. 3c).

Wnt5a promotes osteoclast fusion in vitro

To attain a deeper understanding of the mechanism of Wnt5a action in the process of osteoclastogenesis, in vitro analyses were performed to determine whether Wnt5a has an intrinsic ability to promote osteoclast fusion. MCSF-dependent BMDM were stimulated to fuse in the presence of L cell medium conditioned by cells that were engineered to overexpress Wnt5a (Wnt5a) or control media (conditioned by L cells without Wnt5a overexpression). TRAP-positive (dark color) multinucleated osteoclasts formed after 5 days of RANKL stimulation (Fig. 4a). Osteoclast fusion was stimulated by Wnt5a, both in terms of total incidence (osteoclast frequency per 1000 cells) and in the percent of nuclei fused into osteoclasts (Fig. 4b). In contrast, Wnt5a did not significantly change the nuclei per osteoclast total or total nuclei in osteoclasts (Additional file 1: Figure S7).

Transcripts were analyzed in fusing BMDM cultures after 2 and 5 days of RANKL stimulation to further evaluate the impact of Wnt5a on osteoclast fusion. *Wnt5a* mRNA levels were not altered during the fusion process (Additional file 1: Figure S8). Treatment with Wnt5a did not significantly alter the expression of osteoclast genes (*CTSK* or *TRAP*) or an inhibitor of *osteoclastogenesis* (*OPG*) (Additional file 1: Figure S8). However, Wnt5a promoted the expression of *DCSTAMP* (Fig. 4c), a cell surface molecule that is essential for osteoclast fusion [30]. Consistent with observations in the STIA model, fusing macrophages treated with Wnt5a expressed increased levels of *MMP9* but not *MMP2* (Fig. 4d). In contrast, Wnt5a did not affect the expression of other nuclear factor activating T cells 1c (NFATc1) downstream genes, including *MMP14*, *CLCN7*, *CAR2*, *RCAN2* and *OSCAR*, or *NFATc1* itself (Additional file 1: Figure S9).

Discussion

Wnt5a is elevated in the synovium of RA patients [18], and enhanced Wnt5a secretion by fibroblast-like synoviocytes has been attributed to their persistent activation

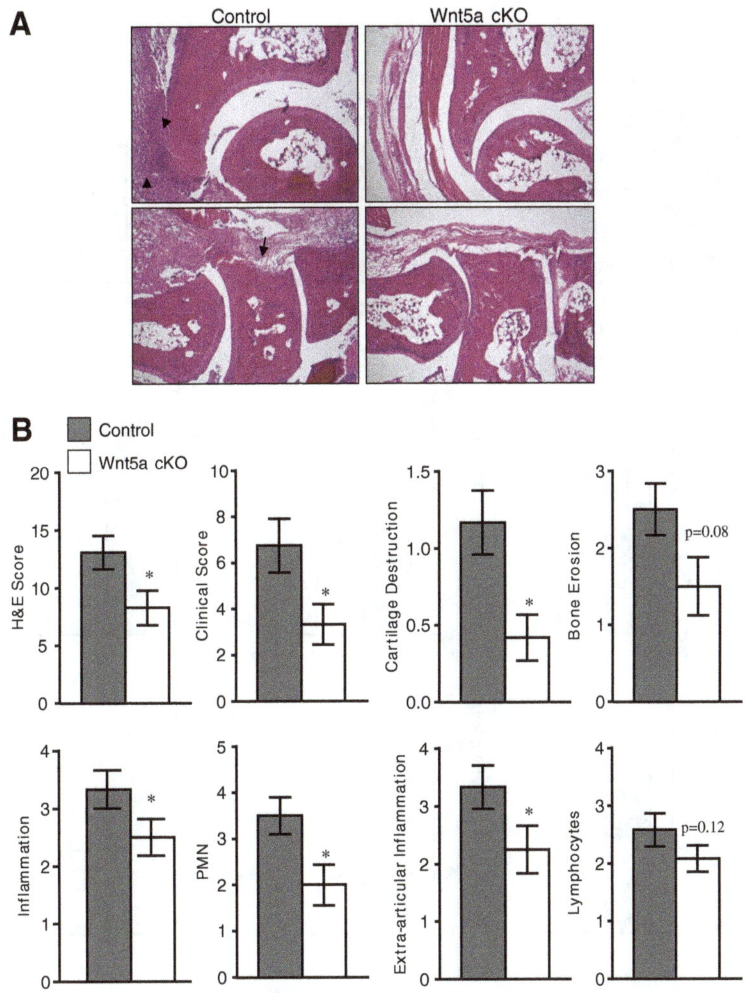

Fig. 2 Whole body inducible Wnt5a knockout (*Wnt5a cKO*) mice develop less severe rheumatoid arthritis (RA) based upon histological analyses. **a** H&E-stained sections from the ankles in control and Wnt5a cKO mice at day 7 after induction of arthritis demonstrate hallmark features of the disease at the tarsotibial joint (*top panels*) and the tarsonavicular joint (*bottom panels*), including expanded pannus formation (*arrowheads*) and destruction pits (*arrow*). **b** Qualitative metrics of the damage induced by RA in control and Wnt5a cKO mice demonstrates reduced overall disease severity (H&E score), clinical score, cartilage destruction, inflammation, polymononuclear (*PMN*) cell infiltration and extra-articular lesions in the joints of Wnt5a cKO mice. $^*P \leq 0.05$

[19]. Thus, we sought to provide genetic evidence for a causal link between Wnt5a and RA development. The present study utilized a mouse model in which ablation of Wnt5a is inducible, thereby avoiding the embryonic lethality of the conventional knockout strain [21]. This inducible ablation model also permits the ablation of Wnt5a proximal to the induction of arthritis, thereby eliminating the confounding effects of Wnt5a in bone development [20] (Additional file 1: Figure S1-S3). Collectively, this study shows that mice deficient for Wnt5a are resistant to development of RA-like disease in the STIA model.

The acute genetic ablation of Wnt5a in the STIA model led to reductions in some markers of inflammation. Based upon histologic analysis, Wnt5a cKO mice exhibited statistically significant reductions in overall inflammatory status, extra-articular inflammation and PMN cell infiltration (Fig. 2). In this regard, it is well-appreciated that neutrophils are important mediators in the development of arthritis [31, 32]. Failure to recruit neutrophils correlates with reduction in the overall progression of disease severity in other models of arthritis [33]. Further, since Wnt5a is described to be chemotactic to neutrophils [34], it is possible that this is a significant component of the mechanism by which Wnt5a cKO mice are protected from the development of STIA.

Using the Wnt5a cKO mouse model, we recently reported that Wnt5a ablation protects against adipose tissue inflammation and systemic metabolic dysfunction that is associated with diminished levels of monocyte chemoattractant protein 1 (MCP-1), IL6 and TNFα in the adipose tissue [10]. Although these cytokines are

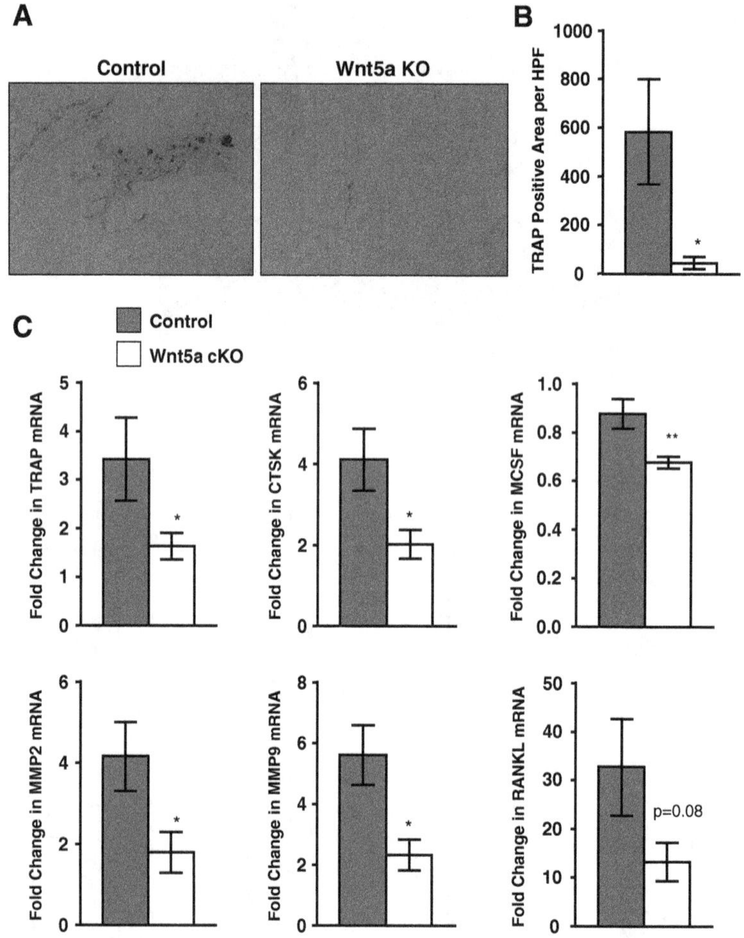

Fig. 3 Whole body inducible Wnt5a knockout (*Wnt5a cKO*) mice have reduced osteoclast activity after induction of arthritis. **a** Tartrate-resistant acid phosphatase (*TRAP*) staining, indicated by *purple color* in control (*left panel*) and Wnt5a cKO (*right panel*), indicates fewer areas of osteoclast activity in the Wnt5a cKO mice at day 7. **b** Quantification of the percent of TRAP-positive area revealed reduced osteoclast activity in the Wnt5a cKO (*white bars*) compared to the controls (*gray bars*). **c** The levels of mRNA for the *TRAP, Cathepsin K* (*CTSK*), *macrophage colony-stimulating factor* (*MCSF*), *matrix metalloproteinase 2* (*MMP2*) and *MMP9* were reduced in the paws from the arthritic Wnt5a cKO mice compared to the arthritic controls. $^*P \leq 0.05$. A trend toward reduced *RANKL* transcript was noted

shared in the pathogenesis of metabolic dysfunction and RA [1, 5], only trends towards reduction of *TNFα*, *IL6*, and *IL1β* transcripts were observed in the arthritic paws from the Wnt5a cKO mice (Additional file 1: Figure S6) as was a trend toward diminished lymphocyte infiltration in the histological sections (Additional file 1: Figure S5). In total, these data are indicative that Wnt5a is one of many modulators of inflammation in the RA model, which can be compensated for by other inflammatory molecules. However, there appears to be a modest and appreciable protection from the inflammation in RA conferred by Wnt5a deficiency. Further, we acknowledge the possibility that Wnt5a has a more profound impact on inflammation in the STIA model at other time points.

In contrast to the increase in Wnt5a expression in the synovium of RA patients [18], we found a reduction in the amount of *Wnt5a* in the joints from mice undergoing STIA. Beyond species differences, there are a number of possible explanations for this discrepancy. First, there was a concurrent increase in the Wnt5a co-receptor *ROR2* (Additional file 1: Figure S1), indicating that reduced amounts of Wnt5a might be sufficient to drive RA pathology. In this regard, Wnt5a is highly glycosylated and is believed to exhibit its effects through short-range paracrine interactions [35, 36]. Thus, localized changes in Wnt5a may be sufficient to modulate RA development, particularly when paired with a concomitant increase in *ROR2*. It should be also noted that our analysis was performed using the entire joint; including fibroblast-like synoviocytes, bone, bone marrow, and extra-articular inflammatory tissue. Indeed, although Wnt5a is reported to be among the most highly expressed Wnt homologs expressed in bone, immunohistochemical analysis demonstrated that it is predominantly expressed

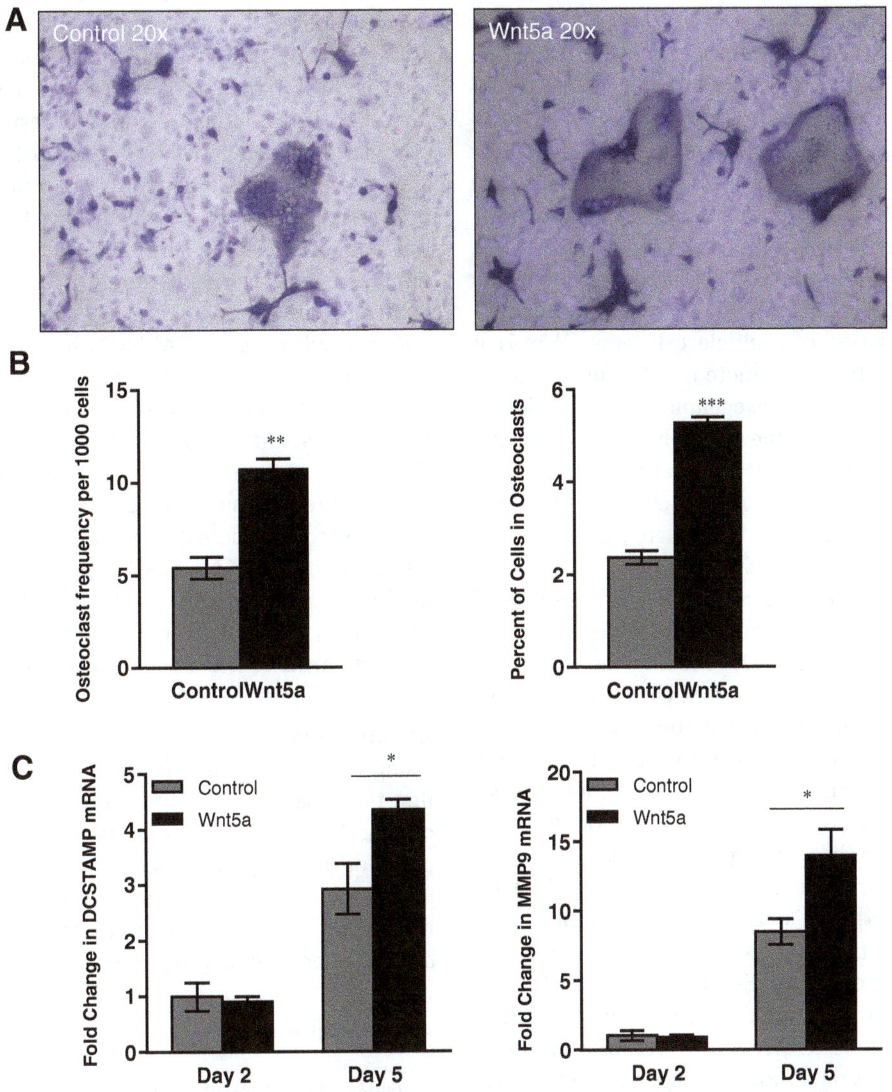

Fig. 4 Wnt5a promotes osteoclast formation through enhanced *dendrocyte-expressed seven transmembrane protein* (*DCSTAMP*) and *matrix metalloproteinase 9* (*MMP9*) expression. Osteoclasts were formed *in vitro* from bone marrow-derived monocytes in L cell conditioned medium (*Control*) or L Wnt5a conditioned medium (*Wnt5a*). Osteoclasts were visualized after 5 days of RANKL stimulation by tartrate-resistant acid phosphatase (TRAP) (*dark color*) and 4′,6-diamidino-2-phenylindole (**a**). Osteoclasts were enumerated by identifying TRAP+ cells with three or more nuclei and expressed as frequency per 1000 cells or by percent of nuclei in osteoclasts (**b**). By both measures, Wnt5a increased the osteoclast formation (**$p \le 0.01$, ***$p \le 0.001$). **c** mRNA isolated from fusing osteoclast cultures at day 2 and day 5 were analyzed for *DCSTAMP* and *MMP9* expression. The levels were increased by Wnt5a treatment. *$P \le 0.05$ for comparison of control and Wnt5a-treated cultures

by osteoblast/osteoclasts and not the osteocyte [20]. Thus, further exploration of Wnt5a in the arthritic space, beyond the synovial tissue, is warranted.

Wnt5a has been functionally implicated in the development of RA by a study that delivered a soluble version of ROR2, a putative Wnt5a receptor, to mice in the collagen-induced arthritis (CIA) model [20]. Although mice receiving the soluble ROR2 were not protected from development of ankle thickness or clinical score, they did exhibit reduced radiographic damage [20], consistent with a reduction in osteoclast activity. Our work supports and extends these observations in several ways. First, using the Wnt5a cKO mouse model we provide direct mouse genetic evidence to support that Wnt5a plays a role in the pathogenesis of RA. Second, the inducible Wnt5a cKO mice were used to ablate Wnt5a immediately prior to the induction of the STIA model, which eliminates the confounding effects of Wnt5a-deficiency on long-term bone development [20, 37–39]. Third, we document an effect of Wnt5a in the STIA model, which recapitulates the initiating events of the disease with a higher penetrance than the CIA model. Notably, the STIA model also avoids the use of adjuvant that can potentially act as a confounder. Finally, our study provides mechanistic detail about the role of Wnt5a in osteoclast fusion.

Macrophage cell fusion is required for the formation of multinucleated osteoclasts that function in the catabolism of bone matrix. Osteoclast formation from myeloid precursors is regulated by a sequence of molecular events involving the cell surface receptors including DCSTAMP, CD36, CD47, TREM2 and E-cadherin [40]. Additionally, osteoclast-specific genes including MMP9, CTSK and TRAP [41], are also required for cell fusion during osteoclastogenesis. Although it has been implicated in differentiation of multiple cell types, Wnt5a is not widely appreciated to promote cellular fusion. In the present study, we find that exogenous Wnt5a added to fusing BMDM enhanced their fusion into osteoclasts and upregulated *DCSTAMP* (Fig. 4), a cell surface molecule essential for formation of osteoclasts in vivo [30]. *MMP9* was also found to be upregulated by Wnt5a in fusing osteoclasts (Fig. 4c). MMP9 has been shown to be critical for the development of arthritis as MMP9 KO mice develop less inflammation and joint destruction in the serum transfer model [42]. MMP9 has also been shown to modulate several aspects of osteoclast function, including enhancement of cell migration, potentiation of cell fusion, and increased bone metabolism [43–46]. Altogether, our data indicate that Wnt5a promotes osteoclast formation, and suggests a possible role of Wnt5a in development of other bone resorption disorders.

Rheumatoid arthritis is associated with cardiometabolic diseases [3, 4], and a growing number of animal studies have investigated this linkage. Assessment of arthritis development in ApoE-deficient mice using the CIA model has led to conflicting reports on the consequences of hypercholesterolemia on promoting arthritis [47, 48]. However, using a modified chronic STIA model, more recent evidence demonstrated that ApoE-deficient mice display aggravated development of arthritis but not an increased plaque burden [49]. Conversely, when placed on an atherogenic diet, K/BxA^{g7} mice display increased plaque burden [50]. The present study suggests that Wnt5a might be a possible common mechanism linking both RA and cardiovascular disease. It has been shown that Wnt5a contributes to increased cardiac dysfunction following ischemia/reperfusion injury [11] and to impaired revascularization in a model of peripheral arterial disease [9]. Moreover, previous research demonstrated that Wnt5a impairs metabolic function at least in part through its role in exacerbating adipose tissue inflammation in the obese state [10, 12]. Wnt5a is markedly upregulated in visceral adipose tissue (VAT) and correlates strongly with indices of inflammation and diabetes mellitus [10, 51]. Despite the existence of "rheumatoid cachexia" in late-stage disease, large scale meta-analysis reveals that obesity is a risk factor for RA that is associated with disease severity [52, 53]. It has been proposed that adipokines, cytokines secreted by adipose tissue, are molecular drivers of both diseases [52, 54]. RA patients exhibit elevated adipokine levels, including leptin, adiponectin, and resistin, in serum or synovial fluid compared to healthy patients [52, 55–57], and these factors frequently correlate with disease progression [58, 59]. Collectively, these observations warrant further study to establish whether Wnt5a functions as a putative nexus target in RA and cardiometabolic diseases.

Recent advances in DMARDs have revolutionized the treatment landscape for RA patients. However, cessation of treatment inevitably leads to relapse. Furthermore, a subset of patients remains refractory to these therapeutics agents. Current treatment modalities focus on inhibition of the inflammatory process and do not directly target osteoclast activity. Based upon the multi-modal influence of Wnt5a on RA etiology, specifically as a modulator of osteoclast activity and inflammation, it may represent a novel target that has potential to modulate both arms of RA disease progression.

Conclusions

Using a genetic model, this study demonstrates for the first time that loss of Wnt5a attenuates the development of RA. Wnt5a functions in two major aspects of RA pathology; through enhancement of some parameters of inflammation and by promoting osteoclast fusion. These results are the first to demonstrate a role of Wnt5a in autoimmune disease progression or in cell-cell fusion.

Additional file

Additional file 1: Figure S1. Gene expression of Wnt5a and ROR2 during the development of STIA. **Figure S2.** Characteristics of the baseline phenotype of control and Wnt5a cKO mice. **Figure S3.** Histology of the baseline phenotype of control and Wnt5a cKO mice. **Figure S4.** Baseline osteoclast phenotype of control and Wnt5a cKO mice. **Figure S5.** Additional histopathological scoring of arthritis in Wnt5a cKO mice. **Figure S6.** Gene expression of cytokines and osteoclast genes in paws of control and Wnt5a cKO mice undergoing STIA. **Figure S7.** Characteristics of fusing osteoclasts in the absence and presence of Wnt5a-treated medium. **Figure S8.** Gene expression of osteoclast markers during BMDM differentiation to osteoclasts. **Figure S9.** Gene expression of NFATa1 markers during BMDM differentiation to osteoclasts. (PDF 4647 kb)

Abbreviations

ANOVA: Analysis of variance; BMDM: Bone marrow-derived macrophages; CAL: Calcitonin receptor; CAR2: Carbonic anhydrase 2; CIA: Collagen-induced arthritis; CLCN7: Chloride voltage-gated channel 7; CTSK: Cathepsin K; DAPI: 4',6-Diamidino-2-phenylindole; DCSTAMP: Dendrocyte-expressed seven transmembrane protein; DMARD: Disease-modifying anti-rheumatic drug; DMEM: Dulbecco's modified Eagle's medium; FBS: Fetal bovine serum; H&E: Hematoxylin and eosin; HPF: High-powered field; HPRT: Hypoxanthine guanine phosphoribosyl transferase; IACUC: Institutional Animal Care and Use Committee; KO: Knockout; MCP1: Monocyte chemoattractant protein 1; MCSF: Macrophage colony-stimulating factor; MMP2: Matrix metalloproteinase 2; MMP9: Matrix metalloproteinase 9; MMP14: Matrix metalloproteinase 14; NFAT1c: Nuclear factor activating T cells 1c; OPG: Osteoprotegerin; OSCAR: Osteoclast-associated immunoglobulin-like receptor; PMN: Polymononuclear; RA: Rheumatoid arthritis; RANKL: Signal receptor activator of nuclear factor-kB ligand; RCAN2: Regulator of calcineurin 2; ROR2: Receptor-tyrosine orphan receptor 2; STIA: Serum transfer-induced arthritis; TNFα: Tumor necrosis factor alpha; TRAP: Tartrate resistant acid phosphatase; Wnt5a: Wingless-type MMTV integration site family, member 5a

Acknowledgements
Not applicable.

Funding
This work was funded by National Institutes of Health (NIH) grants HL120160, HL131006, HL132564, and AG052160 to KW. SM was funded by a T32 grant HL007224. This work was supported by grants from the NIH to CMC (K01AR064313) and HP (AR064546, AR050250, AR054796, AI092490, HL108795), and funds provided to HP by the Mabel Green Myers Chair of Medicine. None of the funding bodies participated in the design of the study or in the collection, analysis, or interpretation of data or in writing the manuscript.

Authors' contributions
SM designed, performed, and analyzed the in vitro and in vivo experiments, and wrote and critically edited the manuscript. MAZ performed and analyzed the in vivo analysis. JJF performed and analyzed the in vivo analysis. JPD performed and analyzed the in vivo analysis. TA performed and analyzed the in vivo analysis. CC performed pathology assessment and analysis of the RA samples. JJ performed pathology assessment and analysis of the RA samples. GKH performed pathology assessment and analysis of the RA samples. FB performed and quantified in vitro analyses and staining. HP provided scientific support and critical editing of the manuscript. KW provided scientific support and critical editing of the manuscript. All authors read and approved the final manuscript and agree to be accountable for all aspects of the work.

Competing interests
The authors declare that they have no competing interests.

Author details
[1]Molecular Cardiology, Whitaker Cardiovascular Institute, Boston University School of Medicine, 700 Albany Street, W-611, Boston, MA 02118, USA. [2]Division of Rheumatology, Department of Medicine, Northwestern University, Feinberg School of Medicine, 240 E. Huron Street, McGaw M338 Chicago, IL, USA. [3]University of Rochester Medical Center, School of Medicine and Dentistry, 601 Elmwood Ave, Box 665, Rochester, NY, USA. [4]Renal Section, Boston University School of Medicine, 650 Albany St, Boston, MA, USA. [5]Department of Pathology, Icahn School of Medicine at Mount Sinai, New York, NY 10029, USA.

References

1. Koenders MI, van den Berg WB. Novel therapeutic targets in rheumatoid arthritis. Trends Pharmacol Sci. 2015;36(4):189–95.
2. McInnes IB, O'Dell JR. State-of-the-art: rheumatoid arthritis. Ann Rheum Dis. 2010;69(11):1898–906.
3. del Rincón ID, Williams K, Stern MP, Freeman GL, Escalante A. High incidence of cardiovascular events in a rheumatoid arthritis cohort not explained by traditional cardiac risk factors. Arthritis Rheum. 2001;44(12): 2737–45.
4. Meune C, Touzé E, Trinquart L, Allanore Y. Trends in cardiovascular mortality in patients with rheumatoid arthritis over 50 years: a systematic review and meta-analysis of cohort studies. Rheumatology (Oxford). 2009;48(10):1309–13.
5. Tanaka Y. Current concepts in the management of rheumatoid arthritis. Korean J Intern Med. 2016;31(2):210–8.
6. Niehrs C. The complex world of WNT receptor signalling. Nat Rev Mol Cell Biol. 2012;13(12):767–79.
7. Bretón-Romero R, Feng B, Holbrook M, Farb MG, Fetterman JL, Linder EA, Berk BD, Masaki N, Weisbrod RM, Inagaki E, et al. Endothelial dysfunction in human diabetes is mediated by Wnt5a-JNK signaling. Arterioscler Thromb Vasc Biol. 2016;36(3):561–9.
8. Farb MG, Karki S, Park SY, Saggese SM, Carmine B, Hess DT, Apovian C, Fetterman JL, Bretón-Romero R, Hamburg NM, et al. WNT5A-JNK regulation of vascular insulin resistance in human obesity. Vasc Med. 2016;21(6):489-96.
9. Kikuchi R, Nakamura K, MacLauchlan S, Ngo DT, Shimizu I, Fuster JJ, Katanasaka Y, Yoshida S, Qiu Y, Yamaguchi TP, et al. An antiangiogenic isoform of VEGF-A contributes to impaired vascularization in peripheral artery disease. Nat Med. 2014;20(12):1464–71.
10. Fuster JJ, Zuriaga MA, Ngo DT, Farb MG, Aprahamian T, Yamaguchi TP, Gokce N, Walsh K. Noncanonical Wnt signaling promotes obesity-induced adipose tissue inflammation and metabolic dysfunction independent of adipose tissue expansion. Diabetes. 2015;64(4):1235–48.
11. Nakamura K, Sano S, Fuster JJ, Kikuchi R, Shimizu I, Ohshima K, Katanasaka Y, Ouchi N, Walsh K. Secreted frizzled-related protein 5 diminishes cardiac inflammation and protects the heart from ischemia/reperfusion injury. J Biol Chem. 2016;291(6):2566–75.
12. Ouchi N, Higuchi A, Ohashi K, Oshima Y, Gokce N, Shibata R, Akasaki Y, Shimono A, Walsh K. Sfrp5 is an anti-inflammatory adipokine that modulates metabolic dysfunction in obesity. Science. 2010;329(5990):454–7.
13. Halleskog C, Dijksterhuis JP, Kilander MB, Becerril-Ortega J, Villaescusa JC, Lindgren E, Arenas E, Schulte G. Heterotrimeric G protein-dependent WNT-5A signaling to ERK1/2 mediates distinct aspects of microglia proinflammatory transformation. J Neuroinflammation. 2012;9:111.
14. Blumenthal A, Ehlers S, Lauber J, Buer J, Lange C, Goldmann T, Heine H, Brandt E, Reiling N. The Wingless homolog WNT5A and its receptor Frizzled-5 regulate inflammatory responses of human mononuclear cells induced by microbial stimulation. Blood. 2006;108(3):965–73.
15. Pereira C, Schaer DJ, Bachli EB, Kurrer MO, Schoedon G. Wnt5A/CaMKII signaling contributes to the inflammatory response of macrophages and is a target for the antiinflammatory action of activated protein C and interleukin-10. Arterioscler Thromb Vasc Biol. 2008;28(3):504–10.
16. Rauner M, Stein N, Winzer M, Goettsch C, Zwerina J, Schett G, Distler JH, Albers J, Schulze J, Schinke T, et al. WNT5A is induced by inflammatory mediators in bone marrow stromal cells and regulates cytokine and chemokine production. J Bone Miner Res. 2012;27(3):575–85.
17. Yu CH, Nguyen TT, Irvine KM, Sweet MJ, Frazer IH, Blumenthal A. Recombinant Wnt3a and Wnt5a elicit macrophage cytokine production and tolerization to microbial stimulation via Toll-like receptor 4. Eur J Immunol. 2014;44(5):1480–90.
18. Sen M, Lauterbach K, El-Gabalawy H, Firestein GS, Corr M, Carson DA. Expression and function of wingless and frizzled homologs in rheumatoid arthritis. Proc Natl Acad Sci USA. 2000;97(6):2791–6.
19. Sen M, Chamorro M, Reifert J, Corr M, Carson DA. Blockade of Wnt-5A/frizzled 5 signaling inhibits rheumatoid synoviocyte activation. Arthritis Rheum. 2001;44(4):772–81.
20. Maeda K, Kobayashi Y, Udagawa N, Uehara S, Ishihara A, Mizoguchi T, Kikuchi Y, Takada I, Kato S, Kani S, et al. Wnt5a-Ror2 signaling between osteoblast-lineage cells and osteoclast precursors enhances osteoclastogenesis. Nat Med. 2012;18(3):405–12.
21. Yamaguchi TP, Bradley A, McMahon AP, Jones S. A Wnt5a pathway underlies outgrowth of multiple structures in the vertebrate embryo. Development. 1999;126(6):1211–23.
22. Monach PA, Mathis D, Benoist C. The K/BxN arthritis model. Curr Protoc Immunol. 2008;Chapter 15:Unit 15.22.
23. Scatizzi JC, Hutcheson J, Bickel E, Woods JM, Klosowska K, Moore TL, Haines GK, Perlman H. p21Cip1 is required for the development of monocytes and their response to serum transfer-induced arthritis. Am J Pathol. 2006;168(5): 1531–41.
24. Scatizzi JC, Mavers M, Hutcheson J, Young B, Shi B, Pope RM, Ruderman EM, Samways DS, Corbett JA, Egan TM, et al. The CDK domain of p21 is a suppressor of IL-1beta-mediated inflammation in activated macrophages. Eur J Immunol. 2009;39(3):820–5.
25. Misharin AV, Cuda CM, Saber R, Turner JD, Gierut AK, Haines GK, Berdnikovs S, Filer A, Clark AR, Buckley CD, et al. Nonclassical Ly6C(-) monocytes drive the development of inflammatory arthritis in mice. Cell Rep. 2014;9(2):591–604.

26. Scatizzi JC, Bickel E, Hutcheson J, Haines GK, Perlman H. Bim deficiency leads to exacerbation and prolongation of joint inflammation in experimental arthritis. Arthritis Rheum. 2006;54(10):3182–93.
27. Scatizzi JC, Hutcheson J, Bickel E, Haines GK, Perlman H. Pro-apoptotic Bid is required for the resolution of the effector phase of inflammatory arthritis. Arthritis Res Ther. 2007;9(3):R49.
28. Perlman H, Georganas C, Pagliari LJ, Koch AE, Haines K, Pope RM. Bcl-2 expression in synovial fibroblasts is essential for maintaining mitochondrial homeostasis and cell viability. J Immunol. 2000;164(10):5227–35.
29. Chen W, ten Berge D, Brown J, Ahn S, Hu LA, Miller WE, Caron MG, Barak LS, Nusse R, Lefkowitz RJ. Dishevelled 2 recruits beta-arrestin 2 to mediate Wnt5A-stimulated endocytosis of Frizzled 4. Science. 2003;301(5638):1391–4.
30. Yagi M, Miyamoto T, Sawatani Y, Iwamoto K, Hosogane N, Fujita N, Morita K, Ninomiya K, Suzuki T, Miyamoto K, et al. DC-STAMP is essential for cell-cell fusion in osteoclasts and foreign body giant cells. J Exp Med. 2005;202(3):345–51.
31. Wang B, Zinselmeyer BH, Runnels HA, LaBranche TP, Morton PA, Kreisel D, Mack M, Nickerson-Nutter C, Allen PM, Miller MJ. In vivo imaging implicates CCR2(+) monocytes as regulators of neutrophil recruitment during arthritis. Cell Immunol. 2012;278(1-2):103–12.
32. Wipke BT, Allen PM. Essential role of neutrophils in the initiation and progression of a murine model of rheumatoid arthritis. J Immunol. 2001; 167(3):1601–8.
33. Duffau P, Menn-Josephy H, Cuda CM, Dominguez S, Aprahamian TR, Watkins AA, Yasuda K, Monach P, Lafyatis R, Rice LM, et al. Promotion of inflammatory arthritis by interferon regulatory factor 5 in a mouse model. Arthritis Rheumatol. 2015;67(12):3146–57.
34. Jung YS, Lee HY, Kim SD, Park JS, Kim JK, Suh PG, Bae YS. Wnt5a stimulates chemotactic migration and chemokine production in human neutrophils. Exp Mol Med. 2013;45, e27.
35. Logan CY, Nusse R. The Wnt signaling pathway in development and disease. Annu Rev Cell Dev Biol. 2004;20:781–810.
36. Kurayoshi M, Yamamoto H, Izumi S, Kikuchi A. Post-translational palmitoylation and glycosylation of Wnt-5a are necessary for its signalling. Biochem J. 2007;402(3):515–23.
37. Bellon M, Ko NL, Lee MJ, Yao Y, Waldmann TA, Trepel JB, Nicot C. Adult T-cell leukemia cells overexpress Wnt5a and promote osteoclast differentiation. Blood. 2013;121(25):5045–54.
38. Bilkovski R, Schulte DM, Oberhauser F, Gomolka M, Udelhoven M, Hettich MM, Roth B, Heidenreich A, Gutschow C, Krone W, et al. Role of WNT-5a in the determination of human mesenchymal stem cells into preadipocytes. J Biol Chem. 2010;285(9):6170–8.
39. Wang Y, Li YP, Paulson C, Shao JZ, Zhang X, Wu M, Chen W. Wnt and the Wnt signaling pathway in bone development and disease. Front Biosci (Landmark Ed). 2014;19:379–407.
40. Helming L, Gordon S. Molecular mediators of macrophage fusion. Trends Cell Biol. 2009;19(10):514–22.
41. Long CL, Humphrey MB. Osteoimmunology: the expanding role of immunoreceptors in osteoclasts and bone remodeling. Bonekey Rep. 2012; 1:59-65.
42. Rajasekaran N, Illges H. Matrix Metalloproteinase MMP-9 Promotes K/BxN Serum Induced Arthritis in Mice. Open J Rheumatol Autoimmune Dis. 2014; 4(1):22-8. doi:10.4236/ojra.2014.41003.
43. MacLauchlan S, Skokos EA, Meznarich N, Zhu DH, Raoof S, Shipley JM, Senior RM, Bornstein P, Kyriakides TR. Macrophage fusion, giant cell formation, and the foreign body response require matrix metalloproteinase 9. J Leukoc Biol. 2009;85(4):617–26.
44. Chabot V, Reverdiau P, Iochmann S, Rico A, Sénécal D, Goupille C, Sizaret PY, Sensebé L. CCL5-enhanced human immature dendritic cell migration through the basement membrane in vitro depends on matrix metalloproteinase-9. J Leukoc Biol. 2006;79(4):767–78.
45. Wucherpfennig AL, Li YP, Stetler-Stevenson WG, Rosenberg AE, Stashenko P. Expression of 92 kD type IV collagenase/gelatinase B in human osteoclasts. J Bone Miner Res. 1994;9(4):549–56.
46. Kusano K, Miyaura C, Inada M, Tamura T, Ito A, Nagase H, Kamoi K, Suda T. Regulation of matrix metalloproteinases (MMP-2, -3, -9, and -13) by interleukin-1 and interleukin-6 in mouse calvaria: association of MMP induction with bone resorption. Endocrinology. 1998;139(3):1338–45.
47. Asquith DL, Miller AM, Hueber AJ, Liew FY, Sattar N, McInnes IB. Apolipoprotein E-deficient mice are resistant to the development of collagen-induced arthritis. Arthritis Rheum. 2010;62(2):472–7.
48. Postigo J, Genre F, Iglesias M, Fernández-Rey M, Buelta L, Carlos Rodríguez-Rey J, Merino J, Merino R. Exacerbation of type II collagen-induced arthritis in apolipoprotein E-deficient mice in association with the expansion of Th1 and Th17 cells. Arthritis Rheum. 2011;63(4):971–80.
49. Archer AM, Saber R, Rose S, Shaffer A, Misharin AV, Tsai F, Haines Iii GK, Dominguez S, Eren M, Vaughan DE, et al. ApoE deficiency exacerbates the development and sustainment of a semi-chronic K/BxN serum transfer-induced arthritis model. J Transl Med. 2016;14(1):170.
50. Rose S, Eren M, Murphy S, Zhang H, Thaxton CS, Chowaniec J, Waters EA, Meade TJ, Vaughan DE, Perlman H. A novel mouse model that develops spontaneous arthritis and is predisposed towards atherosclerosis. Ann Rheum Dis. 2013;72(1):89–95.
51. Catalán V, Gómez-Ambrosi J, Rodríguez A, Pérez-Hernández AI, Gurbindo J, Ramírez B, Méndez-Giménez L, Rotellar F, Valentí V, Moncada R, et al. Activation of noncanonical Wnt signaling through WNT5A in visceral adipose tissue of obese subjects is related to inflammation. J Clin Endocrinol Metab. 2014;99(8):E1407–17.
52. Versini M, Jeandel PY, Rosenthal E, Shoenfeld Y. Obesity in autoimmune diseases: not a passive bystander. Autoimmun Rev. 2014;13(9):981–1000.
53. Feng J, Chen Q, Yu F, Wang Z, Chen S, Jin Z, Cai Q, Liu Y, He J. Body mass index and risk of rheumatoid arthritis: a meta-analysis of observational studies. Medicine (Baltimore). 2016;95(8), e2859.
54. Del Prete A, Salvi V, Sozzani S. Adipokines as potential biomarkers in rheumatoid arthritis. Mediators Inflamm. 2014;2014:425068.
55. Otero M, Lago R, Gomez R, Lago F, Dieguez C, Gómez-Reino JJ, Gualillo O. Changes in plasma levels of fat-derived hormones adiponectin, leptin, resistin and visfatin in patients with rheumatoid arthritis. Ann Rheum Dis. 2006;65(9):1198–201.
56. Yoshino T, Kusunoki N, Tanaka N, Kaneko K, Kusunoki Y, Endo H, Hasunuma T, Kawai S. Elevated serum levels of resistin, leptin, and adiponectin are associated with C-reactive protein and also other clinical conditions in rheumatoid arthritis. Intern Med. 2011;50(4):269–75.
57. Olama SM, Senna MK, Elarman M. Synovial/serum leptin ratio in rheumatoid arthritis: the association with activity and erosion. Rheumatol Int. 2012;32(3):683–90.
58. Giles JT, van der Heijde DM, Bathon JM. Association of circulating adiponectin levels with progression of radiographic joint destruction in rheumatoid arthritis. Ann Rheum Dis. 2011;70(9):1562–8.
59. Bokarewa M, Nagaev I, Dahlberg L, Smith U, Tarkowski A. Resistin, an adipokine with potent proinflammatory properties. J Immunol. 2005;174(9): 5789–95.

17

Traditional Chinese medicine formula Bi-Qi capsule alleviates rheumatoid arthritis-induced inflammation, synovial hyperplasia, and cartilage destruction in rats

Kai Wang[1†], Dongmei Zhang[2†], Yan Liu[1], Xuan Wang[1], Jiantong Zhao[1], Tingting Sun[1], Tingting Jin[1], Baoli Li[2] and Janak L. Pathak[3*]

Abstract

Background: Traditional Chinese medicine (TCM) formula Bi-Qi capsule (Bi-Qi) is a commonly prescribed drug to treat rheumatoid arthritis (RA). However, the mechanism of Bi-Qi-mediated amelioration of RA pathogenesis is still a mystery. Collagen induced arthritis (CIA) in rats is an established model that shares many similarities with RA in humans. In this study we investigated the effect of Bi-Qi on the pathogenesis of CIA in rats.

Methods: CIA was developed in Sprague-Dawley (S.D) rats (n = 60, female) and used as a model resembling RA in humans. Rats were treated with a high or moderate dose of Bi-Qi, or methotrexate (MTX). Effects of the treatment on local joint and systemic inflammation, synovial hyperplasia, cartilage destruction, and other main features in the pathogenesis of CIA were analyzed.

Results: Inflamed and swollen ankles and joints were observed in arthritic rats, while Bi-Qi or MTX treatment alleviated these symptoms. Only the Bi-Qi moderate dose decreased RA-induced serum levels of tumor necrosis factor-alpha (TNF-α). Both Bi-Qi and MTX reduced the interleukin (IL)-18 serum level. Protein levels of cartilage oligomeric matrix protein and osteopontin in serum, synovium, and cartilage were elevated in arthritic rats, while Bi-Qi alleviated these effects. Synovial hyperplasia, inflammatory cell infiltration in synovium and a high degree of cartilage degradation was observed in RA, and Bi-Qi or MTX alleviated this effect. Bi-Qi at the moderate dose was the most effective in mitigating CIA-related clinical complications.

Conclusions: Our findings showed that Bi-Qi alleviates CIA-induced inflammation, synovial hyperplasia, cartilage destruction, and the other main features in the pathogenesis of CIA. This provides fundamental evidence for the anti-arthritic properties of Bi-Qi and corroborates the use of Bi-Qi TCM formula for the treatment of RA.

Keywords: Rheumatoid arthritis, Bi-Qi-capsule, Pathogenesis, Inflammation, Synovial hyperplasia, Cartilage destruction, Methotrexate

* Correspondence: j.pathak@tju.edu.cn
[†]Equal contributors
[3]School of Pharmaceutical Science and Technology, Health Sciences Platform, Tianjin University, Tianjin 300072, China
Full list of author information is available at the end of the article

Background

The Bi-Qi capsule is a TCM formula approved by the Chinese Food and Drug Administration to treat rheumatoid arthritis (RA), cervical spondylosis, scapulohumeral periarthritis, and knee osteoarthritis [1–5]. *Radix Salviae miltiorrhizae* (Dan Shen), *Semen strychni* (Ma Qian Zi), *Radix glycyrrhizae* (Gan Cao), Radix *Codonopsis pilosula* (Dang Shen), *Astragalus membranaceus* (Fisch), Bunge (Huang qi), Notoginseng (San Qi), *Rhizoma Ligustici chuanxiong* (Chuan Xiong), *Radix Achyranthis bidentata* (Huai Niu Xi), and *Rhizoma Atractylodis macrocephalae* (Bai Zhu) are Chinese herbal ingredients of the Bi-Qi capsule. Tanshinone IIA sulfonic sodium, salvianolic acid B, glycyrrhizin, brucine, strychnine, cryptotanshinone, and liquiritin are major compounds present in Bi-Qi extract [6, 7]. Tanshinone IIA sulfonic sodium is a water-soluble extract from *Radix et Rhizoma S. miltiorrhizae* with a strong anti-osteoporotic property [8]. Bi-Qi has been shown to have anti-inflammatory and analgesic properties [3]. However, the mechanism of Bi-Qi-mediated amelioration of RA pathogenesis is still a mystery.

RA is a chronic systemic autoimmune disease which primarily involves synovial joint pain, immobility, and stiffness. RA exhibits extreme variation, ranging from mild, self-limiting disease to rapidly progressive arthritis with extra-articular manifestations [9, 10]. Focal marginal articular erosions, subchondral bone loss, periarticular osteopenia, systemic inflammation, and osteoporosis are the main pathologic stages of skeletal remodeling that characterize RA. RA-related systemic complications affect major vital organs including heart, lung, liver, brain, and bone [11]. Unknown etiology and doubtful prognosis are the main challenges to treating RA. RA initially affects freely movable joints such as joints in the hand, shoulder, knee, and hip. Macrophages, plasma cells, and lymphocytes infiltrate the synovium causing synovial hyperplasia. Increased inflammatory immune cells and fibroblast-like synoviocyte infiltration form pannus and small blood vessels that lead to synovium and cartilage destruction [12, 13]. These cells produce various cytokines and chemokines; among these, TNF-α and IL-18 have been reported to play important role in the pathogenesis of RA [14–16]. Inflamed synovium in RA produces larger amounts of osteopontin (OPN) [17, 18]; it is a pro-inflammatory protein with a critical role in leukocyte migration and production of IL-17 from T cells, thereby play a key role in the pathogenesis of RA [17]. The cartilage oligomeric matrix protein (COMP) is an extracellular matrix protein mainly localized to tendon, cartilage, and pericartilage tissues [19]. Serum and synovial fluid COMP levels are reported to be promising RA diagnostic and prognostic markers [19, 20]. Therefore, TNF-α, IL-18, OPN, and COMP are important markers in investigating the pathogenesis of RA.

Nonsteroidal anti-inflammatory drugs, corticosteroids, disease-modifying anti-rheumatic drugs (DMARDs), and biological agents such as anti-TNF-α and anti-IL-6-receptor antibodies are drugs commonly prescribed to treat RA. However, these drugs have adverse side effects such as bone loss, liver failure, respiratory failure, dermatological damage, and risk of infection [21, 22]. Methotrexate (MTX) is the most commonly used DMARD. Due to its perceived efficacy, acceptable safety profile, low cost, and decades of clinical experience, MTX remains the initial preferred drug and is considered to be the gold standard for treatment of RA [23]. Moreover, pathophysiological and genetic differences among patients also limit the therapeutic effects of these drugs in RA treatment. Compared with the aforementioned conventional Western drugs, TCM provides a more flexible approach to treat RA because various combinations, dosages, and compatibility of herbs are modified according to the pathophysiological condition of the individual patient. TCM formulas have been used for 3000 years, with efficacy to treat disease and neutralize the toxic effects of herbal components in the mixture. Many TCM formulas are in use to treat RA. Bi-Qi is the most commonly used effective TCM formula to treat RA with the least adverse effects. However, the mechanism behind Bi-Qi-mediated mitigation of RA pathogenesis has not yet been investigated.

In this study, we aimed to analyze whether Bi-Qi modulates RA-induced inflammation, synovial hyperplasia, and cartilage destruction. We used a CIA rat model that resembles RA in humans. We treated the CIA with Bi-Qi using two different doses or with MTX. MTX was used as a positive control for RA treatment. Interestingly, Bi-Qi at the moderate dose alleviated the pathogenesis of CIA, i.e., local and systemic inflammation, infiltration of immune cells in synovium, synovium hyperplasia, and cartilage destruction. Bi-Qi moderate dose reduced paw swelling and the arthritic score.

Methods

CIA model

The CIA rat model shares many similarities with RA in humans and is widely used for RA-related in vivo studies. Rats are much larger than mice and provide easy visual analysis of the effect of CIA and treatment against CIA in the ankle and joints. Sprague-Dawley (S.D) rats are an established strain for CIA. Female S.D rats (n = 60, 4 weeks old, 150 ± 10 g in weight) were bought from the Animal Center of Tianjin Military Sciences Academy. Ten rats were randomly selected as control (control group), and CIA was developed in the other 50 rats with slight modification to previously described techniques [24, 25]. Briefly, 10 mg of type II freeze-dried collagen was mixed with 0.05 ml acetic acid and was constantly swung for 12 h at 4 °C to obtain a 2 mg/ml collagen solution. The collagen solution was mixed with incomplete Freund adjuvant (1:1 volume ratio) to obtain a collagen emulsion. The collagen emulsion (0.2 ml) was injected into the rat-tail root. Rats in the control group were injected with an equal volume of saline. At day 7, another 0.1 ml of collagen emulsion was injected into the rat-tail root avoiding the original pinholes. Rats in the control group were again injected with equal volume saline. Animals were housed and acclimatized under standard rat chow diet and tap water under climate-controlled conditions (25 °C; 55% humidity, 12-h light/12-h darkness). All procedures followed were in accordance with the ethical standards of Tianjin Medical University Animal Care and Use Committee guidelines. The study protocol was approved by Animal Experimental Ethical Panel of Tianjin Medical University.

Bi-Qi-extract or MTX treatment

After 2 weeks of collagen emulsion treatment, the arthritis score was measured as described previously [26]. Briefly, a score of 0 represents no red skin and swollen joint symptoms, a score of 1 represents red and slightly swollen ankle or foot, a score of 2 represents red and slightly swollen ankle and mid foot, a score of 3 represents red and moderately swollen ankle and metatarsal joint, and a score of 4 represents red and severely swollen whole ankle, foot and foot plantar. In addition, tail erythema and swelling of the forelimb each score 0.5, which makes a total arthritic score of 5. The severity of arthritis was assessed by visual observation by three independent observers. The observers were unaware about the treatment groups. Paw swelling rate was analyzed every 2 days till day 42 using a water displacement method and a plethysmometer (YLS-7B, Ji'nan Yi Yan science and Technology Development Co., Ltd., Jinan, China) as described previously [27]. Paw swelling rate was measured in both hind limb and average per limb was calculated. Among 50 collagen-treated rats, 43 rats developed severe arthritis (arthritic score >4). Forty rats with an arthritis score >4 were randomly selected and divided into four different groups (ten rats in each group): arthritic group, arthritic rats treated with a high dose of Bi-Qi extract (HDBQ group), arthritic rats treated with a moderate dose of Bi-Qi extract (MDBQ group), and arthritic rats treated with MTX (MTX group). MTX is a drug commonly used to treat rheumatoid arthritis [28] and was therefore used as a positive control in this study. Normal saline in the control group and 0.9 g/kg body weight/day Bi-Qi extract in the HDBQ group or Bi-Qi extract 0.6 g/kg body weight/day in the MDBQ group was gavaged for 4 weeks. In the MTX group, MTX 1.67 mg/kg body weight/week was injected subcutaneously into the abdomen. The dose of MTX was chosen based on the literature [29–31]. Since the dose of MTX mentioned in the literature and used in this study was ~ 10-fold higher than clinical dose, we choose 10-fold and 15-fold higher doses of Bi-Qi. In clinical practice diarrhoea is a commonly observed side effect of Bi-Qi. In this study we also noted occasional diarrhoea in Bi-Qi treated rats. Walking gait, mental alertness, hair color, diet, and stool were observed every 2 days as a physiological and behavioral observation. Body weight was measured every week. Two untreated rats in the arthritic group died at week 5 possibly due to disease severity. Therefore, eight rats were randomly selected from each group to analyze the effect of the treatment.

Serum and tissue collection

Once CIA was established, 2 ml blood was collected from inner canthus. After 4 weeks of treatment with Bi-Qi or MTX, the rats were anesthetized using isoflurane. Blood was collected (7–8 ml) from the abdominal aorta and serum was separated within 1 h of blood collection, by centrifugation for 15 min at 1.500 *g*. The serum was stored without preservative at − 80 °C and then thawed just prior to testing. The rats were killed after blood collection, and skin, fascia, and muscles around the ankles were removed. The left ankles (with the bone) were fixed in 4% paraformaldehyde (PFA) for 72 h. The right ankles were quickly frozen in liquid nitrogen.

Histology and immunohistochemistry assessment

The left ankles were decalcified according to the Plank-Rychlo protocol. Synovium was selected at the ankle joint and cartilage was selected on the surface of the trochleae at ankle joint. For proper tissue selection, synovium and cartilage were confirmed by microscopic morphology study. The PFA fixed tissues were dehydrated in an ascending series of ethanol and embedded in paraffin. Tissue sections of 6-μm thickness were prepared using a rotary microtome (Huiwo Science and Technology Co. Ltd., Shenzhen, China). To analyze the pathological morphology of synovium and cartilage, histological sections were stained with hematoxylin and eosin and pictures were taken at magnification × 400 using a light microscope (Olympus, Japan). For semi-quantitative analysis, five random microscopic fields/images from five random images/rat were analyzed by Image Pro Plus 6.0.

Pathological features of the synovial membranes were analyzed by semi-quantification of inflammatory cell infiltration, synovial cell proliferation, and proliferation of fibrous tissue in the synovium. Neutrophil infiltration was classified as 0–2, i.e., 0, no cells; 0.5, 1–5 cells/high power magnification field (HPF); 1, 6–10 cells/HPF; 1.5, 11–15 cells/HPF; or 2, micro abscess. Lymphocyte infiltration was classified as 0–2 based on number of cells present/HPF. Plasma cells infiltration was classified as 0–2, i.e., 0.5, 1–5 cells/HPF; 1, 6–10 cells/HPF; 1.5, 11–15/HPF; or 2, > 15 cells/HPF. Proliferation of fibrous tissue was classified as 0–2 based on the area of fibrous tissue/HPF. Synovial cell proliferation was classified as 0–2, i.e., 0, no synovial cell infiltration in synovium, 0.5: swollen synovium, 1: swollen synovium with few cells infiltration; 1.5, synovial infiltration in two layers of synovium; 2, synovial infiltration in > 3 layers.

The depth of the damage to the cartilage layer was classified as 0–3, i.e., 0, smooth and intact and smooth cartilage layer; 1, superficial damage of cartilage layer; 2, damage to half of the depth of the cartilage layer; 3, damage of full depth of cartilage layer. The range of damage at the cartilage surface was classified as 0–3, i.e., 0, no damage on cartilage surface; 1, focal damage; 2, > 1/3 to < 2/3 of cartilage surface damage; 3, > 2/3 of cartilage surface damage. Similarly proliferation of fibrous tissue was classified as 0–3 based on the degree of proliferation. Furthermore, inflammatory cell infiltration in the cartilage was classified as 0–3 based on the number of infiltrated cells.

COMP and OPN expression

To analyze COMP and OPN expression in synovium tissue, tissue sections were rehydrated and endogenous peroxidase was quenched with 3% H_2O_2 in PBS with 40% methanol. Antigen retrieval was performed by 20-min incubation with 10 mM citrate buffer at room temperature. After blocking of non-specific binding sites with 10% normal goat serum for 1 h, the sections were incubated overnight at 4 °C with mouse-anti-COMP antibody (Boiss antibodies company, Beijing, China) in PBS or mouse anti-OPN antibody (Boster Bioengineering Co.Ltd., Wuhan, China) in PBS. The sections were incubated for 1 h with 1/100 biotinylated secondary rabbit anti-mouse antibody (ZhongshanJinqiao Bioengineering Co. Ltd., Beijing, China) and for 1 h with horseradish peroxidase-labeled streptavidin (Zhongshan Jinqiao Bioengineering Co. Ltd., Beijing, China). For color development, the sections were incubated with DAB reagent (Zhongshan Jinqiao Bioengineering Co. Ltd., Beijing, China) and counterstained with hematoxylin and pictures were taken at × 400 magnification using a light microscope. For semi-quantitative analysis, five random microscopic fields/images from five random images/rat were analyzed by Image Pro Plus 6.0.

Enzyme-linked immunosorbent assay (ELISA) for OPN, COMP, TNF-α and IL-18

Quantification of OPN, COMP, TNF-α and IL-18 in serum samples was performed using ELISA kits (R&D systems) following the manufacturer's protocol. The minimum detection limit was 5 pg/ml for TNF-α, 5.7 pg/ml for OPN, and 10 pg/ml for IL-18 and COMP.

RNA isolation and quantitative real-time PCR analysis

Cartilage tissue (around 10 mg) frozen at – 80 °C was crushed in a mortar in the presence of liquid nitrogen. Total RNA was isolated using Trizol (Sango Biotech Co. Ltd., Shanghai, China). The concentrations of isolated RNAs were determined using a TECAN Infinite® F200 Pro microtiterplate reader (Thermo Fisher Scientific). cDNA synthesis was performed with 6 μl of total RNA in 20 μl of reaction volume using RevertAid First Strand cDNA Synthesis Kit (Sango Biotech Co. Ltd., Shanghai, China) according to the manufacturer's instructions.

Quantitative expression of COMP and OPN was measured using two-step reverse transcription PCR. Real time PCR reactions were performed using 1 μl cDNA and Hotstart Fluo-PCR mix (Sango Biotech Co. Ltd., Shanghai, China) according to the manufacturer's instructions. The determined cycle threshold (CT) values of the target genes were normalized to the relative expression of the housekeeping gene *Gapdh*. The primer sequence for COMP was forward: 5'-GTGGTGCTCA ATCAGGGAAT-3′, reverse: 5′-G AAGCCAGCGTAGT CATCATC-3′; for OPN it was forward: 5'-AAGCGTG-GAAACACACAGC-3′, reverse: 5'-TTTGGAACTCGCC TGACTG-3′; and for GAPDH it was forward: 5'-CAAC TCCTCAAGATTGTCAGCAA-3′, reverse: 5'-GGCATG GACTGTGGTCATG A-3′.

Statistical analysis

Data are presented as mean ± SD. Effects of different treatments were tested using analysis of variance (ANOVA) followed by Sidak's multiple comparison post hoc test. Differences were considered significant if *P* was < 0.05. Statistical analysis was performed using GraphPad Prism 5.01 (GraphPad Software, Inc., La Jolla, CA, USA).

Results

Collagen treatment successfully induced RA, and Bi-Qi treatment alleviated CIA-related symptoms

Collagen treatment for 2 weeks induced RA in the rats. Rat paws were inflamed and small joints were swollen in rats in the arthritic group (Fig. 1a). The moderate-dose Bi-Qi capsule alleviated arthritis-induced paw inflammation and joint swelling more effectively compared to the high dose Bi-Qi capsule (Fig. 1a, b). The paw swelling rate at day 40, 41, and 42 was dramatically reduced in the Bi-Qi moderate dose group compared to the other groups tested (Fig. 1b). Physiological and behavioral observation identified the negative effect of CIA on walking gait, mental alertness, hair color, and diet. Bi-Qi or MTX treatment slightly alleviated this effect (Additional file 1: Table S1). Slightly loose stool was observed in Bi-Qi or MTX treated groups (Additional file 1: Table S1). Rats in the healthy group had higher body weight at different time points compared to all other rats in the treated and untreated arthritic groups (Additional file 1: Table S2). There was no difference in body weight among the treated and untreated rats in the arthritic groups (Additional file 1: Table S2). Physical and behavioral observation showed no adverse effect of Bi-Qi treatment, except occasional diarrhoea.

The arthritic score was > 4 in the arthritic group from week 2 to 6. Three weeks of treatment with Bi-Qi or MTX did not significantly reduce the arthritic score. Interestingly, 4 weeks of high-dose Bi-Qi, moderate-dose Bi-Qi, and MTX treatment reduced the arthritic score by 13%, 22%, and 15% respectively (Table 1).

Bi-Qi alleviated CIA-induced OPN and COMP expression in synovium, cartilage, and serum

Immunohistochemistry images of the synovium clearly indicated greater expression of OPN and COMP protein in the arthritic group compared to the healthy group (Fig. 2). High-dose or moderate-dose Bi-Qi treatment, or

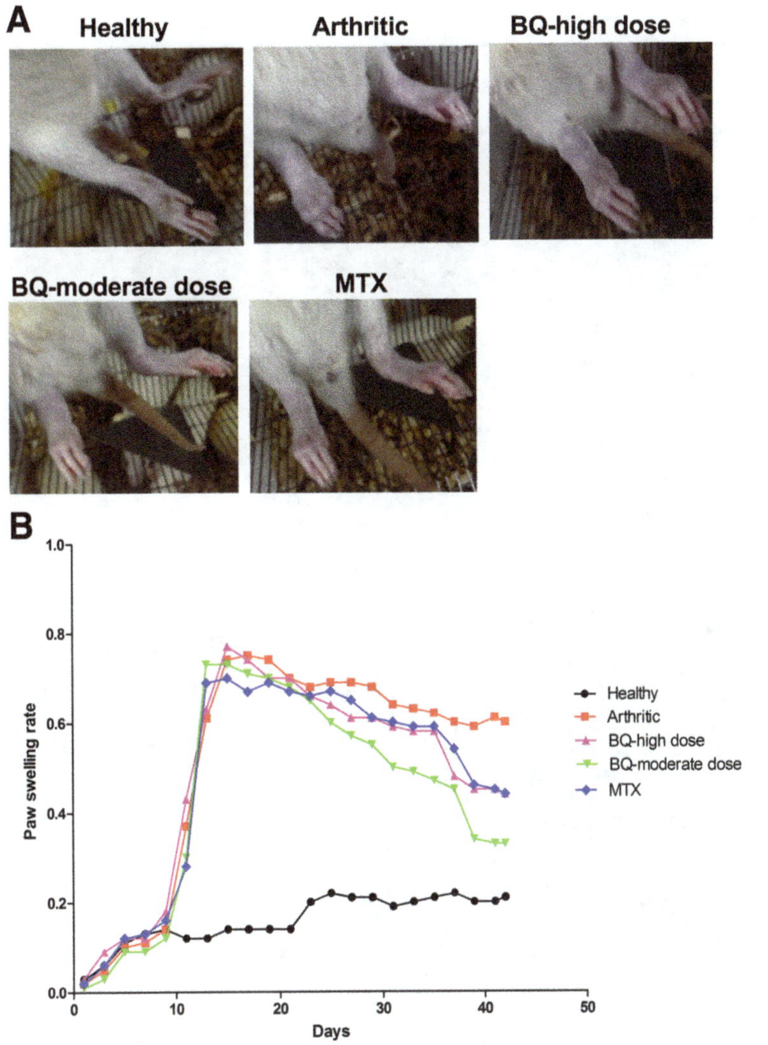

Fig. 1 Bi-Qi capsule or methotrexate (MTX) alleviated paw swelling in collagen induced arthritis (CIA). **a** Representative paws from rats under different treatment conditions at week 6. **b** Quantitative analysis of paw swelling rate. Data shown are the average value/hind limb from eight rats in each group

Table 1 Arthritic score

Group ($n = 8$)	Week 2	Week 3	Week 4	Week 5	Week 6
Healthy	0	0	0	0	0
Arthritic	4.38 ± 0.35	4.50 ± 0.53	4.44 ± 0.32	4.38 ± 0.44	4.25 ± 0.27
BQ high dose	4.44 ± 0.42	4.56 ± 0.42	4.25 ± 0.46	4.13 ± 0.44	3.69 ± 0.37***
BQ moderate dose	4.50 ± 0.46	4.38 ± 0.35	4.19 ± 0.53	3.94 ± 0.32	3.31 ± 0.26****, &
MTX	4.44 ± 0.42	4.44 ± 0.32	4.31 ± 0.26	4.06 ± 0.56	3.63 ± 0.35***

Data are presented as mean ± SD

BQ Bi-Qi capsule, *MTX* methotrexate

Significant effect of treatment compared to arthritic group, ***$P < 0.001$, ****$P < 0.0001$; compared to BQ high-dose and MTX groups, &$P < 0.05$

MTX treatment decreased the arthritis-induced OPN and COMP level in synovium (Fig. 2). Results from quantitative analysis showed that OPN expression in the arthritic synovium was increased by 110% compared to synovium in the healthy group (Fig. 3a). OPN expression was reduced by 27%, 40%, and 29%, respectively in the high-dose Bi-Qi, moderate-dose Bi-Qi, and the MTX groups compared to the arthritic group (Fig. 3a). Moderate dose Bi-Qi reduced OPN expression by 17% compared to high-dose Bi-Qi (Fig. 3a). Similarly, COMP expression was 217% higher in the arthritic synovium compared to that in healthy synovium (Fig. 3b). COMP expression was reduced by 28%, 29%, and 28.5%, respectively, in the high-dose Bi-Qi, moderate-dose Bi-Qi, and MTX groups compared to the arthritic group (Fig. 3b).

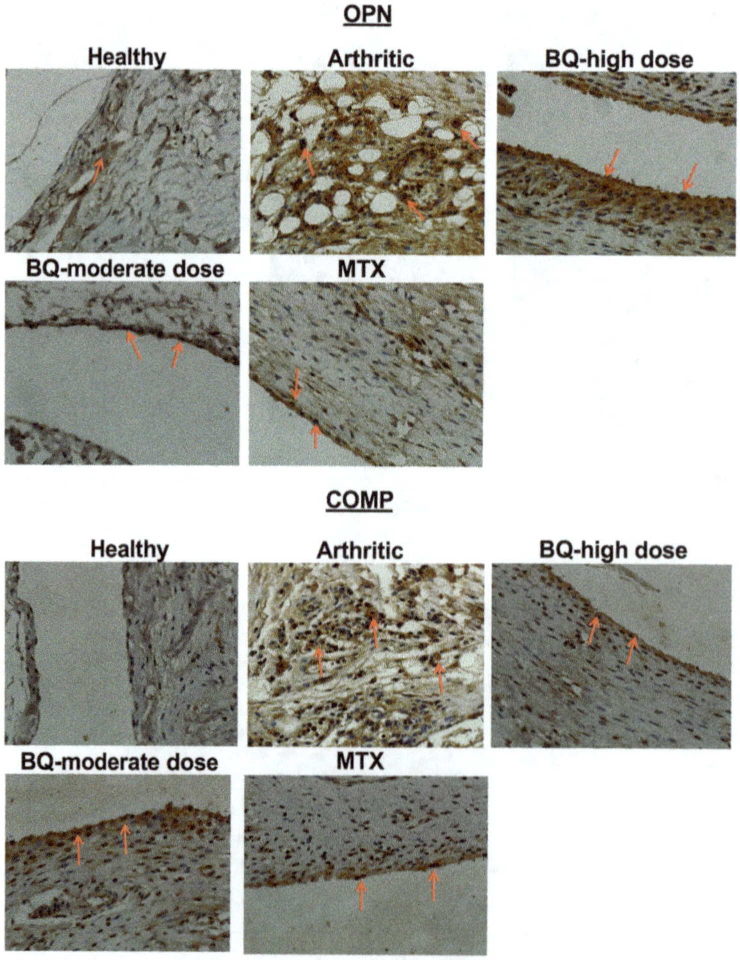

Fig. 2 Collagen-induced arthritis (CIA) enhanced osteopontin (OPN) and cartilage oligomeric matrix protein (COMP) expression in paw joint cartilage, while the Bi-Qi capsule or methotrexate (MTX) treatment reduced this effect. Representative immunohistochemistry images of paw joint synovium with OPN and COMP immunostaining

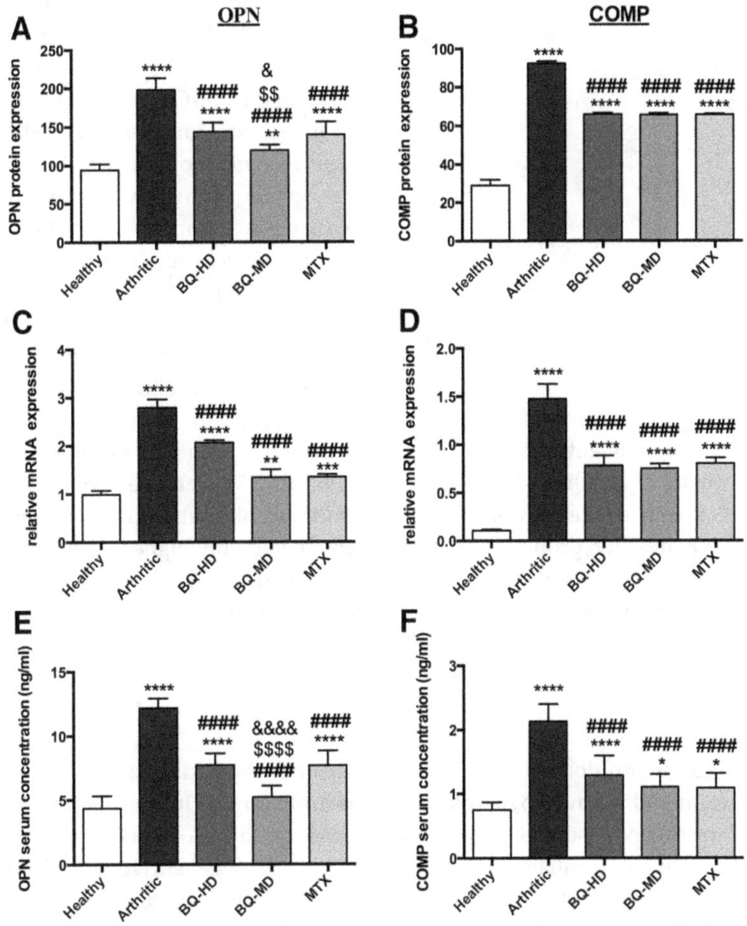

Fig. 3 Bi-Qi capsule (BQ) or methotrexate (MTX) reduced collagen-induced arthritis (CIA)-induced osteopontin (OPN) and cartilage oligomeric matrix protein (COMP) upregulation in serum, and mRNA and protein levels in paw joint tissue. **a, b** OPN and COMP levels in serum. **c, d** OPN and COMP mRNA expression in paw joint cartilage. **e, f** OPN and COMP protein quantification from immunohistochemistry images of paw joint synovium. Data are presented as mean ± SD from eight rats in each group. Significant effect of treatment compared to control: *$^{*}P < 0.05$, $^{**}P < 0.01$, $^{***}P < 0.001$, $^{****}P < 0.0001$*. Significant effect of treatment compared to arthritic group: *$^{\#\#\#\#}P < 0.0001$*. Significant effect of treatment compared to high-dose BQ (BQ-HD): *$^{\$\$}P < 0.01$, $^{\$\$\$\$}P < 0.0001$*. Significant effect of treatment compared to MTX-group: *$^{\&}P < 0.05$, $^{\&\&\&\&}P < 0.0001$. BQ-MD, moderate-dose BQ*

The mRNA expression levels of OPN and COMP were measured in cartilage. OPN expression in arthritic cartilage was 180% higher compared to healthy cartilage. Bi-Qi treatment at high dose, moderate dose, and MTX treatment reduced cartilage OPN expression by 28%, 53%, and 51% respectively, compared to the arthritic group (Fig. 3c). COMP expression in arthritic cartilage was 1400% higher compared to in healthy cartilage. Bi-Qi treatment at high dose, Bi-QI at moderate dose, and MTX treatment reduced cartilage COMP expression by 47%, 49%, and 45%, respectively, compared to the arthritic group (Fig. 3d).

Serum levels of COMP and OPN were measured by ELISA. COMP and OPN serum level in the arthritic group was 184% higher compared to that in the healthy group (Fig. 3e). Bi-Qi high dose, Bi-Qi moderate dose, and MTX treatment reduced serum OPN level by 37%, 57%, and 37%, respectively, compared to the arthritic group. Serum OPN level in the moderate-dose Bi-Qi group was 32% less compared to the high-dose Bi-Qi group (Fig. 3e). Bi-Qi treatment at high dose, Bi-Qi at moderate dose, and MTX treatment reduced serum COMP by 40%, 48%, and 40%, respectively, compared to the arthritic group (Fig. 3f).

Bi-Qi moderate dose decreased arthritis-induced TNF-α and IL-18 serum concentration

Serum concentration of TNF-α was analyzed after 2 weeks of collagen treatment and after 4 weeks of Bi-Qi or MTX treatment. CIA elevated serum TNF-α concentration by 90% and 67% at week 2 and 6, respectively (Table 2). TNF-α serum level was 20% lower in the moderate-dose Bi-Qi group compared to the arthritic group. Bi-Qi treatment at high dose or MTX treatment

Table 2 Serum levels of TNF-α and IL-18

Group (n = 8)	TNF-α (pg/ml)		IL-18 (pg/ml)
	week 2	week 6	week 6
Healthy	22.71 ± 1.79	23.87 ± 5.11	30.28 ± 1.76
Arthritic	43.15 ± 1.57****	39.80 ± 4.38****	38.03 ± 3.35**
BQ-high dose	43.35 ± 1.84****	34.04 ± 5.22**	33.69 ± 4.36
BQ-moderate dose	42.68 ± 2.30****	31.87 ± 2.88*, Δ	32.37 ± 4.20Δ
MTX	43.28 ± 2.29****	33.84 ± 4.39**	32.32 ± 3.61Δ

Data are presented as mean ± SD
BQ Bi-Qi capsule, *MTX* methotrexate
Significant effect of treatment compared to control, $^{**}P < 0.01$, $^{****}P < 0.0001$; compared to arthritic group, $^{\Delta}P < 0.05$

for 4 weeks did not reduce the CIA-induced TNF-α upregulation (Table 2). Serum concentration of IL-18 was measured at after 4 weeks of Bi-Qi or MTX treatment. CIA increased IL-18 serum concentration by 25% at week 6 compared to the healthy group (Table 2). Bi-Qi high-dose treatment for 4 weeks did not affect serum IL-18 level. Bi-Qi treatment at moderate dose or MTX treatment for 4 weeks reduced serum IL-18 level by 17% compared to the arthritic group (Table 2).

Bi-Qi inhibited arthritis-induced infiltration of inflammatory cells in synovium and synovial hyperplasia

Healthy group synovium histology assessment showed an intact layer of synovial cells without inflammatory cell infiltration and synovial hyperplasia (Fig. 4). Disrupted synovial cell layering with inflammatory cell infiltration and synovial hyperplasia were observed in the arthritic group (Fig. 4). Bi-Qi treatment at moderate dose more efficiently alleviated arthritis-induced inflammatory cells infiltration in synovium and synovial hyperplasia compared to Bi-Qi treatment at high dose (Fig. 4).

Quantitative analysis showed that CIA caused a high extent of neutrophil, lymphocyte and plasma cell infiltration in synovium. Bi-Qi moderate-dose treatment reduced neutrophil infiltration by 44% compared to the arthritic group (Table 3). Bi-Qi treatment at high dose or MTX treatment did not affect neutrophil infiltration. Bi-Qi treatment at high or moderate dose reduced lymphocyte infiltration by 38% and 65%, respectively, compared to the arthritic group (Table 3). Bi-Qi treatment at high or moderate dose and MTX treatment reduced plasma cell infiltration by 45%, 62%, and 59%, respectively, compared to the arthritic group. Proliferation of synovial cell and fibrous tissue was remarkably higher in the arthritic group compared to the healthy group. Bi-Qi treatment at moderate dose and MTX treatment reduced synovial cell proliferation by 33% and 44%, respectively, compared to the arthritic group (Table 3).

Bi-Qi treatment alleviated arthritis-induced cartilage destruction and inflammatory cell infiltration in cartilage

Cartilage histology assessment showed a smooth and intact cartilage surface in the healthy group (Fig. 5), while CIA caused deterioration of the cartilage compared to the healthy group, as expected (Fig. 5). Bi-Qi moderate-dose treatment alleviated arthritis-induced cartilage destruction

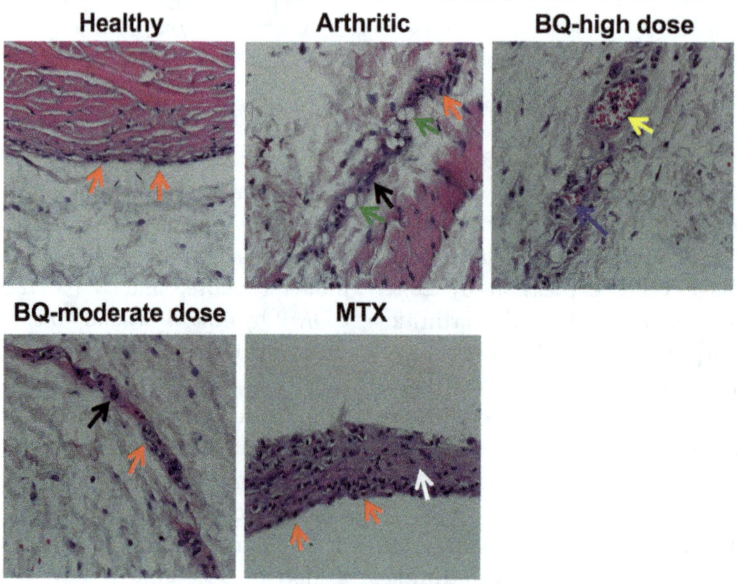

Fig. 4 Bi-Qi capsule (BQ) or methotrexate (MTX) alleviated collagen-induced arthritis (CIA)-induced synovial membrane hyperplasia. Representative histological images of synovial membrane from the paw joint with H&E staining. Red arrow, synoviocyte; black arrow, plasmocyte; green arrow, lymphocyte; yellow arrow, pannus; blue arrow, vascular endothelial cells; white arrow, fibrous tissue growth

Table 3 Pathological feature of synovial membranes

Group (n = 8)	Neutrophil infiltration	Lymphocyte infiltration	Plasma cell infiltration	Synovial cell proliferation	Proliferation of fibrous tissue
Healthy	0	0	0	0	0
Arthritic	1.00 ± 0.46	1.63 ± 0.35	1.81 ± 0.26	1.69 ± 0.37	1.38 ± 0.44
BQ high dose	0.56 ± 0.32	1.00 ± 0.53*	1.00 ± 0.53**	1.19 ± 0.26	0.94 ± 0.42
BQ moderate dose	0.44 ± 0.32*	0.56 ± 0.32***	0.69 ± 0.26****	1.13 ± 0.52*	0.75 ± 0.27*, &
MTX	0.50 ± 0.38	1.06 ± 0.42	0.75 ± 0.38****	0.94 ± 0.32**	1.31 ± 0.37

Data are presented as mean ± SD

BQ Bi-Qi capsule, *MTX* methotrexate

Significant effect of treatment compared to arthritic group, *$P < 0.05$, **$P < 0.01$, ***$P < 0.001$, ****$P < 0.0001$; compared to MTX-group, &$P < 0.05$

more efficiently compared to Bi-Qi high-dose treatment (Fig. 5). Cartilage damage depth and range, proliferation of fibrous tissue, and inflammatory cell infiltration in cartilage were significantly increased in the arthritic group compared to the healthy group (Table 4). Bi-Qi treatment at high or moderate dose and MTX reduced cartilage destruction depth by 52%, 63% and 52%, respectively, compared to the arthritic group. Bi-Qi treatment at high or moderate dose and MTX treatment reduced the extent of cartilage destruction by 55%, 70%, and 64%, respectively, compared to the arthritic group (Table 4). Similarly, Bi-Qi treatment at high or moderate dose and MTX decreased the proliferation of fibrous tissue in cartilage by 50%, 54%, and 50%, respectively, compared to the arthritic group. Moreover, Bi-Qi treatment at high or moderate dose and MTX treatment reduced inflammatory cell infiltration in cartilage by 22%, 54%, and 36%, respectively, compared to the arthritic group (Table 4). The inflammatory cell infiltration rate in the Bi-Qi moderate-dose treatment group was 41% lower compared to Bi-Qi treatment at high dose.

Discussion

Therapies for RA are mostly aimed at reducing the pain, stiffness, and further progression of joint destruction and inflammation. TCM formula-based therapies for RA are popular in China. Combination therapy of TCM formula with DMARDs such as MTX has been reported to be more effective than DMARDs or TCM formula alone [5]. Bi-Qi is one of the commonly prescribed TCM formulas for RA treatment. However, Bi-Qi-mediated modulation of RA pathogenesis has rarely been investigated. In this study, we extensively studied the effect of Bi-Qi on the pathogenesis of CIA, and

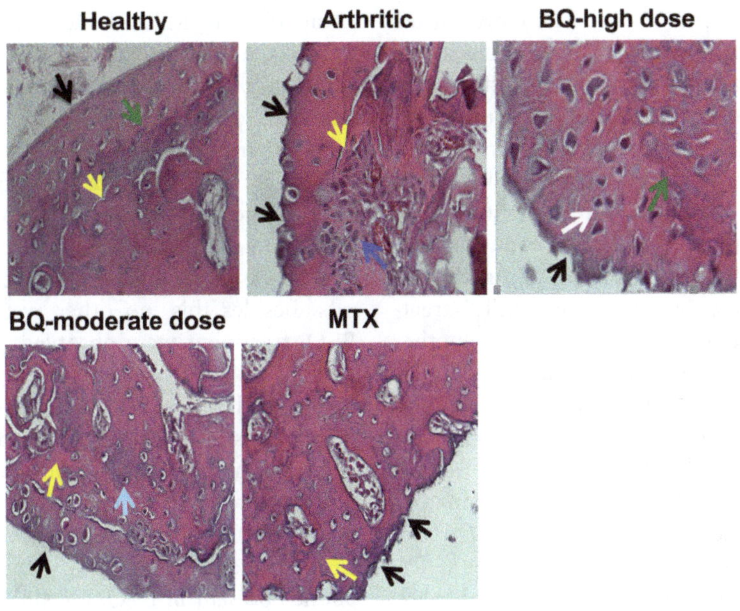

Fig. 5 Bi-Qi capsule (BQ) or methotrexate (MTX) treatment alleviated collagen-induced arthritis (CIA)-induced cartilage destruction. Representative histological images of cartilage from the paw joint stained with H&E. Black arrow, cartilage surface; green arrow, subchondral bone; yellow arrow, bone trabeculae; blue arrow, chondrocytes; white arrow, osteoclast-like cell; light green arrow, osteoblast-like cell

Table 4 Pathological features of cartilage

Group (n = 8)	Cartilage layer damage depth	Cartilage surface damage range	Proliferation of fibrous tissue	Inflammatory cell infiltration
Healthy	0	0	0	0
Arthritic	2.38 ± 0.52	2.50 ± 0.53	2.50 ± 0.53	2.75 ± 0.46
BQ high dose	1.13 ± 0.64****	1.13 ± 0.35****	1.25 ± 0.46***	2.13 ± 0.35*
BQ moderate dose	0.88 ± 0.35****	0.75 ± 0.46****	1.13 ± 0.35****	1.25 ± 0.46****, &
MTX	1.13 ± 0.35****	0.88 ± 0.64****	1.25 ± 0.46***	1.75 ± 0.46***

Data are presented as mean ± SD
BQ Bi-Qi capsule, *MTX* methotrexate
Significant effect of treatment compared to arthritic group, *$P < 0.05$, **$P < 0.01$, ***$P < 0.001$, ****$P < 0.0001$; compared to BQ high-dose group, &$P < 0.05$

MTX treatment was used as a positive control. Bi-Qi alleviated local joint and systemic inflammation, immune cell infiltration to the synovium, synovial hyperplasia and cartilage destruction caused by CIA. The majority of features of CIA pathogenesis were alleviated by treatment with a moderate dose of Bi-Qi. The Bi-Qi treatment at moderate dose alleviated paw swelling, and reduced OPN in serum and synovium, the arthritic score, serum TNF-α, and fibrous tissue proliferation in the synovium more effectively compared to high-dose Bi-Qi. This is the first study to report that Bi-Qi alleviates the majority of RA symptoms in the CIA rat model.

Pro-inflammatory cytokines TNF-α, IL-6, IL-1β, and IL-18 are overexpressed in the joints in RA and play a vital role in the pathogenesis of RA [32, 33]. TNF-α activates the cytokine cascade in the joints in RA via stimulation of pro-inflammatory cytokines and inhibition of anti-inflammatory cytokines [34, 35]. TNF-α upregulation in RA occurs not only in joints and synovial fluid, but also in serum. Although TNF-α inhibitors are available to treat RA, around 30–40% of patients do not respond to this treatment [36–38]. Therefore, partial responders and non-responders to anti-TNF-α constitute a residual group with an unmet clinical need. In this study we found that moderate-dose Bi-Qi but not MTX treatment inhibited a rise in the TNF-α serum level in CIA. Our finding is in accordance with the findings from the clinical study by Nishina and colleagues who reported that MTX treatment is unable to reduce serum TNF-α in patients with early RA [39]. Similarly, we found that both moderate-dose Bi-Qi and MTX treatment slightly alleviated the rise in serum IL-18, another key player in RA pathogenesis. Rooney and colleagues reported that DMARD treatment in patients with RA slightly downregulates serum IL-18, but highly alleviates synovial IL-18 [40]. This indicates that the Bi-Qi might have potential to downregulate the pro-inflammatory cytokines in RA-affected joints.

COMP is a serum marker for disease activity in RA and a potential therapeutic target to treat RA [41]. Clinical studies have shown that DMARDs do not reduce serum COMP in RA [42]. Anti-TNF-α therapy slightly alleviates serum COMP (by 7.5%) in RA after 6 months of treatment [43]. Interestingly, we found that Bi-Qi remarkably reduced serum COMP (by 38%) in CIA. OPN is another protein highly expressed in RA, which regulates cytokine production in macrophages, dendritic cells, and T cells, and thereby activates the inflammation cascade [16, 17]. Clinical studies have shown that DMARDs and anti-TNF-α therapy in RA reduce serum OPN [44]. We found that Bi-Qi treatment at moderate dose remarkably reduced serum OPN (by 57%) in CIA. Moreover, MTX treatment efficiently reduced serum OPN. Bi-Qi treatment greatly reduced COMP and OPN in synovial and joint cartilage. Our results showed that Bi-Qi has the potential to reduce COMP and OPN expression in CIA.

DMARDs and other biological therapies reduce synovial hyperplasia, cartilage destruction, inflammatory cell infiltration, and disease activity score in RA [45]. We found that Bi-Qi treatment at moderate dose reduced the arthritic score, inflammatory cell infiltration, synovial hyperplasia, cartilage destruction, and pannus formation as effectively as MTX treatment. Bi-Qi is very cheap in comparison to MTX. Folic acid is usually prescribed to reduce the adverse effect of MTX. In the field of TCM, the combination of different TCM plant extracts is supposed to synergistically nullify the adverse effect of each other. Bi-Qi has been formulated based on the 3000 years of practice of TCM to minimize the systemic adverse effects. However, Bi-Qi treatment has an adverse effect on the gastrointestinal tract causing diarrhoea, which was occasionally observed in the Bi-Qi-treated rats. Besides this, no other systemic adverse effects of Bi-Qi treatment were observed. However, future studies focused on the possible adverse effect of Bi-Qi in vital organs and systems are highly essential. Among major compounds of Bi-Qi, salvianolic acid B is an antioxidant, glycyrrhizin has anti-autoimmune-reactive properties, brucine is an anti-inflammtory and analgesic compound, Strychnine is a convulsant, and tanshinone IIA is active against oxidative stress [7]. However, many other compounds present in Bi-Qi are still unknown. Identification of all compounds present in Bi-Qi, their metabolism and systemic adverse effects will provide the important insights to corroborate the use of Bi-Qi as a potential therapy for RA. In this study, moderate-dose Bi-Qi more efficiently alleviated CIA-induced inflammation, synovial hyperplasia, and cartilage destruction compared to high-dose Bi-Qi. For a clear explanation of this effect, further studies are needed focusing on the dose-dependent effect of Bi-Qi on molecular and cellular signaling of immune cells involved in RA pathogenesis.

Conclusions

Bi-Qi alleviated local joint and systemic inflammation, synovial hyperplasia and cartilage distruction caused by CIA. Moderate dose Bi-Qi treated the majority of CIA pathogenesis. This provides fundamental evidence for the anti-arthritic properties of Bi-Qi and corroborates the use of Bi-Qi TCM formula for the treatment of RA.

Abbreviations

Bi-Qi: Bi-Qi capsule; CIA: Collagen induced arthritis; COMP: Cartilage oligomeric matrix protein; DMARDs: Disease-modifying anti-rheumatic drugs; ELISA: Enzyme-linked immunosorbent assay; HPF: High-powered field; IL-18: Interleukin-18; MTX: Methotrexate; OPN: Osteopontin; PBS: Phosphate-buffered saline; RA: Rheumatoid arthritis; S.D rats: Sprague-Dawley rats; TCM: Traditional Chinese medicine; TNF-α: Tumor necrosis factor-alpha

Acknowledgements

The authors would like to thank Prof. Matthias Bureik for proofreading the manuscript.

Funding

Not applicable.

Authors' contributions

KW, LB, and JLP designed the study and interpreted the data. YL, XW, JZ, TS, and TJ helped in experiments and data collection. KW and DM performed statistical analysis and drafted the manuscript. All the authors critically reviewed the manuscript. All authors read and approved the final manuscript.

Competing interests

The authors declare that they have no competing interests.

Author details

[1]Department of International Medicine, Geriatric Disease Research Institute, Tianjin Hospital, Tianjin 300211, China. [2]Department of Traditional Chinese Medicine, Tianjin Medical University General Hospital, Tianjin 300070, China. [3]School of Pharmaceutical Science and Technology, Health Sciences Platform, Tianjin University, Tianjin 300072, China.

References

1. Liu W, Zhang L, Xu Z. Clinical observation on treatment of rheumatoid arthritis with biqi capsule. Zhongguo Zhong Xi Yi Jie He Za Zhi. 2006;26(2):157–9.
2. Yu-xuan L, Wen-Wei L, Yu Z, Li-ping W. Clinical and pharmacological research progress of Biqi capsule in nearly three years. Chinese J Tradit Chinese Med. 2011;26(11):2651–3.
3. Liu YX, Zhao Y, Liu J, Guo DL, Chen L, Liu WW. Biqi capsule analgesic effect experimental study on CCI model rats. Chinese J Tradit Chinese Med. 2013;28(6):1737–9.
4. Zhang ZY, Guang-yue X, Sun XW, Hou XH, Xue L. Clinical effect of Biqi capsule in the treatment of knee osteoarthritis. Chinese J Tradit Chinese Med. 2013;28(8):2467–9.
5. Jie HY, Wu QF, Ding ZX. Clinical study of Biqi capsule combined with methotrexate for treatment of rheumatoid arthritis. Zhongguo Zhong Xi Yi Jie He Za Zhi. 2012;32(2):195–8.
6. Liu J, Han FM, Chen Y. Simultaneous determination of brucine, strychnine and salvianolic acid B in Biqi capsule by high performance liquid chromatography. Chin J Anal Chem. 2009;37(4):609–12.
7. Wang QS, Cui YL, Wang YF, Chi W. Effects of compounds from bi-qi capsule on the expression of inflammatory mediators in lipopolysaccharide-stimulated RAW 264.7 macrophages. J Ethnopharmacol. 2011;136(3):480–7.
8. Panwar P, Xue L, Soe K, Srivastava K, Law S, Delaisse JM, Bromme D. An ectosteric inhibitor of cathepsin K inhibits bone resorption in ovariectomized mice. J Bone Miner Res. 2017;32(12):2415–30.
9. Lee DM, Weinblatt ME. Rheumatoid arthritis. Lancet. 2001;358(9285):903–11.
10. Young A, Koduri G. Extra-articular manifestations and complications of rheumatoid arthritis. Best Pract Res Clin Rheumatol. 2007;21(5):907–27.
11. Alam J, Jantan I, Bukhari SNA. Rheumatoid arthritis: recent advances on its etiology, role of cytokines and pharmacotherapy. Biomed Pharmacother. 2017;92:615–33.
12. Aletaha D, Neogi T, Silman AJ, Funovits J, Felson DT, Bingham CO 3rd, Birnbaum NS, Burmester GR, Bykerk VP, Cohen MD, et al. 2010 Rheumatoid arthritis classification criteria: an American College of Rheumatology/ European League Against Rheumatism collaborative initiative. Arthritis Rheum. 2010;62(9):2569–81.
13. McInnes IB, Schett G. The pathogenesis of rheumatoid arthritis. N Engl J Med. 2011;365(23):2205–19.
14. Matsuno H, Yudoh K, Katayama R, Nakazawa F, Uzuki M, Sawai T, Yonezawa T, Saeki Y, Panayi GS, Pitzalis C, et al. The role of TNF-alpha in the pathogenesis of inflammation and joint destruction in rheumatoid arthritis (RA): a study using a human RA/SCID mouse chimera. Rheumatology (Oxford). 2002;41(3):329–37.
15. Volin MV, Koch AE. Interleukin-18: a mediator of inflammation and angiogenesis in rheumatoid arthritis. J Interferon Cytokine Res. 2011;31(10):745–51.
16. Ruth JH, Park CC, Amin MA, Lesch C, Marotte H, Shahrara S, Koch AE. Interleukin-18 as an in vivo mediator of monocyte recruitment in rodent models of rheumatoid arthritis. Arthritis Res Ther. 2010;12(3):R118.
17. Chen GJ, Zhang X, Li RS, Fang L, Niu XY, Zheng YX, He DY, Xu R, Zhang JWZ. Role of osteopontin in synovial Th17 differentiation in rheumatoid arthritis. Arthritis Rheum. 2010;62(10):2900–8.
18. Zhang FJ, Luo W, Li YS, Gao SG, Lei GH. Role of osteopontin in rheumatoid arthritis. Rheumatol Int. 2015;35(4):589–95.
19. Tseng S, Reddi AH, Di Cesare PE. Cartilage oligomeric matrix protein (COMP): a biomarker of arthritis. Biomark Insights. 2009;4:33–44.
20. Liu FX, Wang XJ, Zhang XD, Ren CA, Xin J. Role of serum cartilage oligomeric matrix protein (COMP) in the diagnosis of rheumatoid arthritis (RA): a case-control study. J Int Med Res. 2016;44(4):940–9.
21. Baschant U, Lane NE, Tuckermann J. The multiple facets of glucocorticoid action in rheumatoid arthritis. Nat Rev Rheumatol. 2012;8(11):645–55.
22. Albrecht K, Muller-Ladner U. Side effects and management of side effects of methotrexate in rheumatoid arthritis. Clin Exp Rheumatol. 2010;28(5 Suppl 61):S95–101.
23. Shinde CG, Venkatesh MP, Kumar TM, Shivakumar HG. Methotrexate: a gold standard for treatment of rheumatoid arthritis. J Pain Palliat Care Pharmacother. 2014;28(4):351–8.
24. Trentham DE, Townes AS, Kang AH. Autoimmunity to type II collagen an experimental model of arthritis. J Exp Med. 1977;146(3):857–68.
25. Brand DD, Latham KA, Rosloniec EF. Collagen-induced arthritis. Nat Protoc. 2007;2(5):1269–75.
26. Mossiat C, Laroche D, Prati C, Pozzo T, Demougeot C, Marie C. Association between arthritis score at the onset of the disease and long-term locomotor outcome in adjuvant-induced arthritis in rats. Arthritis Res Ther. 2015;17:184.

25. Brand DD, Latham KA, Rosloniec EF. Collagen-induced arthritis. Nat Protoc. 2007;2(5):1269–75.
26. Mossiat C, Laroche D, Prati C, Pozzo T, Demougeot C, Marie C. Association between arthritis score at the onset of the disease and long-term locomotor outcome in adjuvant-induced arthritis in rats. Arthritis Res Ther. 2015;17:184.
27. Magari K, Miyata S, Ohkubo Y, Mutoh S. Inflammatory cytokine levels in paw tissues during development of rat collagen-induced arthritis: effect of FK506, an inhibitor of T cell activation. Inflamm Res. 2004;53(9):469–74.
28. Pavy S, Constantin A, Pham T, Gossec L, Maillefert JF, Cantagrel A, Combe B, Flipo RM, Goupille P, Le Loet X, et al. Methotrexate therapy for rheumatoid arthritis: clinical practice guidelines based on published evidence and expert opinion. Joint Bone Spine. 2006;73(4):388–95.
29. Liu DY, Lon HK, Wang YL, DuBois DC, Almon RR, Jusko WJ. Pharmacokinetics, pharmacodynamics and toxicities of methotrexate in healthy and collagen-induced arthritic rats. Biopharm Drug Dispos. 2013;34(4):203–14.
30. Le Goff B, Soltner E, Charrier C, Maugars Y, Redini F, Heymann D, Berthelot JM. A combination of methotrexate and zoledronic acid prevents bone erosions and systemic bone mass loss in collagen induced arthritis. Arthritis Res Ther. 2009;11(6):R185.
31. Koyama A, Tanaka A, To H. Daily oral administration of low-dose methotrexate has greater antirheumatic effects in collagen-induced arthritis rats. J Pharm Pharmacol. 2017;69(9):1145–54.
32. McInnes IB, Schett G. Cytokines in the pathogenesis of rheumatoid arthritis. Nat Rev Immunol. 2007;7(6):429–42.
33. Gracie JA, Forsey RJ, Chan WL, Gilmour A, Leung BP, Greer MR, Kennedy K, Carter R, Wei XQ, Xu D, et al. A proinflammatory role for IL-18 in rheumatoid arthritis. J Clin Invest. 1999;104(10):1393–401.
34. Firestein GS. Evolving concepts of rheumatoid arthritis. Nature. 2003; 423(6937):356–61.
35. Choy EH, Panayi GS. Cytokine pathways and joint inflammation in rheumatoid arthritis. N Engl J Med. 2001;344(12):907–16.
36. Maini RN, Feldmann M. How does infliximab work in rheumatoid arthritis? Arthritis Res. 2002;4(Suppl 2):S22–8.
37. Prajapati R, Plant D, Barton A. Genetic and genomic predictors of anti-TNF response. Pharmacogenomics. 2011;12(11):1571–85.
38. Thomson TM, Lescarbeau RM, Drubin DA, Laifenfeld D, de Graaf D, Fryburg DA, Littman B, Deehan R, Van Hooser A. Blood-based identification of non-responders to anti-TNF therapy in rheumatoid arthritis. BMC Med Genet. 2015;8:26.
39. Nishina N, Kaneko Y, Kameda H, Kuwana M, Takeuchi T. Reduction of plasma IL-6 but not TNF-alpha by methotrexate in patients with early rheumatoid arthritis: a potential biomarker for radiographic progression. Clin Rheumatol. 2013;32(11):1661–6.
40. Rooney T, Murphy E, Benito M, Roux-Lombard P, FitzGerald O, Dayer JM, Bresnihan B. Synovial tissue interleukin-18 expression and the response to treatment in patients with inflammatory arthritis. Ann Rheum Dis. 2004;63(11):1393–8.
41. El Defrawy AO, Gheita TA, Raslan HM, El Ansary MM, El Awar AH. Serum and synovial cartilage oligomeric matrix protein levels in early and established rheumatoid arthritis. Z Rheumatol. 2016;75(9):917–23.
42. Benucci M, Meacci F, Manfredi M, Gobbi FL, Infantino M, Ricci C, Sarzi-Puttini P, Atzeni F. Can tocilizumab decrease cartilage oligomeric matrix protein levels and disease activity in patients with long-standing rheumatoid arthritis? Curr Rheumatol Rev. 2014;10(2):131–5.
43. Kawashiri SY, Kawakami A, Ueki Y, Imazato T, Iwamoto N, Fujikawa K, Aramaki T, Tamai M, Nakamura H, Origuchi T, et al. Decrement of serum cartilage oligomeric matrix protein (COMP) in rheumatoid arthritis (RA) patients achieving remission after 6 months of etanercept treatment: comparison with CRP, IgM-RF, MMP-3 and anti-CCP Ab. Joint Bone Spine. 2010;77(5):418–20.
44. Ji HI, Lee SH, Song R, Yang HI, Lee YA, Hong SJ, Kim S, Park YB, Lee SK, Yoo MC, et al. Serum level of osteopontin as an inflammatory marker does not indicate disease activity or responsiveness to therapeutic treatments in patients with rheumatoid arthritis. Clin Rheumatol. 2014;33(3):397–402.
45. Vieira-Sousa E, Gerlag DM, Tak PP. Synovial tissue response to treatment in rheumatoid arthritis. Open Rheumatol J. 2011;5:115–22.

Structural cartilage damage attracts circulating rheumatoid arthritis synovial fibroblasts into affected joints

Jan Hillen[1,2], Christiane Geyer[3], Marianne Heitzmann[1], Denise Beckmann[1], Annika Krause[1], Ina Winkler[3], Hermann Pavenstädt[5], Christoph Bremer[3,4], Thomas Pap[1] and Adelheid Korb-Pap[1*]

Abstract

Background: Rheumatoid arthritis synovial fibroblasts (RASFs) are known to travel via the bloodstream from sites of cartilage destruction to new locations where they reinitiate the destructive processes at distant articular cartilage surfaces. In this study, we examined the role of interleukin (IL)-1-induced cartilage changes and their chemotactic effect on RASF transmigratory capacity.

Methods: To investigate synovial fibroblast (SF) transmigration through endothelial layers, we used a modified Boyden chamber with an endothelioma cell layer (bEnd.5) as a barrier and IL-1-treated murine cartilage explants as a chemotactic stimulus for SFs from human tumor necrosis factor–transgenic (hTNFtg) mice. We injected recombinant IL-1 or collagenase into knee joints of wild-type mice, followed by tail vein injection of fluorescence-labeled hTNFtg SFs. The distribution and intensity of transmigrating hTNFtg SFs were measured by fluorescence reflectance imaging with X-ray coregistration. Toluidine blue staining was performed to evaluate the amount of cartilage destruction.

Results: Histomorphometric analyses and in vivo imaging revealed a high degree of cartilage proteoglycan loss after intra-articular IL-1 and collagenase injection, accompanied by an enhanced in vivo extravasation of hTNFtg SFs into the respective knee joints, suggesting that structural cartilage damage contributes significantly to the attraction of hTNFtg SFs into these joints. In vitro results showed that degraded cartilage was directly responsible for the enhanced transmigratory capacity because stimulation with IL-1-treated cartilage, but not with IL-1 or cartilage alone, was required to increase hTNFtg SF migration.

Conclusions: The present data indicate that structural cartilage damage facilitates the migration of arthritic SF into affected joints. The prevention of early inflammatory cartilage damage may therefore help prevent the progression of rheumatoid arthritis and its spread to previously unaffected joints.

Keywords: Rheumatoid arthritis, Synovial fibroblasts, Transmigration, In vivo imaging, Mouse model

Background

Rheumatoid arthritis (RA) is a chronic inflammatory disorder that leads to symmetrical polyarthritis characterized by synovial inflammation, cartilage destruction, and bone erosions [1, 2]. Research in recent years has identified synovial fibroblasts (SFs) in the lining layer of the hyperplastic synovial membrane as key player in the destructive process in RA [3]. SFs actively contribute to joint destruction by their secretion of matrix-degrading enzymes and inflammatory cytokines [3–6]. This aggressive phenotype is unique for SFs obtained from patients with RA (RASFs) [7]. Interestingly, RASFs retain their destructive potential in the absence of an inflammatory environment, as demonstrated by studies using mice with severe combined immunodeficiency (SCID) [8, 9]. In a recently published study using this SCID mouse model, it was shown that RASFs are more than just resident, immobile cells within the destructive synovial

* Correspondence: korba@uni-muenster.de
[1]Institute of Experimental Musculoskeletal Medicine, University Hospital Muenster, Albert-Schweitzer-Campus 1, D3, 48149 Muenster, Germany
Full list of author information is available at the end of the article

pannus. They have been suggested to contribute to the spreading of disease by their ability to leave cartilage destruction sites, migrate via the bloodstream, and reinitiate the destructive process at distant articular cartilage surfaces [10].

Because the ability of RASFs to enter and leave the bloodstream was demonstrated in a SCID mouse coimplantation model, it must be at least in part independent on a stimulated immune system. This suggests that not only cytokines implicated in immune processes but also other signals attract RASFs to cartilage surfaces and facilitate their transmigration at sites of extravasation. In this context, structural changes occurring in the articular cartilage early in the course of RA might be of importance as such signal for the diapedesis of RASFs. At present, very little is known about the early pathological changes within articular cartilage during RA, although it is widely agreed that biocellular changes precede the onset of arthritis development [11, 12]. Also, several lines of evidence suggest that cartilage damage, and particularly the loss of proteoglycans, precedes the attachment and activation of SFs at least in animal models of RA [13, 14].

On the basis of these data, we hypothesized that, in addition to alterations in the immune response, early cartilage damage is one important factor contributing to joints being affected by RA and potentially in the spread of the disease by attracting activated SFs into previously unaffected joints. The aim of this study was to substantiate this hypothesis by investigating the role of cartilage changes in mediating the transmigratory capacity of RASFs in a modified Boyden chamber assay and in an in vivo mouse model using fluorescent cell trackers. We obtained SFs from the human tumor necrosis factor–transgenic (hTNFtg) mouse model of RA and used interleukin (IL)-1 for the induction of intra-articular (IA) cartilage damage because it has been shown to initiate and mediate cartilage degradation in a mouse model of RA without affecting synovial inflammation [14–16].

Methods

Animals

C57BL/6 wild-type (WT) mice aged 12 weeks were used for the IA injection of cytokines and subsequent intravenous (IV) application of SFs. The injected SFs were obtained from mice heterozygous for the transgene of 3′-modified human soluble tumor necrosis factor-α (hTNFtg line Tg197, genetic background C57BL/6). These mice were generated and kindly provided by Dr. George Kollias and his group (Alexander Fleming Biomedical Sciences Research Center, Vari, Greece) [17]. For in vivo imaging and joint injections, inhalational anesthesia (Vetland Medical Sales and Services, Louisville, KY, USA) was performed by using 2.5% isoflurane with an oxygen flow rate of 1.0 L/minute. For ex vivo imaging and preparation of murine tissue, the animals were killed by cervical dislocation. The mice were bred in the animal facility at the University Hospital Muenster under standard conditions, and all animal procedures were approved by the local ethics committee.

Tissues and cells

SFs were isolated from the hind paws of WT and hTNFtg mice. The skin and surrounding tissue of the hind paw were removed, and the synovial tissue was exposed to enzymatic digestion as previously described [18]. Cells were then cultured in DMEM (Sigma-Aldrich, Steinheim, Germany) at 37 °C in a 5% CO_2 atmosphere. The medium was supplemented with 10% fetal calf serum (FCS; Biochrom, Berlin, Germany), 100 U/ml penicillin, and 10 μg/ml streptomycin (PAA Laboratories, Pasching, Austria). Cells at passages 3–5 were used for all experiments.

Isolation of murine femoral hip cartilage was performed as previously described [13]. In short, WT mice were killed at an age of 4–5 weeks, hip joints were dissected, and cartilage caps were isolated aseptically. Cartilage tissue was then cultivated in high-glucose DMEM containing 10% FCS, 100 U/ml penicillin, and 10 μg/ml streptomycin (PAA Laboratories, Pasching, Austria), 10 mM HEPES, and 50 μg/500 ml ascorbic acid for 24 h at 37 °C in a 5% CO_2 atmosphere.

In vitro transmigration assay

To study the effects of cytokines and cartilage on the transmigration of SFs, an in vitro transmigration assay using a modified Boyden chamber was established (Fig. 1). For this purpose, cells from the blood-brain barrier (brain endothelioma 5 cell line [b.End5]), known for the formation of close tight junctions [19], were seeded and grown to confluence on a laminin-coated porous membrane (8-μm Transwell©; Sigma-Aldrich). Where indicated, the endothelium was stimulated by adding 50 ng/ml recombinant murine TNF-α (R&D Systems, Wiesbaden, Germany) into the upper compartment to facilitate the transmigration. TNF-α was removed after 4 h, and the SFs were seeded onto the endothelial layer in the upper compartment. Depending on the assay, the lower compartment was filled with medium alone (10% FCS gradient between the compartments) or with different stimulating agents such as 10 ng/ml recombinant murine IL-1β (R&D Systems), murine cartilage hip joint explants (three cartilage hip caps per well), or 50 ng/ml monocyte chemoattractant protein (MCP)-1 (R&D Systems), which were added to study their chemotactic effects on SFs. After a transmigration time of 16 h the SFs that had successfully migrated through the b.End5 layer were trypsinized from the basal layer and counted

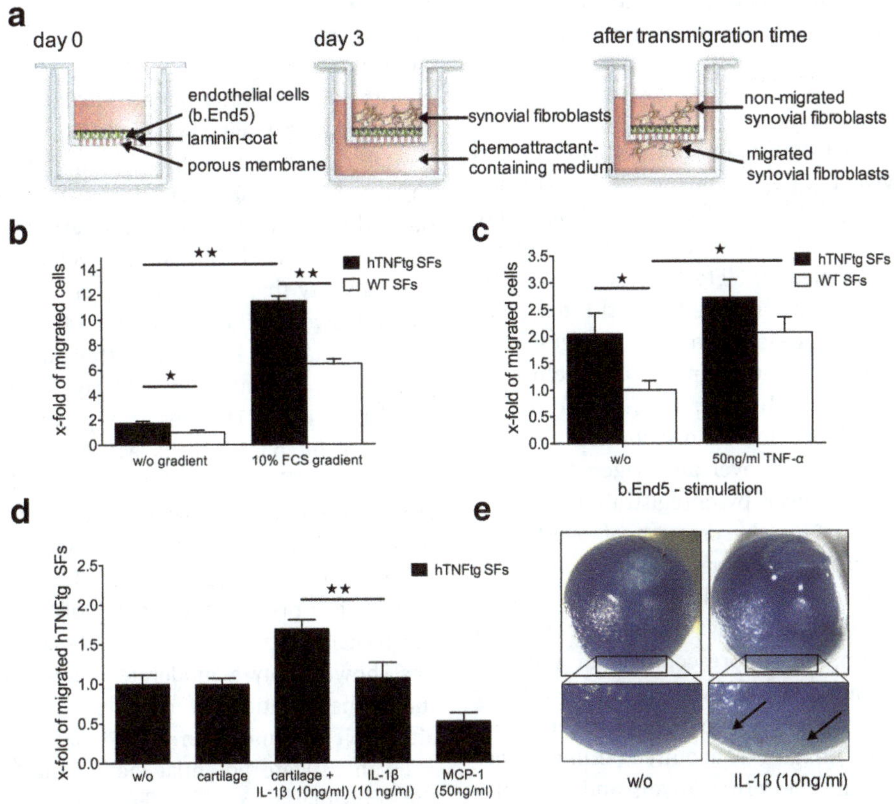

Fig. 1 Cartilage coincubation with interleukin (IL)-1 stimulates transmigration of human tumor necrosis factor–transgenic (hTNFtg) synovial fibroblasts (SFs). **a** Schematic overview showing a modified Boyden chamber with a brain endothelioma 5 cell line (b.End5) layer on a laminin-coated porous membrane. SFs were seeded onto the b.End5 layer into the upper compartment, whereas the lower compartment contained different chemoattractant media. **b** Quantification of transmigrated SFs shows the significantly increased transmigration rate of hTNFtg SFs compared with SFs derived from WT mice (WTSFs), particularly when a fetal calf serum (FCS) gradient was generated. **c** Quantification of transmigrated SFs through an endothelial cell layer. hTNFtg SFs showed a significantly higher transmigratory capacity than WTSFs when migrating through an unstimulated b.End5 endothelium. TNF-α stimulation of the b.End5 layer prior to the seeding of SFs further increased the transmigration of both hTNFtg SFs and WTSFs, showing a significant increase for WTSFs. **d** Coincubation of murine cartilage explants with IL-1β in the lower compartment significantly increased the transmigration of hTNFtg SFs. In contrast, neither cartilage nor IL-1β alone was sufficient to enhance the transmigratory capacity of hTNFtg SFs. **e** Representative images of cartilage hip caps showing IL-1-induced proteoglycan loss (*arrows*) via toluidine blue staining. The values represent the mean ± SEM of at least three independent experiments consisting of duplicates as *x*-fold of (**b**) migrated WTSFs without gradient, (**c**) migrated WTSFs without b.End5 stimulation, or (**d**) migrated hTNFtg SFs without chemoattractant medium. $^{*}p < 0.05$, $^{**}p < 0.01$, Student's *t* test. *MCP-1* Monocyte chemoattractant protein-1

using the CASY© cell counter (Roche Innovatis, Bielefeld, Germany). In vitro transmigration assays using different chemoattractant substrates were performed in duplicate in at least three independent experiments.

Intra-articular cytokine injections

For the administration of cytokines, a volume of 5 μl containing 10 ng of recombinant murine IL-1β (R&D Systems) [15] in PBS or 5 μl of collagenase type IV (Worthington Biochemical Corp., Lakewood, NJ, USA) was administered by IA injection into the right knees as previously described [20]. Briefly, the region of the knee joint was shaved and disinfected. The joint was flexed at 90 degrees to provide access to the joint cavity at the lower pole of the patella. The injection was performed by puncturing the knee joint laterally from the patellar ligament using a 32-gauge microneedle (Hamilton AG, Bonaduz, Switzerland). The left knee joint was treated with the same volume of PBS to serve as a control. After the procedure, the animals were left for 48 h prior to IV injection of SFs to incubate the cartilage with the corresponding cytokine/PBS. For all IA injections, a stereomicroscope was used (Stemi 2000-C; Carl Zeiss Microscopy, Oberkochen, Germany).

Fluorescent dyes for cell tracking

The lipophilic cell labeling solution 1,1′-dioctadecyl-3,3,3′,3′-tetramethylindotricarbocyanine iodide (DiR; Life Technologies, Carlsbad, CA, USA) was used to label SFs in vitro prior to their IV injection. The labeling was performed following the manufacturer's instructions. To reduce dye transfer in vivo, cells were washed gently five times with PBS after being labeled, followed by overnight incubation and further washing before IV application.

In vivo fluorescence imaging

In vivo fluorescence reflectance imaging (FRI) was carried out with the in vivo FX PRO Imaging Station (Bruker BioSpin MRI GmbH, Ettlingen, Germany). Mice were shaved using clippers and hair removal cream. A quantity of 1×10^6 DiR-labeled hTNFtg SFs (100 μl of PBS with 50 U/ml heparin) was injected into the tail veins of WT mice using a 26-gauge needle. Images were taken at different time points, namely 0 h (before IV application) and 3 h, 6 h, 8 h, 24 h, 48 h, and 96 h after IV application. The fluorochrome distribution and signal intensity were measured over an image acquisition time of 30 seconds, followed by coregistration of x-ray and white light images for the creation of overlay/fusion images. The excitation light was set to 730 nm using an appropriate bandpass filter. According to an emission maximum of the DiR dye in the near-infrared spectrum at 790 nm, the fluorescent signal was detected using a 750-nm filter–equipped, high-sensitivity (4 million pixels) cooled charge-coupled device camera. After the last in vivo image was acquired, animals were killed for the removal of internal organs and the ablation of muscles and soft tissue from the skeleton, respectively. These samples were then imaged again separately to reduce interference and absorption by overlaying tissue sections. For the tissue distribution of hTNFtg SF (Fig. 2), WT mice were analyzed ($n = 3$), whilst for histological quantification and for the SF transmigration after IA cytokine injection (Figs. 3 and 4), at least three independent experiments were performed in each case. For the IL-1 and collagenase experiments, 16 and 9 mice were used, respectively.

Histology and histomorphometric analysis

Knee joints of the WT mice were fixed in formalin (4%) overnight at 4 °C, decalcified in 10% ethylenediaminetetraacetic acid (Sigma-Aldrich) for 8 weeks and embedded in paraffin. For the evaluation of the articular cartilage and proteoglycan content, paraffin-embedded sections of the joints were stained with toluidine blue. The total amount of cartilage and the percentage of destained cartilage as a sign of proteoglycan loss were quantified as previously described [13].

Statistical analysis

Data are expressed as mean ± SEM. Differences between the mean values of the groups were compared using an unpaired, two-tailed Student's t test. p Values below 0.05 were considered statistically significant.

Results

SFs can cross endothelial barriers

To evaluate the general ability of SFs to migrate through endothelial junctions, an in vitro transmigration assay was established (Fig. 1a). First, we wanted to study potential differences in the transmigration rate between hTNFtg SFs and SFs derived from WT mice (WTSFs) independent of the presence of a barrier. Although only at very low levels, hTNFtg SFs showed a higher transmigration capacity than WTSFs (Fig. 1b) (+72% vs WTSF, $p < 0.05$). However, the generation of a 10% FCS gradient led to a massive increase of transmigrated SFs of both genotypes, particularly of hTNFtg SFs (Fig. 1b) (+77.5% vs WTSF, $p < 0.01$). Next, we performed these experiments using b.End5 cells as an endothelial cell layer. Although WTSFs as well as hTNFtg SFs were able to cross the endothelial barrier, the migratory potential of hTNFtg SFs was significantly higher (Fig. 1c) (+104% vs WTSFs, $p < 0.05$). Stimulation of the endothelial layer with TNF-α prior to the seeding of SFs further increased the transmigration of both cell types. Whereas hTNFtg SFs showed only a moderate increase (+34%, $p = 0.22$), the transmigration of WTSFs increased significantly after TNF-α stimulation (+106%, $p < 0.05$).

To investigate potential factors that further stimulate the transmigration of hTNFtg SFs through the endothelium in vitro, we investigated the role of articular cartilage as a chemoattractant for hTNFtg SFs. On the basis of the established function of IL-1 in inducing structural cartilage damage [14], IL-1β and murine cartilage explants were placed either alone or together into the lower compartment of the chamber. Neither IL-1 nor cartilage alone was sufficient to increase the transmigratory capacity of hTNFtg SFs (Fig. 1d). Interestingly, the coincubation of cartilage together with IL-1 led to a significant augmentation of hTNFtg SF transmigration through the endothelial layer into the lower compartment (+69.8% vs control, $p < 0.01$). As a control, cartilage hip caps were stained with toluidine blue, which revealed clearly destained areas following IL-1 incubation (Fig. 1e).

Following the evidence that preincubation of cartilage caps with IL-1 was an essential step in inducing SF transmigration, we also tested MCP-1, a known chemoattractant for SFs [21] as a transmigratory stimulus. For this purpose, MCP-1 was placed into the lower chamber (50 ng/ml); however, in contrast to the IL-1 experiments, MCP-1 did not stimulate SF transmigration (−49.5% vs control) (Fig. 1d).

hTNFtg SFs migrate into joints within hours following their IV injection in vivo

To investigate the sites at which hTNFtg SFs leave the bloodstream and the time course of this process, we established an in vivo transmigration model. Therefore,

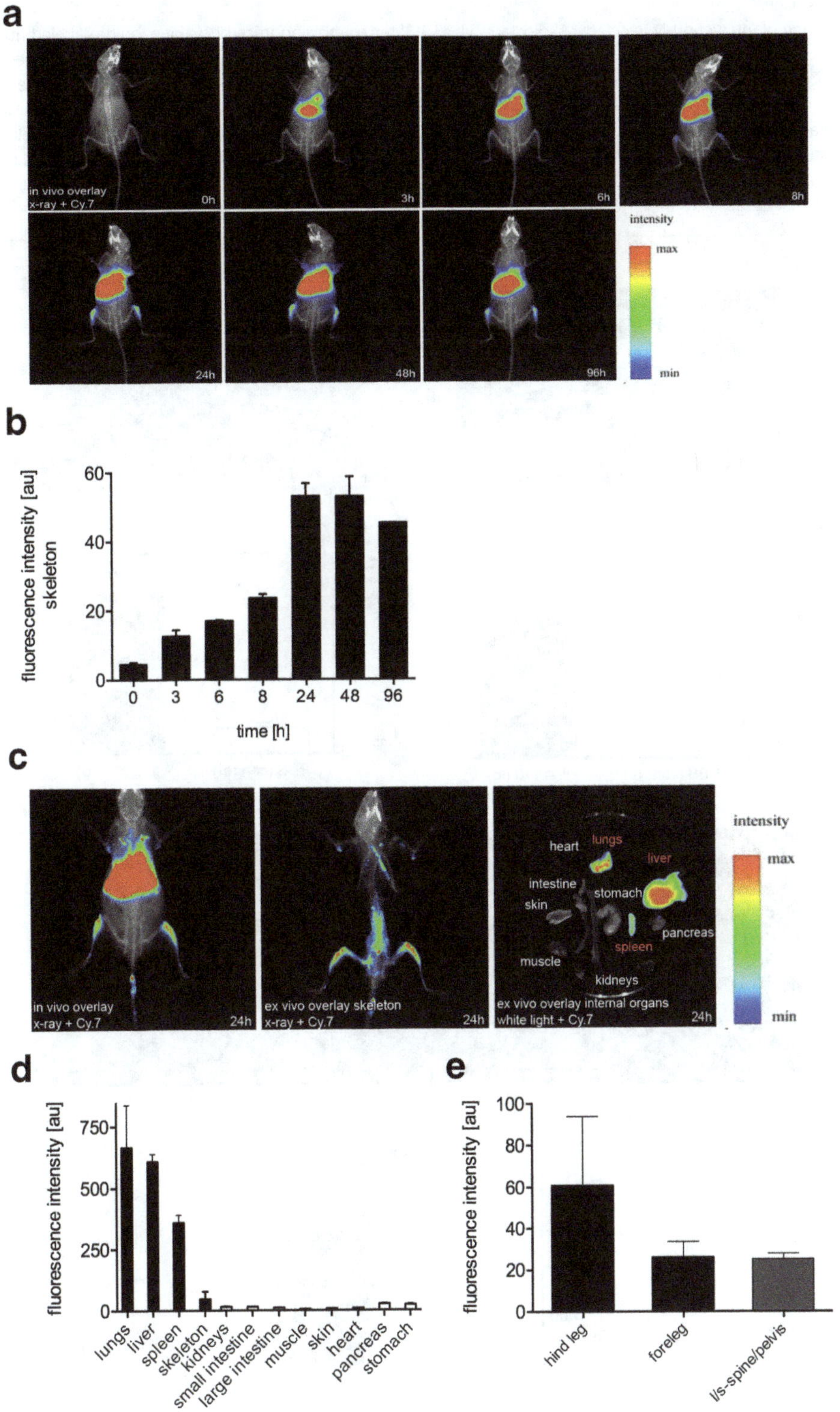

Fig. 2 (See legend on next page.)

(See figure on previous page.)
Fig. 2 Tissue extravasation of intravenously injected 1,1′-dioctadecyl-3,3,3′,3′-tetramethylindotricarbocyanine iodide–labeled human tumor necrosis factor–transgenic (hTNFtg) synovial fibroblasts (SFs). **a** In vivo coregistration of X-rays and fluorescent signals (cyanine 7 [Cy.7] spectrum) showed an accumulation of hTNFtg SFs in the articular and periarticular zones of the hind legs and liver over time. **b** Quantification of fluorescent signals revealed an increase in intensity up to 24 h after intravenous (IV) injection of hTNFtg SFs in the regions of interest, such as the juxta-articular areas of femora and tibiae. **c–e** In vivo and ex vivo fusion images of the skeleton and internal organs with quantification of the fluorescent signals. At the time of maximal hTNFtg SF tissue extravasation 24 h after IV injection, detailed preparation and imaging of the different tissues revealed cells additionally in the lungs, liver, spleen, and the lower part of the spinal column and forelegs. The values represent the mean ± SEM for three animals. *l/s* lumbosacral

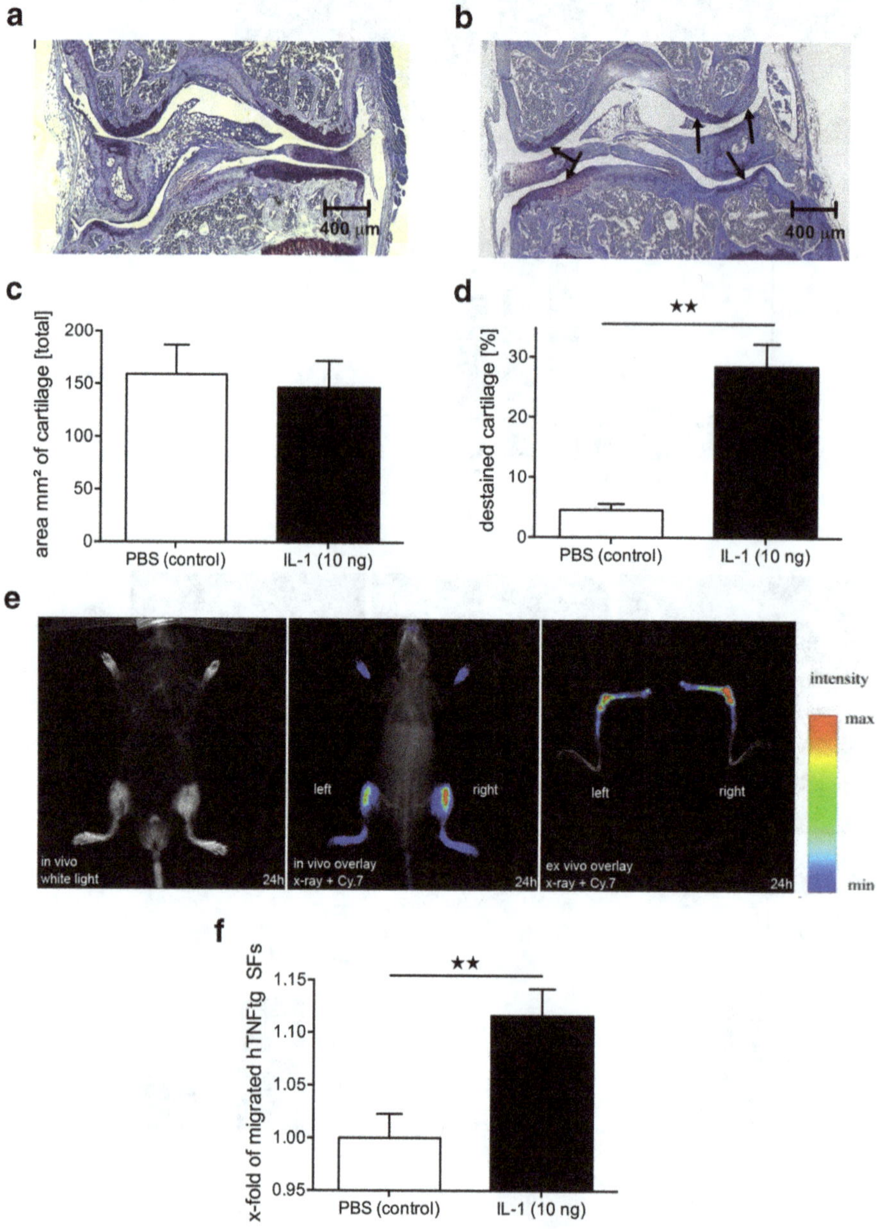

Fig. 3 Interleukin (IL)-1-induced depletion of proteoglycans attracts human tumor necrosis factor–transgenic (hTNFtg) synovial fibroblasts (SFs) in vivo. **a–d** Wild type mice received simultaneous intra-articular injections of (**a**) PBS into the left and (**b**) IL-1 into the right knee joints. Forty-eight hours after injection, the cartilage of IL-1-treated knees revealed a significant loss of proteoglycans, as indicated by a higher percentage of destained cartilage (*arrows*) visualized by toluidine blue staining compared with control joints, whereas the total cartilage area was not affected (**c**, **d**). In contrast, the total amount of cartilage was equal in both groups. Scale bar = 400 µm. Mean ± SEM values are shown. ** $p < 0.01$, $n = 4$. **e** and **f** Intravenous injection of 1,1′-dioctadecyl-3,3,3′,3′-tetramethylindotricarbocyanine iodide–labeled hTNFtg SFs 48 h after intra-articular application of PBS/IL-1 showed significantly increased homing into the IL-1 pretreated knee joint. The values represent mean ± SEM for 12 animals. ** $p < 0.01$. *Cy.7* Cyanine 7

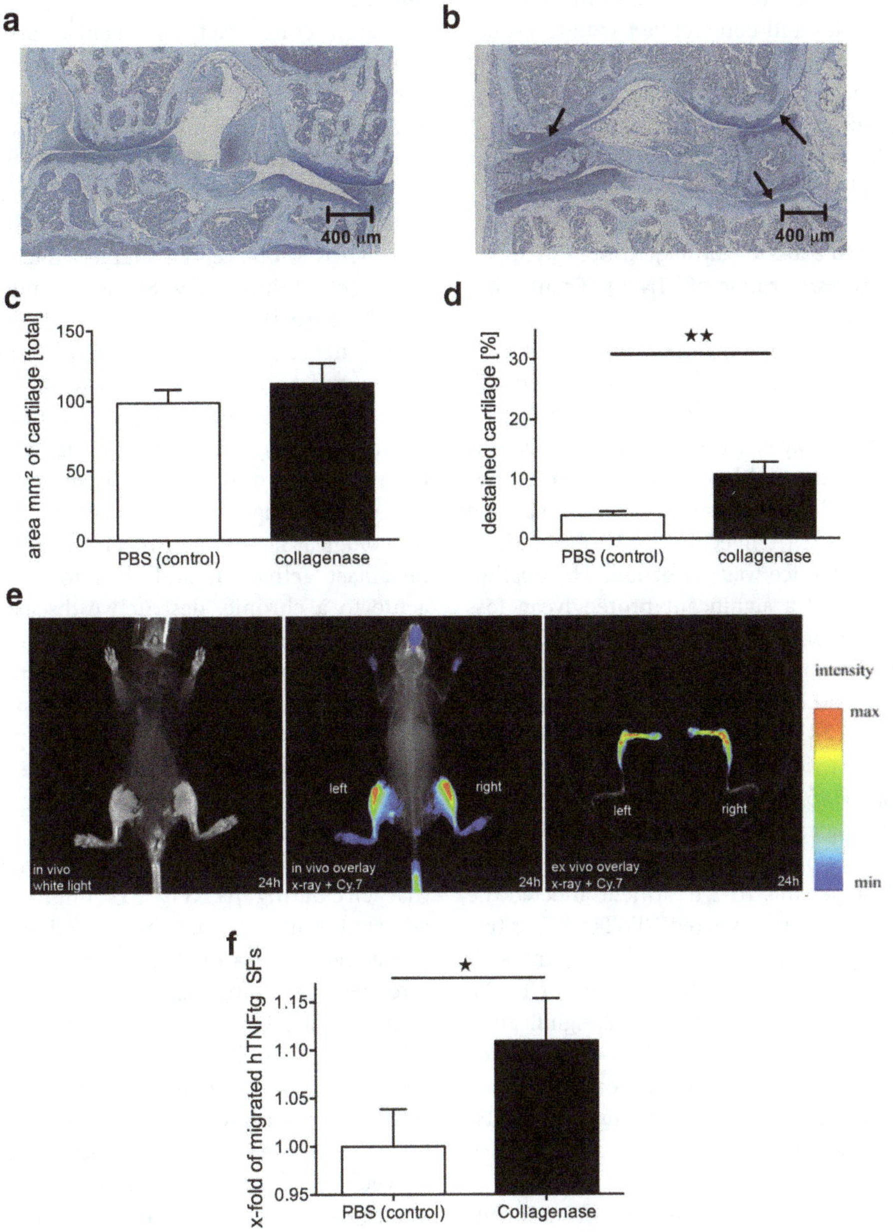

Fig. 4 Intra-articular collagenase injection attracts human tumor necrosis factor-transgenic (hTNFtg) synovial fibroblasts (SFs) into knee joints. **a**–**d** Wild-type mice received simultaneous intra-articular injections of (**a**) PBS into the left and (**b**) bacterial collagenase into the right knee joints. **c** and **d** After 48 h, quantification of toluidine blue staining showed a significant proteoglycan loss (*arrows*) without affecting the total cartilage area. Scale bar = 400 μm, $n = 4$. **e** and **f** Subsequent intravenous injection of 1,1′-dioctadecyl-3,3,3′,3′-tetramethylindotricarbocyanine iodide–labeled hTNFtg SFs showed increased fluorescence intensity in the collagenase-pretreated right knee joint in comparison to the control left knee joint ($n = 5$). The values represent the mean ± SEM. * $p < 0.05$, ** $p < 0.01$. *Cy.7* Cyanine 7

hTNFtg SFs were stained with a lipophilic dye (DiR), followed by IV application and subsequent detection of the emitted fluorescent signal using an FRI chamber [22]. In vivo imaging revealed a strong signal associated with the large joints and adjacent bones of the hind legs (Fig. 2a). hTNFtg SFs homed into these areas within hours (3 h = 12.61 AU, 6 h = 17.00 AU, 8 h = 23.53 AU), showing the highest accumulation at only 24 h (53.06 AU) after IV application (Fig. 2b). After this time point, no further qualitative redistribution of the hTNFtg SFs to other tissues took place, and an apparent decay of the fluorescent signal was observed only several days after IV application (48 h = 53.03 AU, 96 h = 45.32 AU). For detailed analyses, the internal organs were removed

24 h after IV injection of hTNFtg SFs, and the skeleton was freed from muscles and connective tissue to reduce the absorption of the signal by overlying tissue sections (Fig. 2c). Ex vivo images showed hTNFtg SFs also in the lungs (665.22 AU), liver (608.50 AU), spleen (358.62 AU), spinal column (25.2 AU), and forelegs (26.3 AU) of the animals (Fig. 2d and e).

IL-1 treatment leads to a loss of cartilage proteoglycans and stimulates the transmigration of hTNFtg SFs into the respective joint in vivo

On the basis of observations obtained from the in vitro transmigration assay showing that IL-1β-mediated cartilage changes stimulate the transmigration of hTNFtg SFs through an endothelial layer, we were interested in the role of predamaged joint cartilage as a chemoattractive stimulus for hTNFtg SF extravasation into the affected joint. Therefore, a single IA injection of 10 ng of IL-1β into knee joints of WT mice was performed. Histopathological analyses revealed a significant proteoglycan loss 48 h after IL-1 injection (Fig. 3a, b). The amount of destained cartilage indicating proteoglycan depletion was significantly higher in IL-1-treated knees compared with control knees (PBS) (28.5% vs 4.6%, $p < 0.01$) (Fig. 3d), whereas there was no significant difference in the total amount of cartilage (146.8 mm^2 vs 159.0 mm^2, $p = 0.08$) (Fig. 3c). No histological signs of inflammation were detected after IA injection of either IL-1 or PBS.

To determine whether this IL-1 treatment affected the attraction of hTNFtg SFs, we injected hTNFtg SFs intravenously following pretreatment of one knee joint with IL-1 and the other with PBS. Twenty-four hours after IV injection of hTNFtg SFs, FRI revealed a significantly increased homing of hTNFtg SFs into IL-1-treated knee joints compared with the PBS-treated control joints (+11.6%, $p < 0.01$) (Fig. 3e, f). Furthermore, ex vivo sagittal images of the joints showed a prominent signal in the knee joints, the distal femur, and the proximal tibia (Fig. 3e).

Because IL-1 not only induces cartilage damage but also constitutes an important inflammatory cytokine with the ability to affect chondrocytes or resident SFs in the joint in multiple ways, we also induced cartilage damage directly by collagenase application in vivo. In line with our IL-1 studies, we injected a single dose of 5 μl of collagenase solution into WT murine knee joints. Similar to the effects observed with IL-1, we found a significant collagenase-induced destaining of the articular cartilage, indicating proteoglycan loss (10.7% vs 3.5%, $p < 0.01$), whereas no differences in the total cartilage area were detected (111.72 mm^2 vs 103.86 mm^2). Twenty-four hours after DiR-labeled hTNFtg SF injection, an increased signal intensity indicating SF accumulation was detected in the collagenase-treated knee joints compared with the control knee joints (+10.9%, $p < 0.05$) (Fig. 4e, f).

Discussion

Research conducted in recent years has revealed a number of mechanisms, such as abundant secretion of proinflammatory cytokines and proteases, that together perpetuate the inflammatory response in joints of patients with RA [23]. However, the ultimate cause of RA, as well as the changes during early stages of the disease that lead to the dissemination of arthritis to previously unaffected joints, remains largely unclear. In addition to systemic autoimmunity, SFs are of interest in this context because recent data derived from a SCID mouse model demonstrated SFs' ability to migrate long distances and to reinitiate cartilage destruction at distant sites of subcutaneously implanted human cartilage [10]. Moreover, there is increasing evidence that in the course of disease, not only does cartilage purely suffer damage but early changes to the cartilage in addition to immunological factors and mechanisms also contribute to fibroblast activation and thus to the switch from an acute to a chronic, destructive disease. In fact, several lines of evidence suggest that cartilage damage precedes the activation of SFs at least in animal models of RA, such as the hTNFtg mouse, and that prevention of IL-1-induced cartilage damage significantly alters the behavior of SFs in the course of this RA-like disease [13, 14].

In this study, we established an in vivo transmigration assay to visualize the tissue extravasation of hTNFtg SFs in a time-dependent manner. We found that circulating hTNFtg SFs migrate into joints and adjacent bones within hours following IV injection. Once the process of diapedesis from the bloodstream into the joint compartments was overcome, no significant quantitative or qualitative redistribution into other tissues took place. This emphasizes the primary function of SFs as resident cells in contrast to leukocytes that continuously recirculate between blood and lymphoid tissues as part of their function in immune surveillance [24]. Nevertheless, the attraction to and passaging of SFs at the endothelium-joint border requires close interactions between hTNFtg SFs and endothelial cells.

In vitro and in vivo studies of SFs and synovial endothelium from patients with RA have shown enhanced expression of adhesion molecules, including E-selectin, vascular cell adhesion molecule VCAM-1, integrin $\alpha_1\beta_1$ (VLA-1), intercellular adhesion molecule ICAM-1, or junctional adhesion molecule JAM-C, resulting from the abundant secretion of TNF-α, because a therapeutic blockade with monoclonal antibodies effectively reduces the expression of these molecules [25–31]. In line with this, we found that the capability of SFs to break endothelial barriers in vitro is stimulated by the presence of TNF-α. Thus, both the endogenous expression in SFs (hTNFtg SFs vs WTSFs) and exogenous stimulation of endothelial cells with this cytokine led to an enhanced transmigratory capacity. This suggests an important role for TNF-α in the induction of adhesion molecules that are necessary for the transmigration of SFs through endothelial cell layers, although specific binding partners for this interaction are yet to be determined. However, hTNFtg SFs were also able to leave the bloodstream at sites of healthy, noninflamed joints of WT mice. This implies that chemoattractants other than TNF-α are also involved in this process. Interestingly, the joint compartments represent the only specific site of hTNFtg SF tissue extravasation because the transendothelial migration into liver, lungs, and spleen is most likely a result of their physiological function to purify and store cells from the blood.

Numerous data have shown that IL-1, another key cytokine in RA, mediates cartilage and bone degradation in RA [13, 16, 32]. In line with these data, we found that IL-1-induced proteoglycan depletion in cartilage hip caps as well as in knee joints of WT mice resulted in an increased transmigration of hTNFtg SFs in vitro and in vivo. In vitro only the coincubation of cartilage together with IL-1, but not IL-1 or cartilage alone, was able to stimulate the transmigration of hTNFtg SFs. The resulting notion that structural damage induced by IL-1 significantly contributes to the observed effects of IL-1 is also supported by our experiments in which the IA injection of collagenase resulted in effects similar to those seen with IL-1 treatment.

On the basis of these observations, we hypothesized that factors released from the joint cartilage as a result of cartilage damage are the important mediators that attract SFs into the joint and that structural cartilage damage increases the chemotactic effect on the transmigration of SFs. Although the exact nature of these factors remains to be established, there are a number of different possible mechanisms by which cartilage damage such as that induced by our experimental procedures as well as in patients with RA may lead to the attraction of fibroblasts into joints. These include the release of cartilage degradation products; the release of soluble factors that are bound to the extracellular matrix and get released as cartilage is degraded [33]; the release of small, leucine-rich proteoglycans and other potential damage-associated molecular pattern molecules that can directly stimulate fibroblast-like cells via Toll-like receptors; and perhaps also direct secretion of chemokines, cytokines, growth factors, and by chondrocytes. Moreover, some of these effects may be direct, whereas others may be indirect in that factors released from cartilage stimulate neighboring cells in the synovial membrane, which in turn attracts fibroblasts from the circulation [34, 35]. Our in vitro studies using MCP-1 failed to demonstrate an enhancing effect of this chemokine on SF transmigration, but there are a variety of other chemokines that may well play a role in this process. Also, it needs to be emphasized that most likely it is not only one single factor that mediates the trafficking of fibroblasts into predamaged joints, but that several of the aforementioned mechanisms contribute to this process.

Conclusions

Currently, not much is known about pathological changes that initiate and drive the progression of RA in very early stages of the disease, despite a consensus that there are molecular and cellular alterations, including changes in cartilage structure, that precede the onset of synovitis in RA [33–38]. Furthermore, why certain joints are more likely to be affected than others remains almost completely unexplored, although there are some data derived from microanatomical studies suggesting that mechanically exposed areas in joints are more prone to developing synovitis [39, 40]. In the present study, we provide evidence that structural cartilage changes that may be present in very early phases of the disease facilitate the homing of SFs and thus promote the spread and progression of RA. On the basis of these data, we suggest that changes in cartilage homeostasis are not only a result but also a potential trigger of joint destruction in RA. As a result, early treatment of cartilage degradation may help prevent the progression of RA and its spread to previously unaffected joints. Although many questions about the responsible molecules and pathways remain unanswered, we hope that our demonstration of SF homing into predamaged joints in this work will stimulate further research in this area and eventually help to solve the conundrum of disease pattern and effects on joints in RA.

Abbreviations

b.End5: Brain endothelioma 5 cell line; Cy.7: Cyanine 7; DiR: 1,1'-dioctadecyl-3,3,3',3'-tetramethylindotricarbocyanine iodide; FCS: Fetal calf serum; FRI: Fluorescence reflectance imaging; hTNFtg: Human tumor necrosis factor–transgenic; IA: Intra-articular; ICAM-1: Intercellular adhesion molecule 1; IL-1: Interleukin-1; IV: Intravenous; JAM-C: Junctional adhesion molecule, C variant; MCP-1: Monocyte chemoattractant protein-1; RA: Rheumatoid arthritis; RASF: Rheumatoid arthritis synovial fibroblast; SCID: Severe combined immunodeficiency; SF: Synovial fibroblast; VCAM-1: Vascular cell adhesion molecule; VLA-1: integrin $\alpha_1\beta_1$; WT: Wild type

Acknowledgements

The authors thank Stefan Butz and Dietmar Vestweber for providing b.End5 cells.

Funding

This project was supported by the 'Deutsche Gesellschaft für Rheumatologie' and the 'Bundesministerium für Bildung und Forschung (Impam 01EC1008D).

Authors' contributions

JH made substantial contributions to the study design, data acquisition and analysis/interpretation of the in vitro experiments, participated in the in vivo imaging studies, and drafted the manuscript. CG made substantial contributions to the study conception as well as to data acquisition and analyses of the in vivo imaging studies. MH made substantial contributions to the study conception and data interpretation of the in vitro experiments. DB made substantial contributions to the study design as well as to data acquisition and analysis/interpretation of the in vitro experiments and helped to revise the manuscript. AK made substantial contributions to data acquisition and analysis of histology and helped to revise the manuscript. IW made substantial contributions to the study design, data acquisition, and analyses. HP made substantial intellectual contributions to the study conception and interpretation of the in vitro data. CB made substantial intellectual contributions to the study conception and data interpretation of the in vivo experiments. TP made substantial intellectual contributions to the study conception and data interpretation, helped to draft and revise the manuscript for important intellectual content, and approved the final version to be published. AKP made substantial intellectual contributions to the study conception and coordination, data acquisition, and data analysis/interpretation; performed the statistical analysis; drafted and revised the manuscript for important intellectual content; and approved the final version to be published. All authors read and approved the final manuscript.

Authors' information

JH holds an MD degree, CG holds a PhD degree, MH holds a PhD degree, DB holds a Dipl-Biol degree, AK has an MTA certification, IW has an MTA certification, HP is a university professor and holds an MD degree, CB is a professor and holds an MD degree, TP is a university professor and holds an MD degree, and AKP holds an MD degree.

Competing interests

The authors declare that they have no competing interests.

Author details

[1]Institute of Experimental Musculoskeletal Medicine, University Hospital Muenster, Albert-Schweitzer-Campus 1, D3, 48149 Muenster, Germany. [2]Department of Anesthesiology, Intensive Care and Pain Medicine, University Hospital Muenster, Muenster, Germany. [3]Interdisciplinary Centre for Clinical Research, University Hospital Muenster, Muenster, Germany. [4]Department of Radiology, St. Franziskus Hospital GmbH Muenster, Muenster, Germany. [5]Department of General Internal Medicine, Nephrology, Hypertension Diseases and Rheumatology, University Hospital Muenster, Muenster, Germany.

References

1. McInnes IB, Schett G. The pathogenesis of rheumatoid arthritis. N Engl J Med. 2011;365(23):2205–19.
2. Schett G, Gravallese E. Bone erosion in rheumatoid arthritis: mechanisms, diagnosis and treatment. Nat Rev Rheumatol. 2012;8(11):656–64.
3. Bottini N, Firestein GS. Duality of fibroblast-like synoviocytes in RA: passive responders and imprinted aggressors. Nat Rev Rheumatol. 2013;9(1):24–33.
4. Cunnane G, FitzGerald O, Hummel KM, Youssef PP, Gay RE, Gay S, et al. Synovial tissue protease gene expression and joint erosions in early rheumatoid arthritis. Arthritis Rheum. 2001;44(8):1744–53.
5. Pap T, Shigeyama Y, Kuchen S, Fernihough JK, Simmen B, Gay RE, et al. Differential expression pattern of membrane-type matrix metalloproteinases in rheumatoid arthritis. Arthritis Rheum. 2000;43(6):1226–32.
6. Westhoff CS, Freudiger D, Petrow P, Seyfert C, Zacher J, Kriegsmann J, et al. Characterization of collagenase 3 (matrix metalloproteinase 13) messenger RNA expression in the synovial membrane and synovial fibroblasts of patients with rheumatoid arthritis. Arthritis Rheum. 1999;42(7):1517–27.
7. Wunrau C, Schnaeker EM, Freyth K, Pundt N, Wendholt D, Neugebauer K, et al. Establishment of a matrix-associated transepithelial resistance invasion assay to precisely measure the invasive potential of synovial fibroblasts. Arthritis Rheum. 2009;60(9):2606–11.
8. Müller-Ladner U, Kriegsmann J, Franklin BN, Matsumoto S, Geiler T, Gay RE, et al. Synovial fibroblasts of patients with rheumatoid arthritis attach to and invade normal human cartilage when engrafted into SCID mice. Am J Pathol. 1996;149(5):1607–15.
9. Pap T, Aupperle KR, Gay S, Firestein GS, Gay RE. Invasiveness of synovial fibroblasts is regulated by p53 in the SCID mouse in vivo model of cartilage invasion. Arthritis Rheum. 2001;44(3):676–81.
10. Lefèvre S, Knedla A, Tennie C, Kampmann A, Wunrau C, Dinser R, et al. Synovial fibroblasts spread rheumatoid arthritis to unaffected joints. Nat Med. 2009;15(12):1414–20.
11. Nishimura K, Sugiyama D, Kogata Y, Tsuji G, Nakazawa T, Kawano S, et al. Meta-analysis: diagnostic accuracy of anti-cyclic citrullinated peptide antibody and rheumatoid factor for rheumatoid arthritis. Ann Intern Med. 2007;146(11):797–808.
12. Kokkonen H, Mullazehi M, Berglin E, Hallmans G, Wadell G, Ronnelid J, et al. Antibodies of IgG, IgA and IgM isotypes against cyclic citrullinated peptide precede the development of rheumatoid arthritis. Arthritis Res Ther. 2011;13(1):R13.
13. Korb-Pap A, Stratis A, Mühlenberg K, Niederreiter B, Hayer S, Echtermeyer F, et al. Early structural changes in cartilage and bone are required for the attachment and invasion of inflamed synovial tissue during destructive inflammatory arthritis. Ann Rheum Dis. 2012;71(6):1004–11.
14. Zwerina J, Redlich K, Polzer K, Joosten L, Kronke G, Distler J, et al. TNF-induced structural joint damage is mediated by IL-1. Proc Natl Acad Sci U S A. 2007;104(28):11742–7.
15. Dudler J, Renggli-Zulliger N, Busso N, Lotz M, So A. Effect of interleukin 17 on proteoglycan degradation in murine knee joints. Ann Rheum Dis. 2000;59(7):529–32.
16. van de Loo AA, van den Berg WB. Effects of murine recombinant interleukin 1 on synovial joints in mice: measurement of patellar cartilage metabolism and joint inflammation. Ann Rheum Dis. 1990;49(4):238–45.
17. Keffer J, Probert L, Cazlaris H, Georgopoulos S, Kaslaris E, Kioussis D, et al. Transgenic mice expressing human tumour necrosis factor: a predictive genetic model of arthritis. EMBO J. 1991;10(13):4025–31.
18. Armaka M, Gkretsi V, Kontoyiannis D, Kollias G. A standardized protocol for the isolation and culture of normal and arthritogenic murine synovial fibroblasts. Protoc exch. 2009. doi:10.1038/nprot.2009.102
19. Yang T, Roder KE, Abbruscato TJ. Evaluation of bEnd5 cell line as an in vitro model for the blood–brain barrier under normal and hypoxic/aglycemic conditions. J Pharm Sci. 2007;96(12):3196–213.
20. van der Kraan PM, Vitters EL, van Beuningen HM, van de Putte LB, van den Berg WB. Degenerative knee joint lesions in mice after a single intra-articular collagenase injection: a new model of osteoarthritis. J Exp Pathol (Oxford). 1990;71(1):19–31.
21. García-Vicuña R, Gómez-Gaviro MV, Domínguez-Luis MJ, Pec MK, González-Alvaro I, Alvaro-Gracia JM, et al. CC and CXC chemokine receptors mediate migration, proliferation, and matrix metalloproteinase production by fibroblast-like synoviocytes from rheumatoid arthritis patients. Arthritis Rheum. 2004;50(12):3866–77.
22. Eisenblatter M, Ehrchen J, Varga G, Sunderkotter C, Heindel W, Roth J, et al. In vivo optical imaging of cellular inflammatory response in granuloma formation using fluorescence-labeled macrophages. J Nucl Med. 2009; 50(10):1676–82.
23. McInnes IB, Schett G. Cytokines in the pathogenesis of rheumatoid arthritis. Nat Rev Immunol. 2007;7(6):429–42.
24. Vestweber D. Adhesion and signaling molecules controlling the transmigration of leukocytes through endothelium. Immunol Rev. 2007;218:178–96.
25. Foster W, Carruthers D, Lip GY, Blann AD. Inflammatory cytokines, endothelial markers and adhesion molecules in rheumatoid arthritis: effect of intensive anti-inflammatory treatment. J Thromb Thrombolysis. 2010;29(4):437–42.
26. Gonzalez-Gay MA, Garcia-Unzueta MT, De Matias JM, Gonzalez-Juanatey C, Garcia-Porrua C, Sanchez-Andrade A, et al. Influence of anti-TNF-α infliximab therapy on adhesion molecules associated with atherogenesis in patients with rheumatoid arthritis. Clin Exp Rheumatol. 2006;24(4):373–9.
27. Koch AE, Burrows JC, Haines GK, Carlos TM, Harlan JM, Leibovich SJ. Immunolocalization of endothelial and leukocyte adhesion molecules in human rheumatoid and osteoarthritic synovial tissues. Lab Invest. 1991;64(3):313–20.
28. Luo SF, Fang RY, Hsieh HL, Chi PL, Lin CC, Hsiao LD, et al. Involvement of MAPKs and NF-κB in tumor necrosis factor α-induced vascular cell adhesion

molecule 1 expression in human rheumatoid arthritis synovial fibroblasts. Arthritis Rheum. 2010;62(1):105–16.
29. Morales-Ducret J, Wayner E, Elices MJ, Alvaro-Gracia JM, Zvaifler NJ, Firestein GS. α4/β1 integrin (VLA-4) ligands in arthritis: vascular cell adhesion molecule-1 expression in synovium and on fibroblast-like synoviocytes. J Immunol. 1992;149(4):1424–31.
30. Müller-Ladner U, Elices MJ, Kriegsmann JB, Strahl D, Gay RE, Firestein GS, et al. Alternatively spliced CS-1 fibronectin isoform and its receptor VLA-4 in rheumatoid arthritis synovium. J Rheumatol. 1997;24(10):1873–80.
31. Rabquer BJ, Pakozdi A, Michel JE, Gujar BS, Haines III GK, Imhof BA, et al. Junctional adhesion molecule C mediates leukocyte adhesion to rheumatoid arthritis synovium. Arthritis Rheum. 2008;58(10):3020–9.
32. van de Loo FA, Joosten LA, van Lent PL, Arntz OJ, van den Berg WB. Role of interleukin-1, tumor necrosis factor α, and interleukin-6 in cartilage proteoglycan metabolism and destruction: effect of in situ blocking in murine antigen- and zymosan-induced arthritis. Arthritis Rheum. 1995;38(2):164–72.
33. Sherwood J, Bertrand J, Nalesso G, Poulet B, Pitsillides A, Brandolini L, et al. A homeostatic function of CXCR2 signalling in articular cartilage. Ann Rheum Dis. 2015;74(12):2207–15.
34. Pap T, Korb-Pap A. Cartilage damage in osteoarthritis and rheumatoid arthritis—two unequal siblings. Nat Rev Rheumatol. 2015;11(10):606–15.
35. Korb-Pap A, Bertrand J, Sherwood J, Pap T. Stable activation of fibroblasts in rheumatic arthritis—causes and consequences. Rheumatology (Oxford). 2016;55 Suppl 2:ii64–7.
36. Miese F, Buchbender C, Scherer A, Wittsack HJ, Specker C, Schneider M, et al. Molecular imaging of cartilage damage of finger joints in early rheumatoid arthritis with delayed gadolinium-enhanced magnetic resonance imaging. Arthritis Rheum. 2012;64(2):394–9.
37. Herz B, Albrecht A, Englbrecht M, Welsch GH, Uder M, Renner N, et al. Osteitis and synovitis, but not bone erosion, is associated with proteoglycan loss and microstructure damage in the cartilage of patients with rheumatoid arthritis. Ann Rheum Dis. 2014;73(6):1101–6.
38. Rantapää-Dahlqvist S, de Jong BA, Berglin E, Hallmans G, Wadell G, Stenlund H, et al. Antibodies against cyclic citrullinated peptide and IgA rheumatoid factor predict the development of rheumatoid arthritis. Arthritis Rheum. 2003;48(10):2741–9.
39. Tan AL, Tanner SF, Conaghan PG, Radjenovic A, O'Connor P, Brown AK, et al. Role of metacarpophalangeal joint anatomic factors in the distribution of synovitis and bone erosion in early rheumatoid arthritis. Arthritis Rheum. 2003;48(5):1214–22.
40. Brawer AE, Goel N. The onset of rheumatoid arthritis following trauma. Open Access Rheumatol. 2016;8:77–80.

Th17 and CD24^{hi}CD27^{+} regulatory B lymphocytes are biomarkers of response to biologics in rheumatoid arthritis

Sarah Salomon[1†], Caroline Guignant[2†], Pierre Morel[3], Gauthier Flahaut[2], Clément Brault[2], Clément Gourguechon[2], Patrice Fardellone[1], Jean-Pierre Marolleau[3], Brigitte Gubler[2] and Vincent Goëb[1*]

Abstract

Background: The aim was to describe the regulatory B and T cells (Breg and Treg) and T helper 17 (Th17) lymphocytes before and under treatment with biologic drugs, and to assess their potential predictive value as biomarkers of response in rheumatoid arthritis (RA).

Methods: This was a non-randomised, single-centre, prospective study. Patients with active RA (American College of Rheumatology (ACR)/European League Against Rheumatism (EULAR) 2010) who required the initiation or switch to any biologic drug except rituximab were included. The main judgement criterion was the frequency and absolute number of CD24^{hi}CD27^{+} Breg and CD24^{hi}CD38^{hi} T2/Breg cells, CD25^{hi}CD127^{low} Treg and CD45RA^{-}CD161^{+}CCR6^{+} Th17 cells measured at inclusion in both patients and controls, and after 1, 3 and 6 months of treatment (M1, M3 and M6) in patients with RA, and compared with the M6 response to treatment (EULAR response and Disease Activity Score in 28 joints (DAS28) remission).

Results: Thirty-one patients with RA and 17 controls were included. There was a reduction in T2/Breg frequency at M0 in patients ($p < 0.001$) and absolute numbers ($p = 0.014$) and in immunopositive vs. immunonegative RA ($p = 0.016$). DAS28 remission at M6 was associated with increased frequency of Treg ($p = 0.01$). A higher level of CD24^{hi}CD27^{+} Breg at baseline was associated with DAS28 remission at M6 ($p = 0.04$) and a good EULAR response at M6 for abatacept-treated patients ($p = 0.01$). A lower M0 level of Th17 was associated with a good EULAR response at M6 ($p = 0.007$), notably under anti-cytokine drugs ($p = 0.048$).

Conclusions: Altogether, these data, although preliminary, suggest that phenotyping of T and B cells has potential value for the stratification of biologic drugs, notably with respect to choosing between abatacept and anti-cytokine blockade.

Keywords: Rheumatoid arthritis, Biomarker, Lymphocyte, Th17, Breg, Treg, Response, Remission, Abatacept, Anti-TNF

Background

The development of different targeted immunotherapies and treatment strategies (treat to target (T2T) and tight control) has allowed significant improvement in the prognosis of rheumatoid arthritis (RA), and long-lasting clinical remission may now be a consideration [1]. Approximately one third of patients, however, experience primary non-response or insufficient response to these different drugs [2, 3]. The search for biomarkers that could predict response to biologic drugs is therefore crucial, in order to ensure that the treatment chosen will be sufficiently effective to halt the progress of the disease, whilst avoiding prescribing patients ineffective, potentially deleterious (leading to infectious or neoplastic complications, etc.) and expensive treatment [4].

Different lymphocyte subpopulations play a major role in the physiopathology of RA, such as regulatory T cells (Treg), T helper 17 (Th17) cells and regulatory B lymphocytes (Breg). In the physiological condition,

* Correspondence: goeb.vincent@chu-amiens.fr
†Equal contributors
[1]Rheumatology Department & EA 4666, Amiens University Hospital, University of Picardie-Jules Verne, Amiens, France
Full list of author information is available at the end of the article

CD4 + $CD25^{hi}FoxP3^{+}$ regulatory T cells constitute 5–10% of the population of $CD4^{+}$ T lymphocytes in the blood [5]. A functional deficit in Treg with a reduction of their suppressive activity has been observed in RA [6]. A loss of Treg capacity to suppress effector $CD4^{+}CD25^{-}$ T cells has been observed, prior to anti-TNF treatment for active RA, and a recovery of this defect was observed in patients who respond clinically to anti-TNF drugs with a quantitative increase in Treg frequencies post treatment [6]. Moreover, the quantitative restoration of the Treg upon achieving remission with anti-TNF has been associated with greater probability of long-term remission [7]. An increase in T lymphocytes, and Treg in particular, was furthermore recorded after the use of abatacept, a biologic drug that reproduces the physiological inhibitor role of CTLA4 [8].

The identification of the Th17 lymphocytes, a subpopulation of $CD4^{+}$ T-lymphocytes that produces the highly proinflammatory cytokine IL-17 [9, 10], opened the way for new understanding of the physiopathological and new treatment options (secukinumab or ixekizumab) for RA [11, 12]. Th17 cells are characterised by considerable plasticity (interconversion with Th1 cells), which themselves can also develop into Th17 under some pathophysiological circumstances [13–16]. An inverse correlation between blood Th17 and anti-citrullinated peptide antibodies (ACPA) levels has been observed in patients with RA [17], illustrating the interrelationship between this subpopulation and humoral immunity in this autoimmune rheumatism. The role of Th17 appears to be particularly relevant during the onset of RA and later may be influenced by treatments, increasing under methotrexate (MTX) [18] and decreasing in patients that do not respond to infliximab [19].

B lymphocytes and humoral immunity also play a key role in RA, notably with ACPA and rheumatoid factor (RF) production [20]. Breg, by analogy to Treg, represent a subpopulation of B cells that have immune-regulating properties [21] and play a role in peripheral tolerance [22], mainly via the substantial secretion of IL-10 [22, 23]. Discrepancies in the phenotype of human Breg have been described [24–28], although the most commonly accepted is the inclusion of putative Breg within the immature transitional T2 population (CD19+$CD24^{hi}CD38^{hi}$). Additional regulatory properties have been described in the memory B cells $CD24^{hi}CD27^{+}$ phenotype (also producing IL-10) [29]. These cells are reported to be able to inhibit the proliferation of $CD4^{+}$ T cells differentiating between Th1 and Th17 cells, producing different proinflammatory cytokines. Although they are reported to be quantitatively and functionally altered in patients with active RA (reduction of their capacity to induce both Treg from CD4+ and prevent the conversion of Treg into Th17 cells) [30, 31], a recent report observed that a high baseline level of Breg appeared to be predictive of a clinical European League Against Rheumatism (EULAR) response at 3 months upon anti-TNF treatment [25].

Thus, the main aim of our study was to describe the different lymphocyte subpopulation frequencies in RA (regulatory B and T cells and Th17 lymphocytes) before and under biologic drugs, in order to test the correlation with subsequent response to the drug received and to identify potential biomarker value that could be used to predict therapeutic response.

Methods

Patients and controls

Patients who met the American College of Rheumatology (ACR)/EULAR 2010 criteria for RA [32] with active disease despite receiving a conventional synthetic or biologic disease-modifying antirheumatic drug (DMARD) and who required the initiation or a switch to any biologic drug except rituximab, in association with MTX, were prospectively included in this study. The exclusion criteria were the use of corticosteroid therapy, concurrent or within the last 3 months, at a dose of more than 10 mg/day or treatment with other immunosuppressive therapy than MTX. At least five half-lives were required before changing the treatment if a biologic drug was previously used. Adult patients with a confirmed "mechanical" pathologic condition (osteoporosis, osteoarthritis, etc.) who did not have a personal medical history of neoplastic, inflammatory or infectious diseases were included as controls. All patients and controls signed a consent form to participate in this study, approved by the medical ethics committee of Amiens University hospital, France (number 2015-000833-64).

Different parameters were gathered at inclusion (month 0 (M0)): history and treatments, body mass index (BMI), disease activity evaluated by calculation of the Disease Activity Score in 28 joints (DAS28) and the Health Assessment Questionnaire (HAQ), the erosive nature of the RA (evaluated on radiographs of both hands and feet), the autoimmune status (RF and ACPA assessed by anti-cyclic citrullinated peptide (anti-CCP2 tests)), complete blood count (CBC), measurement of C-reactive protein (CRP) and erythrocyte sedimentation rate (ESR). Patients underwent the same clinical and biological monitoring at 1 (M1), 3 (M3) and 6 months (M6) following treatment.

Analysis of lymphocyte subpopulations by flow cytometry

Flow cytometry (CMF) was used to conduct lymphocyte phenotyping of fresh blood (Navios A80706, 3 lasers, 10 colours) at M0 in patients and controls and then at M1, M3 and M6 in patients only. We used standard protocols developed under routine immunology hospital services with a view to be able to transfer data into clinical practice with limited additional work. The following monoclonal antibodies conjugated with a fluorochrome were used for the

B cell phenotyping: CD19-AA750 (APC-AlexaFluor750), CD24-PC5.5 (phycoerythrin-cyanine) and CD27-PC7, CD38-APC (allophycocyanin). The following antibodies were used for T cell phenotyping: CD3-AA750, CD4-PB, CD45RA-FITC, CD62L-ECD, CD25-PC5.5, CD161-PC7, CD127-AA700 and CCR6(CD196)-APC. All the antibodies came from Beckmann-Coulter® (except CCR6-APC from BioLegend®). At least 20,000 cells were analysed for each sample.

The T and B cell populations were identified on the single-parameter expression of CD3 and CD19, respectively, combined with scatter (gating strategies are described in Fig. 1). Regulatory B cells were defined as $CD19^{+}CD24^{hi}CD38^{hi}$ further referred to as T2/Breg. We also assessed the $CD19^{+}CD24^{hi}CD27^{+}$ subpopulations. Treg were identified as the $CD4 + CD25^{hi}CD127^{low}$ subpopulation as previously described [33]. Th17 cells were identified as subpopulation $CD45RA{+}CD161^{+}CCR6^{+}$ within the $CD3 + CD4^{+}$ T cell gate. The results were expressed as percentage of the parental lineage gate and absolute value per millimeter cubed.

Statistical analysis

The characteristics of patients and controls were recorded as a percentage for the category-based variables and as the median and 25th and 75th percentiles (interquartile range (IQR)) for continuous variables. The differences in percentage or absolute value of the lymphocyte subpopulations were evaluated using the parametric t test, the non-parametric Mann–Whitney or Wilcoxon tests for matched data, or the Friedman test for multiple comparisons. Correlation between the different lymphocyte subpopulations was evaluated using the Spearman test. The general linear model (GLM) and MIXED procedures were used for the repetitive analysis models. We used $p < 0.05$ as the significance threshold for the statistical tests, corrected by the number of tests carried out, where necessary. The statistical analyses were carried out using the Statistical Package for Social Sciences (SPSS) and Statistical Analysis System (SAS) 9.3 software.

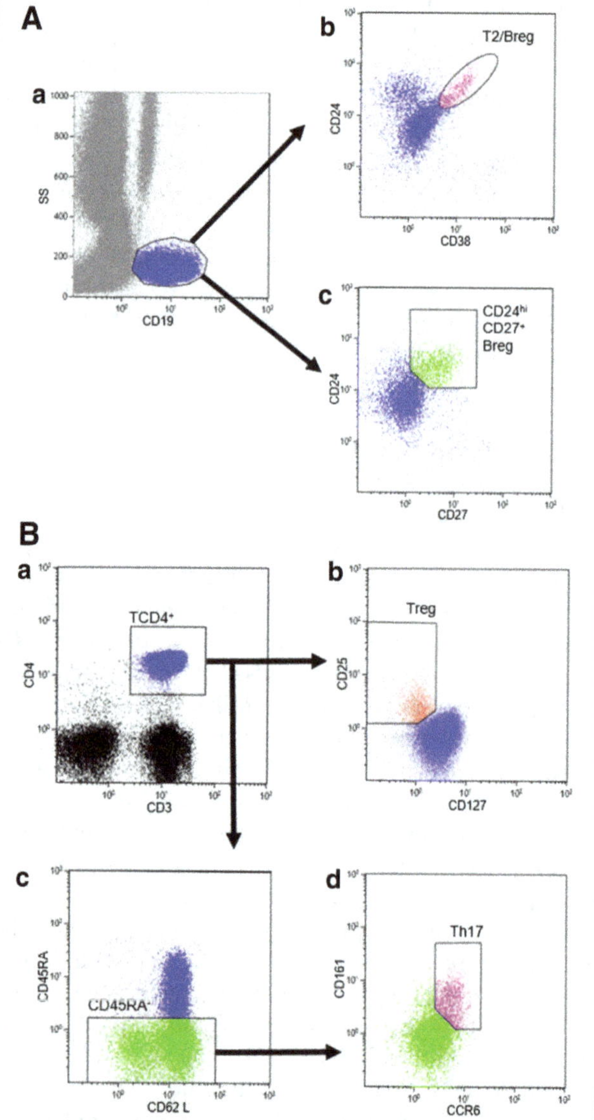

Fig. 1 Analysis of lymphocyte subpopulations by flow cytometry: gating strategy. **A** Gating strategy for B lymphocytes; **a** expressed as a single parameter of CD19 and scatter; **b** T2/Breg ($CD24^{hi}CD38^{hi}$); **c** $CD24^{hi}CD27^{+}$ Breg. **B** Gating strategy for T lymphocytes; **a** $CD3^{+}CD4^{+}$; **b** Treg ($CD25^{hi}CD127^{low}$); **c** $CD4^{+}45RA^{-}$; **d** Th17 ($CD45RA^{-}CD161^{+}CCR6^{+}$). *Breg* B regulatory cells, *Treg* T regulatory cells, *Th17* T helper 17

Results

Baseline characteristics of patients and controls

Table 1 gives the demographic and clinical characteristics of the 31 patients and 17 controls, included prospectively between November 2014 and October 2015. No statistically significant difference was observed. Two patients left the study at M1 and three left at M6.

Baseline lymphocyte subpopulations levels in patients and controls

We compared the frequencies of lymphocyte subpopulations in patients before the use of biologic drugs with those in controls (Table 2). The only statistically significant differences were in T2/Breg cells, which were lower in patients, both in frequency (%, $p < 0.01$) and in absolute numbers ($p < 0.05$), and Th17 frequency ($p < 0.05$).

Association between the immunologic and radiographic status of patients and their lymphocyte subpopulations at baseline

We compared the frequencies of lymphocyte subpopulations before the use of biologic drugs in patients with positive (n = 23) or negative (n = 8) RF, positive (n = 25)

Table 1 Baseline characteristics of patients and controls

		Patients with RA (n = 31)	Control group (n = 17)	*p*
Women		58.1% (n = 18)	41.2% (n = 7)	0.367
Age		57 (48–61)[a]	41 (29–68)[a]	0.131
BMI (kg/m2)		25.8 (22.2–33)[a]	24.0 (22.16–26.30)[a]	0.343
Medical history of smoking		48.4% (n = 15)	23.5% (n = 4)	0.127
Consumption (packets per year)		20 (11–28)[a]	0 (0–5)[a]	0.094
Recent RA ≤2 years		32.3% (n = 10)	-	
Antibodies				
RF+		74.2% (n = 23)	-	
ACPA+		80.6% (n = 25)	-	
Structural damage (erosions)		41.9% (n = 13)	-	
NSAID		12.9% (n = 4)	-	
Corticoids		54.8% (n = 17)	-	
Median dosage (mg/day)		5 (5–6)[a]	-	
Methotrexate		64.5% (n = 20)	-	
Median dose (mg/week)		15 (10–20)[a]	-	
Initiation (1st line of biomedicine)		54.8% (n = 17)	-	
Abatacept		38.7% (n = 12)	-	
Tocilizumab		19.4% (n = 6)	-	
Anti-TNF drugs	Golimumab	16.1% (n = 5)	-	
	Etanercept	22.6% (n = 7)	-	
	Certolizumab	3.2% (n = 1)	-	
ESR (mm)		14 (6–31)[a]	-	
CRP (mg/L)		7.9 (3.0–23.2)[a]	-	
DAS28		4.24 (3.70–5.32)[a]	-	
DAS28-CRP		4.42 (3.69–5.11)[a]	-	
HAQ		1.63 (1–2)[a]	-	

[a]Results expressed as median and 25th and 75th percentiles. The Mann–Whitney test was used for quantitative variables; the Fisher exact test was used for other variables (male/female, tobacco precursor). *RA* rheumatoid arthritis, *BMI* body mass index, *RF* rheumatoid factor, *ACPA* anti-citrullinated peptide antibodies, *ESR* erythrocyte sedimentation rate, *CRP* C-reactive protein, *DAS28* Disease Activity Score in 28 joints, *HAQ* Health Assessment Questionnaire, *NSAID* nonsteroidal anti-inflammatory drugs

or negative (n = 6) ACPA and with or (n = 13) or without (n = 18) structural damage. There was an association between the presence of RF and lower absolute numbers of T2/Breg ($p = 0.016$) with a median of 10.99/mm^3 (8.12–16.58) for RF$^+$ patients vs. 23.1/mm^3 (16.03–24.74) for RF$^-$ patients. No further association was found between other lymphocyte subpopulations and ACPA or radiographic status.

Correlation between lymphocyte subpopulation levels in patients and controls

We tested potential correlation between T2/Breg, Treg and Th17 frequencies or absolute values, in controls and patients at different time points during treatment. In controls (n = 17), there was a trend toward correlation between the absolute number of Treg and T2/Breg ($r = 0.500$, $p = 0.041$) and between Treg and Th17 cells ($r = 0.740$ and $p = 0.001$).

In patients at baseline (n = 31), the positive correlation between absolute numbers of Treg and Th17 cells was confirmed ($r = 0.579$, $p = 0.001$) and between CD24^{hi}CD27$^+$ B cells and Th17 cells ($r = 0.375$, $p = 0.037$). At M1, there was positive correlation between absolute numbers of Treg and Th17 cells ($r = 0.466$, $p = 0.011$) and at M6 ($r = 0.497$ and $p = 0.010$); between absolute values of T2/Breg and Th17 cells at M1 ($r = 0.385$ and $p = 0.039$) and at M3 in percentage values ($r = 0.383$ and $p = 0.040$) and positive correlation between absolute values of CD24^{hi}CD27$^+$ Breg and Th17 cells only at M1 ($r = 0.513$ and $p = 0.004$).

Evolution of lymphocyte subpopulations levels under biologic drugs

We compared the evolution of the lymphocyte subpopulations in patients between M0 (n = 31), M1 (n = 29), M3 (n = 26) and M6 (n = 26). We observed a difference

Table 2 Initial lymphocyte subpopulations levels in patients with RA and controls

Lymphocyte populations	Patient group (n = 31)	Control group (n = 17)	p
Lymphocytes			
(%)	23.8 (17.0–30.0)	18.6 (13.6–28.5)	0.413
(/mm3)	1600 (1300–2000)	1700 (1050–1950)	0.974
B lymphocytes			
(%)	11.1 (8.2–17.6)	10.0 (7.3–14.4)	0.651
(/mm3)	156 (95–278)	151 (122–195)	0.957
TCD4+			
(%)	53.5 (47.0–60.9)	51.7 (44.8–58.1)	0.779
(/mm3)	723 (569–1081)	739 (549–955)	0.821
T2/Breg			
(%)	8.5 (5.9–10.5)	13.8 (10.9–15.6)	<0.001**
(/mm3)	13 (9–22)	17 (14–31)	0.014*
CD24hiCD27$^+$ Breg			
(%)	16.3 (13.1–28.6)	18.8 (11.9–24.5)	0.612
(/mm3)	33 (20–45)	23 (19–34)	0.185
Treg			
(%)	6.4 (4.9–8.1)	7.1 (6.3–8.3)	0.223
(/mm3)	49 (35–65)	56 (44–68)	0.371
Th17			
(%)	19.6 (13.2–22.7)	23.4 (18.6–28.4)	0.036*
(/mm)	77 (45–97)	76 (51–135)	0.539

Total lymphocytes, B lymphocytes, T2/B regulatory cells (Breg), CD24^{hi}CD27$^+$ Breg, T regulatory cells (Treg) and T helper 17 (Th17) observed in patients with rheumatoid arthritis (RA) and controls in absolute value (cells per mm^3) and percentage; expressed in median and IQR; difference observed between the two groups as per the Mann-Whitney test. *$p < 0.05$. **$p < 0.001$

only in Treg percentage between the four measurement times ($p = 0.048$). No significant evolution between the different treatment duration was observed for percentage or for absolute numbers in any of the other subsets (Table 3).

We then compared the evolution of the lymphocyte subpopulations according to the type of treatment received: (1) abatacept, an "anti-costimulation" treatment (n = 12) vs. "anti-cytokine" (n = 19) comprising anti-TNF (n = 13) and tocilizumab (n = 6) and then (2) anti-TNF drug (n = 13) vs. abatacept and tocilizumab (n = 18). We observed that Treg frequencies significantly decreased over time under abatacept ($p < 0.001$), from a M0 median of 6.37% (5.26–7.23) to 4.68% (4.32–5.70) at M6; while the frequencies of Treg increased under anti-TNF drugs between M0 and M6 ($p = 0.005$), from a median of 6.49 (4.77–8.49) to 7.13 (6.69–7.95).

Baseline levels and evolution of lymphocyte subpopulations in patients according to the DAS28 remission at M6

We attempted to determine whether the initial level of the different lymphocyte subpopulations studied was associated with DAS28 remission at M6. We dichotomised patients who achieved DAS28 remission (Fig. 2, dark grey box plot (n = 7)), or not (white box plot, (n = 19)) at M6. We then observed the evolution of these different populations at M1, M3 and M6. A higher baseline frequency of CD24^{hi}CD27$^+$ B cells was associated with DAS28 remission at M6 ($p = 0.04$) (Fig. 2a) with a median of 24.13% (20.04–27.34) for the patients in remission at M6 vs. 15.66% (12.31–27.72) for the others. The Treg increased during treatment in patients achieving DAS28 remission at M6 (p = 0.01), their median increasing from 4.76% (4.21–7.89) at M0 to 6.90% (6.43–7.22) at M6 (Fig. 2b).

Baseline levels and evolution of lymphocyte subpopulations in patients according to the EULAR response at M6

We repeated this analysis with respect to achieving a good response (n = 9) or not (n = 17) using EULAR criteria at M6. A higher baseline frequency of CD24^{hi}CD27$^+$ B cells was associated with a good EULAR response at M6 but this was not statistically significant ($p = 0.130$), with a median of 26.79% (8.13–28.64) at M0 in patients with a good EULAR response at M6 vs. 14.22% (11.66–22) in the others.

Table 3 Evolution of lymphocyte subpopulations levels in patients with RA under biologic drugs

Lymphocyte populations	Patients M0 (n = 31)	Patients M1 (n = 29)	Patients M3 (n = 29)	Patients M6 (n = 26)	*p* (6 months)
Lymphocytes					
(%)	23.8 (18.2–29.9)	29.8 (17.9–36.7)	28.9 (22.9–33.4)	29.55 (20.95–36.8)	0.140
(/mm)	1600 (1300–2000)	1600 (1300–2200)	1900 (1500–2300)	1550 (1300–1900)	0.117
B lymphocytes					
(%)	11.07 (8.28–16.05)	11.60 (8.94–17.47)	12.42 (8.44–15.96)	10.365 (8.38–14.52)	0.077
(/mm3)	156.15 (95.5–270.2)	201.57 (143.02–314.80)	192.63 (122.65–260.56)	180.66 (119.86–255.99)	0.989
T2/Breg					
(%)	8.46 (5.95–10.35)	6.43 (4.31–9.92)	8.54 (6.35–12.5)	9.35 (5.93–12.65)	0.099
(/mm)	12.75 (8.88–21.15)	13.47 (8.85–24.43)	15.29 (9.06–28.36)	15.81 (8.40–22.83)	0.489
$CD24^{hi}CD27^{+}$ Breg					
(%)	16.34 (13.2–27.71)	18.53 (15.02–31.61)	20.16 (14.81–30.26)	23.33 (14.02–33.00)	0.246
(/mm3)	33.26 (20.1–43.84)	34.87 (23.29–65.00)	35.22 (22.38–66.29)	35.54 (17.28–55.98)	0.813
Treg					
(%)	6.37 (4.91–7.98)	5.41 (4.36–7.06)	5.54 (4.63–6.85)	6.38 (4.87–7.02)	0.048*
(/mm3)	49.40 (37.6–62.52)	40.36 (30.60–60.24)	47.7 (35.89–65.28)	51.20 (34.97–66.14)	0.702
Th17					
(%)	19.57 (13.4–22.48)	19.0 (12.87–24.39)	19.01 (14.63–23.90)	19.50 (14.40–25.85)	0.928
(/mm3)	76.85 (49.1–96.77)	76.4 (47.75–112.7)	77.10 (61.80–113.43)	77.27 (65.66–91.44)	0.958

Total lymphocytes, B lymphocytes, T2/B regulatory cells (Breg), $CD24^{hi}CD27^{+}$ Breg, T regulatory cells (Treg) and T helper 17 (Th17) cells observed in absolute value (cells/mm^3) and percentage (%) at different stages of the treatment, i.e. M0 (n = 31), M1 (n = 29), M3 (n = 29) and M6 (n = 26) and the difference observed; expressed as median and IQR, Kruskall – Wallis test. *RA* rheumatoid arthritis. $^{*}p < 0.05$

A trend was observed in favour of a higher frequency of $CD24^{hi}CD27^{+}$ B cell in percentage at each of the treatment duration time points in patients with a good EULAR response at M6 vs. the others ($p = 0.07$) (Fig. 2c).

A lower frequency of Th17 cells before treatment was significantly associated with a good EULAR response at M6 ($p = 0.007$) with a median of 13.73% (12.1–19.57) at M0 in patients with a good EULAR response at M6 vs. 20.66% (17.92–26.16) in the others. An identical trend was observed in absolute numbers ($p = 0.06$) with a Th17 median of 13.73/mm^3 (12.1–19.57) for patients with a good response at M6 vs. 20.66/mm^3 (17.92–26.16) for the others. Likewise, a significantly lower frequency of Th17 cells was recorded at each treatment duration time point in patients with a good EULAR response at M6 vs. the others ($p = 0.009$), and the same trend was observed in absolute numbers ($p = 0.06$) (Fig. 2d).

The initial level of T2/Breg and Treg cells was not associated with good EULAR response at M6. Finally, there was no significant difference in the evolution of the other lymphocyte subpopulations under treatment, whether the patient did or not have a good EULAR response at M6.

Baseline lymphocyte subpopulations levels according to type of biologic drugs used

We analysed out data again with respect to good EULAR response at M6, according to the type of biologic drug received, i.e. abatacept (n = 10), anti-cytokine (anti-TNF drugs and tocilizumab, (n = 16)) or anti-TNF drugs only (n = 10). The proportion of patients with a good EULAR response at M6 was 4/10 with abatacept, 2/6 with tocilizumab and 3/10 with anti-TNF drugs.

A high frequency of $CD24^{hi}CD27^{+}$ B cells was associated with a good EULAR response at M6 under abatacept ($p = 0.01$) (Fig. 3a), with a median of 26.79% (10.29–30.43) for patients with good response vs. 13% (10.32–15.19). The initial level of the other lymphocyte subpopulations was not associated with this response. A low initial level of Th17 cells was associated with a good EULAR response at M6 with the use of anti-cytokine (Fig. 3b, $p = 0.048$) with a median of 13.73% (12.1–21.13) in patients with good response vs. 20.62% (18.55–25.08) in the others. The initial level of the other lymphocyte subpopulations was not associated with this response.

Discussion

Our data describe the effects of biologic drugs on B cells ($CD24^{hi}CD27^{+}$ Breg and T2/Breg), Treg and Th17 subsets, immuno-regulating lymphocyte subpopulations, involved in numerous autoimmune pathologic conditions such as RA. In our study, participants were representative of the patients commonly encountered in clinical practice (2/3 women, median age approximately 60 years). One third of the RA had developed within the previous 2 years.

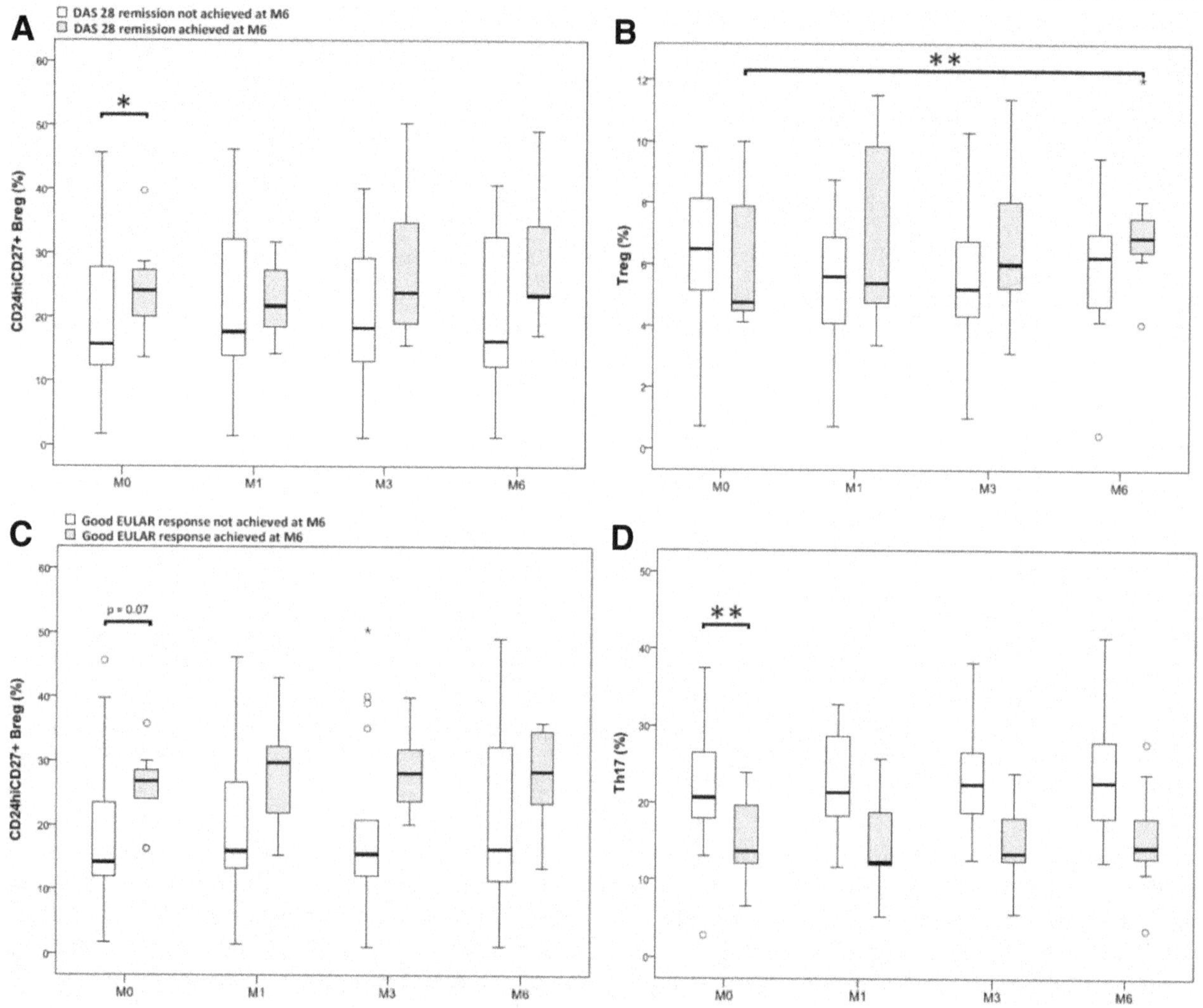

Fig. 2 Baseline levels and evolution of lymphocyte subpopulations in patients with rheumatoid arthritis according to Disease Activity Score in 28 joints (*DAS28*) remission or European League Against Rheumatism (*EULAR*) response at month (M)6. **a** Baseline levels and evolution of $CD24^{hi}CD27^{+}$ B regulatory cells (*Breg*) in percentage between M0 and M6 in the patients who achieved DAS 28 remission (n = 7) or not (n = 19) at M6. **b** Initial levels and evolution of T regulatory cells (*Treg*) in percentage between M0 and M6 in the patients who achieved DAS28 remission (n = 7) or not (n = 19) at M6. **c** Initial levels and evolution of $CD24^{hi}CD27^{+}$ Breg in percentage between M0 and M6 in patients who achieved good EULAR response at M6 (n = 9) or not (n = 17). **d** Baseline levels and evolution of T helper 17 (Th17) cells in percentage between M0 and M6 in patients who achieved good EULAR response at M6 (n = 9) or not (n = 17). Results in box plots are median and IQR; difference observed between the two groups was assessed by the Mann-Whitney test at M0 and the general linear model (GLM) procedure and MIXED SAS for repetitive analyses. *$p < 0.05$, **$p < 0.01$

The median DAS28 was 4.24 and 3/4 of the subjects had immunopositive (RF and/or CCP+) RA and almost 50% of them had erosive RA.

In our study, T2/Breg cells were significantly reduced, both in percentage and in absolute numbers, in patients compared with controls. Other studies report a quantitative decrease in Breg in patients with RA compared to healthy control subjects and in patients with active RA compared with inactive disease [30, 31]. This lymphocyte subpopulation may therefore represent an objective biomarker of the activity of the disease. Moreover, we observed positive correlation in absolute numbers between T2/Breg and Treg cells in controls but not in patients, both at inclusion and during treatment, which may reflect dysfunction of the T2/Breg-Treg cell balance in RA. The T2/Bregs were also lower in patients with RF, as described in another study [30], in which negative correlation was observed between Bregs and RF and ACPA levels. There is no consensus as yet on the role of these antibodies in RA, but it has been proven that their presence is a marker of poor prognosis. Our data showing lower T2/Breg levels in patients with RA compared to controls, and in RF^{+} patients with RA, may therefore indicate a "protective" role.

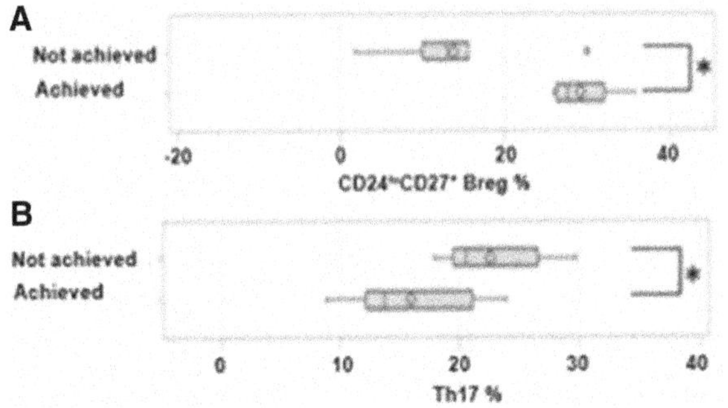

Fig. 3 Baseline lymphocyte subpopulation levels according to the European League Against Rheumatism (*EULAR*) response at month 6 (*M6*) by type of biologic drug. **a** Comparison of baseline levels of $CD24^{hi}CD27^{+}$ B regulatory cells (*Breg*) in percentage, between the patients who achieved a good EULAR response at M6 (n = 4) or not (n = 6) under abatacept. **b** Comparison of T helper 17 cell (*Th17*) levels in percentage at M0 between patients who achieved good EULAR response at M6 (n = 5) or not (n = 11) under anti-cytokine treatment; box-plots show median and IQR; difference observed between the two groups using the *t* test. $^{*}p < 0.05$

DAS28 remission at M6 was associated with significantly higher $CD24^{hi}CD27^{+}$Breg frequency at baseline. Likewise, higher $CD24^{hi}CD27^{+}$ Breg frequency was initially observed in patients who had a good EULAR response at M6 (although not significant). The literature suggests that higher pre-treatment levels of $CD24^{hi}CD27^{+}$ Breg and T2/Breg may be predictive of a good EULAR response at 3 months with anti-TNF treatment [25]. A retrospective study of patients with RA receiving abatacept, showed that the level of $CD24^{hi}CD27^{+}$ Breg prior to treatment was not significantly different between patients who were EULAR responders and non-responder patients at M6 [34], whereas our results showed that a high initial level of $CD24^{hi}CD27^{+}$ Breg is significantly associated with a good EULAR response at M6 under abatacept. Therefore, $CD24^{hi}CD27^{+}$ Breg, that were higher at M0 in patients with DAS28 remission and in patients with good EULAR responses at M6, may represent a predictive biomarker for response to treatment, notably with abatacept. Finally, the activity of the disease (evaluated by DAS28) correlated negatively with the proportion of T2/Breg cells (and $CD5^{+}CD1d^{hi}$ [25] and IL-10 + $CD5Cd1d^{hi}$ and IL-10^{+}TIM-1^{+} [30, 31]) which also suggest a potential of this subset for disease monitoring.

Several studies reported more Treg in healthy subjects than in patients with early RA, but others reported similar levels [35–37]. Our data showed no significant difference in Treg at baseline between the patients and the controls, most likely due to the small number of participants in our current work, as we previously identified significant differences with larger numbers of subjects [38]. Whereas the frequency of Treg cells was similar at baseline in patients treated with the different drugs (anti-TNF, tocilizumab and abatacept), we observed a decrease in Tregs under abatacept but an increase under anti-TNF drugs. As previously described [6, 7], this may be partly explained by the removal of the repression exerted by this major proinflammatory cytokine on these cells.

In our study, the pre-treatment level of Treg was not predictive of DAS28 remission or EULAR response at M6. However, we observed a significant evolution of Treg under biologic drugs, with a recovery of these cells in patients with DAS28 remission at M6. Their level is described in the literature as being higher in drug-naive patients with early disease, who will achieve remission with MTX [38] and recovery of these cells under anti-TNF drugs was associated with a greater probability of long-term remission on anti-TNF drugs [7]. Other authors also report an increase in Treg over the course of anti-TNF [6] and abatacept [8] treatment only in patients with a good response. Treg may therefore represent an efficient biomarker for monitoring patients but not for predicting their personal response.

Th17 cell levels were significantly lower in patients than in the control group. Another study, however, described elevated levels of Th17 cells in RA, but only in patients with recent onset of disease [18]. There is a large amount of literature on such quantification with major discrepancies due to the use of different techniques (with or without a polarization-inducing condition) and the use of different phenotypes to identify Th17 cells [39, 40]. We did not find any association between the level of Th17 cells and the presence or absence of ACPA, although inverse correlation between the frequency of Th17 cells in the blood and the ACPA level had been previously described [17]. In addition, there was positive correlation between the absolute numbers of $CD24^{hi}CD27^{+}$ Breg and Th17 cells in patients with RA at baseline, but not in the controls. This was no longer observed after 3 and 6 months of treatment. This would therefore suggest initial pathologic correlation in RA, which disappeared over the course of a biology-modifying treatment such as a biologic drug.

Reduction in Th17 cells under MTX [18] and increase in non-response to infliximab [19] have been described In our study, patients with a good EULAR response at M6 had a significantly lower frequency of Th17 cells compared with moderate responders or non-responders, both at inclusion and at all the treatment points. A small proportion of Th17 cells at baseline was associated with a good EULAR response at M6 under anti-cytokine treatments but not under abatacept. The levels also did not evolve under treatment, whether the patients responded or not, which possibly reflects a lack of implication of this cell population in RA at late stages of the disease continuum (i.e. DMARD-resistant, biologic-drug-naive), which appears to contribute to the explanation of the disappointing results with treatments targeting IL-17 in clinical trials among patients with established RA [41]. In contrast, the positive correlation between the absolute numbers of Treg and Th17 cells, both in the controls and in the patient groups is likely to reinforce the hypothesis of an early role of Th17 cells in establishing chronicity [18]. It should finally be noted that low levels of Th17 cells may have predictive value for response to "anti-cytokine" treatments.

Conclusions

This work aimed to establish pilot data using routine immunology hospital services protocols towards describing the evolution of different lymphocyte subpopulations in patients with RA under biologic drugs with different mechanisms of action, and assessing whether there is correlation between their levels and the later therapeutic response. Whereas, to date, only RF and ACPA are used to attempt to stratify patients for personalised treatment, $CD24^{hi}CD27^{+}$ B cells and Th17 cells may offer predictive value as biomarkers of therapeutic response under biologic drugs and may be able to guide clinicians in their choice of a tailored treatment. If validated, our data would suggest the prescribing of abatacept if the patient has high baseline levels of $CD24^{hi}CD27^{+}$ B cells, whereas a low initial level of Th17 cells may guide the choice of an anti-cytokine. As this was a pilot study, it remains crucial that our results are confirmed on a wider scale before being used to guide our therapeutic strategies.

Abbreviations

ACPA: Anticitrullinated peptide antibody; ACR/EULAR: American College of Rheumatology/European League Against Rheumatism; BMI: Body mass index; Breg: Regulatory B lymphocytes; CMF: Flow cytometry; CRP: C-reactive protein; DAS28: Disease Activity Score in 28 joints; DMARD: Disease-modifying antirheumatic drug; ESR: Erythrocyte sedimentation rate; HAQ: Health Assessment Questionnaire; IL: Interleukin; MTX: Methotrexate; PBMC: Peripheral blood mononuclear cell; RA: Rheumatoid arthritis; RF: Rheumatoid factor; T2T: Treat to target; Th17: T helper type 17 cell; TNF: Tumour necrosis factor; Treg: regulatory T cells

Acknowledgements

The authors want to thanks the patients included in this study, Dr Germain Jelin and Dr Marie Fechtenbaum (Amiens university Hospital) for their help in the follow up of the patients and Dr Frédérique Ponchel (University of Leeds, UK) for her critical reading of the manuscript.

Funding

This study is fully academic and funding was only provided by the University of Picardy Jules-Verne (Amiens, France).

Authors' contributions

SS contributed to the conception and design of the study, participated in the performance of the statistical analyses, was responsible for the analysis of the blood samples, contributed to the acquisition of patient material and data and also drafted the manuscript. CG contributed to conception and design of the study, participated in the performance of the statistical analyses and drafted the manuscript. PM was the main contributor to the statistical analyses. GF, CB, CG, PF, JPM and BG contributed to the conception and design of the study and in patient assessments. VG contributed to the conception and design of the study, participated in the performance of the statistical analyses, is responsible for patient assessments and drafted the manuscript. All authors read, critically reviewed and approved the final version to be submitted for publication.

Competing interests

The authors declare that they have no competing interests for this work.

Author details

[1]Rheumatology Department & EA 4666, Amiens University Hospital, University of Picardie-Jules Verne, Amiens, France. [2]Immunology laboratory & EA 4666, Amiens University Hospital, University of Picardie-Jules Verne, Amiens, France. [3]Hematology laboratory & EA 4666, Amiens University Hospital, University of Picardie-Jules Verne, Amiens, France.

References

1. Smolen JS, Aletaha D, McInnes IB. Rheumatoid arthritis. Lancet. 2016;S0140-6736:30173–8.
2. Smolen JS, Landewé R, Breedveld FC, Buch M, Burmester G, Dougados M, et al. EULAR. Recommendations for the management of rheumatoid arthritis with synthetic and biological disease-modifying antirheumatic drug. Ann Rheum Dis. 2014;73:492–509.
3. Stoffer MA, Schoels M, Smolen JS, et al. Evidence for treating rheumatoid arthritis to target: results of a systematic literature search update. Ann Rheum Dis. 2016;75:16–22.
4. Daïen CI, Morel J. Predictive factors of response to biological disease modifying antirheumatic drugs: towards personalized medicine. Mediators Inflamm. 2014;2014:386148.
5. Ponchel F, Burska AN, Hensor EM, Raja R, Campbell M, Emery P, Conaghan PG. Changes in peripheral blood immune cell composition in osteoarthritis. Osteoarthritis Cartilage. 2015;23:1870–8.
6. Ehrenstein MR, Evans JG, Singh A, et al. Compromised function of regulatory T-cells in rheumatoid arthritis and reversal by anti-TNF-alpha therapy. J Exp Med. 2004;200:277–85.
7. Saleem B, Keen H, Goeb V, Parmar R, Nizam S, Hensor EM, Churchman SM, Quinn M, Wakefield R, Conaghan PG, Ponchel F, Emery P. Patients with RA in remission on TNF blockers: when and in whom can TNF blocker therapy be stopped? Ann Rheum Dis. 2010;69:1636–42.
8. Bonelli M, Göschl L, Blüml S, Karonitsch T, Hirahara K, Ferner E, Steiner CW, Steiner G, Smolen JS, Scheinecker C. Abatacept (CTLA-4Ig) treatment reduces T cell apoptosis and regulatory T cell suppression in patients with rheumatoid arthritis. Rheumatology. 2016;55:710–20.
9. Harrington LE, Hatton RD, Mangan PR, Turner H, Murphy TL, Murphy KM, et al. Interleukin 17-producing CD4+ effector T cells develop via a lineage distinct from the T helper type 1 and 2 lineages. Nat Immunol. 2005;6:1123–32.
10. Park H, Li Z, Yang XO, Chang SH, Nurieva R, Wang YH, et al. A distinct lineage of CD4 T cells regulates tissue inflammation by producing interleukin 17. Nat Immunol. 2005;6:1133–41.
11. Sundrud MS, Trivigno C. Identity crisis of Th17 cells: many forms, many functions, many questions. Semin Immunol. 2013;25:263–72.
12. Calderón-Gómez E, Bassolas-Molina H, Mora-Buch R, Dotti I, Planell N, Esteller M, Gallego M, Martí M, Garcia-Martín C, Martínez-Torró C, Ordás I, Singh S, Panés J, Benítez-Ribas D, Salas A. Commensal-specific CD4+ cells from patients with Crohn's disease have a T-helper 17 inflammatory profile. Gastroenterology. 2016;S0016–5085:34576.
13. Mc Innes IB, Schett G. The pathogenesis of rheumatoid arthritis. N Engl J Med. 2011;365:2205–19.
14. Furst DE, Emery P. Rheumatoid arthritis pathophysiology: update on emerging cytokine and cytokine-associated cell targets. Rheumatology (Oxford). 2014;53:1560–9.
15. Komatsu N, Okamoto K, Sawa S, et al. Pathogenic conversion of Foxp3+ T cells into TH17 cells in autoimmune arthritis. Nat Med. 2014;20:62–8.
16. Alunno A, Manetti M, Caterbi S, Ibba-Manneschi L, Bistoni O, Bartoloni E, Valentini V, Terenzi R, Gerli R. Altered immunoregulation in rheumatoid arthritis: the role of regulatory T cells and proinflammatory Th17 cells and therapeutic implications. Mediators Inflamm. 2015;2015:751793.

17. Kotake S, Nanke Y, Yago T, Kawamoto M, Kobashigawa T, Yamanaka H. Ratio of circulating IFNγ (+) "Th17 cells" in memory Th cells is inversely correlated with the titer of anti-CCP antibodies in early-onset rheumatoid arthritis patients based on flow cytometry methods of the Human Immunology Project. Biomed Res Int. 2016;2016:9694289.
18. Kotake S, Nanke Y, Yago T, Kawamoto M, Kobashigawa T, Yamanaka H. Elevated ratio of Th17 cell-derived Th1 Cells (CD161(+)Th1 Cells) to CD161(+)Th17 cells in peripheral blood of early-onset rheumatoid arthritis patients. Biomed Res Int. 2016;2016:418602.
19. Talotta R, Berzi A, Atzeni F, Batticciotto A, Clerici M, Sarzi-Puttini P, Trabattoni D. Paradoxical expansion of Th1 and Th17 lymphocytes in rheumatoid arthritis following infliximab treatment: a possible explanation for a lack of clinical response. J Clin Immunol. 2015;35:550–7.
20. Klareskog L, Amara K, Malmström V. Adaptive immunity in rheumatoid arthritis: anticitrulline and other antibodies in the pathogenesis of rheumatoid arthritis. Curr Opin Rheumatol. 2014;26:72–9.
21. Berthelot JM, Jamin C, Amrouche K, Le Goff B, Maugars Y, Youinou P. Regulatory B cells play a key role in immune system balance. Joint Bone Spine. 2013;80:18–22.
22. Mauri C, Bosma A. Immune regulatory function of B cells. Annu Rev Immunol. 2012;30:221–41.
23. Rosser EC, Blair PA, Mauri C. Cellular targets of regulatory B cell-mediated suppression. Mol Immunol. 2014;62:296–304.
24. Iwata Y, Matsushita T, Horikawa M, Dilillo DJ, Yanaba K, Venturi GM, Szabolcs PM, Bernstein SH, Magro CM, Williams AD, Hall RP, St Clair EW, Tedder TF. Characterization of a rare IL-10-competent B-cell subset in humans that parallels mouse regulatory B10 cells. Blood. 2011;117:530–41.
25. Daien CI, Gailhac S, Mura T, Rachel A, Combe B, Hahne M, Morel J. Regulatory B10 cells are decreased in patients with rheumatoid arthritis and are inversely correlated with disease activity. Arthritis Rheumatol. 2014;66:2037–46.
26. Rosser EC, Mauri C. Regulatory B cells: origin, phenotype, and function. Immunity. 2015;42:607–12.
27. Bouaziz JD, Calbo S, Maho-Vaillant M, et al. IL-10 produced by activated human B cells regulates CD4(+) T-cell activation in vitro. Eur J Immunol. 2010;40:2686–91.
28. Garraud O, Borhis G, Badr G, Degrelle S, Pozzetto B, Cognasse F, Richard Y. Revisiting the B-cell compartment in mouse and humans: more than one B-cell subset exists in the marginal zone and beyond. BMC Immunol. 2012;13:63.
29. Van de Veen W, Stanic B, Wirz OF, Jansen K, Globinska A, Akdis M. Role of regulatory B cells in immune tolerance to allergens and beyond. J Allergy Clin Immunol. 2016;138:654–65.
30. Flores-Borja F, Bosma A, Ng D, Reddy V, Ehrenstein MR, Isenberg DA, Mauri C. CD19 + CD24hiCD38hi B cells maintain regulatory T cells while limiting TH1 and TH17 differentiation. Sci Transl Med. 2013;5:173ra23.
31. Ma L, Liu B, Jiang Z, Jiang Y. Reduced numbers of regulatory B cells are negatively correlated with disease activity in patients with new-onset rheumatoid arthritis. Clin Rheumatol. 2014;33:187–95.
32. Aletaha D, Neogi T, Silman AJ, Funovits J, Felson DT, Bingham CO, et al. Rheumatoid arthritis classification criteria: an American College of Rheumatology/European League Against Rheumatism collaborative initiative. Ann Rheum Dis. 2010;69:1580–8.
33. Saison J, Demaret J, Venet F, Chidiac C, Malcus C, Poitevin-Later F, Tardy JC, Ferry T, Monneret G. CD4 + CD25 + CD127- assessment as a surrogate phenotype for FOXP3+ regulatory T cells in HIV-1 infected viremic and aviremic subjects. Cytometry B Clin Cytom. 2013;84:50–4.
34. Gazeau P, Devauchelle-Pensec V, Pochard P, Pers JO, Saraux A, Renaudineau Y, Cornec D. Abatacept efficacy in rheumatoid arthritis is dependent upon baseline blood B-cell levels. Rheumatology. 2016;55:1138–40.
35. Lawson CA, Brown AK, Bejarano V, et al. Early rheumatoid arthritis is associated with a deficit in the CD4 + CD25high regulatory T-cell population in peripheral blood. Rheumatology (Oxford). 2006;45:1210–7.
36. Van Amelsfort JM, Jacobs KM, Bijlsma JW, et al. CD4 + CD25+ regulatory T-cells in rheumatoid arthritis: differences in the presence, phenotype, and function between peripheral blood and synovial fluid. Arthritis Rheum. 2004;50:2775–85.
37. Boissier MC, Assier E, Falgarone G, et al. Shifting the imbalance from Th1/Th2 to Th17/Treg: the changing rheumatoid arthritis paradigm. Joint Bone Spine. 2008;75:373–5.
38. Ponchel F, Goëb V, Parmar R, El-Sherbiny Y, Boissinot M, El Jawhari J, Burska A, Vital EM, Harrison S, Conaghan PG, Hensor E, Emery P. An immunological biomarker to predict MTX response in early RA. Ann Rheum Dis. 2014;73:2047–53.
39. Aerts NE, De Knop KJ, Leysen J, Ebo DG, Bridts CH, Weyler JJ, Stevens WJ, De Clerck LS. Increased IL-17 production by peripheral T helper cells after tumour necrosis factor blockade in rheumatoid arthritis is accompanied by inhibition of migration-associated chemokine receptor expression. Rheumatology (Oxford). 2010;49:2264–72.
40. Miao J, Zhang K, Lv M, Li Q, Zheng Z, Han Q, Guo N, Fan C, Zhu P. Circulating Th17 and Th1 cells expressing CD161 are associated with disease activity in rheumatoid arthritis. Scand J Rheumatol. 2014;43:194–201.
41. Genovese MC, Durez P, Richards HB, Supronik J, Dokoupilova E, Mazurov V, Aelion JA, Lee SH, Codding CE, Kellner H, Ikawa T, Hugot S, Mpofu S. Efficacy and safety of secukinumab in patients with rheumatoid arthritis: a phase II, dose-finding, double-blind, randomised, placebo controlled study. Ann Rheum Dis. 2013;72:863–9.

Molecular alterations in skeletal muscle in rheumatoid arthritis are related to disease activity, physical inactivity, and disability

Kim M. Huffman[1*], Ryan Jessee[1], Brian Andonian[1], Brittany N. Davis[2], Rachel Narowski[3], Janet L. Huebner[1], Virginia B. Kraus[1], Julie McCracken[1], Brian F. Gilmore[4], K. Noelle Tune[5], Milton Campbell[1], Timothy R. Koves[1], Deborah M. Muoio[1], Monica J. Hubal[6] and William E. Kraus[1]

Abstract

Background: To identify molecular alterations in skeletal muscle in rheumatoid arthritis (RA) that may contribute to ongoing disability in RA.

Methods: Persons with seropositive or erosive RA ($n = 51$) and control subjects matched for age, gender, race, body mass index (BMI), and physical activity ($n = 51$) underwent assessment of disease activity, disability, pain, physical activity and thigh muscle biopsies. Muscle tissue was used for measurement of pro-inflammatory markers, transcriptomics, and comprehensive profiling of metabolic intermediates. Groups were compared using mixed models. Bivariate associations were assessed with Spearman correlation.

Results: Compared to controls, patients with RA had 75% greater muscle concentrations of IL-6 protein ($p = 0.006$). In patients with RA, muscle concentrations of inflammatory markers were positively associated ($p < 0.05$ for all) with disease activity (IL-1β, IL-8), disability (IL-1β, IL-6), pain (IL-1β, TNF-α, toll-like receptor (TLR)-4), and physical inactivity (IL-1β, IL-6). Muscle cytokines were not related to corresponding systemic cytokines. Prominent among the gene sets differentially expressed in muscles in RA versus controls were those involved in skeletal muscle repair processes and glycolytic metabolism. Metabolic profiling revealed 46% higher concentrations of pyruvate in muscle in RA ($p < 0.05$), and strong positive correlation between levels of amino acids involved in fibrosis (arginine, ornithine, proline, and glycine) and disability ($p < 0.05$).

Conclusion: RA is accompanied by broad-ranging molecular alterations in skeletal muscle. Analysis of inflammatory markers, gene expression, and metabolic intermediates linked disease-related disruptions in muscle inflammatory signaling, remodeling, and metabolic programming to physical inactivity and disability. Thus, skeletal muscle dysfunction might contribute to a viscous cycle of RA disease activity, physical inactivity, and disability.

Keywords: Gene expression, Metabolomics, Satellite cells, Fibrosis, Inflammation

Background

Despite a vast array of pharmacologic agents available to treat rheumatoid arthritis (RA), management is often complicated by insufficient treatment response, drug toxicity and contraindications, poor access to care and/or medications, and/or damage that predates medical intervention. These barriers lead to or are accompanied by systemic manifestations, disease-associated co-morbidities, chronic pain, physical inactivity, dysmobility, and poor physical function. Thus, further advances in RA care require identification of factors contributing to persistent deficiencies in quality of life and physical function, despite access to excellent anti-rheumatic medications.

Importantly, inactivity and muscle wasting are two important contributors to RA-related morbidity and mortality. Approximately half of patients with RA do not perform even a single bout of weekly physical exercise [1]. The sedentary lifestyle common to patients

* Correspondence: Huffm007@mc.duke.edu
[1]Department of Medicine, Duke Molecular Physiology Institute, Duke School of Medicine, Durham, NC, USA
Full list of author information is available at the end of the article

with RA gives rise to physical deconditioning and muscle atrophy, both of which are associated with osteoporosis, impaired immune function, glucose intolerance, insulin resistance, loss of independence, and increased mortality [2].

In addition to physical inactivity, other factors that likewise promote muscle loss and disability in patients with RA include inadequate protein ingestion, glucocorticoid treatment, and pro-inflammatory cytokines, all resulting in reduced myocyte protein synthesis and increased protein degradation [2, 3]. Inflammation can impact normal muscle turnover and responses to injury, both of which require an exquisitely coordinated remodeling process involving activation, proliferation and differentiation of muscle stem cells—also known as satellite cells. These processes are mediated largely by signals from intramuscular immune cells: neutrophils, regulatory T cells, pro-inflammatory M1 macrophages, and anti-inflammatory M2 macrophages.

The established roles of inflammation in both skeletal muscle remodeling and RA pathophysiology raise obvious questions regarding the potential interplay between muscle dysfunction and RA morbidity. Whereas the link between pro-inflammatory cytokines and muscle dysfunction has been investigated intensely in the context of diseases such as diabetes and cancer cachexia, this topic has remained surprisingly unexplored in RA. In the current study we sought to identify molecular perturbations in muscle specimens from individuals with RA, and to test the hypothesis that skeletal muscle inflammatory markers and derangements in tissue remodeling might contribute to metabolic decline and disability in these patients. Herein, we report that disease-activity-related muscle inflammatory markers are related to physical inactivity, and moreover, that disrupted skeletal muscle repair processes are associated with greater disability. These findings support a model in which skeletal muscle deterioration contributes to a vicious cycle of disease activity, muscle inflammatory signaling and disrupted remodeling, physical inactivity, and disability in patients with RA.

Methods

Design and participants

This was a cross-sectional investigation of individuals with RA and matched controls collected from the Durham, NC area. The RA group met the following criteria: (1) RA diagnosis meeting American College of Rheumatology 1987 criteria [4]; (2) seropositive disease (positive rheumatoid factor or anti-cyclic citrullinated peptide) or evidence of erosions on hand or foot imaging; (3) no medication changes within the three months prior to study enrollment; and (4) daily prednisone use ≤5 mg. Healthy participants without a diagnosis of RA, without joint pain, and without joint swelling lasting more than a week were matched to individual participants with RA by gender, race, age within 3 years, and body mass index (BMI) within 3 kg/m^2. Exclusions included current pregnancy, type 2 diabetes mellitus, and known coronary artery disease. Further specific details on questionnaires and measurement protocols have previously been described [5]. This study was in compliance with the Helsinki Declaration and was approved by the Duke University Institutional Review Board.

Assessments of both groups included questionnaires, physical exams for disease status, fasting blood collection, intravenous glucose tolerance tests for insulin sensitivity, 7 days of accelerometer-measured physical activity, computed tomography (CT) imaging of abdomen and thigh, and *vastus lateralis* muscle biopsies [5]. Disability (health assessment questionnaire-disability index (HAQ-DI) and co-morbidities (co-morbidity index) were assessed by previously published questionnaires [6, 7]. Disease activity assessed by the disease activity score in 28 joints (DAS-28) was determined from a patient-completed visual analog scale, physician-determined numbers of tender and swollen joints, and erythrocyte sedimentation rate [8]. Plasma concentrations of inflammatory markers and cytokines were determined by immunoassay [5] and nuclear magnetic resonance (NMR) spectroscopy (GlycA) [9]. Insulin sensitivity was determined using Bergman's minimal model [10] and concentrations of glucose and insulin (glucose: Beckman-CoulterDXC600; insulin: electrochemiluminscent assay from Meso Scale Discovery) at each of 29 time points during the intravenous glucose tolerance test.

Physical activity was measured with 7 days of accelerometry. After completing assessments, accelerometers (RT3, Stayhealthy, Inc., Monrovia, CA, USA) were provided to participants. Participants also received a pre-addressed and postage-applied box for return and directions for wearing on the waist above the right knee during waking hours for 7 days. Accelerometer data were evaluated for validity and non-wear time, and categorized into metabolic equivalents (METs) as previously described [11]. After data cleaning, valid data were available for 41 persons with RA and 31 controls. Time spent exercising was defined as the sum of time spent performing activity at METs equal to or greater than 3. CT scan analyses were performed using OsiriX (Pixmeo) to determine adipose and muscle tissue size and muscle tissue density (greater tissue density is indicative of less inter-muscular adipose tissue) [5]. Standard Bergstrom needle muscle biopsies were performed on the *vastus lateralis* in the fasting state; participants consumed only water during the 12 hours overnight

Table 1 Participant characteristics

Variable	All participants ($n = 102$)	Rheumatoid arthritis ($n = 51$)	Matched controls ($n = 51$)
Age (years)	54.2 (12.5)	54.8 (13.2)	53.8 (11.9)
BMI (kg/m^2)	30.0 (6.4)	30.3 (7.5)	29.6 (5.1)
Waist circumference (cm)	94.1 (15.2)	94.9 (16.8)	92.9 (13.3)
Race			
Caucasian	74 (72.6%)	36 (70.6%)	38 (74.5%)
African American	27 (26.5%)	14 (27.5%)	13 (25.5%)
Pacific Islander	1 (1.0%)	1 (2.0%)	0
Gender			
Female	72 (70.6%)	36 (70.6%)	36 (70.6%)
Male	30 (29.4%)	15 (29.4%)	15 (29.4%)
Physical activity (kCal/day)	557.1 (280.8)	517.7 (279.4)	609.1 (278.7)
Physical activity (MET-hr/day)	5.4 (2.6)	4.9 (2.5)	6.0 (2.5)
Disease duration (months)	NA	138.9 (136.3)	NA
HAQ-disability index	0.46 (0.6)	0.68 (0.7)*	0.00 (0.0)
Comorbidity index	1.2 (1.2)	1.6 (1.1)*	0.6 (0.9)
DAS-28 mean (SD)	NA	3.0 (1.4)	NA
Remission (DAS-28 < 2.6)		19 (40%)	
Low activity (DAS-28 2.6 3.2)		8 (17%)	
Moderate activity (DAS-28 3.2 5.1)		16 (33%)	
High activity (DAS-28 > 5.1)		5 (10%)	
Rheumatoid factor positive	NA	42/47 (89.4%)	NA
Anti-cyclic citrullinated antibody positive	NA	21/22 (95.6%)	NA
Erosions present on radiographs	NA	21/38 (55.2%)	NA
Medication use	NA		
Etanercept		10 (19.6%)	NA
Infliximab		2 (3.9%)	NA
Adalimumab		5 (9.8%)	NA
Abatacept		5 (9.8%)	NA
Methotrexate		39 (76.5%)	NA
Leflunomide		1 (2.0%)	NA
Sulfasalazine		0	NA
Hydroxychloroquine		10 (19.6%)	NA
Nonsteroidal anti-inflammatory agents		18 (35.3%)*	1 (4.0%)
Prednisone (<5.0 mg/day)		13 (25.5%)	NA
Systemic inflammation			
hsCRP (mg/L)	3.0 (3.9)	3.7 (4.9)*	2.4 (2.9)
IL-1beta (pg/mL)	0.23 (5.3)	0.22 (4.1)	0.17 (6.4)
IL-6 (pg/mL)	4.9 (2.8)	8.9 (2.9)*	2.7 (1.6)
IL-8 (pg/mL)	8.2 (2.1)	8.9 (1.8)	7.5 (2.3)
TNF-alpha (pg/mL)	13.7 (2.3)	19.9 (2.4)*	9.5 (1.7)
IL-18 (pg/mL)	408.3 (1.4)	440.6 (1.3)	379.3 (1.4)
Adiposity and muscle tissue			
Abdominal total adipose area (cm^2)	427.9 (181.0)	408.4 (199.5)	447.3 (160.2)
Abdominal subcutaneous adiposity (cm^2)	303.3 (143.7)	304.5 (154.2)	302.1 (133.9)

Table 1 Participant characteristics *(Continued)*

Abdominal visceral adiposity (cm^2)	124.6 (93.2)	104.0 (77.1)*	145.2 (103.6)
Abdominal liver density (Hu)	59.0 (11.6)	59.7 (10.6)	58.2 (12.9)
Thigh total area (cm^2)	249.6 (65.4)	248.8 (73.6)	251.7 (57.1)
Thigh total adipose area (cm^2)	250.2 (66.0)	134.3 (65.8)	110.9 (68.0)
Thigh subcutaneous adiposity (cm^2)	122.6 (67.6)	122.6 (62.7)	113.8 (54.0)
Thigh inter-muscular adiposity (cm^2)	11.3 (7.4)	11.7 (6.7)	11.0 (8.1)
Thigh muscle area (cm^2)	119.6 (35.1)	114.5 (37.1)	125.4 (32.1)
Thigh muscle density (Hu)	54.0 (8.1)	50.7 (6.2)	55.4 (6.8)
Skeletal muscle inflammatory markers			
IL-1β (pg/mL/mg)	0.035 (0.084)	0.037 (0.093)	0.033 (0.069)
IL-6 (pg/mL/mg)	0.012 (0.010)	0.014 (0.010)*	0.008 (0.007)
IL-8 (pg/mL/mg)	0.139 (0.178)	0.169 (0.211)	0.097 (0.106)
TNF-α (pg/mL/mg)	0.012 (0.015)	0.014 (0.016)	0.010 (0.014)
TLR4 (pg/mL/mg)	0.891 (0.666)	0.859 (0.692)	0.937 (0.625)

Data are presented as means (SD) for continuous variables and number (percentages) of participants for dichotomous variables. Data that were not normally distributed (systemic inflammatory markers and cytokines) are presented as geometric means (SD). Physical activity data reflect rheumatoid arthritis (RA) (n = 41) and controls (n = 31) with valid data. *BMI* body mass index, *MET* metabolic equivalents, *HAQ* health assessment questionnaire, *DAS-28* disease activity score with 28-joint count, *hsCRP* high sensitivity C-reactive protein, *IL* interleukin, *TNF* tumor necrosis factor, *Hu* Houndsfield units, *TLR* toll-like receptor
*$p < 0.05$ for comparison with matched controls

prior to the biopsy [12]. Tissue was flash frozen in liquid nitrogen and stored at −80 ° C.

Skeletal muscle inflammatory marker measurements

Flash frozen muscle samples (5–10 mg) were homogenized in a buffer consisting of 1% Nonidet-P40, 1 mM EDTA, 150 mM NaCl, and 20 mM Tris-Cl for ELISA-based measures of muscle (m) interleukin (IL)-1β, mIL-6, mIL-8, m-tumor necrosis factor (TNF)-α (MSD 4-plex; K15053D-1) and m-toll like receptor (TLR)-4 (Abnova; KA1238). Assays were performed according to the manufacturers' directions except for the addition of a 30-minute, room temperature, blocking step with 5% BSA followed by three PBS-T washes. Concentrations were normalized to starting masses. Spike-and-recovery assays for all analytes achieved 80–100% recovery confirming lack of assay interference by muscle homogenates. For each cytokine, the mean intra-assay and inter-assay coefficients of variation were: mIL-1β 8.5%, 13.2%; mIL-6 3.5%, 1.5%; mIL-8 4.0%, 4.0%; mTNF-α 8.4%, 10.4%; and mTLR-4 1.7% (only one plate was used for analyses).

Gene expression analyses

Muscle samples were selected for gene expression analyses in an effort to span the range of RA disease activity seen in the larger sample; these corresponded to the following DAS-28 categories: remission ($n = 7$), low ($n = 4$), moderate ($n = 6$), and high activity ($n = 3$). For each RA muscle sample, the corresponding sample from a control matched by age, gender, and BMI was included.

For RNA preparation, flash frozen muscle samples (20–30 mg) were homogenized in 1 mL TRIzol® (Thermo Fisher Scientific, Inc, Waltham, MA, USA). Biotinylated total RNA was generated using the Illumina TotalPrep RNA amplification kit (Life Technologies, Grand Island, NY, USA); 200 nanograms of RNA were used for the kit. The quality of the RNA was determined using the Bioanalyzer RNA Nano chip assay (Agilent, Santa Clara, CA, USA). Quantification of the RNA was determined using the Quant-iT RiboGreen RNA Assay Kit. The Human HT-12v3 Expression BeadChip (Illumina, San Diego, CA, USA) was used for quantitative whole genome RNA profiling. Biotinylated RNA (750 ng) was hybridized to the BeadChip and washed; Cy3-SA was then introduced to the hybridized samples and the BeadChips scanned on the Illumina iScan system according to manufacturer's protocol. Quality control was performed using the Illumina GenomeStudio tools.

Gene expression fold-differences between groups were compared in Partek Genomics Suite (Partek, Inc.; St. Louis, MO, USA). For pathway analyses, differentially expressed genes ($p < 0.02$) were evaluated using the Ingenuity Pathway Analysis software (IPA, www.ingenuity.com). IPA identified the canonical pathways containing the greatest number of significant, differentially expressed genes in the dataset. IPA also generated novel networks of related genes and molecules based on the relationships present in the current literature.

Table 2 Skeletal muscle inflammatory marker correlations in patients with rheumatoid arthritis

Variable	Muscle IL-6	Muscle IL-8	Muscle TNF-α	Muscle IL-1β	Muscle TLR-4
Age (years)	−0.07	0.05	0.09	−0.09	**−0.29***
BMI (kg/m²)	0.24	−0.05	−0.23	−0.10	−0.25
Disease activity (DAS28)	0.23	**0.30***	0.14	**0.35***	−0.01
Disability (HAQ-DI)	**0.33***	0.19	0.09	**0.33***	0.12
Pain (VAS)	0.15	0.17	**0.29***	**0.39***	**0.47***
Prednisone use (yes = 1)	0.14	−0.05	0.00	0.01	−0.01
DMARD use (yes = 1)	−0.04	−0.07	**−0.30**	0.21	0.08
Biologic use (yes = 1)	−0.25	**−0.37***	0.21	**−0.33***	0.01
Comorbidity index	0.17	0.12	0.17	0.26	−0.08
Plasma hsCRP (mg/L)	0.20	0.07	0.11	−0.03	−0.17
Plasma IL-1β (pg/mL)	0.01	−0.07	−0.07	−0.14	−0.12
Plasma IL-6 (pg/mL)	−0.03	0.11	0.12	−0.01	−0.10
Plasma IL-8 (pg/mL)	−0.11	0.06	0.11	0.14	0.02
Plasma TNF-α (pg/mL)	**−0.37***	−0.15	0.02	−0.23	−0.08
Plasma IL-18 (pg/mL)	−0.08	−0.12	−0.02	−0.24	0.06
GlycA (μmol/L)	**0.41***	**0.38***	−0.06	0.07	−0.21
HOMA	0.11	0.04	−0.06	−0.10	−0.07
Insulin sensitivity (10^{-5}·min^{-1}/(pmol/L))	−0.20	−0.19	−0.06	−0.09	−0.18
Fasting insulin (mU/L)	0.13	0.09	−0.13	−0.06	−0.06
Visceral adiposity (cm²)	0.11	0.01	−0.28	0.03	−0.23
Abdominal subcutaneous adiposity (cm²)	0.21	0.06	−0.19	−0.06	−0.19
Total abdominal adiposity (cm²)	0.19	0.07	−0.24	−0.06	−0.28
Thigh muscle density (Hu)	−0.04	−0.10	0.06	0.16	**0.28***
Thigh inter-muscular adiposity (cm²)	0.12	0.01	−0.08	−0.11	−0.12
Thigh subcutaneous adiposity (cm²)	**0.31***	−0.07	−0.11	−0.09	−0.11
Exercise (min/day)	**−0.40***	**−0.38***	−0.05	**−0.38***	−0.11
Physical activity (MET h/day)	**−0.33***	−0.26	0.10	**−0.35***	−0.15

Data are shown as Spearman correlation coefficients. *BMI* body mass index, *DAS-28* disease activity score with 28 joint count, *HAQ-DI* health assessment questionnaire disability index, *VAS* visual analog scale, *DMARD* disease-modifying anti-rheumatic drug (methotrexate, leflunomide, hydroxychlorquie), *biologic* biologic DMARD (adalimumab, etanercept, infliximab, abatacept), *hsCRP* high-sensitivity C-reactive protein, *IL* interleukin, *TNF* tumor necrosis factor, *HOMA* homeostasis model assessment, *Hu* Houndsfield units, *MET* metabolic equivalent, *TLR* toll-like receptor. *$p < 0.05$ for Spearman correlation

Table 3 Canonical pathways implicated in gene expression in muscle in rheumatoid arthritis

Pathway	Dataset genes[a] in pathway (*n*)	Total genes in pathway (*n*)	*Z*-score	*p* value
Wnt/Ca + pathway	5	55	0	0.006
Netrin signaling	4	39	NaN	0.008
Glycolysis	3	24	NaN	0.013
Atherosclerosis signaling	7	121	NaN	0.013
Altered T and B cell signaling in rheumatoid arthritis	5	81	NaN	0.023
Methionine degradation to homocysteine	2	16	NaN	0.043
PI3K signaling in B lymphocytes	6	123	−0.816	0.043
April mediated signaling	3	38	NaN	0.044
B cell activating factor signaling	3	40	NaN	0.049

[a]Dataset genes were those differentially expressed between 20 patients with rheumatoid arthritis and 20 age, gender, and body mass index matched controls ($p < 0.02$). *NaN* Not a number

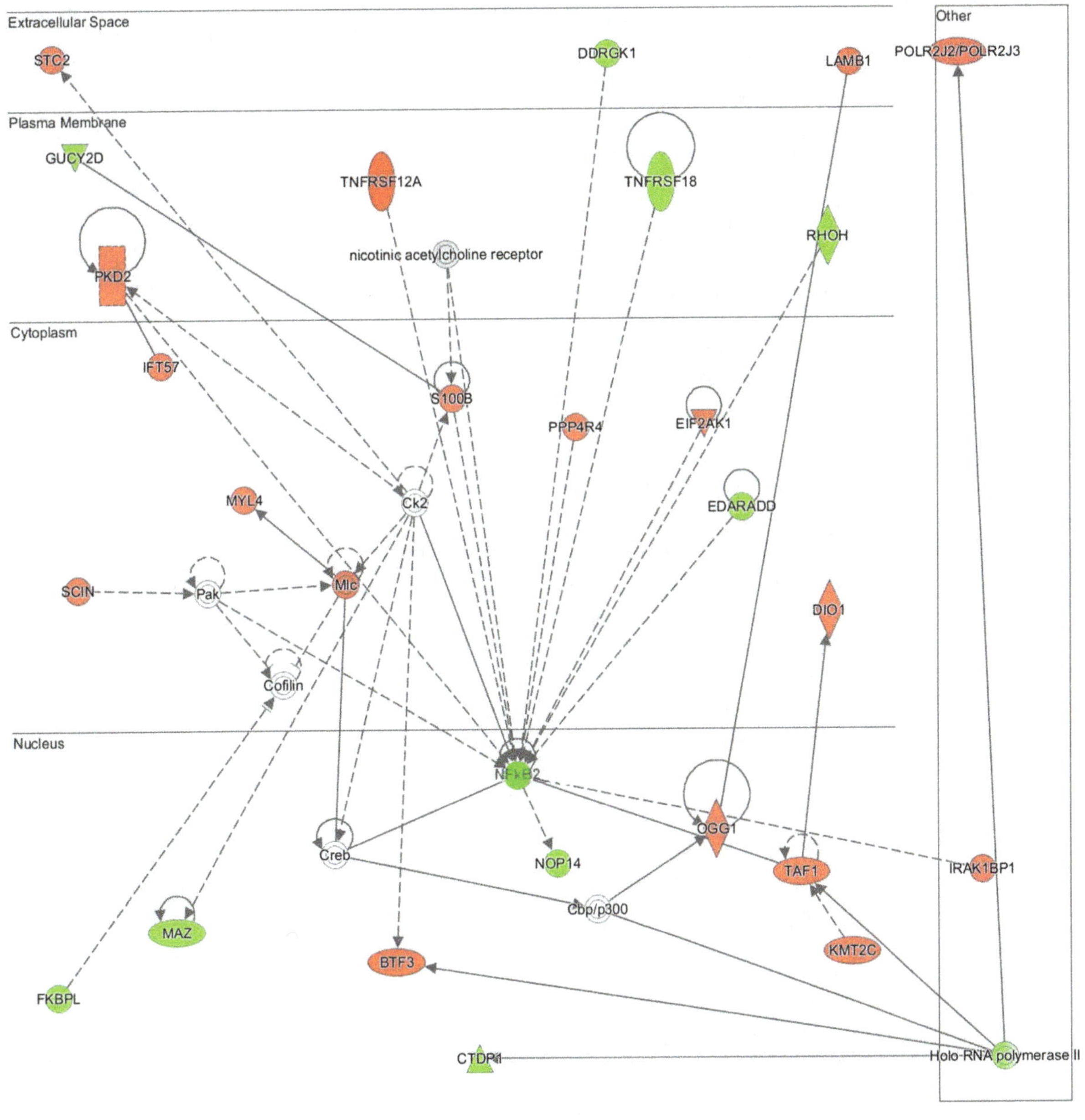

Fig. 1 Novel network identified by muscle gene expression in rheumatoid arthritis (RA): gene expression was determined in muscle from 20 persons with RA and 20 controls matched by age, gender, and body mass index. The network shows connections between genes with differential expression in RA relative to control muscle. Genes in *red* were upregulated and genes in *green* were downregulated in muscle in RA

Skeletal muscle metabolic intermediate measurements

Metabolites were measured in muscle from all participants (n = 102). Flash frozen muscle biopsies weighing approximately 25 mg were diluted 20 times (wt:vol) in ice-cold 50% acetonitrile containing 0.3% formate and homogenized for 120 sec in a TissueLyser II (Qiagen) at 30 Hz. Amino acids, organic acids, and acylcarnitines were analyzed using stable isotope dilution techniques in the Duke Molecular Physiology Metabolomics Core. Amino acids and acylcarnitine measurements were made by flow injection tandem mass spectrometry (MS) as previously described [13, 14]. The data were acquired using a Micromass Quattro Micro liquid chromatography (LC)-MS system running MassLynx 4.0 software (Waters Corporation, Milford, MA, USA). Organic acids were quantified using methods described previously [15]

Table 4 Novel network genes

Gene ID	Gene name	RA vs. CONTROL	
		Fold change	*p* value
BTF3	Basic transcription factor 3	1.11	0.003
CTDP1	CTD (carboxy-terminal domain, RNA polymerase II, polypeptide A) phosphatase, subunit 1	−1.04	0.006
DDRGK1	DDRGK domain containing 1	−1.07	0.02
DIO1	Deiodinase, iodothyronine, type I	1.03	0.005
EDARADD	EDAR-associated death domain	−1.06	0.007
EIF2AK1	Eukaryotic translation initiation factor 2-alpha kinase 1	1.05	0.007
FKBPL	FK506 binding protein like	−1.06	0.003
GUCY2D	Guanylate cyclase 2D, membrane (retina-specific)	−1.04	0.004
IFT57	Intraflagellar transport 57	1.04	0.01
IRAK1BP1	Interleukin-1 receptor-associated kinase 1 binding protein 1	1.02	0.02
KMT2C	Lysine (K)-specific methyltransferase 2C	1.03	0.01
LAMB1	Laminin, beta 1	1.11	0.02
MAZ	MYC-associated zinc finger protein (purine-binding transcription factor)	−1.03	0.008
MYL4	Myosin, light chain 4, alkali; atrial, embryonic	1.02	0.01
NFkB2	Nuclear factor of kappa light polypeptide gene enhancer in B-cells 2 (p52/p100)	−1.06	0.003
NOP14	NOP14 nucleolar protein	−1.08	0.008
OGG1	8-Oxoguanine DNA glycosylase	1.03	0.002
PKD2	Polycystic kidney disease 2 (autosomal dominant)	1.05	0.02
POLR2J2/POLR2J3	Polymerase (RNA) II (DNA directed) polypeptide J3	1.08	0.004
PPP4R4	Protein phosphatase 4, regulatory subunit 4	1.03	0.006
RHOH	Ras homolog family member H	−1.06	0.002
S100B	S100 calcium binding protein B	1.02	0.02
SCIN	Scinderin	1.04	0.001
STC2	Stanniocalcin 2	1.04	0.008
TAF1	TAF1 RNA polymerase II, TATA box binding protein (TBP)-associated factor, 250 kDa	1.04	0.02
TNFRSF12A	Tumor necrosis factor receptor superfamily, member 12A; TNF-like weak inducer of apoptosis (TWEAK) receptor	1.24	0.01
TNFRSF18	Tumor necrosis factor receptor superfamily, member 18	−1.02	0.005

employing Trace Ultra GC coupled to ISQ MS operating under Xcalibur 2.2 (Thermo Fisher Scientific, Austin, TX, USA). All data are expressed as picomoles/mg tissue.

Statistical analyses

Accounting for the repeated measures in matched participants, patients with RA and controls were compared using mixed models. Muscle inflammatory molecules and metabolic intermediates were logarithmically transformed prior to group comparisons. Bivariate associations were assessed with Spearman correlation. Gene expression fold-changes were compared in Partek using analysis of variance (ANOVA). All other statistical analyses were performed using SAS 9.4 (SAS, Cary, NC). All data are available from the corresponding author upon reasonable request.

Results

Clinical measures and skeletal muscle inflammatory markers

As shown in Table 1, persons with RA were well-matched to controls by age, gender, and BMI. Patients with RA were recruited based on the inclusion criteria

Table 5 Genes with the greatest differences in expression between patients with rheumatoid arthritis (RA) and controls

Gene ID	Gene name and description	Fold change	*p* value
Upregulated in RA			
OTUD1	OUT deubiquitinase 1: removes ubiquitin molecules with probable signaling regulatory role	1.50	0.035
FEZ2[a]	Fasciculation and elongation protein zeta 2 (zygin II): reduces autophagy [32]; associated with reduced cardiorespiratory fitness [33]	1.40	0.005
PITX1[a]	Paired-like homeodomain 1: promotes muscle atrophy [34]	1.37	0.046
RNU4ATAC	RNA, U4atac small nuclear (U12-dependent splicing): codes for component of the minor spliceosome [35, 36]	1.36	0.045
ABRA[a]	Actin binding Rho activating protein: promotes myoblast differentiation and myotube maturation [24]	1.33	0.031
RCAN1[a]	Regulator of calcineurin 1: regulates fiber type patterning during differentiation	1.32	0.019
CITED2[a]	Cbp/p300-interacting transactivator, with Glu/Asp-rich carboxy-terminal domain, 2: promotes stem cell maintenance [22, 23]; prevents myofibril degradation [37]	1.32	0.027
VGLL2[a]	Vestigial-like family member 2: expressed in myotubes [27]	1.30	0.035
MYF6[a]	Myogenic factor 6 (herculin): promotes myoblast terminal differentiation [29]	1.27	0.033
RPL36AL	Ribosomal protein L36a-like: ribosomal protein with ability to terminate translation in certain situations [38]	1.27	0.011
Downregulated in RA			
FBP2[b]	Fructose-1,6 bisphosphatase 2: promotes glycogen storage [39, 40]; protects mitochondria from Ca2+ -induced injury [41]	−1.42	0.013
MYLK4[a]	Myosin light chain kinase family, member 4: reduced expression associated with cardiomyopathies [42]	−1.37	0.024
ZFP36[ac]	ZFP36 ring finger protein; encodes tristetraprolin (TTP): reduces inflammation and prevents satellite cell activation [20]	−1.36	0.023
DDIT4[a]	DNA damage-inducible transcript 4; also known as protein regulated in development and damage response 1 (REDD-1): promotes autophagy, with reduced expression associated with exercise intolerance [43]	−1.34	0.023
MIDN[b]	Midnolin: regulates neurogenesis [44]; reduces pancreatic glycolysis in low glucose states [45]	−1.32	0.017
SLC2A5[b]	Solute carrier family 2 (facilitated glucose/fructose transporter), member 5: performs facilitative fructose uptake into muscle [46]	−1.31	0.041
SLC25A25[b]	Solute carrier family 25 (mitochondrial carrier; phosphate carrier), member 25: promotes anti-atherosclerotic macrophage ATP production [47]; promotes muscle ATP production and physical endurance [48]	−1.30	0.013
RRAD[a]	Ras-related associated with diabetes: increases myoblast proliferation and promotes myotube formation [30]	−1.30	0.044
ZBTB16[bc]	Zinc ring finger and BTB domain containing 16: suppresses autoreactive T cells and inflammation [21]; promotes adaptive thermogenesis and mitochondrial capacity [49]	−1.27	0.050
SMTNL2	Smoothelin-like 2: associated with myotube formation [50]	−1.22	0.008

[a]Genes associated with muscle remodeling, satellite cell maturation, or exercise intolerance. See Additional file 1 for more details. [b]Genes associated with metabolism
[c]Genes associated with immune and inflammatory responses

described and without respect to physical activity levels, body mass or body composition; similarly controls were included upon matching a patient with RA by age, gender, and BMI. Despite this, patients with RA and controls were similar with respect to physical activity levels, abdominal and thigh adipose depot size, muscle area, and muscle density [5, 11]. In those with RA, there was more comorbidity, disability, and systemic inflammation; specifically, greater serum concentrations of high sensitivity C-reactive protein (hs-CRP), IL-6, and TNF-α ($p < 0.05$ for all) [5]. When skeletal muscle inflammatory markers were compared, there was approximately two times greater concentrations of the muscle cytokines, mIL-6 ($p = 0.006$) and mIL-8 in RA ($p = 0.059$) (Table 1).

Akin to disease activity, RA muscle inflammatory markers exhibited variation across a broad range (Table 1). Muscle inflammatory marker concentrations were positively associated with disease activity (mIL-1β, mIL-8), disability (mIL-1β, mIL-6), and pain (mIL-1β, mTNF-α, mTLR-4) ($p < 0.05$ for all) (Table 2). Muscle cytokines, mIL-1β and mIL-8, were negatively correlated with use of biological agents; mTNF-α was negatively correlated with use of non-biological disease-modifying therapy ($p < 0.05$ for all) (Table 2). Importantly, there were no correlation between muscle inflammatory marker concentrations and prednisone treatment.

In addition to disease-related factors, muscle cytokine concentrations (mIL-1β, mIL-6, and mIL-8) were negatively associated with exercise minutes ($p < 0.05$ for all) (Table 2). Higher mIL-1β and mIL-6 concentrations were associated with less total physical activity (total METs; $p < 0.05$ for both) (Table 2). Although, both mIL-6 and mIL-8 were positively correlated with the systemic inflammatory marker, GlycA ($p < 0.05$ for both) (Table 2),

Table 6 Genes involved in skeletal muscle anabolic, catabolic, and inflammatory pathways

Gene ID	Gene name	Rheumatoid arthritis vs. control	
		Fold change	*p* value
Ubiquitin-proteasome pathway			
MuRF1	Muscle RING-finger protein-1	−1.02	0.25
MuRF2	Muscle-specific RING finger-2	−1.01	0.47
FbxO32	F-box protein 32	1.02	0.88
FbxO40	F-box protein 40	−1.03	0.37
Autophagy-lysozyme pathway			
Atg5	Autophagy related 5	−1.01	0.77
Atg7	Autophagy related 7	−1.09	0.13
NAF1	Nuclear assembly factor 1 ribonucleoprotein	−1.03	0.12
Lamp2	Lysosomal-associated membrane protein 2	−1.03	0.65
IGF1/Akt signaling pathway			
IGF1	Insulin-like growth factor 1	1.00	0.85
Akt1	V-Akt murine thymoma viral oncogene homolog 1	1.00	0.92
Akt2	V-Akt murine thymoma viral oncogene homolog 2	−1.04	0.41
Rptor	Regulatory associated protein of MTOR, complex 1	1.02	0.45
Rictor	RPTOR independent companion of MTOR, complex 2	1.01	0.54
FoxO1	Forkhead box O1	−1.07	0.34
FoxO3	Forkhead box O3	−1.09	0.39
TGFbeta/Myostatin signaling pathway			
ActRIIIB	ARP3 actin-related protein 3 homolog B	1.02	0.69
FST	Follistatin	−1.02	0.30
NFkB signaling pathways			
IKBKB	Inhibitor of kappa light polypeptide gene enhancer in B cells, kinase beta	−1.08	0.17
IKBKAP	Inhibitor of kappa light polypeptide gene enhancer in B cells, kinase complex-associated protein	1.001	0.43
TRAF6	TNF receptor-associated factor 6, E3 ubiquitin protein ligase	1.02	0.37
TRADD	TNFRSF1A-associated via death domain	−1.02	0.46
Bcl3	B-Cell CLL/lymphoma 3	−1.02	0.32
TRAF2	TNF receptor-associated factor 2	−1.00	0.95
TRAF5	TNF receptor-associated factor 5	1.01	0.37
MAPK8	Mitogen-activated protein kinase 8	−1.01	0.32
NFkB1	Homo sapiens nuclear factor of kappa light polypeptide gene enhancer in B cells 1 (p105/p50)	−1.00	0.97
NFkB2	Homo sapiens nuclear factor of kappa light polypeptide gene enhancer in B cells 2 (p52/p100)	−1.06	0.003

muscle inflammatory marker concentrations were not related to insulin sensitivity or systemic cytokine concentrations.

Skeletal muscle gene expression

To better understand the etiology of RA muscle inflammatory markers, we compared RA ($n = 20$) and control ($n = 20$) skeletal muscle gene expression: 1939 genes were significantly upregulated or downregulated in RA samples ($p < 0.05$); 445 genes were identified when using a more stringent definition of significance ($p < 0.02$).

To identify other relationships between differentially expressed RA muscle genes, pathway analyses were performed using IPA, which has thousands of canonical pathways onto which our experimental gene expression differences were overlaid. Of those canonical pathways, IPA identified several pathways impacted by differential gene expression in muscle in RA ($p < 0.05$) (Table 3). Except for glycolysis and methionine degradation, these canonical pathways were identified because of reduced RA muscle gene expression for nuclear factor (NF)-kβ2, both nuclear factor of activated T cells (NFAT)5 and NFATC4, or all three. Also, none of the canonical

Table 7 Skeletal muscle metabolic intermediate concentrations

	Rheumatoid arthririts (*n* = 51)		Controls (*n* = 50)	
	Mean	SD	Mean	SD
Amino acids				
Glycine	1012.669	304.568	1042.875	360.089
Alanine	2781.241	876.247	2735.464	820.802
Serine	773.987	190.246	777.726	286.455
Proline	502.861	179.5	528.023	222.984
Valine	291.82	75.004	300.739	99.003
Leucine/isoleucine	659.544	197.996	663.116	233.404
Methionine	54.167	14.36	55.372	17.48
Histidine	488.821	164.605	548.187	276.048
Phenylalanine	77.739	22.414	80.155	27.759
Tyrosine	80.962	23.249	88.815	32.052
Aspartate/asparagine	100.518	62.088	144.672	198.704
Glutamate/glutamine	2096.524	658.272	2359.04	878.482
Ornithine	212.338	85.775	184.849	69.873
Citrulline	69.446	39.718	75.05	50.441
Arginine	431.024	182.215	394.565	149.594
Organic acids				
Lactate	22862.683	9246.29	20956.576	8926.553
Pyruvate	1168.544*	604.675	803.474	539.098
Succinate	48.143	35.538	41.793	29.968
Fumarate	70.313	26.403	62.708	25.253
Malate	521.019	205.905	476.648	198.079
alphaKetoglutarate	144.24	143.952	113.438	118.669
Citrate	41.677	33.591	36.853	24.096
Acylcarnitines				
Free carnitine: C0	3369.034	1006.646	3631.978	1243.598
C2	455.175	288.39	485.702	312.966
C3	5.206	2.024	5.019	2.018
C4/Ci4	3.541	4.994	3.008	2.594
C5:1	1.033	0.397	1.03	0.41
C5	1.667	1.15	2.246	5.666
C4OH	2.789	2.231	2.378	1.778
C6	3.58	3.882	2.956	2.855
C5OH	0.676	0.363	0.65	0.343
C3DC	0.793	0.356	0.809	0.292
C4DC/Ci4DC	2.439	1.424	2.547	1.192
C8:1	0.531	0.328	0.532	0.252
C8	0.942	0.904	0.826	0.694
C5DC	1.528	1.043	1.43	0.727
C8:1OH/C6:1 DC	0.216	0.129	0.204	0.123
C6DC/C8OH	0.353	0.239	0.388	0.226
C10:3	0.067	0.047	0.067	0.034

Table 7 Skeletal muscle metabolic intermediate concentrations *(Continued)*

C10:2	0.05	0.03	0.063	0.041
C10:1	0.261	0.253	0.239	0.164
C10	0.655	0.6	0.58	0.48
C7DC	0.108	0.079	0.088	0.049
C8:1 DC	0.087	0.073	0.093	0.051
C10OH:C8DC	0.305	0.253	0.31	0.21
C12:2	0.052	0.034	0.052	0.035
C12:1	0.364	0.281	0.366	0.287
C12	1.359	1.073	1.31	1.125
C12:2OH/C10:2 DC	0.075	0.045	0.064	0.04
C12:1OH/C10:1 DC	0.224	0.178	0.202	0.114
C12OH/C10DC	0.441	0.472	0.417	0.382
C14:3	0.078	0.052	0.073	0.054
C14:2	1.126	1.025	0.902	0.83
C14:1	2.726	2.354	2.449	2.232
C14	4.156	3.277	3.781	3.373
C14:3OH/C12:3 DC	0.032	0.025	0.028	0.022
C14:2OH/C12:2 DC	0.174	0.121	0.143	0.081
C14:1OH/C12:1 DC	0.704	0.538	0.701	0.431
C14OH/C12DC	0.502	0.525	0.487	0.381
C16:3	0.198	0.164	0.157	0.103
C16:2	1.533	1.201	1.199	0.948
C16:1	6.736	5.227	5.751	3.973
C16	20.041	15.253	17.878	12.497
C16:3OH/C14:3-DC	0.053	0.038	0.045	0.024
C16:2OH/C14:2 DC	0.477	0.336	0.412	0.248
C16:1OH/C14:1 DC	1.306	1.077	1.256	0.834
C16OH/C14DC	1.18	1.265	1.229	1.059
C18:3	1.463	0.982	1.354	0.925
C18:2	20.561	15.909	17.722	13.495
C18:1	46.521	37.117	40.451	28.311
C18	11.278	8.401	10.817	8.203
C18:3OH/C16:3 DC	0.186	0.158	0.168	0.101
C18:2OH/C16:2 DC	1.357	1.235	1.323	1.177
C18:1OH/C16:1 DC	2.683	2.889	2.844	2.749
C18OH/C16DC	0.695	0.68	0.732	0.523
C20:4	2.023	1.801	1.778	1.872
C20:3	0.63	0.597	0.57	0.431
C20:2	0.308	0.271	0.261	0.164
C20:1	0.554	0.484	0.485	0.409
C20	0.369	0.4	0.329	0.308
C20:3OH/C18:3 DC	0.075	0.059	0.074	0.056
C20:2OH/C18:2 DC	0.053	0.034	0.05	0.03
C20:1OH/C18:1 DC	0.071	0.062	0.062	0.046

Table 7 Skeletal muscle metabolic intermediate concentrations *(Continued)*

C20OHC18DC/C22:6	0.212	0.248	0.198	0.206
C22:5	0.264	0.299	0.247	0.277
C22:4	0.241	0.279	0.193	0.158
C22:3	0.064	0.057	0.056	0.044
C22:2	0.051	0.035	0.044	0.025
C22:1	0.069	0.05	0.065	0.038
C22	0.059	0.049	0.062	0.046

Data are shown as means and standard deviations (pmol/mg tissue). Metabolic intermediates were measured in muscle homogenates. Group comparisons between muscle from patients with rheumatoid arthritis and from controls were performed using logarithmically transformed metabolic intermediates and mixed models. Prefix *C* denotes acylcarnitines followed by carbon number and degree of unsaturation. Suffixes *OH* and *DC* denote hydroxyl and dicarboxyl groups, respectively. $^*P < 0.05$ for comparison with matched controls

pathways was predicted to be activated or inhibited by gene expression differences in muscle in RA (*Z*-scores < |2|) (Table 3) [16].

In addition to canonical networks, pathway analyses generate novel networks connecting differentially regulated molecules based on published associations. The IPA-generated novel network with the highest connection score depicted significant differences in expression of genes associated with connective tissue, dental, and dermatological diseases (Fig. 1; Table 4). The prominent pathway connections in muscle in RA were centered on regulation of the NF-kB complex, specifically NF-kB2. These were in the setting of differential regulation of genes in muscle repair and glycolysis.

To augment traditional pathway analyses, we evaluated the 20 genes with the largest muscle expression differences in RA and control samples (Table 5) and examined gene members of well-established skeletal muscle anabolic, catabolic, and inflammatory pathways (Table 6). The top 20 upregulated and downregulated genes by fold difference were associated with muscle remodeling, satellite cell maturation, exercise intolerance, and/or energy metabolism; for these genes, the range of differences in expression was 20–50% (Table 5). Except for NF-kB2, there was no differential expression of canonical genes involved in skeletal muscle anabolic, catabolic, or inflammatory pathways (Table 6).

Skeletal muscle metabolic intermediates

When concentrations of skeletal muscle metabolic intermediates were compared between RA ($n = 51$) and controls ($n = 51$), muscle pyruvate concentrations were 46% greater in muscle in RA than in controls ($p < 0.001$) (Table 7). There were no significant differences in the concentrations of muscle amino acids, other organic acids, or acylcarnitines in RA compared to controls (Table 7). However, several muscle amino acids and acylcarnitines were related to RA disease activity and disability. For instance, greater concentrations of glycine, serine, aspartate/asparagine, and ornithine and lower muscle concentrations of alanine and fumarate were related to greater disease activity ($p < 0.05$) (Table 8). Greater muscle concentrations of glycine, proline, ornithine, arginine, and aspartate/asparagine were related to greater disability ($p < 0.05$) (Fig. 2); in contrast, lower concentrations of several long-chain unsaturated acylcarnitines were related to greater disease activity and disability ($p < 0.05$) (Table 8).

Discussion

Here, we report that in RA, skeletal muscle exhibits molecular alterations in inflammatory markers, transcriptional profiles, and metabolic signatures. Both at protein and transcriptional levels, muscle had a pro-inflammatory phenotype in RA. Additionally, differential gene expression in muscle in RA was indicative of dysregulation of muscle repair, promotion of glycolysis, and poor mitochondrial function. Upregulated glycolysis and mitochondrial inefficiency were supported by greater muscle concentrations of the glycolytic end-product pyruvate in RA. Further, disease activity and disability were related to lesser concentrations of long-chain acylcarnitines and greater concentrations of amino acid precursors for muscle fibrosis. Taken together, these alterations in proteins, gene expression, and metabolic intermediates were indicative of muscle in RA in a state of chronically activated, yet dysregulated remodeling with increased glycolysis, mitochondrial inefficiency, and fibrotic material (Fig. 2).

This represents the first report of significant markers of inflammation in muscle in RA. The clinical importance of these molecules is demonstrated by the significant association of several muscle cytokines with RA disease activity, disability, pain, and physical inactivity. The IPA-generated novel network centered on downregulation of NF-kB2, a protein that promotes non-canonical NF-kB signaling and opposes inflammatory signaling [17]. Downregulation of NF-kB2 would be predicted to favor coordinated upregulation of pro-inflammatory NF-kB signaling in muscle in RA. We were unable to determine if the muscle cytokines and pro-inflammatory transcripts in RA were derived from myocytes, inflammatory cells, or other cellular sources. Interestingly, muscle cytokine concentrations did not reflect those measured in circulation, suggesting these disease-associated inflammatory markers stem from local rather than systemic events.

Based on the strong relationships between muscle inflammatory markers and disability, pain and physical

Table 8 Relationships between rheumatoid arthritis clinical features and muscle metabolic intermediates

	Disease activity	Disability	Pain	Exercise (min/d)	Physical activity (MET h/d)
Amino acids					
Glycine	0.33[b]	0.50[a]	0.23	0.11	0.02
Alanine	-0.31[b]	0.03	-0.01	0.11	0.08
Serine	0.31[b]	0.20	0.17	-0.03	-0.01
Proline	0.20	0.36[a]	0.09	0.05	0.08
Valine	0.12	0.11	-0.04	0.05	-0.01
Leucine/isoleucine	0.09	0.18	-0.01	-0.08	-0.16
Methionine	0.07	0.16	-0.17	-0.01	-0.04
Histidine	-0.08	-0.02	-0.12	0.23	0.19
Phenylalanine	-0.06	-0.04	-0.21	0.06	0.04
Tyrosine	-0.06	0.08	-0.13	0.13	0.14
Aspartate/asparagine	0.34[b]	0.36[a]	0.20	-0.13	-0.12
Glutamate/glutamine	0.20	0.24	0.06	-0.12	-0.04
Ornithine	0.32[b]	0.39[a]	0.14	-0.21	-0.20
Citrulline	0.08	0.21	0.13	-0.02	0.13
Arginine	0.27	0.45[a]	0.24	-0.26	-0.27
Organic acids					
Lactate	-0.09	-0.18	-0.06	-0.09	-0.12
Pyruvate	-0.22	-0.22	-0.21	0.16	0.05
Succinate	0.03	-0.01	0.15	-0.06	-0.12
Fumarate	-0.34[b]	-0.24	-0.15	0.05	-0.01
Malate	-0.28	-0.14	0.04	-0.01	-0.07
alphaKetoglutarate	-0.22	-0.03	-0.03	0.27	0.18
Citrate	0.17	0.23	0.29	0.05	0.14
Acylcarnitines					
Free carnitine: C0	-0.10	0.19	0.10	0.04	0.08
C2	-0.07	0.08	0.07	-0.22	-0.02
C3	-0.05	0.10	-0.01	0.10	0.00
C4/Ci4	-0.02	-0.13	-0.20	0.09	0.16
C5:1	0.15	0.09	0.06	-0.10	0.05
C5	0.01	0.05	-0.24	0.14	0.10
C4OH	0.11	0.09	0.11	-0.11	-0.04
C6	0.05	-0.10	-0.24	0.30	0.29
C5OH	-0.24	0.04	0.14	0.14	0.25
C3DC	-0.17	0.13	0.03	-0.02	0.10
C4DC/Ci4DC	0.02	0.28[b]	0.05	-0.32[b]	-0.23
C8:1	-0.10	-0.05	-0.15	-0.07	0.00
C8	0.01	-0.11	-0.13	0.16	0.13
C5DC	0.19	0.20	0.03	-0.12	-0.11
C8:1OH/C6:1 DC	0.11	0.21	0.12	-0.05	-0.11
C6DC/C8OH	-0.02	0.03	-0.10	0.08	0.11
C10:3	0.02	0.15	0.15	-0.10	-0.09
C10:2	0.00	0.06	-0.05	-0.14	-0.20
C10:1	-0.09	-0.09	-0.08	0.19	0.11

Table 8 Relationships between rheumatoid arthritis clinical features and muscle metabolic intermediates *(Continued)*

C10	-0.05	-0.12	-0.13	0.15	0.14
C7DC	0.04	0.13	0.06	-0.20	-0.20
C8:1 DC	-0.17	-0.03	-0.13	-0.06	-0.09
C10OH:C8DC	-0.08	0.00	-0.15	0.06	0.07
C12:2	0.04	-0.01	-0.08	-0.24	-0.26
C12:1	-0.14	-0.12	-0.13	0.14	0.12
C12	-0.20	-0.22	-0.19	0.20	0.19
C12:2OH/C10:2 DC	-0.19	-0.03	-0.14	0.06	0.00
C12:1OH/C10:1 DC	-0.19	-0.07	-0.16	0.15	0.18
C12OH/C10DC	-0.16	0.03	-0.13	0.13	0.14
C14:3	-0.14	-0.09	-0.15	0.19	0.20
C14:2	-0.22	-0.17	-0.22	0.27	0.26
C14:1	-0.18	-0.16	-0.17	0.21	0.21
C14	-0.25	-0.21	-0.26	0.24	0.22
C14:3OH/C12:3 DC	-0.05	0.08	-0.01	-0.03	0.12
C14:2OH/C12:2 DC	-0.12	-0.03	-0.20	0.04	0.03
C14:1OH/C12:1 DC	-0.24	-0.11	-0.19	0.14	0.17
C14OH/C12DC	-0.13	0.03	-0.14	0.16	0.17
C16:3	-0.28	-0.19	-0.22	0.26	0.27
C16:2	-0.34[b]	-0.26	-0.26	0.35[a]	0.33[b]
C16:1	-0.28	-0.22	-0.17	0.22	0.18
C16	-0.27	-0.20	-0.19	0.17	0.18
C16:3OH/C14:3-DC	-0.16	-0.10	-0.03	0.11	0.19
C16:2OH/C14:2 DC	-0.26	-0.16	-0.19	0.12	0.10
C16:1OH/C14:1 DC	-0.25	-0.09	-0.21	0.10	0.12
C16OH/C14DC	-0.17	0.04	-0.08	0.10	0.12
C18:3	-0.43[a]	-0.36[a]	-0.19	0.20	0.19
C18:2	-0.40[a]	-0.39[a]	-0.19	0.23	0.18
C18:1	-0.33[b]	-0.32[b]	-0.15	0.15	0.13
C18	-0.21	-0.13	-0.12	0.06	0.09
C18:3OH/C16:3 DC	-0.29	-0.06	-0.02	0.18	0.18
C18:2OH/C16:2 DC	-0.31[b]	-0.06	-0.08	0.12	0.14
C18:1OH/C16:1 DC	-0.22	0.02	-0.04	0.06	0.07
C18OH/C16DC	-0.18	0.03	-0.08	-0.03	0.00
C20:4	-0.28	-0.30[b]	-0.12	0.26	0.27
C20:3	-0.29[b]	-0.37[a]	-0.11	0.18	0.17
C20:2	-0.25	-0.20	-0.14	0.11	0.14
C20:1	-0.25	-0.16	-0.11	0.07	0.08
C20	-0.18	-0.04	-0.09	-0.02	-0.01
C20:3OH/C18:3 DC	0.09	0.21	-0.01	-0.14	-0.08
C20:2OH/C18:2 DC	-0.16	-0.15	0.06	-0.14	-0.14
C20:1OH/C18:1 DC	-0.03	0.18	-0.03	0.00	0.04
C20OHC18DC/C22:6	-0.16	0.00	-0.09	-0.05	-0.08
C22:5	-0.28	-0.20	-0.14	0.15	0.09
C22:4	-0.22	-0.24	-0.06	0.07	0.09

Table 8 Relationships between rheumatoid arthritis clinical features and muscle metabolic intermediates *(Continued)*

C22:3	-0.03	-0.11	0.01	-0.06	-0.03
C22:2	0.13	-0.01	-0.06	0.09	0.24
C22:1	0.06	0.01	-0.12	0.28	0.36
C22	-0.02	-0.06	0.00	0.03	0.10

Data are shown as Spearman correlation coefficients. [a]Significant relationships ($p < 0.05$) to all red and green color and [b]Significant relationships r ≥ |0.35| to all bright red and green

inactivity, we suspected that increased intramuscular cytokines may be indicative of a disrupted muscle remodeling process. In fact, muscle gene expression alterations in RA were consistent with promotion of satellite cell differentiation and upregulation of several facets of the normally well-coordinated process of muscle remodeling. For instance, muscle in RA was characterized by downregulation of ZFP36, the gene that encodes tristetraprolin (TTP), which reduces inflammation by destabilizing pro-inflammatory cytokine transcripts [18, 19] and prevents satellite cell activation by destabilizing myogenic regulatory factor, MyoD, mRNA [20]. Thus, the reduction in ZFP36 expression in muscle in RA would be expected to promote pro-inflammatory cytokine production and satellite cell activation.

Other gene expression changes also suggest both chronic activation and temporal dysregulation of muscle remodeling. For instance, downregulation of ZBTB16 would promote inflammation and proliferation of autoreactive T cells [21]. In contrast to the reduced ZFP36 expected to promote satellite cell activation, the increased CITED2 would be expected to reduce satellite cell activation [22, 23]. Increased expression of ABRA, RCAN1, VGLL2, MYF6 and decreased expression of RRAD would promote differentiation of satellite cells [24–30]. More descriptions of differentially expressed genes are provided in Additional file 1.

Gene expression alterations indicative of glycolysis promotion and poor mitochondrial function were supported by greater muscle concentrations of the glycolytic end-product pyruvate in RA. Further, disease activity and disability were related to lower concentrations of fatty-acid-derived long-chain acylcarnitines. One plausible explanation for this relationship is that fewer long-chain acylcarnitines indicate less oxidative metabolism and fewer mitochondria, consistent with a glycolytic phenotype. RA disease activity and disability were also related to higher concentrations of amino acid precursors for muscle fibrosis. M2-type macrophages contain arginase, which metabolizes arginine to ornithine [31]. Ornithine is converted to proline, which provides a substrate for resident fibroblasts to generate collagen. In addition to proline, collagen formation also requires

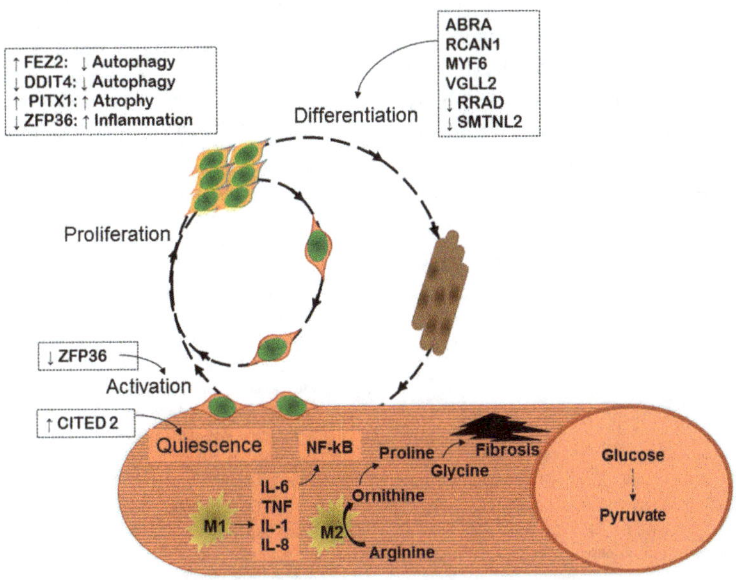

Fig. 2 Schematic depiction of muscle injury repair showing potential impact of cytokine, gene expression, and amino acids on satellite cell activation, macrophage function, and fibrosis in muscle from patients with rheumatoid arthritis (RA). Boxes show gene IDs for genes differentially regulated in patients with RA and in controls. See Table 3 for gene descriptions

glycine; glycine and proline each account for a third of the collagen amino acids. While collagen is critical for extracellular matrix production, in the setting of a chronically activated remodeling process, excess collagen production leads to fibrosis [31]. Thus, the relationships between these amino acids and disease activity and disability may indicate a fibrotic process in muscle associated with active disease that contributes to RA-associated disability.

There were several limitations to this study. RA medication regimens were not uniform among participants, and effects of these medications on skeletal muscle are unclear. Twenty-five percent of patients with RA used prednisone at low doses, which is not expected to have significant myopathic effects; despite this, they had significant alterations in muscle inflammatory markers and systemic inflammation relative to controls. Without histopathologic assessment or single cell isolations, we were unable to determine the cellular source of muscle cytokines, transcripts, or metabolites. Our findings indicate that either RA medication regimens or the RA disease process itself alters skeletal muscle inflammatory molecules, transcriptional profiles, and metabolic pathways.

Conclusions

Taken together, these alterations in pro-inflammatory cytokines, gene expression, and metabolic intermediates are indicative of RA muscle in a state of chronically activated, yet dysregulated remodeling, with increased glycolysis, mitochondrial inefficiency, and fibrosis. It is very likely these changes contribute to the ongoing issues of exercise intolerance and disability in persons with RA. Future work should be directed at understanding whether these deficits may be mitigated by combining pharmacologic treatment with physical activity, to reduce inflammatory signaling and/or fibrosis while promoting skeletal muscle efficiency. Therefore, to improve the lives of patients with RA, future work should be directed toward understanding the role of skeletal muscle in RA, and interactions between treatment regimens, physical activity, and influences of skeletal muscle on the clinical status in RA.

Abbreviations

BMI: body mass index; BSA: bovine serum albumin; DAS-28: disease activity score; DMARD: disease modifying anti-rheumatic drugs; ELISA: enzyme-linked immunosorbent assay; HAQ-DI: health assessment questionnaire-disability index; HOMA: homeostasis model assessment; hsCRP: high sensitivity C-reactive protein; Hu: Houndsfield units; IL: interleukin; IPA: Ingenuity Pathway Analysis; LC: liquid chromatography; m: muscle; MET: metabolic equivalent; MS: mass spectrometry; NaN: not a number; NF-kβ: nuclear factor-kβ; NMR: nuclear magnetic resonance; PBS: phosphate-buffered saline; RA: rheumatoid arthritis; TLR: toll-like receptor; TNF-α: tumor necrosis factor-alpha; TTP: tristetraprolin; VAS: visual analog scale

Acknowledgements

Not applicable.

Funding

This work was supported by NIH/NIAMS K23AR054904; a pilot project part of NIH/NIA P30AG028716; an Early Career Development Award from the Central Society of Clinical Research; and an ACR-REF/ASP Junior Career Development Award in Geriatric Medicine funded via Atlantic Philanthropies, ACR-REF, John A. Hartford Foundation and ASP. LipoScience, Inc. (now LabCorp) provided GlycA determinations at no cost.

Authors' contributions

KMH, RJ, BA, BND, and MJH contributed to the data analysis and data interpretation, and wrote the manuscript. RN, JLH, JM, BFG, KNT, and MC participated in acquisition of data and laboratory studies, and reviewed/edited the manuscript. VBK, TRK, DMM, and WEK participated in conceptual design and data interpretation, and reviewed/edited the manuscript. All authors read and approved the manuscript.

Competing interests

The authors declare that they have no competing interests.

Author details

[1]Department of Medicine, Duke Molecular Physiology Institute, Duke School of Medicine, Durham, NC, USA. [2]Biomedical Engineering, Duke University, Durham, NC, USA. [3]Harvard University School of Law, Boston, MA, USA. [4]Department of Surgery, Duke School of Medicine, Durham, NC, USA. [5]Department of Emergency Medicine, Indiana University, Indianapolis, IN, USA. [6]George Washington University, Washington, DC, USA.

References

1. Lee J, Dunlop D, Ehrlich-Jones L, Semanik P, Song J, Manheim L, Chang RW. Public health impact of risk factors for physical inactivity in adults with rheumatoid arthritis. Arthritis Care Res (Hoboken). 2012;64:488–93.
2. Kotler DP. Cachexia. Ann Intern Med. 2000;133:622–34.
3. Glass DJ. Skeletal muscle hypertrophy and atrophy signaling pathways. Int J Biochem Cell Biol. 2005;37:1974–84.
4. Arnett FC, Edworthy SM, Bloch DA, McShane DJ, Fries JF, Cooper NS, Healey LA, Kaplan SR, Liang MH, Luthra HS, et al. The American Rheumatism Association 1987 revised criteria for the classification of rheumatoid arthritis. Arthritis Rheum. 1988;31:315–24.
5. AbouAssi H, Tune KN, Gilmore B, Bateman LA, McDaniel G, Muehlbauer M, Huebner JL, Hoenig HM, Kraus VB, St Clair EW, et al. Adipose depots, not disease-related factors, account for skeletal muscle insulin sensitivity in established and treated rheumatoid arthritis. J Rheumatol. 2014;41:1974–9.
6. Rigler SK, Studenski S, Wallace D, Reker DM, Duncan PW. Co-morbidity adjustment for functional outcomes in community-dwelling older adults. Clin Rehabil. 2002;16:420–8.
7. Bruce B, Fries JF. The Stanford health assessment questionnaire: dimensions and practical applications. Health Qual Life Outcomes. 2003;1:20.
8. Prevoo ML, van 't Hof MA, Kuper HH, van Leeuwen MA, van de Putte LB, van Riel PL. Modified disease activity scores that include twenty-eight-joint counts. Development and validation in a prospective longitudinal study of patients with rheumatoid arthritis. Arthritis Rheum. 1995;38:44–8.
9. Bartlett DB, Connelly MA, AbouAssi H, Bateman LA, Tune KN, Huebner JL, Kraus VB, Winegar DA, Otvos JD, Kraus WE, Huffman KM. A novel inflammatory biomarker, GlycA, associates with disease activity in rheumatoid arthritis and cardio-metabolic risk in BMI-matched controls. Arthritis Res Ther. 2016;18:86.
10. Bergman RN, Ider YZ, Bowden CR, Cobelli C. Quantitative estimation of insulin sensitivity. Am J Physiol. 1979;236:E667–77.

11. Huffman KM, Pieper CF, Hall KS, St Clair EW, Kraus WE. Self-efficacy for exercise, more than disease-related factors, is associated with objectively assessed exercise time and sedentary behaviour in rheumatoid arthritis. Scand J Rheumatol. 2015;44:106–10.
12. Bergstrom J. Percutaneous needle biopsy of skeletal muscle in physiological and clinical research. Scand J Clin Lab Invest. 1975;35:609–16.
13. An J, Muoio DM, Shiota M, Fujimoto Y, Cline GW, Shulman GI, Koves TR, Stevens R, Millington D, Newgard CB. Hepatic expression of malonyl-CoA decarboxylase reverses muscle, liver and whole-animal insulin resistance. Nat Med. 2004;10:268–74.
14. Wu JY, Kao HJ, Li SC, Stevens R, Hillman S, Millington D, Chen YT. ENU mutagenesis identifies mice with mitochondrial branched-chain aminotransferase deficiency resembling human maple syrup urine disease. J Clin Invest. 2004;113:434–40.
15. Jensen MV, Joseph JW, Ilkayeva O, Burgess S, Lu D, Ronnebaum SM, Odegaard M, Becker TC, Sherry AD, Newgard CB. Compensatory responses to pyruvate carboxylase suppression in islet beta-cells. Preservation of glucose-stimulated insulin secretion. J Biol Chem. 2006;281:22342–51.
16. Kramer A, Green J, Pollard Jr J, Tugendreich S. Causal analysis approaches in Ingenuity Pathway Analysis. Bioinformatics. 2014;30:523–30. 510.1093/bioinformatics/btt1703. Epub 2013 Dec 1013.
17. Cubillos-Zapata C, Hernandez-Jimenez E, Toledano V, Esteban-Burgos L, Fernandez-Ruiz I, Gomez-Pina V, Del Fresno C, Siliceo M, Prieto-Chinchina P, Perez de Diego R, et al. NFkappaB2/p100 is a key factor for endotoxin tolerance in human monocytes: a demonstration using primary human monocytes from patients with sepsis. J Immunol. 2014;193:4195–202.
18. Geyer BC, Ben Ari S, Barbash S, Kilbourne J, Mor TS, Soreq H. Nicotinic stimulation induces Tristetraprolin over-production and attenuates inflammation in muscle. Biochim Biophys Acta. 2012;1823:368–78.
19. Carballo E, Lai WS, Blackshear PJ. Feedback inhibition of macrophage tumor necrosis factor-alpha production by tristetraprolin. Science. 1998;281:1001–5.
20. Hausburg MA, Doles JD, Clement SL, Cadwallader AB, Hall MN, Blackshear PJ, Lykke-Andersen J, Olwin BB. Post-transcriptional regulation of satellite cell quiescence by TTP-mediated mRNA decay. Elife. 2015;4:e03390. doi:10.7554/eLife.03390.
21. Liu TM, Lee EH, Lim B, Shyh-Chang N. Concise review: balancing stem cell self-renewal and differentiation with PLZF. Stem Cells. 2016;34: 277–87.
22. Kranc KR, Schepers H, Rodrigues NP, Bamforth S, Villadsen E, Ferry H, Bouriez-Jones T, Sigvardsson M, Bhattacharya S, Jacobsen SE, Enver T. Cited2 is an essential regulator of adult hematopoietic stem cells. Cell Stem Cell. 2009;5:659–65.
23. Bhattacharya S, Michels CL, Leung MK, Arany ZP, Kung AL, Livingston DM. Functional role of p35srj, a novel p300/CBP binding protein, during transactivation by HIF-1. Genes Dev. 1999;13:64–75.
24. Lamon S, Wallace MA, Russell AP. The STARS signaling pathway: a key regulator of skeletal muscle function. Pflugers Arch. 2014;466:1659–71.
25. Rybkin II OM, Copeland V, Czubryt MP, Shelton JM, van Rooij E, Richardson JA, Hill JA, De Windt LJ, Bassel-Duby R, et al. Calcineurin is necessary for the maintenance but not embryonic development of slow muscle fibers. Mol Cell Biol. 2005;25:6629–38.
26. Maeda T, Chapman DL, Stewart AF. Mammalian vestigial-like 2, a cofactor of TEF-1 and MEF2 transcription factors that promotes skeletal muscle differentiation. J Biol Chem. 2002;277:48889–98. Epub 42002 Oct 48889.
27. Bonnet A, Dai F, Brand-Saberi B, Duprez D. Vestigial-like 2 acts downstream of MyoD activation and is associated with skeletal muscle differentiation in chick myogenesis. Mech Dev. 2010;127:120–36.
28. Yang Y, Creer A, Jemiolo B, Trappe S. Time course of myogenic and metabolic gene expression in response to acute exercise in human skeletal muscle. 1985) 2005; 98:1745-1752.
29. Ma Z, Sun X, Xu D, Xiong Y, Zuo B. MicroRNA, miR-374b, directly targets Myf6 and negatively regulates C2C12 myoblasts differentiation. Biochem Biophys Res Commun. 2015;467:670–5.
30. Hawke TJ, Kanatous SB, Martin CM, Goetsch SC, Garry DJ. Rad is temporally regulated within myogenic progenitor cells during skeletal muscle regeneration. Am J Physiol Cell Physiol. 2006;290:C379–87.
31. Wehling-Henricks M, Jordan MC, Gotoh T, Grody WW, Roos KP, Tidball JG. Arginine metabolism by macrophages promotes cardiac and muscle fibrosis in mdx muscular dystrophy. PLoS One. 2010;5:e10763.
32. Spang N, Feldmann A, Huesmann H, Bekbulat F, Schmitt V, Hiebel C, Koziollek-Drechsler I, Clement AM, Moosmann B, Jung J, et al. RAB3GAP1 and RAB3GAP2 modulate basal and rapamycin-induced autophagy. Autophagy. 2014;10:2297–309.
33. Su J, Ekman C, Oskolkov N, Lahti L, Strom K, Brazma A, Groop L, Rung J, Hansson O. A novel atlas of gene expression in human skeletal muscle reveals molecular changes associated with aging. Skelet Muscle. 2015;5:35.
34. Pandey SN, Cabotage J, Shi R, Dixit M, Sutherland M, Liu J, Muger S, Harper SQ, Nagaraju K, Chen YW. Conditional over-expression of PITX1 causes skeletal muscle dystrophy in mice. Biol Open. 2012;1:629–39.
35. Merico D, Roifman M, Braunschweig U, Yuen RK, Alexandrova R, Bates A, Reid B, Nalpathamkalam T, Wang Z, Thiruvahindrapuram B, et al. Compound heterozygous mutations in the noncoding RNU4ATAC cause Roifman Syndrome by disrupting minor intron splicing. Nat Commun. 2015;6:8718.
36. Nagy R, Wang H, Albrecht B, Wieczorek D, Gillessen-Kaesbach G, Haan E, Meinecke P, de la Chapelle A, Westman JA. Microcephalic osteodysplastic primordial dwarfism type I with biallelic mutations in the RNU4ATAC gene. Clin Genet. 2012;82:140–6.
37. Tobimatsu K, Noguchi T, Hosooka T, Sakai M, Inagaki K, Matsuki Y, Hiramatsu R, Kasuga M. Overexpression of the transcriptional coregulator Cited2 protects against glucocorticoid-induced atrophy of C2C12 myotubes. Biochem Biophys Res Commun. 2009;378:399–403. 310.1016/j.bbrc.2008.1011.1062.
38. Hountondji C, Bulygin K, Crechet JB, Woisard A, Tuffery P, Nakayama J, Frolova L, Nierhaus KH, Karpova G, Baouz S. The CCA-end of P-tRNA contacts both the human RPL36AL and the A-site bound translation termination factor eRF1 at the peptidyl transferase center of the human 80s ribosome. Open Biochem J. 2014;8:52–67.
39. Tillmann H, Eschrich K. Isolation and characterization of an allelic cDNA for human muscle fructose-1,6-bisphosphatase. Gene. 1998;212:295–304.
40. Rakus D, Maciaszczyk E, Wawrzycka D, Ulaszewski S, Eschrich K, Dzugaj A. The origin of the high sensitivity of muscle fructose 1,6-bisphosphatase towards AMP. FEBS Lett. 2005;579:5577–81.
41. Pirog M, Gizak A, Rakus D. Changes in quaternary structure of muscle fructose-1,6-bisphosphatase regulate affinity of the enzyme to mitochondria. Int J Biochem Cell Biol. 2014;48:55–9.
42. Herrer I, Rosello-Lleti E, Rivera M, Molina-Navarro MM, Tarazon E, Ortega A, Martinez-Dolz L, Trivino JC, Lago F, Gonzalez-Juanatey JR, et al. RNA-sequencing analysis reveals new alterations in cardiomyocyte cytoskeletal genes in patients with heart failure. Lab Invest. 2014;94:645–53.
43. Qiao S, Dennis M, Song X, Vadysirisack DD, Salunke D, Nash Z, Yang Z, Liesa M, Yoshioka J, Matsuzawa S, et al. A REDD1/TXNIP pro-oxidant complex regulates ATG4B activity to control stress-induced autophagy and sustain exercise capacity. Nat Commun. 2015;6:7014.
44. Tsukahara M, Suemori H, Noguchi S, Ji ZS, Tsunoo H. Novel nucleolar protein, midnolin, is expressed in the mesencephalon during mouse development. Gene. 2000;254:45–55.
45. Hofmeister-Brix A, Kollmann K, Langer S, Schultz J, Lenzen S, Baltrusch S. Identification of the ubiquitin-like domain of midnolin as a new glucokinase interaction partner. J Biol Chem. 2013;288:35824–39.
46. Stuart CA, Yin D, Howell ME, Dykes RJ, Laffan JJ, Ferrando AA. Hexose transporter mRNAs for GLUT4, GLUT5, and GLUT12 predominate in human muscle. Am J Physiol Endocrinol Metab. 2006;291:E1067–73.
47. Karunakaran D, Thrush AB, Nguyen MA, Richards L, Geoffrion M, Singaravelu R, Ramphos E, Shangari P, Ouimet M, Pezacki JP, et al. Macrophage mitochondrial energy status regulates cholesterol efflux and is enhanced by anti-miR33 in atherosclerosis. Circ Res. 2015;117:266–78.
48. Anunciado-Koza RP, Zhang J, Ukropec J, Bajpeyi S, Koza RA, Rogers RC, Cefalu WT, Mynatt RL, Kozak LP. Inactivation of the mitochondrial carrier SLC25A25 (ATP-Mg2+/Pi transporter) reduces physical endurance and metabolic efficiency in mice. J Biol Chem. 2011;286:11659–71.
49. Plaisier CL, Bennett BJ, He A, Guan B, Lusis AJ, Reue K, Vergnes L. Zbtb16 has a role in brown adipocyte bioenergetics. Nutr Diabetes. 2012;2:e46.
50. Gordon EA, Whisenant TC, Zeller M, Kaake RM, Gordon WM, Krotee P, Patel V, Huang L, Baldi P, Bardwell L. Combining docking site and phosphosite predictions to find new substrates: identification of smoothelin-like-2 (SMTNL2) as a c-Jun N-terminal kinase (JNK) substrate. Cell Signal. 2013;25: 2518–29.

The relationship between synovitis quantified by an ultrasound 7-joint inflammation score and physical disability in rheumatoid arthritis

Jakub Závada[1*], Petra Hánová[1], Jana Hurňáková[1], Lenka Szczuková[2], Michal Uher[2], Šárka Forejtová[1], Martin Klein[1], Herman Mann[1], Marta Olejárová[1], Olga Růžičková[1], Olga Šléglová[1], Karel Hejduk[2] and Karel Pavelka[1]

Abstract

Background: Restoring normal physical functioning is a major therapeutic aim in the management of rheumatoid arthritis (RA). It is unknown, whether the extent of synovial inflammation quantified by musculoskeletal ultrasound (US) can predict current or future capacity for physical functioning. To answer this question we investigated the longitudinal relationship between physical function assessed by the health assessment questionnaire (HAQ) and the German 7-joint ultrasound score (US7S) in a prospective cohort of patients with RA.

Methods: Patients with RA ($n = 185$ (46 with incident and 139 with prevalent disease) were followed for 30.9 ± 9.1 months. Baseline and annual assessments comprised the disease activity score in 28 joints (DAS28), HAQ and US7S. The US7S includes semiquantitative measurements of synovitis assessed by greyscale (GS) and power Doppler (PD) in seven joints of the clinically dominant hand and foot, which are then aggregated in PD and GS synovitis sum-scores (PDsynSS and GSsynSS). A linear mixed-effect model was used to assess the longitudinal relationship between GSsynSS, PDsynSS and HAQ. We used standard and time-lag models to explore the association between HAQ, and GSsynSS, PDsynSS and DAS28 measured at the same time or at the previous visit 12 months ago, respectively.

Results: When the standard model was applied, in univariate analyses HAQ score was positively associated with GSsynSS and PDsynSS with β coefficients significantly higher in incident than in prevalent disease. In multivariate analysis both synSSs were individually no longer significant predictors of HAQ score. When using the time-lag model, after adjustment for the previous DAS28 or HAQ score, both PDsynSS and GSsynSS were significantly and negatively associated with the current HAQ.

Conclusions: US7 PD and GS synovitis sum-scores alone were positively associated with current functional status reflected by the HAQ in patients with RA, and this relationship was stronger in patients with early disease. When combined with the DAS28 or HAQ, US7 PD and GS synovitis sum-scores were predictive of the change in HAQ score over one year.

Keywords: Rheumatoid arthritis, Ultrasonography, Synovitis, Health assessment questionnaire

* Correspondence: zavada@revma.cz
[1]Institute of Rheumatology, Prague, and Department of Rheumatology, First Faculty of Medicine, Charles University, Na Slupi 4, 12850 Prague, Czech Republic
Full list of author information is available at the end of the article

Background

Rheumatoid arthritis (RA) may lead to substantial functional impairment caused by the combined effect of potentially reversible inflammatory activity and irreversible destructive articular and periarticular damage [1–4]. The main objective of RA management is to prevent and/or reverse the decline of physical functioning by aggressive control of disease activity and thus halting the structural progression.

The currently recommended tight control and treat-to-target RA management strategies are guided by close monitoring of disease activity using composite indexes such as the disease activity score in 28 joints (DAS28), simplified disease activity index (SDAI) or clinical disease activity score (CDAI) [5]. However, clinical disease activity indexes also have several limitations [6]: clinical examination may be poorly reproducible [7, 8] and may fail to capture subclinical synovitis associated with progressive joint damage [9, 10]), especially in the feet [11–13]. Disease activity scores may be falsely increased in some patients without evidence of synovitis due to fibromyalgia [14].

An important question is whether these limitations of conventional disease activity scores may be alleviated by complementing clinical examination with musculoskeletal ultrasound (US), which has been shown to be more sensitive [15–18] and reliable [19–21] in detecting synovitis compared to physical examination. The German US7 score (US7S) has been shown to be a feasible, reliable and sensitive tool for the US examination of inflammatory joint activity in RA [22–24]. The US7S includes seven joints of the clinically dominant hand and foot, consists of five additive sum-scores for synovitis (syn) and tenosynovitis (ten) assessed by greyscale (GS) and power-Doppler (PD), and an erosions score (ES). It is unknown whether an US joint inflammation score may contribute additional prognostic information on measures of functional impairment beyond the standard clinical indexes.

In our longitudinal prospective cohort study, we have systematically performed repeated clinical and US assessments of joint inflammation (using the DAS28 and US7S) and physical function evaluations (using the health assessment questionnaire (HAQ)) in patients with early RA and established RA. The main objectives of the present analysis were to examine the ability of US7S synovitis sum scores (PDsynSS, GSsynSS) to predict the HAQ score measured concurrently or 12 months later, either alone or as an adjunct to the DAS28 (or previous HAQ).

Methods

Patients

Patients with early RA ($n = 46$) newly started on therapy with conventional synthetic disease-modifying drugs (csDMARDs) or glucocorticoids (incident cohort), and 139 patients with established RA (prevalent cohort) were asked to participate in this this study. Diagnosis of RA was based on the American College of Rheumatology/European League against Rheumatism (EULAR) 2010 classification criteria for RA [25]. The patient characteristics are provided in Table 1. All patients were recruited from the outpatient rheumatology clinic at the Institute of Rheumatology in Prague and were followed longitudinally according to a predefined protocol. Informed consent was obtained from all patients before entry into the study. Patients on biological DMARDs were not included in the study, because they are followed separately in the Czech biologics ATTRA registry. During the observation period, patients were routinely treated by their rheumatologist. The study was approved by the Ethics Committee of the Institute of Rheumatology in Prague (Reference number 3560/2010) and was conducted according to the guidelines of the Declaration of Helsinki.

Outcome measurements

The same measures of clinical assessment and US imaging were applied at baseline and every 6 months during the follow-up period. Physical function was assessed by the HAQ [26] at baseline and then annually. For the purpose of this analysis only clinical and US data collected concurrently with the HAQ every 12 months were used. Demographic and anthropometric data collection, and data on rheumatoid factor (RF), and anti-citrullinated protein antibody (ACPA) testing were performed at baseline. Tender and swollen joint counts were carried out on 28 joints by an experienced nurse, in accordance with the EULAR recommendations [27]. C-reactive protein (CRP) was measured in a local laboratory using turbidimetry (Beckman Coulter, CA, USA). For the purpose of this analysis, we have used the DAS28 with CRP (DAS28-CRP) as the main outcome measure of clinical activity.

Ultrasound imaging

The US examinations were performed by eight clinicians who have undergone intermediate to advanced US training. The results of a practical exercise published elsewhere [28] showed moderate interobserver agreement for assessment of PD synovitis, substantial agreement for assessment of GS synovitis, and excellent intrareader agreement. We used the Esaote Mylab 60 equipment (Esaote S.p.A., Genova, Italy) and a linear transducer with an 18-MHz frequency. The power Doppler sensitivity was pre-set (pulse repetition frequency 750 Hz, wall filter 3/5, persistence 4/16, colour flow mapping frequency 7.1 MHz), and no adjustments of the Doppler parameters were allowed.

Table 1 Baseline characteristics

	Total ($N = 185$)	Incident RA ($N = 46$)	Prevalent RA ($N = 139$)	P value
Female (%)	76.8	69.6	79.1	0.066
Age (years)	55.2 (14.0)	51.7 (12.6)	56.4 (14.2)	<0.001*
Disease duration (years)	6.3 (7.7)	0.8 (0.7)	8.1 (8.1)	<0.001*
Symptom duration (years)	7.3 (7.7)	1.5 (1.8)	9.2 (8.0)	<0.001*
BMI	26.7 (4.5)	27.5 (5.2)	26.4 (4.3)	0.020*
RF+ (%)	47.2	43.5	48.5	0.466
ACPA+ (%)	62.9	58.7	64.3	0.952
CRP (mg/l)	7.6 (9.0)	10.5 (12.6)	6.6 (7.1)	0.354
DAS28-CRP	3.7 (1.5)	4.0 (1.5)	3.6 (1.5)	0.192
GSsynSS	6.91 (6.39)	7.70 (5.62)	6.65 (6.61)	0.255
PDsynSS	4.02 (5.20)	5.24 (5.95)	3.61 (4.87)	0.438
GStenSS	0.66 (1.15)	0.78 (1.18)	0.63 (1.14)	0.842
PDtenSS	0.68 (1.63)	0.80 (1.75)	0.63 (1.59)	0.402
Erosions score	1.18 (2.10)	0.46 (1.50)	1.42 (2.21)	<0.001*
HAQ	0.77 (0.73)	0.88 (0.73)	0.74 (0.73)	0.896
Oral glucocorticoids (%)	43.8	41.3	44.6	0.607
csDMARDs (%)	87.0	69.6	92.8	<0.001*

Values are mean (SD) if not stated otherwise. *RA* rheumatoid arthritis, *BMI* body mass index, *RF* rheumatoid factor, *ACPA* anti-citrullinated peptide antibodies, *CRP* C-reactive protein, *DAS28* disease activity score in 28 joints, *GS* greyscale, *PD* power Doppler, *syn* synovitis, *ten* tenosynovitis, *ES* erosions score, *SS* sum-score, *HAQ* health assessment questionnaire, *csDMARDS* conventional synthetic disease-modifying anti-rheumatic drugs. *Significant at $p < 0.05$

The patients were examined according to the German US7 score in the following seven joint areas: wrist, second and third metacarpophalangeal (MCP) and second and third proximal interphalangeal (PIP) and second and fifth metatarsophalangeal (MTP) joints of the hand and foot that clinically was more affected [22]. We used a modification of the original German US7 [29], which is currently used and endorsed by the authors of both the original and modified versions (personal communication with M. Backhaus). In contrast to the original US7, which examines synovitis of the MCP and PIP joints in GS only from the palmar view; we assessed synovitis in GS in this area using both the palmar and the dorsal view. Further, while the original German US7 assesses tenosynovitis/paratenonitis on the second and third finger both from the palmar and dorsal aspect, we assessed tenosynovitis only from the palmar aspect. Synovitis in the GS was scored semiquantitatively (0 = absence, 1 = mild, 2 = moderate, 3 = severe synovitis), as follows: grade 1 = a small hypoechoic/anechoic line beneath the joint capsule; grade 2 = the joint capsule elevated parallel to the joint area; and grade 3 = strong distension of the joint capsule [30].

Synovitis and tenosynovitis were classified semiquantitatively by PD, as follows: grade 0 = no intraarticular color signal; grade 1 = up to three single colour signals or two single signals and one confluent signal in the intraarticular area; grade 2 = greater than grade 1 to <50% of the intraarticular area filled with colour signals; and grade 3 = ≥50% of the intraarticular area filled with colour signals. Tenosynovitis in the GS was registered as absent (0) or present (1). An overall GS and PD signal score was calculated as the sum of GS synovitis, PD synovitis and GS tenosynovitis and PD tenosynovitis with the range of scores of 0–39 for GS synovitis, 0–39 for PD synovitis, 0–5 for GS tenosynovitis and 0–15 for PD tenosynovitis. The ultrasonographers were unaware of each patient's clinical examination and laboratory findings.

Statistical analysis

Differences in baseline variables between the included patients with early ($n = 46$) and established ($n = 139$) RA (incident and prevalent cohorts, respectively) were examined by the Mann-Whitney test (continuous variables) or Fisher's exact test (categorical variables). A linear mixed effects model (LMM) was used to study the longitudinal relationship between the clinical measures of disease activity (DAS28-CRP), US inflammatory score (German US7 scores sum-scores for GS and PD synovitis, GS and PD tenosynovitis, and erosions) as explanatory variables, and physical function (HAQ score) as a dependent variable. Age, sex, rheumatoid factor (RF) and anti-CCP status, body mass index (BMI) and disease duration were also introduced in one of the multivariate models as covariates. All the subsequently described analytical models used in our study were pre-planned.

To explore the influence of current disease activity (assessed either clinically or by US) on the current HAQ score, we used the standard ("current") model. To explore the impact of previous disease activity (assessed either clinically or by US) on the current HAQ score we used a "time-lag" model. In the time-lag model the covariates measured at the previous visit (12 months before) are related to the outcome variable assessed at the current visit. Also, the previous HAQ (assessed at the previous visit 12 months earlier) was added to the model (i.e. the first-order autoregression) to model change in the HAQ score rather than absolute HAQ scores. The proportion of variability in the HAQ scores explained by given covariates or models was assessed using R^2 and compared to each other using analysis of variance (ANOVA).

Participants with missing data on baseline characteristics and parameters of disease activity were included in the analysis by using multiple imputations using the Markov chain Monte Carlo method with 30 imputations obtained after 20 iterations. Variables included in imputation models were all baseline covariates and parameters of disease activity (variables with missing data were imputed and used as predictors, and variables with complete data were used as predictors only). IBM SPSS Statistics version 22 (SPSS Inc., Chicago, IL, USA) was used for the analyses. All P values equal to or less than 0.05 were considered statistically significant.

Results

Descriptive analyses

The baseline characteristics of the whole cohort, and the incident and prevalent cohorts, are shown in Table 1. Most of the patients were female (77%), mean age was 55 years, 47% were RF-positive and 63% ACPA-positive. At the baseline examination, 87% of the patients were taking conventional csDMARDs, and 44% oral glucocorticoids. The patients with early RA were younger (52 vs. 56 years; $P < 0.001$), had significantly shorter disease duration than patients with established disease (0.9 vs. 8.1 years; $P < 0.001$), had significantly lower erosions scores (0.5 vs. 1.4; $P < 0.001$), and were less frequently taking csDMARDs (69 vs. 93%; $P < 0.001$). Mean (SD) length of follow up was 30.9 (9.1) months.

In the whole cohort, the average HAQ scores were relatively stable over the 3-year follow-up period, while both clinical and US parameters of disease activity improved (Additional file 1). However, the evolution of functional and activity measures in time was somewhat different in the incident vs. prevalent cohorts (Additional files 2 and 3). While the mean HAQ scores had dropped during the first year of observation in patients with early RA, there was a steady increasing trend in HAQ scores in patients with established disease. Also, there was a more pronounced decrease in both clinical and US activity parameters in the incident cohort than in the prevalent cohort since the baseline visit.

Cross-sectional associations between ultrasound inflammatory score and physical function (standard or current model)

In univariate analyses (Table 2) the HAQ score was positively associated with GSsyn, PDsyn, PDten and GSten US7 sum-scores with β coefficients significantly higher in patients with incident than in patients with prevalent disease, respectively. However, the proportion of variability of the HAQ score explained by GSsynSS, PDsynSS, GStenSS and PDtenSS was relatively small (R^2 of 2–4% for US7S as compared to R^2 of 41% for DAS28-CRP), and the erosions score was not correlated with HAQ score at all. In a multivariate analysis that included conventional demographic, immunological and clinical variables (Table 3), female gender, age and DAS28-CRP were all significantly and positively associated with HAQ score, while US7 sum-scores were individually no longer significant predictors of HAQ score and the R^2 of the whole model improved only marginally after the addition of US7 items (from 44.7 to 45.9; $P < 0.001$ for improvement in R^2).

Longitudinal associations between ultrasound inflammatory score and physical function (time-lag model)

When applying a time-lag model, in univariate analyses only previous HAQ score and DAS28-CRP, but not the US7 sum-score, was predictive of current HAQ score measured 12 months apart (Table 4). However, in multivariate analyses (Table 5) after adjustment for previous DAS28 and/or previous HAQ score, both previous PDsynSS and GSsynSS were significantly and inversely associated with the current HAQ score. Previous PDsynSS remained a statistically significant predictor of current HAQ score, even in a more extensive multivariate model after adjustment for the most important conventional demographic, immunological and clinical variables (Table 6), and the percent variability of HAQ score explained by this model was substantially improved by the addition of the US7S sum-scores (from 32 to 39%, $P < 0.001$).

Additional analyses

One possible explanation for why previous higher values of PDsynSS are associated (in the multivariate model) with improvement of functional status between the previous and current visit, may be the fact that treatment of RA was escalated between the previous and current visit. To examine this we conducted several analyses with PDsynSS (and DAS28, or HAQ) as exploratory variables

Table 2 Standard (current) model

Predictor	RA	β (95% CI)	*P* value*	*P* value**	Percent variability explained - R^2
DAS28-CRP	all	0.186 (0.157; 0.216)	*<0.001*		41.3
	i	0.234 (0.174; 0.295)	*<0.001*	0.072	
	p	0.171 (0.137; 0.204)	*<0.001*		
GSsynSS	all	0.018 (0.011; 0.026)	*<0.001*		3.2
	i	0.035 (0.020; 0.050)	*<0.001*	*0.013*	
	p	0.013 (0.004; 0.022)	*0.003*		
PDsynSS	all	0.025 (0.015; 0.035)	*<0.001*		3.6
	i	0.038 (0.021; 0.055)	*<0.001*	0.056	
	p	0.018 (0.006; 0.030)	*0.004*		
GStenSS	all	0.048 (0.004; 0.092)	*0.033*		2.4
	i	0.123 (0.039; 0.207)	*0.004*	*0.038*	
	p	0.019 (-0.032; 0.071)	0.460		
PDtenSS	all	0.051 (0.019; 0.082)	*0.002*		2.8
	i	0.100 (0.039; 0.162)	*0.001*	0.064	
	p	0.033 (-0.003; 0.070)	0.073		
ES	all	0.007 (-0.022; 0.036)	0.632		0.3
	i	-0.024 (-0.102; 0.054)	0.549	0.390	
	p	0.013 (-0.019; 0.045)	0.416		

Univariate analyses and interaction with incident (i) or prevalent (p) rheumatoid arthritis (RA). Predicted variable is current health assessment questionnaire (HAQ) score, univariate predictors are current disease activity score in 28 joints using C-reactive protein (DAS28-CRP), sum-scores (SS) for greyscale (GS) and power Doppler (PD) synovitis, GS and PD tenosynovitis (ten), and erosions score (ES). **P* value of significance of given β. ***P* value of significance of difference between incident and prevalent RA. *P*-values higlighted in italics are significant at $p < 0.05$

and escalation of therapy (defined as new/increased use of glucocorticoids or DMARDS within 6 months after the index visit) as a dependent variable (see Additional files 4 and 5). Although in univariate analyses (Additional file 4) all parameters (PDsynSS, DAS28, and HAQ) were positively associated with escalation of therapy within the next 6 months, after adjustment for previous HAQ score or DAS28, previous PDsynSS was no longer an independent predictor of escalation of therapy (Additional file 5).

Table 3 Standard (current) model: multivariate analyses

Predictor	Model without US-7		Model with US-7	
	β (95% CI)	*P* value	β (95% CI)	*P* value
Female	0.211 (0.045; 0.376)	*0.013*	0.208 (0.044; 0.372)	*0.013*
Age (years)	0.149 (0.097; 0.201)	*<0.001*	0.147 (0.096; 0.199)	*<0.001*
BMI	0.008 (-0.007; 0.024)	0.276	0.008 (-0.007; 0.023)	0.291
RF+ or ACPA+	0.029 (-0.115; 0.172)	0.696	0.029 (-0.114; 0.172)	0.691
Prevalent vs. incident RA	-0.048 (-0.209; 0.113)	0.558	-0.050 (-0.212; 0.111)	0.541
DAS28-CRP	0.184 (0.155; 0.213)	*<0.001*	0.202 (0.166; 0.238)	*<0.001*
GSsynSS	-		-0.003 (-0.014; 0.008)	0.595
PDsynSS	-		-0.001 (-0.015; 0.014)	0.916
GStenSS	-		-0.062 (-0.129; 0.006)	0.073
PDtenSS	-		0.018 (-0.032; 0.068)	0.487
Erosions score	-		0.005 (-0.022; 0.032)	0.720
R^2 (% variability explained)	44.7		45.9	
Improved R^2	-		1.1	*<0.001**

Predicted variable is current health assessment questionnaire (HAQ) score. Comparison of models based on demographic, clinical and immunological parameters with or without the German 7-joint ultrasound score (US7) sum-scores (SS). **P* value of significance for improvement of prediction. *BMI* body mass index, *RF* rheumatoid factor, *ACPA* anti-citrullinated peptide antibodies, GS greyscale, *PD* power Doppler, *syn* synovitis, *ten* tenosynovitis, *ES* erosions score. *P*-values higlighted in italics are significant at $p < 0.05$

Table 4 Time-lag model

Predictor	RA	β (95% CI)	*P* value*	*P* value**	Percent variability explained - R^2
Previous DAS28-CRP	all	0.102 (0.062; 0.143)	*<0.001*		29.0
	i	0.072 (-0.008; 0.152)	0.079	0.353	
	p	0.115 (0.069; 0.161)	*<0.001*		
Previous GSsynSS	all	0.003 (-0.006; 0.012)	0.530		7.4
	i	0.000 (-0.019; 0.019)	1.000	0.713	
	p	0.004 (-0.007; 0.015)	0.465		
Previous PDsynSS	all	-0.003 (-0.015; 0.009)	0.605		0.4
	i	-0.001 (-0.021; 0.019)	0.924	0.816	
	p	-0.004 (-0.018; 0.011)	0.595		
Previous GStenSS	all	0.006 (-0.044; 0.056)	0.822		0.7
	i	0.005 (-0.089; 0.099)	0.922	0.972	
	p	0.007 (-0.053; 0.066)	0.825		
Previous PDtenSS	all	-0.005 (-0.041; 0.032)	0.801		0.5
	i	-0.019 (-0.092; 0.054)	0.606	0.655	
	p	0.000 (-0.042; 0.042)	1.000		
Previous ES	all	0.028 (-0.007; 0.062)	0.118		0.4
	i	-0.043 (-0.158; 0.072)	0.462	0.216	
	p	0.033 (-0.004; 0.070)	0.081		
Previous HAQ	all	0.740 (0.676; 0.803)	*<0.001*		63.5
	i	0.627 (0.496; 0.759)	*<0.001*	*0.050*	
	p	0.775 (0.705; 0.846)	*<0.001*		

Univariate analyses and interaction with incident (i) or prevalent (p) rheumatoid arthritis (RA). Predicted variable is current HAQ score, univariate predictors are previous disease activity score in 28 joints using C-reactive protein (DAS28-CRP), sum-scores for greyscale (GS) and power Doppler (PD) synovitis (syn), GS and PD tenosynovitis (ten), and erosions score (ES). **P* value of significance of given β. ***P* value of significance of difference between incident and prevalent RA. *P*-values higlighted in italics are significant at $p < 0.05$

Table 5 Time-lag model: multivariate analyses

Analysis number	Predictor	β (95% CI)	*P* value	Percent variability explained by the model (R^2)
1	Previous HAQ	0.762 (0.698; 0.827)	*<0.001*	64.8
	Previous PDsynSS	-0.017 (-0.027; -0.007)	*0.001*	
2	Previous PDsynSS	-0.025 (-0.039; -0.011)	*<0.001*	32.8
	Previous DAS28	0.156 (0.109; 0.203)	*<0.001*	
3	Previous HAQ	0.703 (0.620; 0.786)	*<0.001*	65.4
	Previous PDsynSS	-0.022 (-0.034; -0.011)	*<0.001*	
	Previous DAS28	0.050 (0.005; 0.096)	*0.029*	
4	Previous HAQ	0.754 (0.690; 0.819)	*<0.001*	64.2
	Previous GSsynSS	-0.009 (-0.017; -0.001)	*0.024*	
5	Previous GSsynSS	-0.012 (-0.023; -0.001)	*0.036*	32.5
	Previous DAS28	0.135 (0.088; 0.183)	*<0.001*	
6	Previous HAQ	0.707 (0.623; 0.792)	*<0.001*	64.5
	Previous GSsynSS	-0.013 (-0.022; -0.004)	*0.006*	
	Previous DAS28	0.039 (-0.007; 0.085)	0.096	

Predicted variable is current health assessment questionnaire (HAQ) score. Predictors used in the six analyses are either previous HAQ score or disease activity score in 28 joints (DAS28) or both, and previous power Doppler (PD) synovitis (SS) or greyscale (GS) syn sum-score (SS) (previous = measured 12 months ago. ES = erosions score. *P*-values higlighted in italics are significant at $p < 0.05$

Table 6 Time-lag model: multivariate analysis, extended model

Predictor	Model without US-7		Model with US-7	
	β (95% CI)	*P* value	β (95% CI)	*P* value
Female	0.182 (-0.007; 0.370)	0.059	0.167 (-0.012; 0.347)	0.068
Age (years)	0.172 (0.113; 0.231)	*<0.001*	0.169 (0.113; 0.226)	*<0.001*
BMI	0.009 (-0.009; 0.026)	0.316	0.007 (-0.010; 0.024)	0.405
RF+ or ACPA+	0.060 (-0.103; 0.224)	0.471	0.052 (-0.106; 0.210)	0.517
Prevalent vs. incident RA	0.026 (-0.156; 0.209)	0.779	0.010 (-0.165; 0.186)	0.910
Previous DAS28-CRP	0.100 (0.061; 0.140)	*<0.001*	0.161 (0.113; 0.208)	*<0.001*
Previous GSsynSS			-0.004 (-0.019; 0.010)	0.563
Previous PDsynSS			-0.021 (-0.040; -0.002)	*0.035*
Previous GStenSS			0.000 (-0.085; 0.085)	0.997
Previous PDtenSS			-0.015 (-0.078; 0.048)	0.643
Previous erosions score			0.012 (-0.022; 0.046)	0.484
R^2 (% variability explained)	32.3		39.1	
Improved R^2			6.8	*<0.001**

Predicted variable is current health assessment questionnaire (HAQ) score. Comparison of models based on baseline demographic, anthropometric and immunological parameters, and previous disease activity score in 28 joints (DAS28) with or without previous German 7-joint ultrasound score (US7) sum-scores (SS) (previous = measured 12 months ago). **P* value of significance for improvement of prediction. *RA* rheumatoid arthritis, *BMI* body mass index, *RF* rheumatoid factor, *ACPA* anti-citrullinated peptide antibodies, *GS* greyscale, *PD* power Doppler, *syn* synovitis, *ten* tenosynovitis. *P*-values higlighted in italics are significant at $p < 0.05$

Discussion

Preservation of physical function represents a fundamental long-term outcome for patients with RA. To our knowledge, this is the first study that systematically examines the longitudinal relationship between an US joint inflammation score and physical function in patients with RA. Several previous studies have informed us on the relationship between the conventional clinical, radiological and laboratory measures of disease activity and HAQ evolution [1–4], but we have lacked deeper knowledge on the impact of synovitis detected by US on the HAQ score.

Musculoskeletal US is increasingly being used to detect and monitor joint inflammation in RA, in both clinical practice and clinical research. Indeed, both GSUS and PDUS have been shown to have greater sensitivity for detecting synovitis as compared with physical examination [9, 10], are more reliable [14–16] and detect response to therapy more rapidly in comparison to various clinical scores [31–34]. Because US examination of all joints and tendons that can be affected in RA would be extremely time consuming, several reduced joint scores for assessing US joint inflammation have been developed. Concentration on a small number of active joint regions reduces examination time, but still retains most of the quantitative information compared to the extended joint scores [35–39]. It is important to stress that we have mainly been examining the relationship between the HAQ score (as a dependent variable), and the DAS28 and US7S synovitis sum-scores (as explanatory variables). This does not mean that we have been comparing only the additive role of ultrasound examination to clinical joint counts. DAS28-CRP is a construct based on a 28-joint count of swollen and tender joints, patient global assessment and CRP. While most patient-reported outcome measures tend to be highly correlated, the representation of the patient global assessment and the number of tender joints in the DAS28 helps to explain a substantial part of the variability in HAQ score. US7S synovitis sum-scores reflect synovitis in the five joints of the clinically dominant hand (wrist, MCP II, III, PIPI II, III) and two joints of the foot (MTP II and V), but synovitis of the wrist is assessed from the dorsal, volar and ulnar aspects, synovitis of the MCP and PIP joints from the dorsal and volar aspects, MTP V from the dorsal and lateral aspects, and MTP II only from the dorsal aspects. Hence, the joints of the hand (11 joint areas) are represented much more than the joints of the foot (3 joint areas) in the sum-scores for PD and GS synovitis.

Using LLM analysis, we applied two main models - a standard (current) model and a time-lag model - in a cohort of patients with RA that included both patients with early and with established RA. While the standard model reflects mainly the cross-sectional relationship between covariates and predicted variables collected at the same time, the time-lag model allows for more longitudinal interpretation of the data. When applying the standard model, the PD and GS synovitis sum-scores were significantly positively correlated with current HAQ score and the relative impact of US-detected synovitis was twice as high in patients with early RA as compared to those with established disease. A similar trend was seen in the tenosynovitis score, while the erosions score was not significantly associated with current HAQ score. This finding is in accordance with other studies showing that the reversible part of the HAQ related to disease activity is higher in early RA, while prolonged duration of the disease increases the part of the HAQ related to irreversible damage caused by structural joint damage [1–4, 40–42].

The magnitude of the effect of the individual US7 sum-scores on HAQ score in univariate analyses was relatively minor (explained percent variability in the HAQ score was in the range of 3 – 5%) and became statistically insignificant when adjustments were made for the conventional clinical and anthropometric variables, although the performance of the whole multivariate model was still slightly better when all US7S sum-scores were entered into the model. These findings suggest that at least in this population of patients with RA, the ultrasound measures included in the US7S were only weakly associated with overall physical functioning as reflected by the HAQ score. This may be partly related to the design of the HAQ itself - although this instrument is capable of detecting small but meaningful changes in function in individual patients [43], it is dominated by effects on large joints such as the hips, knees and shoulders (which are not represented in the US7S), and is relatively insensitive in detecting changes in, for example, hand function, which is mainly represented in the US7S [44, 45].

The results of the time-lag model revealed a somewhat different perspective. Although the univariate analyses relating previous US7 sum-scores to current HAQ score using the time-lag model were non-significant, both PDsynSS and GSsynSS appeared to be significant predictors of current HAQ after adjustment for the previous DAS28 or HAQ score, and previous PDsynSS contributed additional information on current HAQ even in the more extensive multivariate model. This apparent discordance may be explained by the fact that by adding previous HAQ (or DAS28, which is highly correlated with HAQ) into the multivariate model creates an autoregressive model that mainly predicts the change in HAQ score.

Somewhat counterintuitively, higher PDUS and GSUS synovitis scores were longitudinally (when using the time-lag model after adjustment for previous DAS28 or HAQ) associated with improvement (not deterioration) of HAQ. This probably reflects the ability of PDUS and GSUS to discriminate between the activity-driven reversible part of the HAQ and the irreversible part of the HAQ caused by structural damage. The additional analysis on the role of clinical and US-based measures to determine escalation of therapy suggested that the main driver of change was mainly the clinical score, and not the US7S. Although the treating physicians were allowed to see the results of the US assessment, they were not actively encouraged to apply them in their decision-making, because the role of the US-based inflammatory score for treat-to-target strategies was not established. This may mean that the part of the HAQ associated with the impact of synovitis detected by PDUS or GSUS is reversible (either because of change in therapy, or because of spontaneous fluctuation in disease activity), and does not necessarily contribute - at least in the time-frame of one year - to the irreversible part of the HAQ caused by ensuing structural damage. Because patients with longer follow up contributed more data, we compared baseline characteristics between groups of patients who completed one, two or three annual follow-up visits and found no significant trends or differences (Additional file 6).

Our study has several limitations. In our analyses we treated the US7 sum-scores as a linear continuum, equalizing the effect of three joints with a PD or GS signal of 1 to a single joint with a PD or GS signal of 3. This assumption may not be entirely correct, as shown by others [46]. However the primary goal of this analysis was to assess the relationship of one specific US score (US7S) either alone or in combination with conventional clinical tools, and hence we used the US7 sum-scores as designed by its authors. The fact that US examination of patients was performed by different observers may also be a limitation of this study, as US is still considered to be operator-dependent. In order to verify interobserver and intraobserver agreement among arthro-sonographers in this project, we performed a reliability study, which was published elsewhere [28], and showed moderate to excellent results.

Our study also has several strengths. To our knowledge, a true longitudinal analysis of the relationship between an ultrasound inflammation score and physical function, after adjustment for clinical measures of disease activity, has never been published. The most important advantage of longitudinal data analysis, including the LLM method, is that all available data are used, which increases the power to detect subtle relationships. We have analyzed data from 185 patients overall (46 with incident and 139 with prevalent disease) and 522 follow-up visits.

Conclusions

In conclusion, we found that US7 PD and GS synovitis sum-scores alone were positively associated with current functional status reflected by the HAQ score in RA patients, and this relationship was stronger in patients with early disease. However, they contributed little additional information on the current HAQ score, beyond standard clinical measures. When combined with the DAS28, or HAQ, US7 PD and GS synovitis sum-scores were predictive of the change in HAQ score over one year. Based on the multivariate analyses of the time-lag model and taking into the account the results of univariate analyses of the standard model we may assume that US7S sum-scores for synovitis were associated mainly with the reversible activity-related component of HAQ, and may thus help to identify patients with higher chance of functional improvement. Although the interpretation of the results is not straightforward, our study adds further argument to caution against indiscriminate use of more aggressive therapeutic approaches (with the aim of preventing irreversible damage) based on information from the US inflammatory score, beyond standard clinical activity indexes.

Additional files

Additional file 1: Descriptive characteristics of the cohort over time[1]. (DOCX 22 kb)

Additional file 2: Descriptive characteristics of the incident cohort only over time[1]. (DOCX 21 kb)

Additional file 3: Descriptive characteristics of the prevalent cohort only over time[1]. (DOCX 22 kb)

Additional file 4: Prediction of escalation of therapy - univariate analyses (with and without stratification for incident vs. prevalent disease, and low vs. moderate to high disease activity). (DOCX 21 kb)

Additional file 5: Prediction of escalation of therapy - multivariate analyses. (DOCX 24 kb)

Additional file 6: Comparison of baseline variables between groups of patients with one, two and three years of follow up. (DOCX 24 kb)

Abbreviations

ACPA: anti-citrullinated protein antibody; ANOVA: analysis of variance; BMI: body mass index; CDAI: clinical disease activity Score; CRP: C-reactive protein; csDMARDs: conventional synthetic disease modifying drugs; DAS28: disease activity score in 28 joints; ES: erosions score; EULAR: European League against Rheumatism; GS: greyscale; GSsynSS: greyscale synovitis sum-score; HAQ: health assessment questionnaire; LMM: linear mixed-effects model; MCP: metacarpophalangeal; MTP: metacarpophalangeal; PD: power-Doppler; PDsynSS: power-Doppler synovitis sum-score; PIP: proximal interphalangeal; RA: rheumatoid arthritis; RF: rheumatoid factor; SDAI: simplified disease activity score; Syn: synovitis; Ten: tenosynovitis; US: ultrasound; US7S: German 7-joint ultrasound score

Acknowledgements

We would like to thank our study nurse Lada Filipová for her valuable assistance throughout this study.

Funding

This work was supported by a project of the Ministry of Health of the Czech Republic for conceptual development of a research organization, number 023728.

Authors' contributions

JZ designed the study, performed ultrasonography and prepared the first draft of the manuscript. JH, PH, MK, HM, OS, MO, SF and OR performed ultrasonography and revised the manuscript. LS and MU performed statistical analyses and participated in the data interpretation and helped to draft the manuscript. KP and KH contributed to the design of the cohort study and revised the manuscript. All authors have read and approved the final manuscript.

Competing interests

The authors declare that they have no competing interests.

Author details

[1]Institute of Rheumatology, Prague, and Department of Rheumatology, First Faculty of Medicine, Charles University, Na Slupi 4, 12850 Prague, Czech Republic. [2]Institute of Biostatistics and Analyses, Faculty of Medicine, Masaryk University, Brno, Czech Republic.

References

1. Drossaers-Bakker KW, de Buck M, van Zeben D, Zwinderman AH, Breedveld FC, Hazes JM. Long-term course and outcome of functional capacity in rheumatoid arthritis: the effect of disease activity and radiologic damage over time. Arthritis Rheum. 1999;42:1854–60.
2. Kuper HH, van Leeuwen MA, van Riel PL, Prevoo ML, Houtman PM, Lolkema WF, van Rijswijk MH. Radiographic damage in large joints in early rheumatoid arthritis: relationship with radiographic damage in hands and feet, disease activity, and physical disability. Br J Rheumatol. 1997;36:855–60.
3. Welsing PM, van Gestel AM, Swinkels HL, Kiemeney LA, van Riel PL. The relationship between disease activity, joint destruction, and functional capacity over the course of rheumatoid arthritis. Arthritis Rheum. 2001;44:2009–17.
4. Welsing PM, Landewé RB, van Riel PL, Boers M, van Gestel AM, van der Linden S, Swinkels HL, van der Heijde DM. The relationship between disease activity and radiologic progression in patients with rheumatoid arthritis: a longitudinal analysis. Arthritis Rheum. 2004;50:2082–93.
5. Stoffer MA, Schoels MM, Smolen JS, Aletaha D, Breedveld FC, Burmester G, et al. Evidence for treating rheumatoid arthritis to target: results of a systematic literature search update. Ann Rheum Dis. 2016;75:16–22.
6. Dale J, Purves D, McConnachie A, McInnes I, Porter D. Tightening up? Impact of musculoskeletal ultrasound disease activity assessment on early rheumatoid arthritis patients treated using a treat to target strategy. Arthritis Care Res (Hoboken). 2014;66:19–26.
7. Eberl DR, Fasching V, Rahlfs V, Schleyer I, Wolf R. Repeatability and objectivity of various measurements in rheumatoid arthritis: a comparative study. Arthritis Rheum. 1976;19:1278–86.
8. Lassere MN, van der Heijde D, Johnson KR, Boers M, Edmonds J. Reliability of measures of disease activity and disease damage in rheumatoid arthritis: implications for smallest detectable difference, minimal clinically important difference, and analysis of treatment effects in randomized controlled trials. J Rheumatol. 2001;28:892–903.
9. Brown AK, Quinn MA, Karim Z, Conaghan PG, Peterfy CG, Hensor E, et al. Presence of significant synovitis in rheumatoid arthritis patients with disease-modifying antirheumatic drug-induced clinical remission: evidence from an imaging study may explain structural progression. Arthritis Rheum. 2006;54:3761–73.
10. Brown AK, Conaghan PG, Karim Z, Quinn MA, Ikeda K, Peterfy CG, et al. An explanation for the apparent dissociation between clinical remission and continued structural deterioration in rheumatoid arthritis. Arthritis Rheum. 2008;58:2958–67.
11. Cheung PP, Mari K, Devauchelle-Pensec V, Jousse-Joulin S, D'Agostino MA, Chalès G, et al. Predictive value of tender joints compared to synovitis for structural damage in rheumatoid arthritis. RMD Open. 2016;2, e000205.
12. Sheane BJ, Beddy P, O'Connor M, Miller S, Cunnane G. Targeted ultrasound of the fifth metatarsophalangeal joint in an early inflammatory arthritis cohort. Arthritis Rheum. 2009;61:1004–8.
13. Sant'Ana Petterle G, Natour J, Rodrigues da Luz K, Soares Machado F, dos Santos MF, Rocha Correa Fernandes A, et al. Usefulness of US to show subclinical joint abnormalities in asymptomatic feet of RA patients compared to healthy controls. Clin Exp Rheumatol. 2013;31:904–12.

14. Pollard LC, Kingsley GH, Choy EH, Scott DL. Fibromyalgic rheumatoid arthritis and disease assessment. Rheumatology (Oxford). 2010;49:924–8.
15. Backhaus M, Kamradt T, Sandrock D, Loreck D, Fritz J, Wolf KJ, et al. Arthritis of the finger joints: a comprehensive approach comparing conventional radiography, scintigraphy, ultrasound, and contrast enhanced magnetic resonance imaging. Arthritis Rheum. 1999;42:1232–45.
16. Szkudlarek M, Court-Payen M, Strandberg C, Klarlund M, Klausen T, Ostergaard M. Power Doppler ultrasonography for assessment of synovitis in the metacarpophalangeal joints of patients with rheumatoid arthritis: a comparison with dynamic magnetic resonance imaging. Arthritis Rheum. 2001;44:2018–23.
17. Karim Z, Wakefield RJ, Quinn M, Conaghan PG, Brown AK, Veale DJ, et al. Validation and reproducibility of ultrasonography in the detection of synovitis in the knee: a comparison with arthroscopy and clinical examination. Arthritis Rheum. 2004;50:387–94.
18. Weiner SM, Jurenz S, Uhl M, Lange-Nolde A, Warnatz K, Peter HH, et al. Ultrasonography in the assessment of peripheral joint involvement in psoriatic arthritis: a comparison with radiography, MRI and scintigraphy. Clin Rheumatol. 2008;27:983–9.
19. Naredo E, Bonilla G, Gamero F, Uson J, Carmona L, Laffon A, et al. Assessment of inflammatory activity in rheumatoid arthritis: a comparative study of clinical evaluation with grey scale and power Doppler ultrasonography. Ann Rheum Dis. 2005;64:375–81.
20. Dougados M, Jousse-Joulin S, Mistretta F, d'Agostino MA, Backhaus M, Bentin J, et al. Evaluation of several ultrasonography scoring systems of synovitis and comparison to clinical examination: results from a prospective multi-center study of rheumatoid arthritis. Ann Rheum Dis. 2010;69:828–33.
21. Mandl P, Balint PV, Brault Y, Backhaus M, D'Agostino MA, Grassi W, et al. Metrologic properties of ultrasound versus clinical evaluation of synovitis in rheumatoid arthritis: results of a multicenter, randomized study. Arthritis Rheum. 2012;64:1272–82.
22. Backhaus M, Ohrndorf S, Kellner H, Strunk J, Backhaus TM, Hartung W, et al. Evaluation of a novel 7-joint ultrasound score in daily rheumatologic practice: a pilot project. Arthritis Rheum. 2009;61:1194–201.
23. Ohrndorf S, Fischer IU, Kellner H, Strunk J, Hartung W, Reiche B, et al. Reliability of the novel 7-joint ultrasound score: results from an inter- and intraobserver study performed by rheumatologists. Arthritis Care Res (Hoboken). 2012;64:1238–43.
24. Backhaus TM, Ohrndorf S, Kellner H, Strunk J, Hartung W, Sattler H, et al. The US7 score is sensitive to change in a large cohort of patients with rheumatoid arthritis over 12 months of therapy. Ann Rheum Dis. 2013;72: 1163–9.
25. Aletaha D, Neogi T, Silman AJ, Funovits J, Felson DT, Bingham 3rd CO, et al. 2010 rheumatoid arthritis classification criteria: an American College of Rheumatology/European League Against Rheumatism collaborative initiative. Ann Rheum Dis. 2010;69:1580–8.
26. Fries JF, Spitz P, Kraines RG, Holman HR. Measurement of patient outcome in arthritis. Arthritis Rheum. 1980;23:137–45.
27. Scott D, van Riel PL, van der Heijde DM, Studnicka-Benke A. Assessing disease activity in rheumatoid arthritis: the EULAR handbook of standard methods. EULAR: Zürich; 1993.
28. Hurnakova J, Zavada J, Hanova P, Hulejova H, Klein M, Mann H, et al. Serum calprotectin (S100A8/9): an independent predictor of ultrasound synovitis in patients with rheumatoid arthritis. Arthritis Res Ther. 2015;17:252.
29. Backhaus MWS, Werner S, Ohrndorf S, Alraqi S, Crowther S, Dhillon S, et al. Can satisfactory reliability of the 7-joint ultrasound score be attained by inexperienced readers in a single calibration exercise? Results from the biodam program. [abstract]. Arthritis Rheum. 1946;65.
30. Scheel AK, Hermann KG, Kahler E, Pasewaldt D, Fritz J, Hamm B, et al. A novel ultrasonographic synovitis scoring system suitable for analyzing finger joint inflammation in rheumatoid arthritis. Arthritis Rheum. 2005;52:733–43.
31. Taylor PC, Steuer A, Gruber J, Cosgrove DO, Blomley MJ, Marsters PA, et al. Comparison of ultrasonographic assessment of synovitis and joint vascularity with radiographic evaluation in a randomized, placebo controlled study of infliximab therapy in early rheumatoid arthritis. Arthritis Rheum. 2004;50:1107–16.
32. Filippucci E, Iagnocco A, Salaffi F, Cerioni A, Valesini G, Grassi W. Power Doppler sonography monitoring of synovial perfusion at the wrist joints in patients with rheumatoid arthritis treated with adalimumab. Ann Rheum Dis. 2006;65:1433–7.
33. Naredo E, Rodríguez M, Campos C, Rodríguez-Heredia JM, Medina JA, Giner E, et al. Validity, reproducibility, and responsiveness of a twelve-joint simplified power doppler ultrasonographic assessment of joint inflammation in rheumatoid arthritis. Arthritis Rheum. 2008;4:515–22.
34. Iagnocco A, Finucci A, Ceccarelli F, Perricone C, Iorgoveanu V, Valesini G. Power Doppler ultrasound monitoring of response to anti-tumor-necrosis factor alpha treatment in patients with rheumatoid arthritis. Rheumatology (Oxford). 2015;54:1890–6.
35. Hartung W, Kellner H, Strunk J, Sattler H, Schmidt WA, Ehrenstein B, et al. Development and evaluation of a novel ultrasound score for large joints in rheumatoid arthritis: one year of experience in daily clinical practice. Arthritis Care Res. 2012;64:675–82.
36. Mandl P, Kurucz R, Niedermayer D, Balint PV, Smolen JS. Contributions of ultrasound beyond clinical data in assessing inflammatory disease activity in rheumatoid arthritis: current insights and future prospects. Rheumatology. 2014;53:2136–42.
37. Hammer HB, Kvien TK. Comparisons of 7- to 78-joint ultrasonography scores: all different joint combinations show equal response to adalimumab treatment in patients with rheumatoid arthritis. Arthritis Res Ther. 2011;13: R78.
38. Grassi W, Gaywood I, Pande I, Filippucci E. From DAS 28 to SAS 1. Clin Exp Rheumatol. 2012;30:649–51.
39. Ten Cate DF, Luime JJ, Swen N, Gerards AH, De Jager MH, Basoski NM, et al. Role of ultrasonography in diagnosing early rheumatoid arthritis and remission of rheumatoid arthritis - a systematic review of the literature. Arthritis Res Ther. 2013;15:R4.
40. Ødegård S, Landewé R, van der Heijde D, Kvien TK, Mowinckel P, Uhlig T. Association of early radiographic damage with impaired physical function in rheumatoid arthritis: a ten-year, longitudinal observational study in 238 patients. Arthritis Rheum. 2006;54:68–75.
41. Aletaha D, Strand V, Smolen JS, Ward MM. Treatment-related improvement in physical function varies with duration of rheumatoid arthritis: a pooled analysis of clinical trial results. Ann Rheum Dis. 2008;67:238–43.
42. Aletaha D, Smolen J, Ward MM. Measuring function in rheumatoid arthritis: Identifying reversible and irreversible components. Arthritis Rheum. 2006;54: 2784–92.
43. Hawley DJ, Wolfe F. Sensitivity to change of the health assessment questionnaire (HAQ) and other clinical and health status measures in rheumatoid arthritis: results of short-term clinical trials and observational studies versus long-term observational studies. Arthritis Care Res. 1992;5: 130–6.
44. Tanaka E, Saito A, Kamitsuji S, Yamada T, Nakajima A, Taniguchi A, et al. Impact of shoulder, elbow, and knee joint involvement on assessment of rheumatoid arthritis using the American College of Rheumatology Core Data Set. Arthritis Rheum. 2005;53:864–71.
45. Drossaers-Bakker KW, Kroon HM, Zwinderman AH, Breedveld FC, Hazes JM. Radiographic damage of large joints in long-term rheumatoid arthritis and its relation to function. Rheumatology (Oxford). 2000;39:998–1003.
46. Gärtner M, Mandl P, Radner H, Supp G, Machold KP, Aletaha D, et al. Sonographic joint assessment in rheumatoid arthritis: associations with clinical joint assessment during a state of remission. Arthritis Rheum. 2013; 65:2005–14.

Permissions

All chapters in this book were first published in AR&T, by BioMed Central; hereby published with permission under the Creative Commons Attribution License or equivalent. Every chapter published in this book has been scrutinized by our experts. Their significance has been extensively debated. The topics covered herein carry significant findings which will fuel the growth of the discipline. They may even be implemented as practical applications or may be referred to as a beginning point for another development.

The contributors of this book come from diverse backgrounds, making this book a truly international effort. This book will bring forth new frontiers with its revolutionizing research information and detailed analysis of the nascent developments around the world.

We would like to thank all the contributing authors for lending their expertise to make the book truly unique. They have played a crucial role in the development of this book. Without their invaluable contributions this book wouldn't have been possible. They have made vital efforts to compile up to date information on the varied aspects of this subject to make this book a valuable addition to the collection of many professionals and students.

This book was conceptualized with the vision of imparting up-to-date information and advanced data in this field. To ensure the same, a matchless editorial board was set up. Every individual on the board went through rigorous rounds of assessment to prove their worth. After which they invested a large part of their time researching and compiling the most relevant data for our readers.

The editorial board has been involved in producing this book since its inception. They have spent rigorous hours researching and exploring the diverse topics which have resulted in the successful publishing of this book. They have passed on their knowledge of decades through this book. To expedite this challenging task, the publisher supported the team at every step. A small team of assistant editors was also appointed to further simplify the editing procedure and attain best results for the readers.

Apart from the editorial board, the designing team has also invested a significant amount of their time in understanding the subject and creating the most relevant covers. They scrutinized every image to scout for the most suitable representation of the subject and create an appropriate cover for the book.

The publishing team has been an ardent support to the editorial, designing and production team. Their endless efforts to recruit the best for this project, has resulted in the accomplishment of this book. They are a veteran in the field of academics and their pool of knowledge is as vast as their experience in printing. Their expertise and guidance has proved useful at every step. Their uncompromising quality standards have made this book an exceptional effort. Their encouragement from time to time has been an inspiration for everyone.

The publisher and the editorial board hope that this book will prove to be a valuable piece of knowledge for researchers, students, practitioners and scholars across the globe.

List of Contributors

Sho Ishii, Takeo Isozaki, Hidekazu Furuya, Hiroko Takeuchi, Yumi Tsubokura and Tsuyoshi Kasama
Division of Rheumatology, Department of Medicine, Showa University School of Medicine, 1-5-8 Hatanodai, Shinagawa-ku, Tokyo 142-8666, Japan

Katsunori Inagaki
Department of Orthopedic Surgery, Showa University School of Medicine, Tokyo, Japan

Susanna L. Lundström, Dorothea Rutishauser and Roman A. Zubarev
Division of Physiological Chemistry I, Department of Medical Biochemistry and Biophysics, Karolinska Institutet, Scheelesväg 2, SE 17177 Stockholm, Sweden

A. Jimmy Ytterberg
Division of Physiological Chemistry I, Department of Medical Biochemistry and Biophysics, Karolinska Institutet, Scheelesväg 2, SE 17177 Stockholm, Sweden
Rheumatology Unit, Department of Medicine, Karolinska Institutet, Stockholm, Sweden

Aase H. Hensvold, Lars Klareskog and Anca I. Catrina
Rheumatology Unit, Department of Medicine, Karolinska Institutet, Stockholm, Sweden
Rheumatology Unit, Karolinska University Hospital, Stockholm, Sweden

Jeffrey R. Curtis
University of Alabama at Birmingham, Birmingham, AL, USA

Kevin Winthrop
Oregon Health and Science University, Portland, OR, USA

Cathy O'Brien, Matladi N. Ndlovu and Marc de Longueville
UCB Pharma, Brussels, Belgium

Boulos Haraoui
Department of Medicine, Centre Hospitalier de l'Université de Montréal, Montréal, QC, Canada

Leslie R. Harrold and Bernice Gershenson
University of Massachusetts Medical School, Worcester, MA, USA
Pharmacoepidemiology and Outcomes Research, Corrona, 352 Turnpike Road, Suite 325, Southborough, MA 01772, USA

Heather J. Litman, Katherine C. Saunders and Kimberly J. Dandreo
Pharmacoepidemiology and Outcomes Research, Corrona, 352 Turnpike Road, Suite 325, Southborough, MA 01772, USA

Jeffrey D. Greenberg
New York University School of Medicine, New York, NY, USA

Robert Low, Jeffrey Stark, Srihari Jaganathan and Mohamed Yassine
UCB Pharma, Smyrna, GA, USA

Robert Suruki
UCB Pharma, Raleigh, NC, USA

Joel M. Kremer
Albany Medical College, Albany, NY, USA

Kaustav Chowdhury, Prabin Kumar, Uma Kanga and Dipendra Kumar Mitra
Department of Transplant Immunology and Immunogenetics, All India Institute of Medical Sciences (AIIMS), Room No-75, New Delhi 110029, India

Uma Kumar, Soumabha Das, Maumita Kanjilal and Ravi Kiran Basyal
Department of Medicine, All India Institute of Medical Sciences (AIIMS), New Delhi, India

Parashar Ghosh and Geetabali Sircar
Rheumatology Center, Institute of Post Graduate Medical Education and Research (IPGMER), Kolkata, India

Jaydeep Chaudhuri and Santu Bandyopadhaya
Indian Institute of Chemical Biology, Council of Scientific and Industrial Research (CSIR), Kolkata, India

Tsutomu Takeuchi
Keio University School of Medicine, Shinjuku-ku, Tokyo, Japan

Hisashi Yamanaka and Masayoshi Harigai
Tokyo Women's Medical University, Shinjuku-ku, Tokyo, Japan

Ryo Tamamura, Yuichi Kato, Yoshifumi Ukyo and Toshikazu Nakano
Janssen Pharmaceutical K.K., Chiyoda-ku, Tokyo, Japan

Benjamin Hsu
Janssen Research & Development, LLC, Spring House, PA, USA

Yoshiya Tanaka
University of Occupational & Environmental Health Japan, Kitakyushu, Japan

Lucie Andrés Cerezo, Barbora Šumová, Klára Prajzlerová, Karel Pavelka, Jiří Vencovský and Ladislav Šenolt
Institute of Rheumatology, Na Slupi 4, 12850 Prague, Czech Republic
Department of Rheumatology, 1st Faculty of Medicine, Charles University, Prague, Czech Republic

David Veigl
First Orthopaedic Clinic, 1st Faculty of Medicine,Charles University, Prague, Czech Republic

Dres Damgaard and Claus Henrik Nielsen
Institute for Inflammation Research, Center for Rheumatology and Spine Diseases, Copenhagen University Hospital, Rigshospitalet, Copenhagen, Denmark

Kohjin Suzuki, Kohsuke Yoshida, Kenta Kaneshiro, Ayako Nakai, Naonori Hashimoto, Koto Uchida and Akira Hashiramoto
Department of Biophysics, Kobe University Graduate School of Health Sciences, Tomogaoka 7-10-2, Suma-ku, Kobe 654-0142, Japan

Takeshi Ueha and Yoshitada Sakai
Division of Rehabilitation Medicine, Kobe University Graduate School of Medicine, Kobe 650-0017, Japan

Teppei Hashimoto and Yoshiko Kawasaki
Department of Rheumatology, Kobe Kaisei Hospital, Kobe 657-0068, Japan

Nao Shibanuma
Department of Orthopedic Surgery, Kobe Kaisei Hospital, Kobe 657-0068, Japan

Natsuko Nakagawa
Department of Rheumatology, Hyogo Prefectural Kakogawa Medical Center, Kakogawa 675-0003, Japan

Beatrice Bergström, Hans Carlsten and Anna-Karin Hultgård Ekwall
Department of Rheumatology and Inflammation Research, Institute of Medicine, The Sahlgrenska Academy, University of Gothenburg, 405 30 Gothenburg, Sweden
Centre for Bone and Arthritis Research, University of Gothenburg, Gothenburg, Sweden

Lene Terslev
Copenhagen Center for Arthritis Research and Center for Rheumatology and Spine Diseases, Centre of Head and Orthopaedics, Rigshospitalet, Copenhagen, Denmark

Mikkel Østergaard
Copenhagen Center for Arthritis Research and Center for Rheumatology and Spine Diseases, Centre of Head and Orthopaedics, Rigshospitalet, Copenhagen, Denmark
Department of Clinical Medicine, University of Copenhagen, Copenhagen, Denmark

Joe Sexton and Hilde Berner Hammer
Department of Rheumatology, Diakonhjemmet Hospital, Oslo, Norway

R. M. ten Brinck and H. W. van Steenbergen
Department of Rheumatology C1-R, Leiden University Medical Centre, Leiden 2300RC, the Netherlands

A. H. M. van der Helm-van Mil
Department of Rheumatology C1-R, Leiden University Medical Centre, Leiden 2300RC, the Netherlands
Department of Rheumatology, Erasmus Medical Centre, Rotterdam, The Netherlands

Cristiana Barbati, Marta Vomero, Tania Colasanti, Fulvia Ceccarelli, Sara Ferrigno, Annacarla Finucci, Francesca Miranda, Lucia Novelli, Carlo Perricone, Francesca Romana Spinelli, Simona Truglia, Fabrizio Conti, Guido Valesini and Cristiano Alessandri
Arthritis Center, Department of Internal Medicine and Medical Specialties, Sapienza University of Rome, Rome, Italy

Marco Diociaiuti
Technology and health Department, Istituto Superiore di Sanità, Rome, Italy

Chia-Chen Teng and Zachary Burningham
Salt Lake City Veterans Affairs Medical Center, Health Services Research and Development (IDEAS) Center and University of Utah Division of Epidemiology, Salt Lake City, UT, USA

Brian C. Sauer
Salt Lake City Veterans Affairs Medical Center, Health Services Research and Development (IDEAS) Center and University of Utah Division of Epidemiology, Salt Lake City, UT, USA
Salt Lake IDEAS Center, VA; Salt Lake City Health Care System, 500 Foothill Drive Bldg. 182, Salt Lake City, UT 84148-0001, USA

Neil A. Accortt, David Collier and Mona Trivedi
Amgen, Thousand Oaks, CA, USA

Grant W. Cannon
Salt Lake City Veterans Affairs Medical Center, Health Services Research and Development (IDEAS) Center and University of Utah Division of Rheumatology, Salt Lake City, UT, USA

Dana E. Goin
UCSF Benioff Children's Hospital Oakland, Children's Hospital Oakland Research Institute, 5700 Martin Luther King Jr. Way, Oakland, CA, USA
University of California, Berkeley, Berkeley, CA, USA

Mette Kiel Smed
Juliane Marie Center, Copenhagen University Hospital, Rigshospitalet, Copenhagen, Denmark

J. Lee Nelson
Fred Hutchinson Cancer Research Center, Seattle, WA, USA
University of Washington, Seattle, WA, USA

Jørn Olsen
University of California, Los Angeles, Los Angeles, CA, USA
Aarhus University, Aarhus, Denmark

Merete Lund Hetland
DANBIO Registry and Copenhagen Centre for Arthritis Research, Centre for Rheumatology and Spine Diseases (VRR), Rigshospitalet, Glostrup, Denmark
Faculty of Health and Medical Sciences, University of Copenhagen, Copenhagen, Denmark

Nancy A. Shadick, Michael E. Weinblatt, Agnes Zak and Michelle Frits
Division of Rheumatology, Brigham and Women's Hospital, 75 Francis Street, Boston, MA 02115, USA

Daniel H. Solomon
Division of Rheumatology, Brigham and Women's Hospital, 75 Francis Street, Boston, MA 02115, USA
Division of Pharmacoepidemiology, Brigham and Women's Hospital, Boston, MA 02120, USA

Jessica M. Franklin
Division of Pharmacoepidemiology, Brigham and Women's Hospital, Boston, MA 02120, USA

Susan MacLauchlan, Maria A. Zuriaga, José J. Fuster, Fernanda Behzadi, Jennifer Parker Duffen and Kenneth Walsh
Molecular Cardiology, Whitaker Cardiovascular Institute, Boston University School of Medicine, 700 Albany Street, W-611, Boston, MA 02118, USA

Carla M. Cuda and Harris Perlman
Division of Rheumatology, Department of Medicine, Northwestern University, Feinberg School of Medicine, 240 E. Huron Street, McGaw M338 Chicago, IL, USA

Jennifer Jonason
University of Rochester Medical Center, School of Medicine and Dentistry, 601 Elmwood Ave, Rochester, NY, USA

Tamar Aprahamian
Renal Section, Boston University School of Medicine, 650 Albany St, Boston, MA, USA

G. Kenneth Haines III
Department of Pathology, Icahn School of Medicine at Mount Sinai, New York, NY 10029, USA

Index

www.ingramcontent.com/pod-product-compliance
Lightning Source LLC
LaVergne TN
LVHW080659210926
848485LV00003B/399

* 9 7 8 1 6 3 9 2 7 4 7 8 9 *